Target Organ Toxicology Series

Cardiovascular Toxicology

Second Edition

Target Organ Toxicology Series

Series Editors
A. Wallace Hayes, John A. Thomas, and Donald E. Gardner

*Out of print.

Target Organ Toxicology Series

Cardiovascular Toxicology

Second Edition

Editor

Daniel Acosta, Jr., Ph.D.

*Professor, Division of Pharmacology
and Toxicology
College of Pharmacy
University of Texas
Austin, Texas*

Raven Press   New York

Raven Press, Ltd., 1185 Avenue of the Americas, New York, New York 10036

Made in the United States of America

Library of Congress Cataloging-in-Publication Data

Cardiovascular toxicology. — 2nd ed. / editor, Daniel Acosta, Jr.
     p. cm. — (Target organ toxicology series)
  Includes bibliographical references and index.
  ISBN 0-88167-937-2
  1. Cardiovascular toxicology. I. Acosta, Daniel, 1945–
II. Series.
  [DNLM: 1. Cardiovascular Diseases — chemically induced.
2. Cardiovascular System — drug effects. WG 100 C267]
RC677.C37 1992
616.1'07 — dc20
DNLM/DLC
for Library of Congress
                                       92-49691
                                           CIP

9 8 7 6 5 4 3 2 1

Contents

v

Contributing Authors

Daniel Acosta, Jr., Ph.D. *Professor, Department of Pharmacology and Toxicology, University of Texas, College of Pharmacy, Austin, Texas 78712*

H. Richard Adams, D.V.M., Ph.D. *Professor and Chairman, Department of Veterinary Biomedical Sciences, College of Veterinary Medicine, and Dalton Research Center, University of Missouri-Columbia, W116 Veterinary Medicine Building, 1600 Rollins, Columbia, Missouri 65211*

S. Sultan Ahmed, M.D., F.R.C.P.(C), F.A.C.P., F.A.C.C., F.C.C.P. *Professor of Medicine, and Director, Stress Testing, and Co-Director, Catheterization Laboratories, Department of Medicine, University of Medicine and Dentistry of New Jersey, New Jersey Medical School, 185 South Orange Avenue, Newark, New Jersey 07103*

Reynaldo Arceo, M.D. *Department of Toxicology and Pathology, Hoffmann-LaRoche Inc., Nutley, New Jersey 07110*

Domingo M. Aviado, M.D. *President, Atmospheric Health Sciences, 152 Parsonage Hill Road, PO Box 307, Short Hills, New Jersey 07078*

Steven I. Baskin, Pharm D., Ph.D., F.C.P., F.A.C.C., D.A.B.T. *Commander, United States Army Medical Research Institute of Chemical Defense, Aberdeen Proving Ground, Maryland 21010-5425*

Robert E. Beamish, M.D. *Professor, Division of Cardiovascular Sciences, St. Boniface General Hospital Research Center, and Department of Physiology, University of Manitoba, Winnipeg, Canada R2H 2A6*

Irene K. Berezesky, B.A. *Clinical Instructor, Department of Pathology, University of Maryland School of Medicine, and Maryland Institute for Emergency Medical Services Systems, 10 South Pine Street, Baltimore, Maryland 21201*

L. Maximilian Buja, M.D. *Professor and Chairman, Department of Pathology and Laboratory Medicine, University of Texas Health Science Center, and Director, Cardiovascular Pathology Research, Texas Heart Institute, Houston, Texas 77225*

Enrique Chacon, Ph.D. *Department of Pharmacology and Toxicology, The University of Texas, Austin, Texas 78712*

Ken S. Dhalla, D.G.Sc. *Division of Cardiovascular Sciences, St. Boniface Hospital Research Center, and Department of Physiology, University of Manitoba, 351-Tache Avenue, Winnipeg, Manitoba, Canada R2H 2A6*

Naranjan S. Dhalla, Ph.D. *Distinguished Professor and Head, Division of Cardiovascular Sciences, St. Boniface Hospital Research Center, and Department of Physiology, University of Manitoba, 351-Tache Avenue, Winnipeg, Manitoba, Canada R2H 2A6*

Shayne C. Gad, Ph.D., D.A.B.T. *Senior Director, Product Safety, Medical Affairs Technical Services, Becton Dickinson, 21 Davis Drive, Research Triangle Park, North Carolina 27709*

Kathleen A. Havlin, M.D. *Assistant Professor of Medicine, Department of Medicine/Oncology, Temple University Comprehensive Cancer Center, 3322 North Broad Street, PO Box 38346, Philadelphia, Pennsylvania 19140*

Rebecca S. Keller, M.S. *Graduate Research Assistant, Department of Veterinary Biomedical Sciences, College of Veterinary Biomedical Sciences, University of Missouri-Columbia, W116 Veterinary Medicine Building, 1600 Rollins, Columbia, Missouri 65211*

Robert A. Kloner, M.D., Ph.D. *Professor of Medicine, Section of Cardiology, University of Southern California, and Director of Research, Heart Institute, Hospital of the Good Samaritan, 616 S. Witmer, Los Angeles, California 90017*

Paul A. Murray, M.D. *Associate Professor, Department of Anaesthesiology and Critical Care Medicine, Johns Hopkins University School of Medicine, Baltimore, Maryland 21205*

Barbara Naimark, Ph.D. *Assistant Professor, Division of Cardiovascular Sciences, St. Boniface Hospital Research Center, and Department of Physiology, University of Manitoba, 351-Tache Avenue, Winnipeg, Manitoba, Canada R2H 2A6*

Bohuslav Ostadal, M.D. *Director, Institute of Physiology, Czechoslovak Academy of Sciences, Prague, Czechoslovakia*

Janet L. Parker, Ph.D. *Associate Professor, Department of Medical Physiology, School of Medicine, and Dalton Research Center, University of Missouri-Columbia, Columbia, Missouri 65211*

Thomas A. Patrick, B.S. *Department of Medicine, Harvard Medical School, Brigham and Women's Hospital, Boston, Massachusetts 02115, and The New England Regional Primate Research Center, Southborough, Massachusetts 01772*

Karin Przyklenk, Ph.D. *Assistant Professor of Research Medicine, Section of Cardiology, University of Southern California, and Assistant Director of Research, Director of Cardiac Function, Heart Institute, Hospital of The Good Samaritan, Los Angeles, California 90017*

Kenneth S. Ramos, Ph.D. *Associate Professor, Department of Physiology and Pharmacology, College of Veterinary Medicine, Texas A&M University, College Station, Texas 77843-4466*

Timothy J. Regan, M.D., F.A.A.C. *Director, Division of Cardiovascular Diseases, Professor of Medicine, Department of Medicine, University of Medicine and Dentistry of New Jersey, New Jersey Medical School, 185 South Orange Avenue, Newark, New Jersey 07103*

Zadok Ruben, D.V.M., Ph.D. *Department of Toxicology and Pathology, Hoffmann-LaRoche, Inc., 340 Kingsland Street, Nutley, New Jersey 07110*

You-Tang Shen, M.Sc. *Department of Medicine, Harvard Medical School, Brigham and Women's Hospital, Boston, Massachusetts 02115, and The New England Primate Research Center, Southborough, Massachusetts 01772*

Nicholas Sperelakis, Ph.D.   *Professor and Chairman, Department of Physiology and Biophysics, College of Medicine, University of Cincinnati, 231 Bethesda Avenue, Cincinnati, Ohio 45267-0576*

Benjamin F. Trump, M.D.   *Professor and Chairman, Department of Pathology, University of Maryland, and Maryland Institute for Emergency Medical Services Systems, 10 South Pine Street, Baltimore, Maryland 21201*

Stephen F. Vatner, M.D.   *Professor of Medicine, Department of Medicine, Harvard Medical School, Brigham and Women's Hospital, Boston, Massachusetts 02115, and New England Regional Primate Research Center, 1 Pine Hill Drive, Southborough, Massachusetts 01772*

Bernard M. Wagner, M.D.   *Research Professor of Pathology, Department of Pathology, New York University School of Medicine, New York, New York 10016*

John C. Yates, Ph.D.   *Division of Cardiovascular Sciences, St. Boniface General Hospital Research Center, and Department of Physiology, University of Manitoba, Winnipeg, Canada R2H 2A6*

Samir Zakhari, Ph.D.   *Chief, Division of Basic Research, National Institute on Alcohol Abuse and Alcoholism, Parklawn Building, Room 16C-26, 5600 Fishers Lane, Rockville, Maryland 20857*

Preface

The first edition of *Cardiovascular Toxicology,* edited by Ethard W. Van Stee, was published in 1982. Its major objective was to provide information on cardiovascular toxicology for clinicians, public health officials, industrial and experimental toxicologists, and other interested professionals. It fulfilled its goal admirably, and it provided the foundation for the second edition.

The second edition includes many of the same topics as the first edition; however, several new chapters have been added to reflect the growing interest in myocardial injury and toxicity by drugs and chemicals, as well as by cardiovascular diseases associated with myocardial ischemia. Cellular and molecular aspects of cardiovascular toxicity have been emphasized in many of the chapters; these critical examinations of chemically-induced injury to the cardiovascular system provide a better understanding of the mechanism(s) by which chemicals are toxic to the heart and vascular system.

This book is divided into five sections. The first section provides a prologue to the chapters that follow, emphasizing the need to explore biological mechanisms as factors in the toxicity of drugs and chemicals to the cardiovascular system—the role of calcium and oxidative stress in myocardial cell injury. In addition, the use of *in vitro* technology to evaluate the cardiotoxicity of xenobiotics is discussed. The second section highlights the methods used in industry to investigate the acute and chronic toxicity of drugs to the cardiovascular system, as well as the technology employed to assess cardiovascular function in conscious animals. The third section of the book focuses on mechanisms and hypotheses by which myocardial cells may be injured by xenobiotics or ischemic/hypoxic conditions. It provides a cellular and molecular approach to gaining a better understanding of the mechanisms involved in toxic injury to the cardiovascular system.

The last two sections represent major reviews on the toxicity of drugs and chemicals to the myocardium and to the vascular system. For many years, cardiovascular toxicity has referred mainly to myocardial damage, with little reference to vascular injury. The heart and vascular system have been divided into two sections to reflect the general and selective toxicity of xenobiotics to the heart and vascular system. Drugs and chemicals that are examined include antibiotics, anticancer agents, bacterial endotoxins, catecholamines, agents acting on ion channels and pumps, CNS-acting agents, alcohols, solvents and propellants, and environmental tobacco smoke.

We hope that the second edition builds on the interest and respect that was generated by the first edition. This edition will be of interest to students studying to become cardiovascular toxicologists and to the many health professionals involved in the toxicity of drugs and chemicals.

Daniel Acosta, Jr.

SECTION I

Introduction

Cardiovascular Toxicology, Second Edition,
edited by Daniel Acosta, Jr.
Raven Press, Ltd., New York © 1992.

1

Cardiovascular Toxicology

Introductory Notes

*Daniel Acosta, Jr., *Enrique Chacon, and †Kenneth S. Ramos

*Department of Pharmacology and Toxicology, The University of Texas at Austin,
Austin, Texas 78712; and †Department of Veterinary Physiology and
Pharmacology, Texas A&M University, College Station, Texas 77843*

The discipline of cardiovascular toxicology is concerned with the adverse effects of xenobiotics on the heart and circulatory system of living organisms. This volume focuses on four major areas: (a) basic aspects of myocardial cell function and injury, (b) drug-induced cardiotoxicity, (c) vascular toxicity, and (d) methodology. A major consideration in most of these chapters is a better understanding of the mechanistic basis for the toxicity and injury observed in the heart and vascular system after exposure to toxic or injurious stimuli. This brief introduction highlights two biological mechanisms that have generated much interest and research activity over the last several years: calcium homeostasis and oxidative stress. In addition, the use of *in vitro* technology for toxicity evaluation of cardiovascular agents is explored. The reader is directed to those chapters found in the first three sections for more detail and explanation as to the role of calcium, oxidative stress, and other biological mechanisms in the cardiotoxicity of injurious stimuli and agents.

OXIDATIVE STRESS

Oxygen Radicals

If a reactive molecule contains one or more unpaired electrons the molecule is termed a free radical. In recent years, much interest has been focused on the biochemistry of oxygen activation and the biological significance of reactive oxygen species (1). Highly reactive oxygen species are intermediates formed as a normal consequence in a variety of essential biochemical reactions. For example, the univalent step-wise reduction of molecular oxygen to water results in the formation of several potentially toxic intermediates, including superoxide radical anions, hydrogen peroxide, and hydroxyl radicals. Oxidases and the electron transport systems are prime and continuous sources of intracellular reactive oxygen species (2).

Oxidative stress denotes a shift in the prooxidant/antioxidant balance, in favor of the prooxidants, and thus oxidative damage inflicted by reactive oxygen species has been called oxidative stress (1,3). The extent of tissue damage is the result of the balance between the free radicals generated and the antioxidant protective defenses. In other words, the toxic effects of reactive oxygen species are only observed when their rates of formation exceed their rates of inactivation.

Biological Roles of Oxygen Radicals

Radicals are highly reactive and can easily donate an electron or abstract one hydrogen atom from the methylene groups of polyunsaturated fatty acids, which are abundant in membrane phospholipids (4). Under normal conditions, reactive intermediates are rapidly broken down by cellular defensive mechanisms. This rapid inactivation occurs because biological systems contain powerful enzymatic and nonenzymatic antioxidant systems that can protect against the deleterious effects of reactive oxygen species. These defense mechanisms include cytosolic and mitochondrial superoxide dismutases and glutathione peroxidases, catalase that is present in peroxisomes, as well as antioxidants such as beta-carotene, vitamin E, and glutathione (1). However, low levels of reactive oxygen species may escape these cellular defenses and produce damage to DNA, proteins, and unsaturated fats.

Oxygen-derived free radicals are thought to be involved in physiological and pathological changes of the integrity and function of biological systems (5). There is some evidence that free-radical damage contributes and may actually cause some of the problems associated with many chronic health disorders including inflammation, cancer, arteriosclerosis, heart attacks, stroke, and emphysema (6). In addition to these health problems, some drug actions and drug toxicities, as well as the aging process, appear to involve reactive oxygen species (1). The impact of oxidative stress-related toxicities is now being realized as a pathway for potential damage.

Despite our wealth of knowledge concerning the cytotoxic actions of reactive oxygen species, it remains puzzling as to why a cell would produce such a species if it had no other function than to inflict damage to itself. Almost all important metabolic pathways are strictly regulated by different mechanisms. Considering the multiregulatory systems that exist within a cell to maintain an oxidative balance, one might argue that reactive oxygen species may be acting as intracellular messengers. Based on the ability of superoxide to diffuse through membranes and target distant sites, Saran and Bors (7) have suggested that superoxide may serve as a biological messenger. Because of the apparent complexity of the processes underlying cellular entropy, reactive oxygen species may act as intracellular messengers.

CALCIUM HOMEOSTASIS

Calcium as an Intracellular Messenger

The role of calcium in the regulation and control of various cell functions has been an area of productive research during the last several years (8). The calcium messenger system may be considered as an integral function of several systems. The role of calcium as an intracellular messenger is highly influenced by homeostatic mechanisms. All cells contain elaborate systems for the regulation of calcium ions within the cell. Therefore it is not surprising that a great deal of interest has been directed at studying alterations in calcium homeostasis and how such effects may contribute to cell injury (9–11).

Role of Calcium in Cell Injury

Understanding the mechanism of cell injury has been the main quest of toxicologists. Alterations of calcium by toxicants may perturb the regulation of cellular functions beyond the normal range of physiological control. Intracellular calcium overload has been proposed to result in a breakdown of high-energy phosphates (12). Other cytotoxic effects induced by calcium are blebbing of the plasma membrane (13), activation of calcium-dependent phospholipases (14), stimulation of calcium-dependent neutral proteases (15), and calcium-activated DNA fragmentation (16,17). Because of the role of calcium acting as an intracellular messenger, alterations in calcium-mediated processes may be a critical cellular event that may prove to be deleterious to the cell.

MITOCHONDRIA

Cells are continuously engaged in various biochemical reactions. In particular, the synthesis of the major cell components requires energy. The energy to do work is derived from food by way of oxidizing the nutrients and channeling them into the formation of high-energy phosphate compounds such as adenosine triphosphate (ATP). ATP is the immediate energy source to do work for most biological systems and is obtained mainly through the oxidative phosphorylation of adenine dinucleotide diphosphate (ADP). Oxidative phosphorylation (ATP formation) occurs as a function of cellular respiration. Mitochondria possess an inner and outer membrane and are sub-cellular organelles in aerobic eukaryotic cells that are the sites of cellular respiration. In essence, mitochondria are the energy producers within a cell. In a highly energy demanding tissue such as the heart, mitochondria occupy a large proportion of the cell.

Mitochondrial Calcium Transport

Mitochondria contain an elaborate system for regulating calcium transport (Fig. 1). Mitochondrial calcium transport was first discovered by Siekevitz and Potter (18), who found that calcium stimulates the rate of oxygen consumption in isolated rat liver mitochondria. Current understanding for mitochondrial calcium transport has been formulated around an understanding of the chemiosmotic hypothesis and the large internal negative membrane potential (19). The prevailing thesis is that mitochondrial calcium influx occurs by way of a uniport system, while efflux occurs over two separate mechanisms.

Mitochondrial calcium accumulation is an energy-dependent process (19,20). It is well established that mitochondria accumulate calcium against a concentration gradient through a process made energetically possible by respiratory substrate oxidation or ATP hydrolysis (reversal of the ATP synthetase). Hence calcium transport driven by either respiration or ATP hydrolysis occurs at the expense of a common pool of energy maintained by the electrochemical proton gradient. The mechanism required to fulfill the electrogenic uptake of calcium being driven by the membrane potential is a uniporter, that is, the diffusion of an ion down an electrochemical gradient that is not coupled to the transport of any other ion or molecule (21). Due to the bioenergetic requirements for calcium uptake Lehninger (22) proposed that mitochondrial calcium accumulation occurs during state 4 respiration. Jacobus et al. (23) later showed that liver mitochondria would preferably use the available energy pool to accumulate calcium, rather than making ATP, suggesting that calcium uptake occurred as an alternative to oxidative phosphorylation in liver mitochondria. In addition, Jacobus et al. (23) showed that the addition of calcium to isolated respiring mitochondria increased rates of respiration. Jacobus et al. (23) also reported that, in heart mitochondria, calcium accumulation competed with oxidative phosphorylation without increasing respiration rates.

Mitochondrial calcium transport may be affected by different mechanisms. The uniporter has been shown to be reversible (efflux of calcium) upon complete collapse of the mitochondrial membrane potential by the potent uncoupler carbonyl cyanide *p*-chlorophenylhydrazone (CCCP). The energy-dependent accumulation of calcium may be inhibited by various mechanisms grouped into the following four different categories: translocation inhibitors, respiratory inhibitors, uncouplers, and ATPase inhibitors (20).

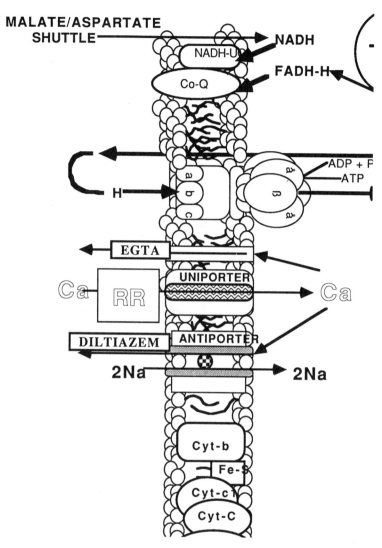

FIG. 1. Mitochondrial inner membrane showing the uptake and release routes for calcium. Mitochondrial calcium accumulation occurs by way of a ruthenium red (RR)-sensitive uniporter at the expense of potential energy stored within the inner membrane. The potential energy stored within the membrane is believed to be generated by the electrochemical proton gradient that exists across the inner mitochondrial membrane. However, upon complete collapse of the membrane potential the uniporter may reverse directions, resulting in a dumping of calcium from the mitochondria (also sensitive to RR). Another pathway for calcium release is the Na^+-dependent antiporter, which can be inhibited by diltiazem. A final calcium release route is the Na^+-independent pathway for calcium release. The Na^+-independent pathway for calcium release has been associated with a reversible permeability change that can be activated by oxidative stress and/or calcium. This permeability transition can be inhibited by the calcium chelator EGTA and the immunosuppressant cyclosporin A.

Translocation inhibitors are agents such as ruthenium red (RR), which essentially block the uniporter without affecting respiration and oxidative phosphorylation. Respiratory inhibitors such as antimycin block electron transport, thereby preventing the establishment of the common pool of energy used to drive calcium uptake. Uncouplers such as CCCP act directly by collapsing the mitochondrial membrane potential. ATPase inhibitors like oligomycin block proton flux through the ATP synthetase, thereby preventing the energy pool driven by the hydrolysis of ATP.

Two types of calcium release mechanisms are currently recognized, namely, the Na^+-dependent (antiporter) and the Na^+-independent pathways. A calcium ion in the mitochondrial matrix is at a lower energy than a calcium ion in the external space. Therefore energy must be supplied to extrude calcium. This energy must be supplied either from ATP hydrolysis, electrochemical potential, or the gradients of other coupled transported ions. It is currently believed that the energy supplied to extrude calcium is provided by the inward transport of two or more Na^+ or two or more H^+ (an antiport system). The antiporter (Na^+-dependent pathway) has been shown to be inhibited by diltiazem (24). A Na^+-independent pathway for calcium release has also been recognized (8).

The Na^+-independent pathway for calcium efflux is believed to occur in the absence of cotransport with any other ion. If calcium efflux by this mechanism is not coupled to the transport of another ion, active transport must be involved because of its ability to transport calcium against its electrochemical gradient. Therefore it is believed that the Na^+-independent pathway for calcium release may be mediated by an active process that uses energy from substrate oxidation (19,25,26). However, the nature of the Na^+-independent pathway for calcium release is controversial (19,27). The consensus appears to be that the Na^+-independent pathway for calcium release is associated with a permeability change within the inner mitochondrial membrane. Riley and Pfeiffer (28) have maintained that this permeability change may be driven by a cyclic deacylation/reacylation of membrane phospholipids. According to their mechanism, oxidation of glutathione displaces the phospholipid deacylation/reacylation cycle toward deacylation with a resultant permeability change. These data support the reports from various laboratories that oxidative stress induces alterations in mitochondrial calcium homeostasis (29). On the other hand, Al-Nassar and Crompton (30,31), as well as Crompton and Costi (27,32), have challenged this hypothesis by showing that permeabilization of the inner mitochondrial membrane may be induced by calcium, inorganic phosphate, and oxidative stress.

Mitochondrial Production of Reactive Oxygen Species

Mitochondria isolated from different tissues such as heart (33,34), liver (35), and lung (36) have been shown to be major producers of superoxide radical anions and hydrogen peroxide. Superoxide anion radicals are essen-

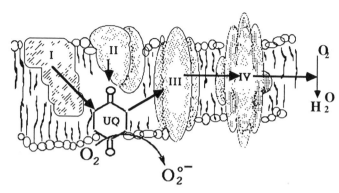

FIG. 2. A model for the arrangement of the mitochondrial electron transport system, showing the components of complexes I, II, III, IV and the sites believed to be involved in the major production of superoxide radical anions ($O_2^{\circ-}$). Superoxide radical anions are believed to be generated between complexes I and III of the respiratory chain. The two major sites proposed for the one-electron reduction of molecular oxygen to superoxide are located at UQ (ubisemiquinone) and a reduced intermediate of complex I (not shown in the schematic). The straight arrows indicate the normal flow of electrons to molecular oxygen, resulting in its four-electron reduction to water.

tial precursors for hydrogen peroxide formation in mitochondria (37,38). Mitochondrial production of superoxide and its by-product, H_2O_2, occurs when electron flux through the respiratory chain is poor, that is, in state 4 respiration (ADP-limited) (37,39). More specifically, the flavoprotein NADH dehydrogenase (40,41) and the ubisemiquinone (42), located between complexes I and III, have been proposed as the two major sites for the production of reactive oxygen species (Fig. 2). Boveris and Cadenas (43), using submitochondrial particles, have suggested that up to 4% of the oxygen consumed during state 4 respiration may escape from the respiratory chain as the partially reduced superoxide radical anion. In particular, superoxide production in isolated mitochondria is maximized when incubated in the presence of antimycin A (39,44). It is generally believed that superoxide produced during mitochondrial respiration is liberated to the matrix side of the mitochondrial membrane. However, superoxide is a rather sluggish reacting radical that has been shown to diffuse through membranes (45–47). Saran and Bors (7) have suggested superoxide to have a lifetime up to 400 nanoseconds and possessing a phospholipid diffusion path length of about 55–3000 nm. Based on the lifetime and diffusion distance of superoxide, Saran and Bors (7) have suggested that oxygen radicals may act as cellular messengers.

HYPOTHESIS: A CASE STUDY WITH DOXORUBICIN

A correlation between mitochondrial calcium and oxidative stress has been suggested, with the majority of the reports concerning an oxidative stress-induced release of calcium via a Na^+-independent pathway (29). Various research laboratories have suggested that a variety of prooxidants may be toxic because of their ability to induce calcium release from mitochondria via an oxidation of pyridine nucleotides. The consensus is that the Na^+-independent pathway for calcium release is associated with an increased permeability of the inner mitochondrial membrane. It is well known that isolated mitochondria become leaky on accumulation of excess calcium, especially in the presence of phosphate. Al-Nassar and Crompton (31) have demonstrated that this calcium release is the result of an increased mitochondrial permeability. Permeabilization is reversed when the calcium concentration is lowered by chelation with EGTA. Their data suggest a reversible, calcium-induced permeability change of the inner mitochondrial membrane. In a subsequent paper, Crompton and Costi (32) proposed that heart mitochondria contain a pore whose permeation state is controlled not only by calcium and phosphate but also by oxidative stress. Olafsdottir et al. (48) have recently reported that an increased intracellular calcium concentration in isolated hepatocytes results in the depletion of mitochondrial glutathione, probably as a result of mitochondrial calcium cycling (49). These observations suggest that alterations in calcium homeostasis may initiate oxidative stress.

A major objective of our laboratory was to investigate the role of mitochondrial calcium overload in the toxicity of doxorubicin and to determine an association, if any, of mitochondrial calcium transport with the formation of superoxide radical anions. This objective was chosen because doxorubicin has been shown to cause a decrease in mitochondrial state 3 respiration, and an increase in state 4 respiration (50,51), to increase the permeability of the inner mitochondrial membrane (51), and to alter the ability of mitochondria to retain large amounts of accumulated calcium (52,53). The inability of the mitochondria to retain accumulated calcium suggests tha doxorubicin may induce mitochondrial calcium cycling. In addition, considering that both mitochondrial calcium accumulation and the formation of reactive oxygen species are processes dependent on state 4 respiration, it is therefore conceivable that an energy dissipation by mitochondrial calcium cycling may be a physiological mechanism by which intracellular reactive oxygen species are made. Our laboratory has proposed that the cardiotoxicity of doxorubicin may involve alterations in mitochondrial calcium homeostasis, as well as the production of intracellular reactive oxygen species (54,55).

The cardiotoxicity of doxorubicin was investigated using a primary culture system of rat myocardial cells, which is an effective and sensitive experimental model for investigating the cytotoxicity of known cardiotoxic agents (56,57). Initial studies, using indirect methods to assess the role of calcium in doxorubicin-induced cell injury, suggested that calcium may be involved in the initiation of oxidative stress. Thus the effects of doxorubicin were investigated in an isolated mitochondrial preparation in attempt to further define a role for calcium in the production of reactive oxygen species. Digitized fluorescence imaging studies were conducted to assess the direct effects of doxorubicin on intracellular calcium homeostasis and relate such changes to alterations in mitochondrial function. The results showed that the mitochondria of cardiac cells appear to be early targets in doxorubicin-induced cell injury.

Doxorubicin is an efficient antineoplastic agent used against human carcinomas, although serious cardiotoxicity limits its clinical use. Various mechanisms have been suggested for the cardiotoxicity of doxorubicin. One theory is an intercalation of the drug between base pairs of DNA helices with the subsequent inhibition of DNA replication and RNA synthesis. The cardiotoxicity has also been related to alterations in intracellular calcium homeostasis. However, the leading hypothesis for the mechanism of doxorubicin-induced cardiotoxicity has been attributed to the production of toxic oxygen radicals. Doxorubicin is believed to generate toxic oxygen radicals by way of a redox cycling. This redox cycling may involve an enzymatic reduction of the parent quinone to a semiquinone, which can then be reoxidized back to the parent quinone by molecular oxygen, resulting in the formation of superoxide radical anions. The enzymatic reduction believed to be responsible for the generation of superoxide by doxorubicin (at the level of the mitochondria) has been suggested to occur between complexes I and II of the respiratory chain (see Fig. 2). Interestingly, the normal production of superoxide by respiring mitochondria has also been localized to occur between complexes I and II of the respiratory chain. Mitochondrial production of reactive oxygen species and the regulation of calcium transport are processes dependent on the electron transport system. The data by our laboratory (54,55) suggest that the production of superoxide by respiring rat heart mitochondria was decreased by either chelating extra-mitochondrial calcium with EGTA or by blocking mitochondrial calcium uptake with ruthenium red (see Fig. 1). Mitochondrial experiments with doxorubicin showed an enhanced stimulation of reactive oxygen species, which was also decreased by calcium chelation or inhibition of calcium uptake. Myocardial cell cultures treated with doxorubicin showed a collapsing mitochondrial membrane potential concurrent with the production of intracellular reactive oxygen species and mitochondrial calcium overload, all of which preceded a rise in cytoxolic calcium and cell death. The relationship between mitochondrial calcium transport and the formation of superoxide suggests that a disruption in mitochondrial calcium homeostasis may be involved in the initiation process of oxidative stress induced by doxorubicin.

There is increasing evidence that oxidative stress induces alterations in mitochondrial calcium homeostasis (29). The data presented by our laboratory suggest that the converse may also exist in that alterations in mitochondrial calcium homeostasis may initiate oxidative stress. The unique energetics of mitochondrial calcium transport among different tissues may provide new insights to the target organ specificity of some drugs. For example, mitochondrial calcium transport in liver mitochondria occurs as an alternative over oxidative phosphorylation; Jacobus et al. (23) demonstrated that state 4 respiration was increased by calcium in liver mitochondria but not in heart mitochondria. In heart mitochondria, the phosphorylation of ADP competed with calcium accumulation without increasing state 4 respiration. The differences in how these tissues regulate mitochondrial calcium transport may affect the outcome of the potential damage imposed by reactive oxygen species. The work presented herein demonstrates that the formation of doxorubicin-induced reactive oxygen species may be dependent on calcium. It is well known that concomitant with the energy-dependent uptake of calcium is the electroneutral release of calcium that provides a continuous cycling of the cation across the inner mitochondrial membrane (58). Loschen et al. (39) have shown that alterations in mitochondrial energy-linked reactions, using respiratory inhibitors with uncouplers, result in H_2O_2 production. Based on these present observations, one cannot clearly say that mitochondrial superoxide production is strictly dependent on calcium uptake or release but the data certainly point to an alteration in energy conservation, possibly as a result of calcium cycling. The data presented by our laboratory suggest either (a) a disruption of a finely regulated calcium/electron transport homeostasis, which results in the formation of superoxide or (b) a calcium-induced increased membrane permeability with the leakage of superoxide from the matrix side of mitochondria. From these results, it becomes evident that the ability to discriminate between mitochondrial calcium transport coupled to the formation of superoxide and calcium-induced mitochondrial permeabilization resulting in an increased leakage of superoxide will provide new insights into the role of reactive oxygen species acting as intracellular messengers and in the cellular injury process.

IN VITRO TECHNOLOGY IN THE EVALUATION OF CARDIOVASCULAR TOXICITY

The detection of cardiovascular injury at the cellular level is beset by many difficulties. The study of cell injury produced by toxins or disease *in vivo* can be complicated by interactions between adjacent cells of different types, neural and hormonal feedback, metabolism of the toxic agent, and a rapidly changing concentration of the agent at the cell–body fluid interface. The use of cell or tissue culture has been advocated as a means of studying the direct effects of drugs or toxicants on isolated cells without the complex interactions of the physiological systems present in the intact animal. Although cultured cells are not perfect test objects, their functional integrity is largely retained; uniform cells of almost any specific type can be studied in almost limitless numbers; the environment, including the concentration of the test agent, is easily maintained; and changes in morphology, function, and biochemistry can be directly observed or measured. The use of cultured cells enables species- and organ-specific toxicity to be studied. The nature of the cultured cell system and the ease of its manipulation may provide an insight into a chemical mechanism that underlies toxicity by measuring a modification of a subcellular macromolecule, enzymatic reaction, or organelle as a sensitive and specific indicator of toxicity.

Many approaches have been made to elucidate the basic mechanisms of heart function and dysfunction. However, no one approach shows the whole picture. Improved testing procedures are needed to detect potential toxicants since the cardiotoxicity produced by several agents has not been detected by preclinical studies in animals (59).

Recently, heart cell culture systems have been advocated as useful models to study myocardial injury and drug-induced cardiotoxicity (60–68). In heart cell culture, the heart is separated into single cells. Isolated cells are grown in a medium composed of amino acids, vitamins, glucose, minerals, and serum. These cells are capable of forming a confluent monolayer. When in contact, cells in culture beat in unison. They are sensitive to drugs and metabolites in a manner similar to the whole heart (69).

Advantages

Primary heart cell cultures offer several advantages over *in vivo* models to study drug-induced cardiotoxicity. Generally, it is not possible to follow the course of myocardial damage using *in vivo* techniques. In contrast, the use of monocyte cultures permits early detection of myocardial injury. Using this model, sequential sampling is facilitated and time-dependent changes can be evaluated.

Primary heart cell cultures can be prepared using a differential pour-off technique that separates muscle cells from nonmuscle cell types (70). This procedure provides a uniform population of myocardial cells maintained under carefully monitored conditions. Therefore complications such as blood flow and hormonal and neuronal factors may be eliminated. In addition, only small amounts of the test compound are required and the concentrations of chemicals to which the cells are exposed are easily manipulated. The time investment and expense required to generate useful information are reduced by using this model.

Disadvantages

The use of heart cell cultures is not without limitations. Several aspects still require refinement. Myocytes in culture may show variable contraction rates and electromechanical uncoupling caused by cell isolation procedures (69). During electromechanical uncoupling, the cells fire action potentials but do not visibly contract. However, simple microscopic examination of the cells is sufficient to reveal the state of the cultures prepared. In addition, the contractile apparatus, namely, the myofibrils, may not be in a highly differentiated state even though the cells may be highly differentiated electrically (69).

Cultured cells revert back to young embryonic states. This limitation can be minimized if the cultures are utilized for toxicity studies shortly after monolayer formation. The metabolism of cultured cells may shift from an aerobic to a more anaerobic state (69). During cell isolation some of the pharmacological receptors may be inactivated. Enzymatic isolation procedures of short duration are thought to minimize the extent of damage. Contaminant cells such as fibroblasts may be present in myocyte cultures. Thus during biochemical determinations, contaminant cells will also be analyzed. Various approaches are currently available to minimize the extent of contamination by cell types other than myocardial cells (70).

There are several problems concerning the use of cultured heart cells. However, if reasonable precautions are taken this model can provide important information not readily available from intact cardiac muscle preparations.

REFERENCES

1. Sies H. Oxidative stress: introductory remarks. In: Sies H, ed. *Oxidative stress.* London: Academic Press; 1985:1–8.
2. Jones DP. The role of oxygen concentration in oxidative stress: hypoxic models. In: Sies H, ed. *Oxidative stress.* London: Academic Press; 1985:151–195.
3. Cadenas E. Oxidative stress and formation of excited species. In: Sies H, ed. *Oxidative stress.* London: Academic Press; 1985:311–330.
4. Kappus H. Lipid peroxidation: mechanisms, analysis, enzymology, and biological relevance. In: Sies H, ed. *Oxidative stress.* London: Academic Press, 1985:273–310.
5. Freeman BA, Crapo JD. Biology of disease. Free radicals and tissue injury. *Lab Invest* 1982;47:412–426.
6. Marx JL. Oxygen free radicals linked to many diseases. *Science* 1987;235:529–531.
7. Saran M, Bors W. Oxygen radicals acting as chemical messengers: a hypothesis. *Free Rad Res Commun* 1989;7:213–220.
8. Carafoli E. Intracellular calcium homeostasis. *Annu Rev Biochem* 1987;56:395–433.
9. Lemasters JJ, Nieminen A-L, Gores GJ, Wray BE, Herman B. Cytosolic free calcium and cell injury in hepatocytes. In: Fiskum G, ed. *Cell calcium metabolism.* New York: Plenum Publishing, 1989:463–470.
10. Trump BF, Berezesky IK, Laiho KV, Osornio AR, Mergner WJ, Smith MW. The role of calcium in cell injury. A review. In: Becker RP, Johari O, eds. *Scanning electron microscopy II.* Chicago: SEM; 1980:437–492.
11. Bellomo G, Orrenius S. Altered thiol and calcium homeostasis in oxidative hepatocellular injury. *Hepatology* 1985;5:876–882.
12. Fleckenstein A, Janke J, Doring HJ, Pachinger O. Ca overload as the determinant factor in the production of catecholamine-induced myocardial lesions. In: Bajusz E, Rona G, eds. *Recent advances in studies on cardiac structure and metabolism.* Baltimore: University Park Press; 1973:455–466.
13. Jewell SA, Bellomo G, Thor H, Orrenius S, Smith MT. Bleb formation in hepatocytes during drug metabolism is caused by disturbances in thiol and calcium homeostasis. *Science* 1982;217:1257–1259.

14. Chien KR, Abrams S, Pfau RG, Farber JL. Prevention by chlorpromazine of ischemic liver cell death. *Am J Pathol* 1977;88:539–548.
15. McConkey DJ, Nicotera P, Hartzell P, Bellomo G, Wyllie AH, Orrenius S. Glucocorticoids activate a suicide process in thymocytes through an elevation of cytosolic calcium concentration. *Arch Biochem Biophys* 1989;269:365–370.
16. Cantoni O, Sestili P, Cattabeni F, Bellomo G, Pou S, Cohen M, Cerutti P. Calcium chelator quin 2 prevents hydrogen-peroxide-induced DNA breakage and cytotoxicity. *Eur J Biochem* 1989;182:209–212.
17. Jones DP, McConkey DJ, Nicotera P, Orrenius S. Calcium-activated DNA fragmentation in rat liver nuclei. *J Biol Chem* 1989;264:6398–6403.
18. Siekevitz P, Potter VR. Biochemical structure of mitochondria I. Intramitochondrial components and oxidative phosphorylation. *J Biol Chem* 1955;215:221–235.
19. Gunter TE, Pfeiffer DR. Mechanisms by which mitochondria transport calcium. *Am J Physiol* 1990;258:C755–C786.
20. Scarpa A. Transport across mitochondrial membranes. In: Giebisch G, Tosteson DC, Ussing HH, eds. *Membrane Transport in Biology.* New York: Springer-Verlag; 1979:263–355.
21. Scarpa A, Azzone GF. The mechanism of ion translocation in mitochondria. 4. Coupling of K efflux with Ca uptake. *Eur J Biochem* 1970;12:328–335.
22. Lehninger AL. Mitochondria and calcium ion transport. *Biochem J* 1970;119:129–138.
23. Jacobus WE, Tiozzo R, Lugi G, Lehninger AL, Carafoli E. Aspects of energy-linked calcium accumulation by rat heart mitochondria. *J Biol Chem* 1975;250:7863–7870.
24. Rizzuto R, Bernardi P, Favaron M, Azzone GF. Pathways for calcium efflux in heart and liver mitochondria. *Biochem J* 1987;246:271–277.
25. Crompton M, Capano M, Carafoli E. The sodium-induced efflux of calcium from heart mitochondria. *Eur J Biochem* 1976;69:453–462.
26. Bernardi P, Azzone GF. Regulation of calcium efflux in rat liver mitochondria. Role of membrane potential. *Eur J Biochem* 1985;134:377–383.
27. Crompton M, Costi A, Hayat L. Evidence for the presence of a reversible calcium-dependent pore activated by oxidative stress in heart mitochondria. *Biochem J* 1987;245:915–918.
28. Riley WW, Pfeiffer DR. The effect of calcium and acyl coenzyme A: lysophospholipid acyl transferase inhibitors on permeability properties of the liver mitochondrial inner membrane. *J Biol Chem* 1986;261:14018–14024.
29. Richter C, Frei B. Ca^{++} release from mitochondria induced by prooxidants. *Free Rad Biol Med* 1988;4:365–373.
30. Al-Nassar I, Crompton M. The reversible Ca^{++}-induced permeabilization of rat liver mitochondria. *Biochem J* 1986;239:19–29.
31. Al-Nassar I, Crompton M. The entrapment of the Ca indicator arsenazo III in the matrix space of rat liver mitochondria by permeabilization and resealing. Na-dependent and independent effluxes of Ca in arsenazo III-loaded mitochondria. *Biochem J* 1986;239:31–40.
32. Crompton M, Costi A. Kinetic evidence for a heart mitochondrial pore activated by Ca^{++}, inorganic phosphate and oxidative stress. *Eur J Biochem* 1988;178:489–501.
33. Boveris A, Chance B. The mitochondrial generation of hydrogen peroxide. *Biochem J* 1973;134:707–716.
34. Loschen G, Flohe L, Chance B. Respiratory chain linked H_2O_2 production in pigeon heart mitochondria. *FEBS Lett* 1971;18:261–264.
35. Boveris A, Oshino N, Chance B. The cellular production of hydrogen peroxide. *Biochem J* 1972;128:617–630.
36. Turrens JF, Freeman BA, Crapo JD. Hyperoxia increases hydrogen peroxide release by lung mitochondria and microsomes. *Arch Biochem Biophys* 1982;217:411–421.
37. Boveris A, Cadenas E. Mitochondrial production of superoxide anions and its relationship to the antimycin insensitive respiration. *FEBS Lett* 1975;54:311–314.
38. Dionisi O, Galeo-Hi T, Terranova T, Azzi A. Superoxide radicals and hydrogen peroxide formation in mitochondria from normal and neoplastic tissues. *Biochim Biophys Acta* 1975;403:292–301.
39. Loschen G, Azzi A, Flohe L. Mitochondrial H_2O_2 formation: relationship with energy conservation. *FEBS Lett* 1973;33:84–88.

40. Krishnamoorthy G, Hinkle PC. Studies on the electron transfer pathway, topography of iron sulphur centers, and sites of coupling in NADH-Q oxidoreductase. *J Biol Chem* 1988;263:17566–17575.
41. Turrens JF, Boveris A. Generation of superoxide anion by the NADH dehydrogenase of bovine heart mitochondria. *Biochem J* 1980;191:421–427.
42. Nohl H, Jordan W. The biochemical role of ubiquinone and ubiquinone-derivatives in the generation of hydroxyl-radicals from hydrogen-peroxide. In: Bors W, Saran M, Tait D, eds. *Oxygen radicals in chemistry and biology*. Berlin: Walter deGruyter; 1984:155–160.
43. Boveris A, Cadenas E. Production of superoxide radicals and hydrogen peroxide in mitochondria. In: Oberley LW, ed. *Superoxide dismutase*. Boca Raton, FL: CRC Press; 1982:15–30.
44. Loschen G, Azzi A, Richter C, Flohe L. Superoxide radicals as precursors of mitochondrial hydrogen peroxide. *FEBS Lett* 1974;42:68–72.
45. Lynch RE, Fridovich I. Permeation of the erythrocyte stroma by superoxide radical. *J Biol Chem* 1978;253:4697–4699.
46. Rumyantseva GV, Weiner LM, Molin YN, Budker VG. Permeation of liposome membranes by superoxide radical. *FEBS Lett* 1979;108:477–480.
47. Takahashi MA, Asada K. Superoxide anion permeability of phospholipid membranes and chloroplast thylakoids. *Arch Biochem Biophys* 1983;226:558–566.
48. Olafsdottir K, Pascoe GA, Reed DJ. Mitochondrial glutathione status during Ca^{++} ionophore-induced injury to isolated hepatocytes. *Arch Biochem Biophys* 1988;263:226–235.
49. Thomas CE, Reed DJ. Effect of extracellular Ca^{++} omission on isolated hepatocytes. II. Loss of mitochondrial membrane potential and protection by inhibitors of uniport Ca^{++} transduction. *J Pharmacol Exp Ther* 1988;254:501–507.
50. Bachmann E, Zbinden G. Effects of doxorubicin and rubidizone on respiratory function and Ca transport in rat heart mitochondria. *Toxicol Lett* 1979;3:29–34.
51. Ferrero ME, Ferrero E, Gaja G, Bernelli-Zazzera A. Adriamycin: energy metabolism and mitochondrial oxidations in the heart of treated rabbits. *Biochem Pharmacol* 1976;25:125–130.
52. Singal PK, Deally CMR, Weinberg LE. Subcellular effects of adriamycin in the heart: a concise review. *J Mol Cell Cardiol* 1987;19:817–828.
53. Sokolove PM, Shinaberry RG. Na-independent release of Ca from rat heart mitochondria. Induction by adriamycin aglycone. *Biochem Pharmacol* 1988;37:803–812.
54. Chacon E, Acosta D. Mitochondrial regulation of superoxide by calcium: an alternate mechanism for the cardiotoxicity of doxorubicin. *Toxicol Appl Pharmacol* 1991;107:117–128.
55. Chacon E, Acosta D. A digitized fluorescence imaging study of mitochondrial calcium increase by doxorubicin in cardiac myocytes. *Biochem J* 1992;281:871–878.
56. Lampidis TJ, Henderson IC, Israel M, Canellos GP. Structural and functional effects of adriamycin on cardiac cells in vitro. *Cancer Res* 1980;40:3901–3909.
57. Ramos K, Combs AB, Acosta D. Cytotoxicity of isoproterenol to cultured heart cells: effects of antioxidants on modifying membrane damage. *Toxicol Appl Pharmacol* 1983;70:317–323.
58. Fiskum G, Lehninger AL. Regulated release of Ca^{++} from respiring mitochondria by $Ca^{++}/2H^+$ antiport. *J Biol Chem* 1979;254:6236–6239.
59. Balazs T, Ferrans VJ. Cardiac lesions induced by chemicals. *Environ Health Perspect* 1978;26:181–191.
60. Ramos K, Acosta D. Prevention by l(-)ascorbic acid of isoproterenol-induced cardiotoxicity in primary cultures of rat myocytes. *Toxicology* 1983;26:81–90.
61. Ramos K, Combs AB, Acosta D. Role of calcium in isoproterenol cytotoxicity to cultured myocardial cells. *Biochem Pharmacol* 1984;33:1989–1992.
62. Acosta D, Combs AB, Ramos K. Attenuation by antioxidants of Na^+/K^+ ATPase inhibition by toxic concentrations of isoproterenol in cultured rat myocardial cells. *J Mol Cell Cardiol* 1984;16:281–284.
63. Acosta D, Ramos K. Cardiotoxicity of tricyclic antidepressants in primary cultures of rat myocardial cells. *J Toxicol Environ Health* 1984;14:137–143.
64. Combs AB, Acosta D, Ramos K. Effects of doxorubicin and verapamil on calcium up-

take in primary cultures of rat myocardial cells. *Biochem Pharmacol* 1985;34:1115–1116.

65. Butler AW, Smith MA, Farrar RP, Acosta D. Ethanol toxicity in primary cultures of rat myocardial cells. *Toxicology* 1985;36:61–70.
66. Welder AA, Smith MA, Ramos K, Acosta D. Cocaine-induced cardiotoxicity *in vitro*. *Toxicol In Vitro* 1988;2:205–213.
67. Mbugua PM, Welder AA, Acosta D. Cardiotoxicity of Jamesoni's mamba venom and its fractionated components in primary cultures of rat myocardial cells. *In Vitro Cell Dev Biol* 1988;24:743–752.
68. Mbugua PM, Welder AA, Acosta D. Cardiotoxicity of Kenyan green mamba venom and its fractionated components in primary cultures of rat myocardial cells. *Toxicology* 1988;52:187–207.
69. Sperelakis N. Cultured heart cell reaggregate model for studying cardiac toxicology. *Environ Health Perspect* 1978;26:243–267.
70. Wenzel DG, Wheatley JW, Byrd GD. Effects of nicotine on cultured little heart cells. *Toxicol Appl Pharmacol* 1970;17:774–785.

SECTION II

Methods

Cardiovascular Toxicology, Second Edition,
edited by Daniel Acosta, Jr.
Raven Press, Ltd., New York © 1992.

2

Acute and Chronic Evaluation of the Cardiovascular Toxicity of Drugs

An Industrial Perspective

Shayne C. Gad

Becton Dickinson and Company, P.O. Box 12016,
Research Triangle Park, North Carolina 27709

Industrial toxicologists have as their prime responsibility the identification of any or all adverse effects associated with compounds or mixtures that their employers intend to commercialize. In almost all cases, toxicologists in industry (though they may possess an individual expertise in one or more target organ systems) must perform as generalists, evaluating a compound for a broad range of adverse effects. Many of the standardized experimental designs that serve for detecting whether such effects are present are regulatorily mandated. This fact and the usual restraints of timing and cost have limited and guided what is done to identify cardiotoxic agents, including the determination that an effect exists, at what dose levels, and occasionally to determine if the effect is reversible.

Compounds with therapeutic potential are the particular domain of interest of the pharmaceutical toxicologist. In this arena, the task becomes considerably more challenging. The challenge occurs because pharmaceutical agents are intended to be administered to a target species (usually humans, except for veterinary drugs) and are intended to have biological effects. Occasionally, the commercial objective is an agent that alters the function of the cardiovascular system. To the pharmaceutical toxicologists, the task of evaluating cardiotoxicity frequently is expanded to identifying and understanding the mechanism of action, the relevance of findings to the target species, and quantitating the therapeutic dose (i.e., the separation between the dose with a desired effect and the higher dose that has an adverse effect). Indeed, the case of detecting cardiovascular toxicity is a function of the underlying mechanism of that toxicity; particularly if we are talking about individuals with preexisting cardiovascular disease.

The basic principles of cardiovascular function and mechanisms of cardiovascular toxicity are presented elsewhere in this book, and in other reviews of cardiovascular toxicity (1,2) and are not addressed here.

Evaluations of cardiotoxicity, with the exception of one special case, tend to be performed by adding measurements and observations to existing "pivotal" test designs. These measures look at alterations in myocardial and vascular structure (pathology, clinical pathology) and function (electrocardiograms, clinical pathology, and clinical observations). Tests focused on the cardiovascular system are designed and executed only if an indication of an effect is found. The special case exception are so called safety pharmacology studies, which seek to look at exaggerated pharmacological effects in rather focused target organ functional studies.

PHARMACOLOGICAL PROFILING

The profiling of the pharmacological effects of a new drug on the cardiovascular system is an essential element in early evaluations and development. Broad assessments of the effects on critical target organ functions (cardiovascular, renal, pulmonary, immune, peripheral and central nervous system) for which no action is intended are often called "safety pharmacology," though other purposes (such as the serendipitous discovery of additional desirable pharmacologic activities—i.e., new therapeutic opportunities) are also served. These assessments are carried out in the therapeutic to near-therapeutic dosage range, for example, from the projected human ED_{50} to perhaps the projected ED_{90}. Such evaluations can reveal other actions that were unintended and undesirable (side effects) or extensions/exaggerations of the intended pharmacology, which are either unacceptable or essential for interpreting results in actual toxicology studies. Such interpretations are more difficult, of course, when the agent is intended to have therapeutic cardiovascular effects. Brunner and Gross (3) and Gilman et al. (4) should be reviewed by anyone undertaking such an effort to ensure familiarity with basic cardiovascular pharmacology.

Focusing on cardiovascular effects, the concerns are both direct (on the heart and vasculature) and indirect (such as on adrenal release) effects in the short term. Accordingly, these studies look at function in the short term (hours to perhaps 3 days). The dog and the rat are generally the model species, with parameters being evaluated including the following:

Physiologic function: blood pressure, electrocardiogram (EKG), blood gases
Biochemistry: enzyme release (LDH, CPK), oxygen consumption, calcium transport, substrate utilization

Several of these (EKG, LDH, and CPK) are also evaluated in traditional "pivotal" safety/toxicology studies at higher doses (up to 100 times the intended human dose) and are discussed in further detail here. Such studies also depend on extensive evaluation of clinical signs to indicate problems.

All of these could also be of concern for nondrug chemical entities but are generally only evaluated to the extent described later under pivotal studies (if at all).

IN VIVO PARAMETER EVALUATIONS IN STANDARD STUDIES

For most new chemical entities, the primary screen for cardiotoxicity in industry consists of selected parameters incorporated into the "pivotal" or systemic toxicity studies of various lengths. These "shotgun" studies (so called because they attempt to collect as much data as possible to identify and crudely characterize toxicities associated with a drug or chemical) are exemplified by the 13-week study shown in Fig. 1.

As shown, a large number of variables are measured, with only a few of them either acting directly or indirectly as predictors of cardiovascular toxicity. These measures are taken at multiple time points and in aggregate compose a powerful tool set for identifying the existence of problems. Their sensitivity and value are limited, however, by several design features incorporated into the pivotal study. First is the limited number of animals (particularly in nonrodent studies—i.e., those that use dogs, primates, etc.) and the number of times that specific measurements are made. Both are limited by cost and logistics, and these limitations decrease the overall power of the study. The second feature is the complications inherent in dealing with background variability in many of these parameters. Though individual animals are typically screened prior to inclusion in a study to ensure that those with unacceptable baselines for parameters of interest (very typically, EKGs, clinical chemistries, and hematologies) are eliminated, clearly some degree of variability must be accepted on grounds of economics or practicality. Proper analysis of the entire data set collected as an integrated whole is the key to minimizing these weaknesses.

Electrocardiograms (EKGs)

Properly employed and analyzed, EKGs represent the most sensitive early indicator of cardiac toxicity or malfunction. Long before the other functional measures (blood pressure or clinical signs) or before the invasive measures (clinical chemistries or histopathology), the EKG should generally reveal that a problem exists.

Deceptively simple in form (see Fig. 2 for examples), EKGs present a great deal of information. Much of this information (amplitudes of the various waves, the lengths of intervals, and the frequency of events—i.e., heart

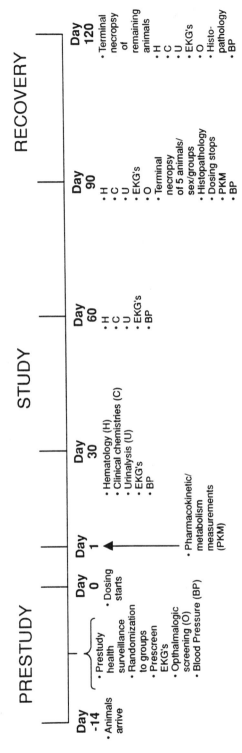

FIG. 1. Line chart for a standard or "pivotal" 13-week toxicity study. Four or more groups of 16 (eight male and eight female) beagle dogs each; Daily dosing (five days a week for chemicals, seven days a week for pharmaceuticals or food additives) at selected dose levels, with one group being controls and receiving only vehicle or sham exposure; Mortality and morbidity checks twice a day, detailed clinical observations at least once a week; function observational battery (FOB; ref. 12) on days 0, 4, 11, 49, and 87; Body weights of every animal on days −7, −1, 0, 4, 7, 11, and weekly thereafter; Food consumption weekly. For the sake of illustration, what is shown is a dog study. The design is the same (except for numbers of animals) for studies conducted in other species (rats, primates, etc.). Dosing is by the appropriate route and frequency (usually, however, once daily in the morning).

rate) is quantitative in nature and can be analyzed by traditional statistical techniques. For this larger portion of the information in EKGs, the problems are that (a) baselines vary significantly from species to species (making interpretation of the relevance of changes seen in some models difficult) and (b) the task of actually collecting the EKGs and then extracting quantitative data from them is very labor intensive. There are now some computer-assisted analysis programs [such as that described in Watkinson et al. (5)] that perform the quantitative aspects of data extraction and analysis well.

There is also a significant amount of information in EKGs that is not quantitative, but rather more of a pattern recognition nature. This requires a learned art and a great deal of experience for the more complex changes.

Interpretation of the underlying causes of changes in EKGs requires a knowledge of cardiac pathophysiology. Sodeman and Sodeman (6) present excellent overviews of this area, and Doherty and Cobbe (7) review the special cases of EKG changes in animal models.

Attention to technique is critical in the proper performance and interpretation of EKGs. Each species has different requirements for the placement and even the type of electrodes employed (8,9). In addition, there are differences in electrocardiographic effects between sedated and nonsedated animals. Additionally, there are rather marked differences in EKGs between species, with the dog having a very labile T wave and the rat ST segment being short to nonexistent (see Fig. 2).

Blood Pressure and Heart Rate

These two traditional noninvasive measures of cardiovascular function have the advantages of being easy and inexpensive to perform. Their chief disadvantage is that they are subject to significant short-term variability, which significantly degrades their sensitivity and reliability. Techniques do exist for minimizing these disadvantages in various animal model species (10,11), and careful attention to general animal husbandry and handling helps.

If EKGs are collected, then it is easy to extract the heart rate from the tracings. Most automated systems will, in fact, perform this calculation as a matter of course. Blood pressure, meanwhile, is attractive because it is a noninvasive measure of vascular function. Techniques for collecting it have improved significantly in recent years.

Neither of these measures is commonly collected in the pivotal or standard safety study, however. If clinical signs, particularly in larger (nonrodent) species indicate that an effect is present, these should readily be added to a study.

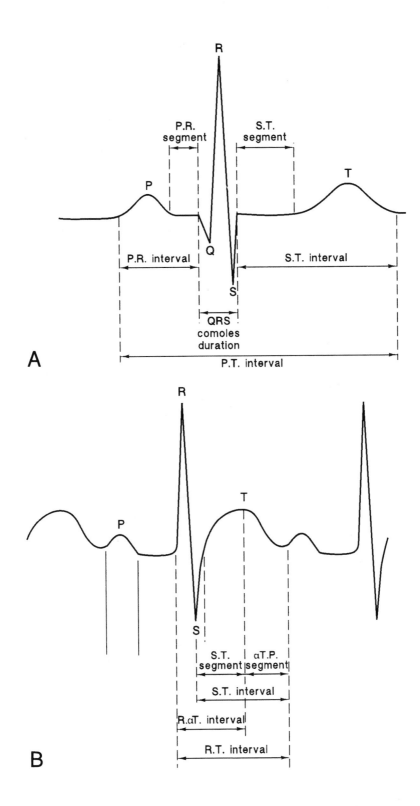

A

B

Clinical Signs

Clinical signs represent the oldest noninvasive assessment of general health and provide in animal studies a crude but broad and potentially very valuable screen for identifying adverse responses. Training, experience, and continuity of the observer are vitally important to having these signs be both meaningful and reliable. A rigorous, regular, and formatted collection of such signs in an objective manner (12) provides an essential component of any systemic toxicity study.

A number of the observations collected in the standard clinical signs measurements either directly or indirectly address cardiovascular function. These include body temperature, the occurrence of cyanosis, flushing, weakness, pulse, and the results of careful palpitation of the cardiac region.

CLINICAL CHEMISTRIES

Traditional systemic or "general" toxicology studies place their greatest reliance for detecting cardiotoxicity on the last two sets of tools presented here—clinical and anatomic pathology. Both of these are invasive and therefore either entail instilling at least some stress in test animals or terminating the animals, but are considered to be reasonably unequivocal in their interpretation. And both require a significant amount of experience/knowledge as to what the normal characteristics of the model species are.

Clinical pathology entails both hematology and clinical chemistry. Here we are interested only in the latter, as cardiovascular toxicity is not generally reflected in the hemogram. Urinalysis is likewise not a useful component of the clinical chemistry screen for detecting cardiotoxicity. Rather, serum levels of selected parameters are of primary interest. During actual myocardial infarction there occurs a leakage of cellular constituents with rapid losses of ions and metabolites, resulting in transient increases in serum concentrations of these parameters. Later, there is a release of specific enzymes and proteins, which are in turn slowly cleared from the plasma. One can broadly classify the measurements made in serum as electrolytes, enzymes, proteins (other than enzymes), and lipids. Analysis of the findings as to their increases and decreases tends to be more powerful when it looks at patterns of changes across several endpoints, such as increases in creatinine phosphokinase (CPK), γ-hydroxybutyrate dehydrogenase (γ-HBDH) and

---

FIG. 2. Stylized EKGs for humans (**A**) and adult rats (**B**). Though there are similarities between species, it is important to be aware of differences here and those that are dependent on age.

lactate dehydrogenase (LDH), and serum glutamic–oxaloacetic transaminase (SGOT).

Though the most important parameters are generally considered to be CPK, γ-HBDH, LDH, and SGOT, each of which is primarily a muscle enzyme (and therefore increased levels of which may be indicative of either skeletal or cardiac muscle damage), it is appropriate to review the entire range of chemistry endpoints.

Electrolytes

Maintenance of the intracellular and extracellular concentrations of cations (sodium, potassium, calcium, magnesium, and zinc) is essential for proper cardiovascular function. Alterations of the concentrations of these cations may result in increased cardiac tissue sensitivity, arrhythmias, or significant adverse changes in vascular permeability. Concentrations of these cations are interrelated, making any significant disturbance of the ionic balance for one cation a consequence for the concentrations of the remaining ions. This interrelationship is observed with cardiac glycosides, which inhibit the sarcolemmal sodium pump Na^+/K^+-ATPase, causing increased intracellular sodium concentration, followed by increases of intracellular calcium and cardiac contractility. Where cardiac output is decreased, disturbances of plasma electrolytes may be due to consequential alterations of renal function, for example, reduced glomerular filtration rate (GFR). GFR may be evaluated by plasma creatinine and urea measurements. In addition, hypernatremia or hyponatremia may be observed in cardiac failure, depending on the volemic state of the animal.

When considering the effects of calcium and magnesium on cardiac function, the concentrations not bound to proteins (free) are more important than the total plasma concentration. Depending on the species, approximately 40% of the total plasma calcium and 30% of the plasma magnesium are bound to proteins. The need to consider plasma free-calcium concentration to protein-bound Ca concentration has been demonstrated by adriamycin-induced cardiotoxicity in rabbits. Hypercalcemia is not apparent when total plasma calcium is measured in adriamycin-treated rabbits, as there is a concomitant reduction of plasma albumin caused by renal toxicity. Increased plasma ionized calcium levels observed in these rabbits may therefore be partly due to the renal dysfunction. Excessive stress and use of restraining procedures during blood collection will markedly affect the potassium, calcium, and magnesium levels. In rodents, the sites used for blood collection and anesthetic techniques will also influence these plasma cation measurements.

Although changes of plasma anion concentrations often follow disturbances of cationic balance, these changes are of lesser significance for cardiac function. Plasma anions (chloride, bicarbonate, and inorganic phosphate) are poor markers of cardiotoxicity, as their plasma concentrations may be altered for many reasons other than those associated with cardiac function.

Osmolality and Acid–Base Balance

Plasma osmolality determinations may be meaningful in conditions such as congestive cardiac failure, where total body sodium concentration and extracellular fluid volume are increased but there is evidence of hyponatremia. Several formulas for the calculation of plasma osmolality from plasma concentrations of sodium, urea, and glucose have been used with humans but have limited applicability with other species, where the component concentrations vary. Acid–base balance determinations can be used to monitor cardiotoxic effects on respiratory and metabolic functions, but the variability due to blood collection procedures on these determinations in small laboratory animals limits their regular use in toxicological studies.

Enzymes

Heart muscle tissue is rich in enzymes but only a few have proved to be useful markers of myocardial damage and congestive cardiac failure. A major limitation on use in animal studies is the relatively short half-life of these markers after damage has occurred. This makes the sampling design shown in Fig. 1 very much a hit-or-miss proposition, particularly as different doses of the same compound will cause damage (and therefore evoke enzyme release) at different times. Additionally, it must be remembered that these enzymes are released by cells that are dead or dying. Damage that is functionally impairing to the organ or organism may not kill enough cells to be detected by this endpoint.

There are also real limits on how many samples may be drawn from smaller animals, particularly when a large enough volume must be drawn for evaluation of all the clinical pathology parameters.

Plasma enzyme activity depends on the enzyme concentrations in different tissues, the mass of damaged tissue, the severity of damage, the molecular size of the enzyme, and the rate of clearance from the plasma. The distribution of enzymes in different tissues varies between species (13,14). Differences between published data for tissue enzyme concentrations in the same species are in part due to the methods used for tissue preparation and sample collection (due to varying levels of physiological stress), extraction of the enzyme, and enzyme measurement. The rate for enzyme removal from the intravascular space varies greatly for individual enzymes and species, as reflected by the differing relative half-lives of each enzyme.

For both CPK and LDH measurements, it is preferable to use plasma rather than serum, owing to the relatively high concentration of these enzymes in platelets—and hence their release into serum during blood coagulation. Plasma samples with visible evidence of hemolysis should not be used due to high enzyme concentrations in erythrocytes. Blood collection procedures may influence plasma enzyme values, particularly in rodents.

Creatine Phosphokinase (CPK)

Creatine phosphokinase has two subunits, B and M, which can form three cytocolic isoenzymes: the dimer consisting of two M (muscle) subunits (CPK-MM) is the "muscle type" isoenzyme, the hybrid dimer (CPK-MB) is the "myocardial type" isoenzyme, and the third dimer (CPK-BB) is the "brain type" isoenzyme. A fourth isoenzyme (CPK_M) is located in the mitochondria of cardiac and other tissues.

Intramuscular injections cause increased plasma CPK activities: however, if blood samples are collected approximately 5 min after injection of an anesthetic agent sufficient to fully anesthetize rats, no effect on CPK is observed. The age of an animal may affect plasma CPK, with activities generally being higher in younger animals. Values also may be affected by stress and severe exercise.

Lactate Dehydrogenase (LDH)

LDH is a cytosolic tetrameric enzyme with five major isoenzymes consisting of M (muscle) and H (heart) subunits; a sixth isoenzyme of C subunits is found in some tissues. The five isoenzymes are numbered according to relative mobility during electrophoretic separation; LDH_1 consists of four H subunits; LDH_5 consists of four identical M units; and LDH_2, LDH_3, and LDH_4 are hybrid combinations of the two subunits (HHHM, HHMM, and HMMM). The distribution of LDH in various tissues is often described as ubiquitous, and variations occur between species. For these reasons and because of the broad normal plasma LDH ranges often encountered in laboratory animals, the plasma total LDH values are often difficult to interpret; separation (and quantification) of plasma LDH isoenzymes therefore is helpful in cardiotoxicity studies.

Plasma α-hydroxybutyrate dehydrogenase (HBD) measurements reflect the activities of LDH_1 and LDH_2 isoenzymes. In seven of ten species examined, tissue HBD activities are highest in cardiac tissue. LDH_5 is the dominant isoenzyme in normal rat and dog plasma, while LDH_1 and LDH_2 are the dominant isoenzymes in plasmas of several primates. Where LDH_5 is the major isoenzyme in the plasma, it may require a considerable increase of LDH_1 before total LDH values change significantly. Some drugs (such as streptokinase) modify the electrophoretic mobility of some LDH isoenzymes.

Serum Glutamic–Oxaloacetic Transaminase (SGOT) and Serum Glutamic–Pyruvic Transaminase (SGPT)

These two enzymes are commonly used as indicators of hepatotoxicity but their plasma activities may also be altered following myocardial damage. Neither of these is tissue specific; in many laboratory animal species, cardiac tissue SGOT concentration is higher than in most other major tissues, whereas cardiac tissue SGPT concentrations vary between species. In the rat, dog, and mouse, hepatic tissue SGPT concentrations are generally higher than that in other major tissues, but hepatic and cardiac tissue concentrations are similar in several primate species. The plasma SGOT/SGPT ratio may be useful in detecting cardiac damage, but the ratios vary with species and often cannot be compared with published data because the ratios are dependent on methods.

There are two isoenzymes of SGOT—cytosolic and mitochondrial isoenzymes; SGPT also has cytosolic and mitochondrial isoenzymes, but SGPT often is commonly believed to be entirely cytosolic owing to the higher proportion of cytosolic to mitochondrial isoenzyme.

Table 1 broadly summarizes these patterns of change for the major classes of damage seen in or confused with cardiac toxicity.

Other Proteins

Plasma albumin acts as a marker of plasma volume following cardiac damage; changes may simply reflect edema or plasma volume differences following congestive cardiac failure. Plasma albumin can be measured by dye-binding methods or more specific immunoassays. Plasma protein electrophoresis can confirm decreased plasma albumin levels and detect changes of other protein fractions. Serial plasma protein electrophoretic measurements may be useful in monitoring inflammatory processes, but changes are not specific for cardiac damage.

Plasma myoglobin can be used as a marker of myocardial damage, but the

TABLE 1. *Differentiation based on serum enzyme findings for major classes of cardiac damage and related/confounding events*

Condition	SGOT	SGPT	CPK	LDH
Myocardial cell death (infarct)	Increased	No change	Increased	Increased
Congestive heart failure (liver congestion)	Increased	Increased	No change	Increased
Muscle necrosis	Increased	No change	Increased	Increased
Lung embolism	No change	No change	Minimal increase	Increased

changes of plasma myoglobin occur more rapidly than those observed for plasma CPK. The myoglobin structure varies between different vertebrates, and the amino acid sequence imparts varying immunogenic properties, preventing the use of some latex agglutination and radioimmunoassay methods with certain species. Again, myoglobinemia may be caused by disease processes other than cardiovascular disorders.

Plasma fibrinogen is a useful measurement, particularly in the assessment of thrombolytic agents and epidosic thrombolysis. Chromogenic substrates designed for human plasma fibrinogen assays do not react identically with samples from other species, and some assays for determining fibrin degradation products do not work with all species.

Lipids

As markers of lipid metabolism, plasma lipids are indicators of potential risks for cardiotoxicity in contrast to some of the preceding markers, which directly or indirectly reflect cardiac tissue damage. In rabbits fed cholesterol-enriched vegetable oil, the relationship between hyperlipidemia and the resulting lesions of the aorta and coronary arteries were demonstrated over 70 years ago. Whereas hypolipidemic agents are designed to prevent atherosclerosis, some drugs may inadvertently moderate or modify metabolic pathways for lipids, lipoproteins, or apolipoproteins (through biliary secretion or lipid surface receptors). Adverse effects on lipid metabolism can be monitored by measuring plasma total cholesterol and triglycerides, with the additional measurements of plasma lipoproteins, total lipids, phospholipids, apolipoproteins, and nonesterified fatty acids.

Plasma lipid patterns vary with age, sex, diet, and the period of food withdrawal prior to collection of blood samples. There are both qualitative and quantitative differences in the lipid metabolism of different laboratory animal species: these occur owing to differences in the rates and routes of absorption, synthesis, metabolism, and excretion. In the rat, ferret, dog, mouse, rabbit, and guinea pig, the major plasma lipoprotein classes are the high-density lipoproteins contrasting to old-world monkeys and humans, where the low-density lipoproteins are the major lipoproteins in plasma.

For a more thorough review of the expected ranges for clinical chemistries in model species and their interpretation, one should consult Loeb and Quimby (17), Evans (18), Wallach (19), or Mikruka and Rawnsley (20).

PATHOLOGY

As with plasma chemistries, major considerations in the use of anatomic pathology as a tool for detecting and evaluating cardiotoxicity are associated with sampling (i.e., how many sections are to be taken and from where). Histopathology is a generally terminal measure [the exception being the use of *in situ* biopsy techniques such as proposed by Fenoglio and Wagner (21)], so the time point for study termination governs whether a lesion will have had time to develop and if its interpretation will not be complicated by subsequent (after the injury of interest) events. Similarly, it is of concern how representative sections will be taken from collected tissues.

The heart shares a primary property with the nervous system, having cells with electrically excitable membranes, a potentially vulnerable target for toxins. These membranes are coupled to an intracellular contraction system and two properties, excitation and contraction, have high energy requirements. The heart has the highest energy demands on a weight basis of any organ in the body and requires a continued supply of oxygen to support aerobic metabolism. Oxygen supply and utilization are therefore another area of vulnerability. To clarify the basic principles of cardiac toxicology, the heart can simply be considered an oxygen-dependent mass of contractile cells driven by excitable membranes that are subject to neurohumoral control. As a result, cardiotoxicity may be caused secondary to alterations in oxygen transport or neurohormonal release.

Cardiotoxicity is a relatively infrequent adverse observation in humans due to the "weeding" out of potential cardiotoxic materials during preclinical testing of drugs. However, a large number of compounds of potential therapeutic value in cardiovascular or neurological disease are administered at high doses to animals in drug development studies and cardiotoxicity may frequently be encountered. The vast majority of effects are acute, transient, functional responses, and reversible if the animal does not die. These functional responses include bradycardia, tachycardia, and various forms of arrhythmia, and like their equivalents in the nervous system these "cardiotoxicities" are generally considered to be exaggerated pharmacological effects.

In many of the best-studied cases of functional abnormalities, the mechanism is related to alterations in the ion shifts across the cell membrane (sarcolemma) that are used in the action potential. Digitalis and related cardiotonic chemicals are probably toxic by inhibiting membrane Na^+, K^+, and Ca^{2+} ATPase, which maintains the normal transcellular gradients of these ions. Other chemicals disturbing ion shifts across the cell membrane are tetrodotoxin, tetraethyl ammonium, and verapamil, which reduce the inflow of Na^+, K^+, and Ca^{2+}, respectively. Other toxins are thought to act on intracellular sites. Heavy metals alter mitochondrial function and may depress the energy production vital to excitation–contraction coupling. The depression of cardiac contractility by halothane may be related in part to inhibition of myosin ATPase activity. Thus there are many potential intracellular mechanisms by which toxins may interfere with excitation–contraction coupling to produce functional abnormalities. Many cardiotoxic agents probably interfere with this process at several sites.

Cardiomyopathy

In contrast to the frequent occurrence of functional effects, relatively few cardiotoxic agents cause structural changes in the heart. When effects are noted, they are usually characterized by degeneration followed by inflammation and repair. These lesions are designated cardiomyopathies. Myocardial (cardiac) necrosis is the most frequently studied cardiomyopathy. In principle, this can result indirectly by disturbance of the blood supply to the myocyte (hypoxic injury) or by direct chemical insult to the myocyte (cytotoxic injury) or by a combination of both effects. The end result, necrosis, is essentially the same, but the location of the lesion may differ. Hypoxic injury tends to affect fairly specific sites, whereas cytotoxic injury may be more widespread.

Bronchodilators and vasodilators are the compounds classically producing site-specific necrosis. One or a few doses of isoproterenol produce acute cardiac necrosis in rat heart with a striking tendency for the subendocardial regions at the apex of the left ventricle. The vasodilator hydralazine acutely produces similar lesions; in beagles, the apex of the left ventricular papillary muscles is the favored site. Continued administration of hydralazine does not increase the incidence or severity of the lesions and the initial acute lesions heal by fibrosis. Such acute cardiomyopathies could easily be missed in long-term studies, unless specific connective tissue stains [such as aniline black, Masson trichromal, van Gieson, or PTAH—see Luna (22) for details] are used to highlight the fibrosis.

The pathogenetic mechanism of this site-specific necrosis is not totally understood, but myocardial hypoxia probably plays an important role. Vasodilation may lower coronary perfusion and tachycardia increases oxygen demand. As the capillary pressure is lowest subendocardially, this area is at most risk to oxygen deprivation. The papillary muscles supporting the forces on the valves have the greatest oxygen requirement and are similarly at risk. The sites of injury are thus consistent with the hypothesis of myocardial hypoxia. Acute cardiac necrosis produced by vasoactive drugs can be considered to be the result of an exaggerated pharmacological effect.

Myocardial hypoxia depletes intracellular high-energy phosphate stores required to maintain membrane ion shifts. Disturbances of Ca^{2+} transport lead to increased cytosolic Ca^{2+}, increasing the ATP breakdown already initiated by hypoxia. Calcium overload ultimately leads to cell death. Histologically, the dead myofibers have homogeneous eosinophilic cytoplasm (hyaline necrosis) and shrunken or fragmented nuclei. The subsequent inflammatory infiltrate consists mainly of macrophages, with healing by fibrosis.

Cytotoxic injury is often chronic in contrast to the acute lesion caused by vasodilators. The lesions resulting from antineoplastic anthracycline antibiotics such as daunorubicin and doxorubicin frequently appear several months after the start of therapy. The clinical picture is generally a chronic congestive cardiomyopathy. Morphologically, the two main features are cardiac dilatation and myofiber degeneration. The degeneration consists of myofibrillar loss, producing lightly stained cells, and vacuolation due to massive dilatation of the sarcoplasmic reticulum. At the ultrastructural level, many cellular components are affected. A similar chronic dose-related cardiomyopathy with congestive failure can be produced in animal models, and in rabbits the lesions tend to be distributed around blood vessels. The pathogenesis of the anthracycline cardiomyopathy is unclear.

Chronic cardiomyopathies can be produced by cobalt and brominated vegetable oils. Cobalt-induced cardiomyopathy was first discovered among heavy beer drinkers in Canada. Vacuolation, swelling, loss of myofibrils, and necrosis occur in experimentally poisoned rats and are found mainly in the left ventricle. Cobalt ions can complex with a variety of biologically important molecules and the potential sites for toxicity are numerous.

The cardiotoxicity of brominated vegetable oils is not characterized by necrosis, but by fat accumulation affecting the whole myocardium. Focal necrosis may occur in the more severely affected hearts. The hearts of rats traeted with brominated cottonseed oil show a dose-related reduction in the ability to metabolize palmitic acid, probably accounting for the accumulation of lipid globules in the myofibers.

Cardiac Hypertrophy

An increase in the mass of heart muscle is occasionally found in toxicity studies. This is usually a compensatory response to an increase in workload of the heart, and in compound-related cases this is usually secondary to effects on the peripheral vasculature. Primary cardiac effects are rare but can be produced by hormones such as growth hormones.

Pigment deposits in the heart are a common feature of aging animals. These aging pigments occur in lysosomes in the perinuclear regions of the sarcoplasm, and in extensive cases the heart appears brown at necropsy. This condition is known as brown atrophy. Food coloring pigment such as Brown FK may also accumulate in a similar manner and in routine hematoxylin and eosin (H&E) sections is impossible to differentiate from the lipofuscin of aging animals.

Vasculature

Chemically induced lesions in blood vessels are uncommon except for local reactions to intravenous injections. Systemic effects generally affect the smaller muscular arteries and arterioles and the various lesions encountered are encompassed by the general diagnosis of arteriopathy.

There are several ways to produce arteriopathy, but the lesions generally follow a similar course. In acute lesions the initial change is hyaline or fibrinoid degeneration of the intima and media. The increased eosinophilia seen histologically may be due to insudation of plasma proteins, necrosis of medial smooth muscle cells, or both. An inflammatory response often follows and the lesion may be described as an acute arteritis. Repair of the lesion is by proliferation of medial myofibroblasts extending into the intima.

The two best-known pathways of vascular injury are hemodynamic changes and immune-complex deposition. Acute arterial injury can result from rapid marked hemodynamic changes produced by the exaggerated pharmacological effects of high doses of vasoactive agents. The bronchodilators and vasodilators producing cardiac necrosis may also cause an arteritis in the dog heart, often in the right atrium. Agents producing vasoconstriction or hypertension such as norepinephrine or angiotensin infusion also produce lesions in small arteries in various regions of the body. Lesions also follow alternating doses of vasodilators and vasoconstrictors. The evidence suggests that a combination of plasma leakage due to physical effects on endothelial cells and acute functional demands on the smooth muscle cell play an important role in the pathogenesis of these acute lesions.

Immune-complex lesions such as vasculitis or hypersensitivity angitis have similar features to hemodynamic lesions but tend to favor small vessels; therefore fibrinoid change may be less conspicuous. In animals, immune-complex lesions are produced most readily by repeated injection of foreign serum proteins.

Arteriopathies dominated by the proliferative component have been reported in women taking oral contraceptives. The lesions consist mainly of fibromuscular intimal thickenings with little or no necrosis or leukocyte infiltrations. Vascular lesions can also be produced in mice chronically dosed with steroid hormones.

Hemorrhage

Blood may escape from vessels because of defects in clotting factors, platelets, or the vessel wall, either singly or in combination. Clotting factor and platelet defects lead to hemorrhage by preventing effective closure of an injured vessel. Hemorrhage due to direct injury of the vessel wall by chemicals is infrequent except as a local toxic effect. The most common form of chemically induced hemorrhage (purpura) is the widespread minor leakages that sometimes occur in the skin and mucous membranes in association with allergic vasculitis.

Hemorrhage is also a common artifact in animals that are dying (agonal artifact) or as a consequence of postmortem techniques. Hemorrhages in the germinal centers of the mandibular lymph node and thymic medulla are observed frequently in rats killed by intraperitoneal injection of barbiturates. These hemorrhages appear as red spots on the surface of the organ. Large areas of hemorrhage may occur in the lungs of rats killed by carbon dioxide inhalation, which may confound the interpretation of inhalation toxicity studies. Pulmonary hemorrhage may also occur in animals killed by physical means such as decapitation or cervical dislocation.

A much more complete discussion of the histopathology of drug and chemically induced cardiac disease can be found in Balazs and Ferrans (23) or Bristow (24).

ANIMAL MODELS

No review of the approaches used to identify and characterize cardiotoxic agents in industry would be complete without consideration of which animal models are used and what their strengths and weaknesses are.

Table 2 presents a summary of baseline values for the common parameters associated with cardiovascular toxicity in standard toxicity studies. These are presented for the species that see a degree of regular use in systemic toxicity studies (the rat, mouse, dog, miniature swine, rabbit, guinea pig, ferrets, and two species of primates).

Major considerations in the use of the standard animal models to study cardiovascular toxicity are summarized as follows (15):

Rat	Very resistant to development of artherosclerosis; classic model for studying hypertension, as some strains are easily induced
Rabbit	Sensitive to microvascular constriction induced by release of epinephrine and norepinephrine
Dog	Resistant to development of artherosclerosis
Swine	Naturally developing high incidence of artherosclerosis; for this reason, a preferred model for study of the disease
Primates	The rhesus is sensitive to the development of extensive artherosclerosis following consumption of high-cholesterol diets

More details on species, handling characteristics, and experimental techniques can be found in Gad and Chengelis (16). There are also some special considerations when sudden cardiac death is a potential concern (25).

IN VITRO MODELS AND THEIR USE

In vitro models, at least as screening tests, have been with us in toxicology for some 20 years now. The last 5–10 years have brought a great upsurge in interest in such models. This increased interest is due to economic and animal welfare pressures, as well as technological improvements. This is par-

TABLE 2. *Baseline (normal) values for parameters potentially related to cardiac toxicity*

Species	HR (beats/minute)	BP (systolic/diastolic)	CPK ($\pm$ U/L)	SGOT ($\pm$ U/L)	LDH ($\pm$ U/L)	SGPT ($\pm$ IU/L)
Rat	350–400	116/90	5.6 $\pm$ 1.3	200 $\pm$ 152	106 $\pm$ 78	42.2 $\pm$ 3.0
Mouse	300–750	113/81	3.7 $\pm$ 1.5	350 $\pm$ 108		98 $\pm$ 22
Dog (beagle)	100–130	148/100	1.2 $\pm$ 1.1	31 $\pm$ 7	68 $\pm$ 37.85	21.7 $\pm$ 8.4
Primate (cynomolgus rhesus)	150–300	159/127	2.06–6.3 22–53	26.1 $\pm$ 9.4 27 $\pm$ 7	100–446 43–426	14.5 $\pm$ 8 42.1 $\pm$ 21.2
Rabbit	120–300	110/80	1.76	44 $\pm$ 26	104.8 $\pm$ 30	35 $\pm$ 16
Ferret	200–255	152/117		95 $\pm$ 52	608 $\pm$ 45.6	208 $\pm$ 217
Guinea pig	260–400	77/47	0.95 $\pm$ 0.2	48 $\pm$ 9.5		44.6 $\pm$ 7.0
Swine	58–86	128/95		8.2 $\pm$ 21.6	96–160	9–17

Notes: $\pm$ Values are one standard deviation. HR, heart rate; BP, blood pressure.
References: 15 and 16.

ticularly true in industry, and cardiotoxicity is one area where *in vitro* systems have found particularly attractive applications.

As predictive systems of the specific target organ toxicity case of cardiotoxicity, any *in vitro* system having the ability to identify those agents with a high potential to cause damage in a specific target organ at physiological concentrations would be extremely valuable.

The second use of *in vitro* models is largely specific. This is to serve as tools to investigate, identify, and/or verify the mechanisms of action for selective target organ toxicities. Such mechanistic understandings then allow one to know if such toxicities are relevant to humans (or to conditions of exposure to humans), to develop means to either predict such responses while they are still reversible or to develop the means to intervene in such toxicosis (i.e., first aid or therapy), and finally to potentially modify molecules of interest to avoid unwanted effects while maintaining desired properties (particularly important in drug design). Such uses are not limited to studying chemicals, drugs, and manufactured agents; they can also be used in the study of such diverse things as plant, animal, and microbial toxins, which may have commercial, therapeutic, or military applications or implications (26) due to their cardiotoxicity.

There is currently much controversy over the use of *in vitro* test systems. Will they find acceptance as "definitive test systems," or only be used as preliminary screens for such final tests? Or, in the end, will they not be used at all? Almost certainly, all three of these cases will be true to some extent. Depending on how the data generated are to be used, the division between the first two is ill defined at best.

Before trying to definitively answer these questions in a global sense, each of the endpoints for which *in vitro* systems are being considered should be overviewed and considered against the factors outlined to this point.

Substantial potential advantages exist in using an *in vitro* system in toxicological testing. These advantages include isolation of test cells or organ fragments from homeostatic and hormonal control, accurate dosing, and quantitation of results. It should be noted that, in addition to the potential advantages, *in vitro* systems *per se* also have a number of limitations that can contribute to their not being acceptable models. Findings from an *in vitro* system that either limit their use in predicting *in vivo* events or make them totally unsuitable for the task include wide differences in the doses needed to produce effects or differences in the effects elicited.

Tissue culture has the immediate potential to be used in two very different ways by industry. First, it has been used to examine a particular aspect of the toxicity of a compound in relation to its toxicity *in vivo* (i.e., mechanistic or explanatory studies). Second, it has been used as a form of rapid screening to compare the toxicity of a group of compounds for a particular form of response. Indeed, the pharmaceutical industry has used *in vitro* test systems in these two ways for years in the search for new potential drug entities: as screens and as mechanistic tools.

Mechanistic and explanatory studies are generally called for when a traditional test system gives a result that is either unclear or for which the relevance to the real life human exposure is doubted. *In vitro* systems are particularly attractive for such cases because they can focus on very defined single aspects of a problem or pathogenic response, free of the confounding influence of the multiple responses of an intact higher level organism. Note, however, that first one must know the nature (indeed the existence) of the questions to be addressed. It is then important to devise a suitable model system that is related to the mode of toxicity of the compound.

One must consider what forms of markers are to be used to evaluate the effect of interest. Initially, such markers have been exclusively either morphological (in that there is a change in microscopic structure), observational (is the cell/preparation dead or alive or has some gross characteristic changed), or functional (does the model still operate as it did before). Recently, it has become clear that more sensitive models do not just generate a single end point type of data, but rather a multiple set of measures, which in aggregate provide a much more powerful set of answers.

There are several approaches to *in vitro* cardiotoxicity models. The oldest is that of the isolated organ preparation. Perfused and superfused tissues and organs have been used in physiology and pharmacology since the late 19th century. There is a vast range of these available, and a number of them have widely been used in toxicology [Mehendale (27) presents an excellent overview]. Almost any endpoint can be evaluated, and these are closest to the *in vivo* situation and therefore generally the easiest to extrapolate or conceptualize from. Those things that can be measured or evaluated in the intact organism can largely also be evaluated in an isolated tissue or organ preparation. The drawbacks or limitations of this approach are also compelling, however.

An intact animal generally produces one tissue preparation. Such a preparation is viable generally for a day or less before it degrades to the point of being useless. As a result, such preparations are useful as screens only for agents that have rapidly reversible (generally pharmacologic or biochemical) mechanisms of action. They are superb for evaluating mechanisms of action at the organ level for agents that act rapidly—but not generally for cellular effects or for agents that act over a course of more than a day.

The second approach is to use tissue or organ culture. Such cultures are attractive due to maintaining the ability for multiple cell types to interact in at least a near physiologically manner. They are generally not as complex as the perfused organs but are stable and useful over a longer period of time, increasing their utility as screens somewhat. They are truly a middle ground between the perfused organs and the cultured cells.

The third and most common approach is that of cultured cell models. These can be either primary or transformed (immortalized) cells, but the former have significant advantages in use as predictive target organ models

TABLE 3. *Representative in vitro test systems for cardiovascular toxicity*

System[a]	Endpoint	Evaluation	References
Coronary artery smooth muscle cells (S)	Morphological evaluation: vacuole formation	Correlates with *in vivo* results	29
Isolated perfused rabbit or rat heart (M,S)	Functional: operation, electrophysiological, biochemical, and metabolism	Long history of use in physiology and pharmacology	27
Isolated superfused atrial and heart preparations (S,M)	Functional: operational and biochemical	Correlation with *in vivo* findings for antioxidants	30,31
Myocytes (S,M)	Functional and morphological	Correlates well with *in vivo* results on a local concentration basis	32,33

[a]Letters in parentheses indicate primary employment of system: (S), screening system; (M), mechanistic tool.

(28). Such cell culture systems can be utilized to identify and evaluate interactions at the cellular, subcellular, and molecular level on an organ- and species-specific basis (28). The advantages of cell culture are that single organisms can generate multiple cultures, the cultures are stable and useful for protracted periods of time, and effects can be studied very precisely at the cellular and molecular level. The disadvantages are that isolated cells cannot mimic the interactive architecture of the intact organ and will respond over time in a manner that becomes decreasingly representative of what happens *in vivo*. An additional concern is that, with the exception of hepatocyte cultures, the influence of systemic metabolism is not factored in unless extra steps are taken. Any such cellular systems would be more likely to be accurate and sensitive predictors of adverse effects if their function and integrity were evaluated while they were operational.

A wide range of target-organ-specific models have already been developed and utilized. Their incorporation into a library type approach requires that they be evaluated for reproducibility of response, ease of use, and predictive characteristics under the intended conditions of use. These evaluations are probably at least somewhat specific to any individual situation. Table 3 presents an overview of representative systems for cardiovascular toxicity. Not mentioned in these tables are any of the new coculture systems in which hepatocytes are "joined up" in culture with a target cell type to produce a metabolically competent cellular system.

SUMMARY

Presented here is an overview of current approaches and the state of the art for detecting and characterizing cardiotoxicity in industrial toxicology studies. This is a field that as yet, even in pharmaceutical companies, is not considered separate from the general case characterization of systemic toxicity. It depends on some very fixed tool sets to deal with both functional and structural toxicities. When the entire suite of methodology as presented here is employed, it has performed very well (as judged by cardiotoxicity not being a frequent finding for products properly used and/or handled in humans). However, incremental improvements are underway in the field, utilizing some of the technologies presented elsewhere in this volume.

REFERENCES

1. Van Stee EW. Cardiovascular toxicology: foundations and scope. In Van Stee EW, ed. *Cardiovascular toxicology*. New York: Raven Press; 1982:1–34.
2. Balazs T, Hanig JP, Herman EH. Toxic responses of the cardiovascular system. In: Klaassen CD, Amdur MO, Doull J, eds. *Casarett and Doull's toxicology: the basic science of poisons*. New York: Macmillan 1986:387–411.
3. Brunner H, Gross F. Cardiovascular pharmacology. In Zbinden G, Gross F, eds. *Pharmacologic methods in toxicology*. Oxford: Pergamon Press; 1979:63–99.
4. Gilman AG, Rall JW, Nies AS, Taylor P. *The pharmacological basis of therapeutics*. New York: Pergamon Press; 1990:749–896.
5. Watkinson WP, Brice MA, Robinson KS. A computer-assisted electrocardiographic analysis system: methodology and potential application to cardiovascular toxicology. *J Toxicol Environ Health* 1985;15:713–727.
6. Sodeman WA, Sodeman TM. *Pathologic physiology*. Philadelphia: Saunders; 1979.
7. Doherty JD, Cobbe SM. Electrophysiological changes in animal model of chronic cardiac failure. *Cardiovasc Res* 1990;24:309–316.
8. Atta AG, Vanace PW. Electrocardiographic studies in the *Macaca mulatta* monkey. *Ann NY Acad Sci* 1960;85:811–818.
9. Hamlin R. Extracting "more" from cardiopulmonary studies on beagle dogs. In: Gilman MR, ed. *The canine as a biomedical model*. Bethesda, MD: American College of Toxicology and LRE; 1985:9–15.
10. Vatner SF, Patrick TA, Murray PA. Monitoring of cardiovascular dynamics in conscious animals. In Van Stee EW, ed. *Cardiovascular toxicology*. New York: Raven Press; 1982:35–55.
11. Garner D, Laks MM. New implanted chronic catheter device for determining blood pressure and cardiac output in the conscious dog V. *Physiology* 1985;363:H681–685.
12. Gad SC. A neuromuscular screen for use in industrial toxicology. *J Toxicol Environ Health* 1982;9:691–704.
13. Clampitt RB, Hart RJ. The tissue activities of some diagnostic enzymes in ten mammalian species. *J Comp Pathol* 1978;88:607–621.
14. Lindena J, Sommerfeld U, Hopfel C, Traukschold I. Catalytic enzyme activity concentration in tissues of man, dog, rabbit, guinea pig, rat and mouse. *J Clin Chem Clin Biochem* 1986;24:35–47.
15. Calabrese EJ. *Principles of animal extrapolation*. New York: Wiley; 1983.
16. Gad SC, Chengelis CP. *Animal models in toxicology*. New York: Marcel Dekker; 1991.
17. Loeb WF, Quimby FW. *The clinical chemistry of laboratory animals*. New York: Pergamon Press; 1989.
18. Evans GO. Biochemical assessment of cardiac function and damage in animal species. *J Appl Toxicol* 1991;11:15–22.
19. Wallach J. *Interpretation of diagnostic tests*. Boston: Little, Brown & Company; 1978.
20. Mitruka BM, Rawnsley HM. *Clinical biochemical and hematological reference values in normal experimental animals*. New York: Masson; 1977.
21. Fenoglio JJ, Wagner BM. Endomyocardial biopsy approach to drug-related heart disease. In: Hayes AW, ed. *Principles and methods of toxicology*. New York: Raven Press; 1989:649–658.

22. Luna Lee G. *Manual of histologic staining methods of the Armed Forces Institute of Pathology.* New York: McGraw-Hill; 1968.
23. Balazs T, Ferrans JJ. Cardiac lesions induced by chemicals. *Environ Health Perspect* 1978;26:181–191.
24. Bristow MR. *Drug-induced heart disease.* New York: Elsevier; 1980.
25. Chan PS, Cervoni P. Current concepts and animal models of sudden cardiac death for drug development. *Drug Dev Res* 1990;19:199–207.
26. Werdan K, Melnitzki SM, Pilz G, Kapsner T. The cultured rat heart cell: a model to study direct cardiotoxic effects of *Pseudomonas* endo- and exotoxins. In: *Second Vienna shock forum.* New York: Alan R Liss; 1989:247–251.
27. Mehendale HM. Application of isolated organ techniques in toxicology. In: Hayes AW, ed. *Principles and methods of toxicology.* New York: Raven Press; 1989:699–740.
28. Acosta D, Sorensen EMB, Anuforo DC, Mitchell DB, Ramos K, Santone KS, Smith MA. An in vitro approach to the study of target organ toxicity of drugs and chemicals. *In Vitro Cell Dev Biol* 1985;21:495–504.
29. Ruben Z, Fuller GC, Knodle SC. Disobutamide-induced cytoplasmic vacuoles in cultured dog coronary artery muscle cells. *Arch Toxicol* 1984;55:206–212.
30. Gad SC, Leslie SW, Brown RG, Smith RV. Inhibitory effects of dithiothreitol and sodium bisulfite on isolated rat ileum and atrium. *Life Sci* 1977;20:657–664.
31. Gad SC, Leslie SW, Acosta D. Inhibitory actions of butylated hydroxytoluene (BHT) on isolated rat ileal, atrial and perfused heart preparations. *Toxicol Appl Pharmacol* 1979;48:45–52.
32. Leslie SW, Gad SC, Acosta D. Cytotoxicity of butylated hydroxytoluene and butylated hydroxyanisole in cultured heart cells. *Toxicology* 1978;10:281–289.
33. Low-Friedrich I, Bredow F, Schoeppe W. *In vitro* studies on the cardiotoxicity of chemotherapeutics. *Exp Chemotherapy* 1990;36:416–421.

Cardiovascular Toxicology, Second Edition,
edited by Daniel Acosta, Jr.
Raven Press, Ltd., New York © 1992.

3

Monitoring of Cardiovascular Dynamics in Conscious Animals

Stephen F. Vatner, Thomas A. Patrick, You-Tang Shen,
and *Paul A. Murray

*Departments of Medicine, Harvard Medical School, Brigham & Women's Hospital,
Boston, Massachusetts 02115; and New England Regional Primate Research
Center, Southborough, Massachusetts 01772; *Current address: Johns Hopkins
University School of Medicine, Baltimore, Maryland 21205*

The extent to which exposure to occupational and environmental toxic substances is related to the etiology of cardiovascular disease has become a matter of increasing public health concern (1,2). Environmental factors, such as smoking, are now well established as risk factors in the development of cardiovascular disease. However, the mechanisms involved remain largely unexplained. Moreover, the effects of other environmental agents on the cardiovascualar system remain largely speculative (1). This paucity of empirical information concerning environmental effects on the cardiovascular system may be due to the lack of appropriate experimental animal models in which precise measurements of cardiovascular function can be monitored over an extended period of time.

The goal of this chapter is to describe a number of physiological monitoring techniques that have been utilized routinely in our laboratory for the chronic and continuous assessment of cardiovascular function in conscious animals. The measurements of intravascular and intracardiac pressures, dimensions, and blood flows represent the fundamental cardiovascular measurements and are stressed in this chapter. The type of experimental model described offers a number of benefits, which makes it particularly well suited for the assessment of the effects of toxic substances on cardiovascular dynamics. First, utilizing conscious animals avoids the confounding influence of anesthesia (which itself is a toxic substance) on cardiovascular function. Second, both the direct and possibly reflex-mediated effects of toxic agents on cardiovascular function can be examined in these intact, conscious animal models. Third, implanted instrumentation permits the assessment of both acute cardiovascular effects of putative toxic substances and effects resulting from chronic exposure. And finally, the cardiovascular effects of toxic agents can be reevaluated following the induction of experimental disease states, for example, myocardial ischemia, cardiac hypertrophy, and cardiac failure.

It is recognized that cardiovascular research utilizing conscious, chronically instrumented animals is both time consuming and costly. It is therefore important to examine the benefits of this experimental model in more detail. Most important, general anesthesia alters virtually every aspect of circulatory function, including heart rate, the level of myocardial contractile state, vascular resistances in regional beds (3,4), and, particularly, the control of these parameters by the autonomic nervous system (5). Therefore responses to normal physiological stimuli, to commonly used pharmacological agents, and to environmental factors may be quite different in healthy, conscious animals as compared to anesthetized animals or isolated organs. Studies using conscious animals as experimental models have uncovered important quantitative and qualitative differences from traditionally held concepts that were derived from studies in anesthetized animals. These differences have been shown in diverse areas such as baroreceptor control of the circulation (6–10), chemoreceptor control (11–13), the influence of increasing cardiac frequency on myocardial contractility (Bowditch phenomenon) (14), increasing afterload on cardiac function (Anrep effect) (15), increasing preload (16–18), hemorrhage (19,20), and the effects of catecholamines (21–23), cardiac glycosides (24–26), and morphine sulfate (27). It is important to note that autonomic reflex control of the circulation can be depressed not only with pentobarbital and halothane anesthesia, but also with α-chloralose (13), an anesthetic agent often thought to actually enhance neural reflex control of the circulation.

TECHNIQUES FOR MEASUREMENT OF CARDIOVASCULAR PARAMETERS

Arterial and Ventricular Pressures

Miniature solid-state pressure transducers can be used routinely for chronic measurement of arterial pressure, as well as pressure in the left (28) (Fig. 1) and right ventricles (29) (Fig. 2). These transducers, which were originally developed by Van Citters and Franklin (30), have been used in our laboratory for more than two decades (31–34) in studies involving maximal exercise in unrestrained, conscious dogs (35), lambs and sheep (36), and primates (31,33). Solid-state pressure transducers offer a number of advantages over commonly used fluid-filled catheter–strain gauge manometer systems for use in chronic implants. The most important of these are (a) wide frequency response (i.e., 1.2 kHz); (b) high sensitivity, which facilitates their use with radiotelemetry systems; and (c) relative freedom from signal distortion that occurs in fluid-filled systems from catheter clotting or kinking, or acceleration effects upon the fluid system. A pressure transducer must have a high-frequency response in order to reproduce accurately the rapidly changing phases of a pressure signal, such as the leading edge of systole in left or right ventricular pressure. Furthermore, the time derivative of ventricular pressure (dP/dt) is often used as an index of cardiac contractility, and to obtain this parameter by analog differentiation, the higher frequency components of the pressure signal must be preserved (Figs. 1 and 2). The upper frequency limit of the implanted solid-state pressure transducer is 1.2 kHz, whereas the frequency response of the catheter–manometer system in chronic animal preparations is typically no greater than 20 Hz and can be even lower if the catheter is clotted or kinked. Moreover, unless the fluid system is properly damped, waveform distortions can occur as a result of oscillations in the catheter–transducer system. On the other hand, overdamping limits the frequency response of the system and prevents accurate detection of changes in the pressure waveform.

The pressure transducer used in our laboratory is a small (5–7 mm diameter, 1 mm thickness), hermetically sealed, cylindrical chamber with a titanium diaphragm, on the back of which are bonded four silicon strain gauge elements arranged in a Wheatstone bridge configuration (Konigsberg Instruments Models P5 and P7, Pasadena, CA). The transducer senses pressure changes as a deformation of the diaphragm, which in turn unbalances the bridge and generates an offset signal proportional to the applied pressure. This signal is subsequently amplified and recorded as an analog reproduction of the pressure wave. Each transducer undergoes an initial *in vitro* calibration prior to surgical implant, during which time the linearity, sensitivity, zero offset voltage, and temperature stability of the transducer are assessed. During each experiment, the solid-state transducers are cross-calibrated *in vivo* against a strain gauge transducer connected to fluid-filled, chronically implanted catheters positioned in the aorta, right ventricle, and left atrium. Arterial pressure can be measured by implanting the solid-state transducer in the thoracic or abdominal aorta through a 1–2 cm longitudinal incision closed by interrupted sutures. The right ventricular transducer can be inserted through a stab wound in the midanterior free wall of the right ventricle, and the left ventricular transducer is most often inserted through a stab wound in the apex of the left ventricle. The ventricular transducers are secured by purse string sutures. As with all implants of this type, the transducer leads are exteriorized through the chest wall and routed subcutaneously to the interscapular area of the animal. The exteriorized transducer leads are protected by shrink tubing and a tear-resistant nylon vest (dogs, sheep). In intractable animals (e.g., primates), the wires are not externalized but are buried subcutaneously until the time of the experiment.

Several features of the solid-state pressure transducer make it preferable

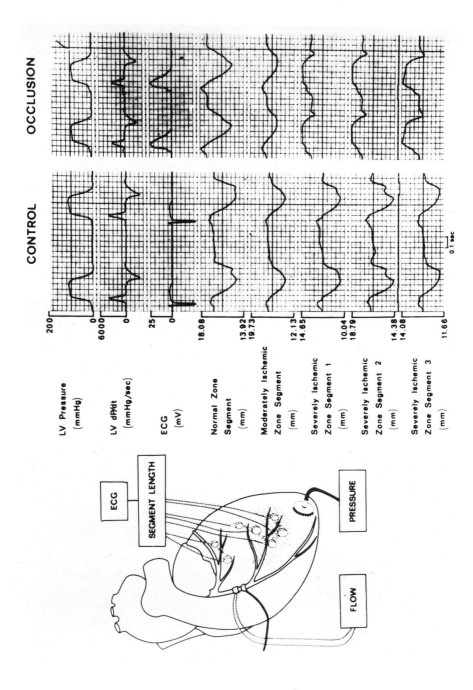

for use in experiments involving radiotelemetry of the pressure signal, although alternative systems using catheters and external strain gauges are available (37). Fluid-filled pressure transducers are larger in size and quite fragile and, as noted above, are susceptible to distortion artifacts in the pressure signal. Moreover, the fluid-filled transducer has a voltage output approximately six times lower than that of a solid-state transducer (0.05 mV/cmHg/V excitation versus 0.3 mV/cmHg/V excitation, respectively). This imposes more stringent requirements on the design of the associated electronic circuitry for signal conditioning and telemetry. Additionally, the lower sensitivity of the fluid-filled gauge results in increased power consumption to achieve similar transducer signal levels. For these reasons (power requirements, size, stability, and maintenance), the solid-state pressure transducers are well suited to investigations in which the mobility of the animal is of primary importance.

The major disadvantages of implantable solid-state pressure transducers for use in chronic implants are drift in zero offset and sensitivity. These problems become critical because it is impossible at the time of the experiment to calibrate the implanted transducer in terms of absolute pressure. Because the unit is sealed at the factory, a zero offset occurs with varying altitude as well as with normal fluctuations in barometric pressure. It becomes necessary therefore to cross-calibrate these transducers with a calibrated system when experiments are conducted, either with a fluid-filled catheter-strain gauge manometer system or a solid-state catheter–tipped manometer.

During an experiment, the implanted, miniature gauge is excited by a constant DC voltage (5 V), and the output voltage (typically 0–30 mV, for 0–200 mm Hg range) generated by the applied pressure is preamplified by an instrumentation amplifier with a frequency response from 0 to 2 kHz. The signal is recorded on magnetic tape and displayed on a standard strip chart recorder. An electronic calibration of the overall pressure-measuring system, exclusive of the transducer, is made at the start and at the end of an experiment by substituting a transducer simulator consisting of a precision resistive divider network for the pressure probe. Bridge imbalance, as would

---

FIG. 1. The techniques for measuring regional myocardial function, flow, and electrocardiograms (ECG) in conscious dogs with regional myocardial ischemia are depicted. A miniature pressure gauge was implanted in the left ventricle (LV) to measure pressure and dP/dt. A coronary flow probe and hydraulic occluder were implanted on a branch of the coronary artery to occlude the vessel and to confirm the occlusion. Multiple pairs of miniature piezoelectric crystals were implanted in the potentially ischemic zone and normal zone to measure regional segment length shortening and electrograms from the same transducers. The panels at the left show typical phasic waveforms prior to occlusion (*left panel*), and then after coronary occlusion (*right panel*). Note that coronary occlusion induced only mild changes in left ventricular pressure and dP/dt but caused striking ST segment elevation and reversal of normal systolic shortening to paradoxical bulging in the severely ischemic zones. From ref. 28, with permission.

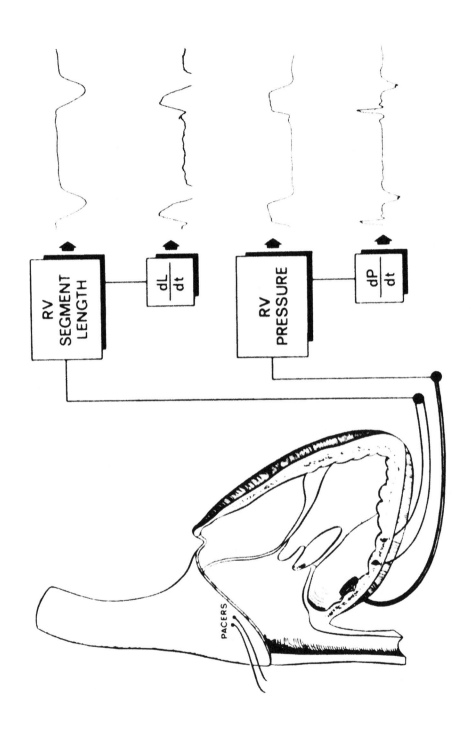

be caused by an applied pressure, is thereby simulated by changing the values of the resistors in the calibration network and monitoring the offset voltage produced. These electrical reference levels can be converted to mm Hg by referring to the most recent *in vitro* or *in vivo* calibration of the transducer. Any drift in the amplifier, transducer excitation power source, tape recorder, or strip chart oscillograph during the course of the experiment can be corrected by frequent electrical calibration of the system in this manner. However, the most accurate method of calibration is to simultaneously compare the output of the implanted solid-state pressure transducer with a calibrated catheter–strain gauge manometer. Blood pressure can be varied transiently with vasoactive agents (intravenous nitroglycerin, phenylephrine) to achieve a wide range of calibration points for comparison. This procedure overcomes the problem of changes that may have occurred in the solid-state transducer's transfer function since the last *in vitro* calibration. In our experience, this procedure should be repeated approximately every week for arterial implants, but daily cross-calibration is necessary for experiments in which small variations in zero pressure level are critical (e.g., measurement of intracardiac end-diastolic pressure).

Although there are many problems associated with the measurement of pressures in animals with long-term chronic implants, it is clear that the inherent advantages of the solid-state transducer make it very attractive. Reduction in size of the transducer and cable would allow application to experiments using smaller animals, for example, smaller primate studies and fetal preparations. Whereas smaller transducers (3–4 mm diameter) do exist, the larger units are both more sensitive and more stable.

Blood Flow Measurements

The ultrasonic and electromagnetic techniques for measuring phasic blood flows in conscious animals are indirect; that is, blood flow *per se* is not measured. Rather, the effects of moving blood on induced wave energy are transduced to obtain a signal that is proportional to blood flow. The signals obtained are subject to certain acceptable errors and are a valid measure of flow only within a range of operating conditions. The signal obtained is usually small and its use depends on appropriate amplification and simultaneous rejection of extraneous signals. Each technique has both advantages and disadvantages that direct its application to particular flow measurements and experimental protocols. Two different ultrasonic approaches, the pulsed-

---

FIG. 2. Schematic diagram of implanted ultrasonic crystals and pressure gauge in the right ventricle and typical waveforms of right ventricular (RV) segment length, velocity, pressure, and dP/dt. From ref. 29, with permission of the American Heart Association, Inc.

Doppler and transit-time methods, will be compared with the electromagnetic technique in the following discussion.

Doppler Ultrasonic Flow Technique

The Doppler principle for velocity measurement of blood flow, in its various implementations, is an important component in conscious animal instrumentation. The advantage of lightweight, long-lasting transducers and the accurate and stable zero that is independent of the transducer or implant conditions greatly facilitate this technique's use.

Three implementations of the principle of measurement are discussed, the nondirectional, continuous wave (CW) method, the directional, continuous wave method, and the pulsed, directional method. All use the common principle that ultrasound reflected from a target (e.g., the moving blood cells) exhibits a shift in frequency proportional to the velocity of the target. Ultrasound is directed diagonally into the bloodstream, and a part of this energy is reflected from moving blood cells. The shift in frequency caused by this process provides an average of the instantaneous velocity profile across the vessel lumen and is determined by extracting the frequency difference between transmitted and reflected sonic waves.

The fact that at zero velocity no Doppler shift exists results in a capability for determination of true zero flow at any time by electrical calibration, without the necessity for mechanical occlusion of the vessel. This is an important advantage over the other ultrasonic technique in use (the transit-time flowmeter) as well as the electromagnetic flow measurement technique, in that accurate and stable zero determinations can be made at any time without manipulating the vessel under study. A measure of volume flow is determined by knowledge of the average velocity and internal cross-sectional area of the vessel. The relationship between velocity and volume flow has been demonstrated repeatedly and confirmed by means of timed collection of blood (38,39) and by simultaneous comparison on a left circumflex coronary artery (40), as shown in Fig. 3. This figure shows an almost identical response to a 15-sec coronary artery occlusion by hydraulic occluder, in that the reactive hyperemia is equally depicted by both the electromagnetic and CW Doppler flowmeters. At autopsy, the vessels have been consistently observed to be firmly adherent to the flow transducers through a fibrous scar, which minimizes changes in the cross-sectional area of the blood vessel within the measurement area, thus ensuring a stable scale factor for the measurement.

The flow transducers are made of lightweight materials, most commonly hinged polystyrene half shells or cast epoxy rings with a small gap to allow the transducer to be placed on the vessel. The function of the transducer is to hold the piezoelectric crystals that generate and detect the ultrasound and to constrain the diameter of the vessel for accurate volume flow determina-

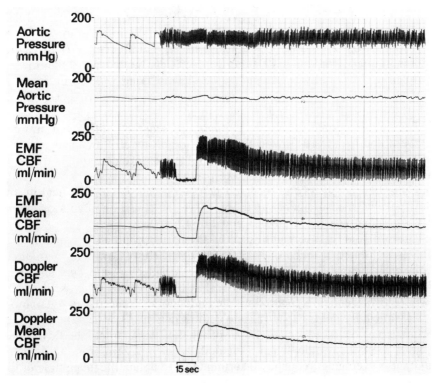

FIG. 3. The effect of a 15-sec occlusion of the left circumflex coronary artery in a conscious, chronically instrumented dog on phasic and mean aortic pressure, phasic and mean coronary blood flow (CBF) measured simultaneously with an electromagnetic flowmeter (EMF), and adjacent Doppler ultrasonic flowmeter. Note the similarity of the waveform and the conformation of the reactive hyperemic response as measured by the two systems. From ref. 40, with permission.

tion. Electrical connections to the crystals are made with silver plated, stranded copper wire, with an implant lifetime of greater than 6 months. For longer chronic implants, stranded stainless steel wire has been successfully employed.

The primary disadvantage of the Doppler ultrasonic flowmeter is that the Doppler effect measures velocity. Volume flow must be determined by *in vivo* calibrations or by measuring the cross-sectional area of the vessel within the lumen. While this has not been a problem for chronic implants, it does raise serious concerns for acute measurements in which turbulence or relative movement of the probe and the vessel can distort the flow waveform. Moreover, measurement of blood flow in a stenotic vessel may also lead to disruption of the normal velocity profile and inaccurate volume flow determinations.

The continuous wave, nondirectional Doppler flowmeter, as developed by Franklin et al. (41), has been used in our laboratory for the measurement of coronary (8,11,22,25,42) (Fig. 3), cerebral (12), renal, mesenteric, and iliac blood flows (43–47). These flowmeters are small (1 in. × 3 in. × 5 in.), lightweight, battery-powered units that use a radiofrequency (RF) carrier that is frequency modulated by the Doppler signal to telemeter the flow information. The ability to telemeter the signals along with aortic pressure enables experiments with intractable animals, as well as experiments in which free-ranging exercise is to be studied.

The nondirectional flowmeter is unable to sense the difference between forward and backward flow in the vessel, reporting all flow measurements in one direction. This is a disadvantage in the measurement of blood flow in arteries in which flow reversals take place, such as the iliac artery. Additionally, the quality of the received Doppler signal is more critical in low flow velocity measurement situations, since the detection of spurious noise causes a positive shift in the perceived flow.

This problem has been addressed by the implementation of a quadrature, phase-shift detector technique (48) to provide the CW flowmeter with direction-sensing capability. This approach uses a detector with dual channels, which introduces a differential phase shift of 90° between the oscillator inputs of two identical synchronous demodulators. While the two detectors see identical frequency spectra, one audio signal leads or lags the other depending on flow direction. A simple phase detector extracts the flow direction, while either audio signal is demodulated by a zero-crossing detector and pulse-averaging frequency discriminator, to obtain the magnitude of the flow velocity. An instrument based on this design (L & M Instruments, Daly City, CA) has been used in the measurement of iliac blood flow in our laboratory. This unit has relatively large power requirements and necessitates the use of shielded, coaxial cables from the flow transducer to the electronics to eliminate most of the electrically coupled, nonshifted signals. This feature makes the flow transducers more difficult to fabricate. Additionally, telemetry is more difficult, since two audio channels must be transmitted, instead of the one for the nondirectional system, or the bidirectional detector must be implemented in the telemetry system, instead of the receiver.

Both CW flowmeters just discussed are very susceptible to pulse interference, which precludes their use with transit-time dimension measurements (as described later). This problem has been circumvented by the development of the pulsed-Doppler flowmeter (49,50), which sends a repetitive burst of ultrasound diagonally into the bloodstream and senses the Doppler-shifted return energy at a moment in time that can be related to a position within the blood vessel. Additionally, it is practical to synchronize this flowmeter to other instruments, and the range-sensing capability of the design makes it practical to measure either the instantaneous average velocity across the vessel or to make simultaneous measurements of the velocity in several areas within the vessel, and thus determine the velocity profile of blood flow (49,50). The pulse-Doppler instrument in primary use in our laboratory is a 10-MHz directional device, with large area piezocrystals to average the instantaneous velocity of flow across the vessel. Figure 4 depicts simultaneous measurements from four peripheral vascular beds (51) (coronary, renal, mesenteric, iliac), along with aortic root blood flow measured with an electromagnetic flowmeter. Commonly available flow transducers use small, 20-MHz crystals, which are used to focus the measurement at the center-stream of the flow. This requires that the velocity profile be assumed and can result in underestimation of blood flow if the velocity profile changes from parabolic to blunt, as in reactive hyperemia with temporary occlusion of coronary arteries.

Ultrasonic Transit-Time Determination of Flow Velocity

The measurement of the change in velocity of ultrasound waves propagated through a moving medium predates the development of the Doppler shift flowmeter. This technique, also developed by Franklin (52), uses opposed pairs of piezoelectric crystals acting alternately as transmitters and receivers. Since the ultrasound moves through the blood, any movement of the blood will change the velocity of the ultrasound. By alternately transmitting upstream and then downstream, a difference in the transit time of the sound may be determined, thus measuring blood velocity. The differential transit times that are to be measured can be as small as 10 nsec at maximum velocity, thus putting severe constraints on the design of the measurement electronics. This technique does not rely on a tight fit of the transducer, as does the electromagnetic sensor (discussed later); consequently, zero stability and performance at low vascular pressures are better than with that measurement technique.

A more recent implementation (Transonic Systems, Inc., Ithaca, NY) uses transducer crystals with a reflector to increase the path length, and thus increase the transit-time difference for a given velocity (53). The transit time of the sound is spatially averaged over the cross section of the lumen, thus enabling the instrument to be calibrated in terms of volume flow. This transducer design uses a flat metal reflector on one side of the artery, with both piezocrystals mounted at an angle in an epoxy shell, which fits on the other side of the artery. This transducer geometry uses two passes of the ultrasound at complementary angles through the lumen of the vessel, which reduces errors due to implant angle differences between the flowprobe and the vessel. Although the transducer design is larger and heavier than either the Doppler or the electromagnetic types, implantation and stable flow measurements are still routinely possible. This design does not require a tight fit in order to function, but for optimum use the transducer should be allowed to stabilize on the artery by the growth of connective tissue, prior to its operation.

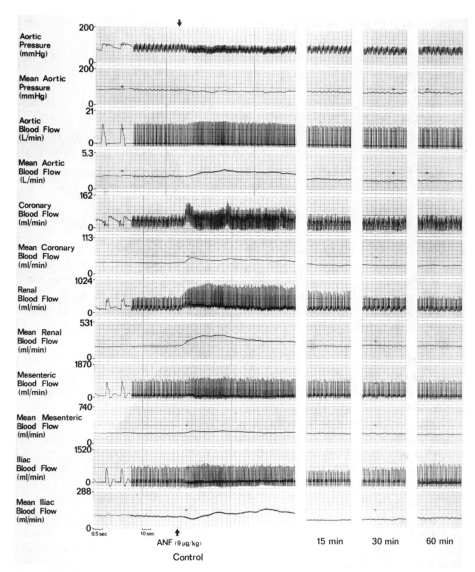

FIG. 4. Effects of bolus injection of atrial natriuretic factor (ANF) (9 µg/kg) via a catheter in left atrium on phasic and mean measurements of aortic pressure and aortic, coronary, renal, mesenteric, and iliac blood flows in a conscious intact dog at time of injection and at 15, 30, and 60 min during recovery period. Note that ANF reduced mean aortic pressure and markedly increased blood flow in all vascular beds during initial period, indicating a fall in vascular resistance. Blood flow in all beds, except kidney, fell below baseline during late recovery period, indicating a rise in vascular resistance. From ref. 51, with permission of the American Physiological Society.

In theory, zero velocity should result in a zero time difference, with primary stability of zero determined by the electronic design. In practice, zero flow offset and gain can be affected by nonuniform tissue density within the measurement area of the transducer, such as growth of fatty tissue, thus causing a static change in the speed of sound being measured. Additionally, if the probe axis does not align properly with the flow axis, a position-related zero flow offset can be observed. A third problem occurs with sensitivity changes if the probe is placed axially on a curved artery. Since the velocity vectors measured by the probe are at a different angle than that assumed by calibration on a straight test section, a reduction in apparent sensitivity of as much as 25% has been observed. Implantation on large arteries such as the aorta of dogs (18–24 mm) results in performance with minimum zero offset ($\pm 5\%$); however, somewhat larger zero offsets can be experienced with smaller probes, since alignment is more of a problem. In use, stable flow sensitivity and little change in the zero offset are typical with chronic implants in our laboratory, after the 2–3 weeks time required to allow the growth of stabilizing connective tissue. Transducers have been functional for over 4 months in long-term studies of cardiac output in rhesus monkeys (Fig. 5).

The transit-time flowmeter is a pulsed, sampling device, and therefore it can be synchronized to work simultaneously with ultrasonic dimension measurements. Its pulse transmission duration (20 μsec), however, is incompatible with the pulsed-Doppler design (pulse repetition rate of 10–16 μsec), thus not allowing mixed instrumentation models with these instruments. Telemetry of these signals has not yet been demonstrated, since the electronics for this device are more complex than either the electromagnetic or Doppler devices.

Electromagnetic Flow Technique

This technique (54,55) is an adaptation of Faraday's law of magnetic induction, using the principle that when flowing blood (a moving conductor) crosses a magnetic field induced through a blood vessel, a voltage is generated that is proportional to the blood velocity, the magnetic field strength, and the length of the moving conductor. If the magnetic field strength is constant, the signal from this measurement is considered to be proportional to volume flow.

Advantages of the electromagnetic flowmeter include an ability to sense direction for flow and a relative insensitivity to changes in velocity profile. The directional flow-sensing ability is important in experiments involving measurement of blood flow where a component of the flow is retrograde (56) (Fig. 6) (e.g., ascending aortic blood flow, iliac artery blood flow). The insensitivity to velocity profile is important when, for example, coronary blood flow is measured in the presence of a partial coronary artery stenosis.

The instrument we use (17,19,35) was developed by Fryer and Sandler

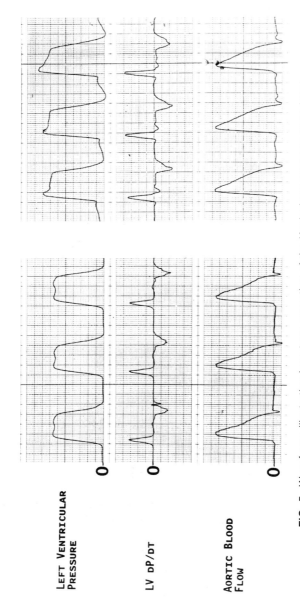

LEFT VENTRICULAR PRESSURE

LV dP/dT

AORTIC BLOOD FLOW

FIG. 5. Waveforms illustrating long-term operation of the Konigsberg pressure transducer and the Transonic, transit-time flowmeter in the *left panel* (4 months), and another Konigsberg pressure transducer and electromagnetic flowmeter in the *right panel* (6 months), implanted in two rhesus monkeys. Both the flow meters and the Konigsberg pressure gauges were operating normally after this length of time.

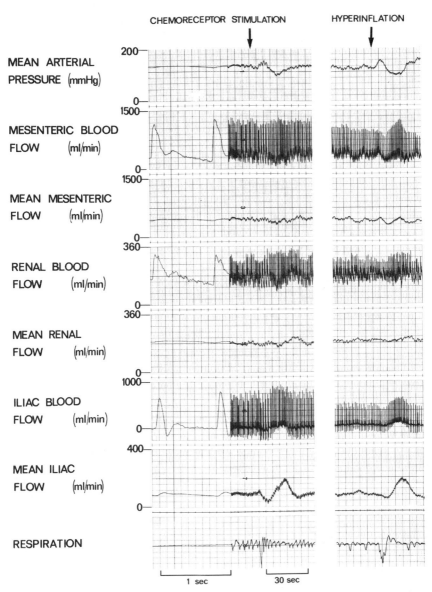

CHEMORECEPTOR STIMULATION   HYPERINFLATION

MEAN ARTERIAL PRESSURE (mmHg)

MESENTERIC BLOOD FLOW (ml/min)

MEAN MESENTERIC FLOW (ml/min)

RENAL BLOOD FLOW (ml/min)

MEAN RENAL FLOW (ml/min)

ILIAC BLOOD FLOW (ml/min)

MEAN ILIAC FLOW (ml/min)

RESPIRATION

1 sec   30 sec

FIG. 6. The effects of carotid chemoreceptor stimulation with nicotine in a conscious dog on mean arterial pressure, phasic and mean mesenteric, renal, and iliac blood flows, and respiration as monitored with a pneumatic cuff are depicted. The continuous wave Doppler ultrasonic technique was used to measure renal blood flow, and the electromagnetic flow technique was used to measure mesenteric and iliac blood flows. During spontaneous respiration (*left panel*), chemoreceptor stimulation elicited an initial bradycardia and reduction in iliac flow with an increase in depth and rate of respiration. Following the respiratory changes, there was tachycardia and a striking increase in iliac flow. There were only minor changes in flow in the renal and mesenteric beds. During controlled respiration (*right panel*), chemoreceptor stimulation elicited a greater increase in mean arterial pressure, bradycardia, and marked reductions in flow in all beds, but the tachycardia and later increase in iliac flow were not observed. From ref. 56, with permission of the American Heart Association, Inc.

(57) and exists in both a bench model for routine laboratory use and a miniature, battery-powered unit suitable for telemetry purposes. The probes used in our laboratory (Zepeda Instruments, Seattle, WA) are relatively light in weight. As long as no degradation of the probes occurs due to the penetration of body fluids, the signals are stable in chronic preparations. Moreover, the flowmeter used for telemetry is both lightweight and simple to use and does not consume an inordinate amount of power. Figure 5 shows waveforms from the aorta of a rhesus monkey after 6 months implantation, indicating that long-term performance of this technique is feasible.

A major disadvantage of the electromagnetic flowmeter is the variability in the electrical zero, making it necessary to establish zero flow mechanically by means of temporary vessel occlusion with a hydraulic occluder. Additionally, the transducers are more massive than the ultrasonic Doppler transducers, which increases the incidence of kinking or occlusion of small vessels (e.g., coronary artery). Finally, the large excitation currents required to establish adequate electrical signals can cause significant localized heating of the vessel and must be chosen with care to minimize vessel damage.

Flowmeter Summary

The three flow measurement techniques discussed above all have advantages and disadvantages, and thus their complementary use in chronic animal instrumentation has been beneficial to work in our laboratory. The Doppler transducers have the lowest mass and exhibit excellent zero flow stability. These factors recommend this technique to a large number of experimental designs, especially with telemetry. The transit-time flow measurement technique, although the most cumbersome to implant, provides direct calibration in terms of volume flow, and zero stability is acceptable with time, although it might be important to establish the exact relationship between occlusive zero and electrical zero after the transducer has stabilized on the artery. The electromagnetic flowmeter employs transducers, which are the most critical of fit to the artery for proper operation, but can be calibrated in terms of volume flow and, with occlusive zero determinations, can be a useful tool for flow measurement. Finally, both the pulsed-Doppler and the transit-time flowmeters may be synchronized to work simultaneously with ultrasonic dimension gauges, but not with each other. The electromagnetic flowmeter operates at a much lower frequency (400 Hz) than the ultrasonic devices and thus may be used simultaneously with dimension measurements without synchronization.

Ventricular Dimensions

The ultrasonic transit-time dimension gauge, as originally described by Rushmer et al. (58) and developed by Patrick and co-workers (33,59), can be used for the measurement of left ventricular internal diameter, right and left ventricular wall thickness, and right and left ventricular regional segment length (10,29,60–63) (Figs. 1, 2, and 7). This technique uses pairs of small piezoelectric transducers operating in the frequency ranges of 3–7 MHz, depending on the application. In operation, a burst of sound from one transducer propagates to the second transducer. If the speed of sound is known in the intervening medium (1.58×10^6 mm/sec for blood), the separation of the transducers can be determined by measuring the transit time of the sound. This one-way, two-transducer technique contrasts with the ultrasonic echo technique used clinically in cardiac diagnosis. The pulse–echo technique uses a single transducer to emit ultrasound, which is then reflected from the internal structures of the body. Even though the two-transducer technique is invasive and is limited to a discrete straight-line measurement, the capability for enhanced and more discrete reception of the ultrasonic signal can radically improve the accuracy and resolution of dimension measurements. This permits the detection of more subtle changes in regional function as compared with the pulse–echo technique.

In operation, the dimension gauge measures the acoustic transit time of bursts of ultrasound (center frequencies ranging from 3 to 7 MHz) propagated between two piezoelectric crystals placed on opposing surfaces of the left ventricular cavity (internal diameter), or placed on opposing surfaces of the right or left ventricular free walls (wall thickness), or multiple pairs of piezoelectric crystals inserted into the free walls of the right or left ventricles approximately 1–2 cm apart (segmental length). The transit-time dimension gauge can be synchronized to measure up to 12 simultaneous dimensions, thus allowing a multiple assessment of regional myocardial function (Fig. 1). The signals can also be differentiated to obtain the rate of myocardial fiber shortening, an index of regional cardiac function (Figs. 1 and 2). In addition, the intramyocardial electrogram from each of the transducers can be assessed, using the standard limb lead arrangements as an indifferent reference (Fig. 1).

The transit-time dimension gauge provides electrical pulses at a 1 kHz rate to one of the crystals, thus inducing the crystals into shock-induced, burst mode vibration. A wideband amplifier senses the propagated ultrasonic bursts received by the opposing crystal. Rectangular voltage pulses are generated, the duration of which is equivalent to the transit time of the acoustic bursts. These are time averaged to produce a voltage proportional to ventricular dimensions. The instantaneous dimensions are determined by sampling at a 1 kHz rate and filtering the output signals with a low-pass filter to 100 Hz. This bandwidth is adequate to assess velocities of contraction by utilizing an analog differentiator. The instrument timing is controlled by a 1 MHz crystal oscillator. Calibration pulses at 1 μsec intervals are generated to ensure the accuracy of the complete data measurement system. Multiple channels are accommodated by interleaving the transit-time measurements in a time-division multiplex mode.

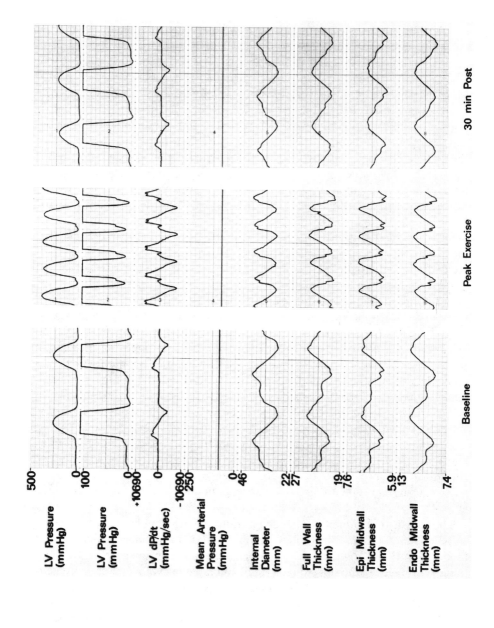

The theoretical resolution of the ultrasonic dimension technique is one-quarter wavelength, with the wavelength being determined by the thickness of the crystal. To achieve improved resolution, it is necessary to use thin, high-frequency piezoelectric crystals when possible. We are currently using 7 MHz crystals (0.3 mm thick and 2.0 mm in diameter) for myocardial segment length determination because transducer separation is typically 1 cm and the signal strength is not adversely affected by this distance. At the other extreme, transducers used for the measurement of ventricular diameter are 3 MHz crystals (0.7 mm thick and 3–4 mm in diameter) because the distance measured is in the 3–4 cm range, and attenuation of the sound is greater, being proportional to both distance and frequency.

The transducers used to measure ventricular dimensions are fabricated from 3–4 mm disks of a thickness-mode resonant, 3 MHz piezoelectric material (lead zirconate–titanate, LTZ-2; Transducer Products, Torrington, CT). Stranded copper wires (AWG 29, 51 strands no. 46) with PVC insulation are carefully soldered, using minimum heat, to each surface of the disk, with the wire leads extending axially from the crystal to facilitate insertion through a stab wound into the ventricle. A polystyrene foam pad is cemented to the back side of each crystal, and a bead of epoxy is placed on the active surface to form an acoustic lens that reduces the directionality of the transducers. The transducers are underdamped with a measured Q of approximately 3. Transducers for wall thickness determination are smaller, with a 2 mm diameter, 5 MHz crystal used for the endocardial surface. A similar transducer with a small dacron patch is sutured to the epicardium to complete the implant. To measure regional subendocardial and subepicardial wall thickness, an additional crystal is implanted in the midwall (61). A short (6 cm) length of small, very flexible, twisted pair stainless steel wire is used to connect these crystal elements to the regular transducer wire. This adds flexibility and strength to the wiring in the vicinity of the moving myocardium. Myocardial segment transducers are fabricated in a similar fashion to the wall thickness transducers, with stainless steel extensions for flexibility. For long-term implants, epoxy is used as a protective agent for the piezoelectric element and as a lens to increase the sonic beam width. If intramyocardial electrograms are desired, a plastic casting resin is used because the development of the sensed electrical voltage requires a "leaky" or less than perfect insulator for the piezoelements. However, this in turn means that transducer lifetime expectancies are somewhat shorter.

FIG. 7. Representative recordings of the measurements of left ventricular (LV) pressure, LV end-diastolic pressure, LV dP/dt, mean arterial pressure, LV internal diameter, full wall thickness, and subepicardial (EPI) and subendocardial (ENDO) wall thicknesses in a dog with LV hypertrophy at baseline, peak exercise, and 30 min after cessation of exercise. There was impairment in subendocardial wall thickening at peak exercise, which persisted into recovery, whereas subepicardial wall thickness increased normally during exercise. From ref. 61, with permission of the American Heart Association, Inc.

A number of features of the present instrument enhance its use. Transformer coupling of both the transmitting and the receiving transducers minimizes the interaction with other implanted transducers and provides safety from power-line induced fibrillation. Resistive damping of these transformers, where small distances are measured, has minimized the ringing associated with the initiating electrical voltage for each sonic burst. This voltage, a 300 V, 0.2 μsec pulse generated by avalanche transistor breakdown, has an extremely wide energy spectrum and is difficult to control when used in proximity to wide-band receiver amplifiers with 60 db of gain. The amplifiers are differential in design to reduce common mode interference and recover from overload within 1 μsec, thus allowing measurements as small as 3 mm to be made routinely. The signal detector or transit-time determinator is a high speed (20-nsec) comparator, which is adjusted to detect the leading edge of the second half-cycle of a received signal, thus enhancing the accuracy and reproducibility of measurement over other designs that use envelope detectors. An inhibit circuit prevents premature mistriggering on noise or instrument artifacts. The previously mentioned calibration pulses are substituted for the signal, resulting in highly accurate, repeatable calibration of the system at any time.

Vascular Dimensions

The study of the elastic properties of the aortic wall is fundamental for the understanding of the coupling between the heart and peripheral circulation, the characteristics of vascular mechanoreceptors, and the pathogenesis of important disease states, such as atherosclerosis and hypertension. Moreover, the concept of large vessel coronary artery vasoconstriction as a possible mechanism for Prinzmetal's variant angina (64), as well as typical angina pectoris and myocardial infarction (65,66), underline the importance of making direct continuous measurements of peripheral vascular dimensions.

The design of the transit-time dimension gauge has recently been modified to permit the measurement of both large (59) and small (67,68) (Fig. 8) vessel dimensions. These modifications involve refinement of the electronics as well as construction of smaller transducers. The transducers (1 mm × 3 mm) are constructed from 7 MHz piezoelectric material, with stainless steel wiring and a thin coat of epoxy. To minimize mass loading of the vessel and to facilitate alignment at surgery, these transducers have been constructed without lenses, although a small dacron patch is attached to the back of the transducer with epoxy for stabilization purposes. The transducers are implanted on opposing sides of the vessel and secured with 5-0 or 6-0 suture material. Resistive loading is used to minimize the instrument ringing artifact. The inhibit pulse is shortened to be adjustable over the range of 0.5–10 μsec, and the sensitivity of the postdetection amplifiers is increased to compensate for the smaller signal developed by the shorter transit time. These

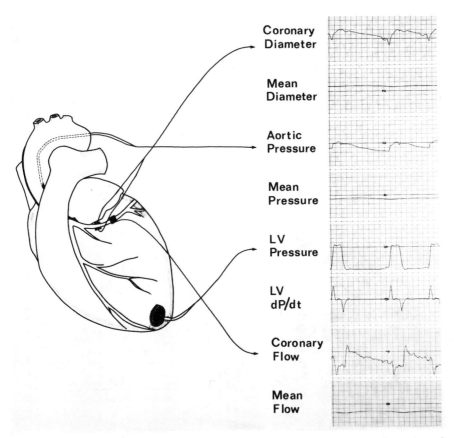

FIG. 8. Schematic diagram of techniques used to assess epicardial coronary dimensions. A pair of miniature ultrasonic crystals was implanted across a diameter of the left circumflex coronary artery to measure phasic and mean coronary diameter. A Millar microtip manometer was advanced to the aortic root to measure phasic and mean aortic pressures. A miniature pressure gauge was implanted in the left ventricle (LV) to measure left ventricular pressure and dP/dt. An electromagnetic flow transducer was implanted on the left circumflex coronary artery to measure phasic and mean coronary blood flow. From ref. 68, with permission.

modifications result in an instrument that is stable enough to resolve 0.05-mm changes in the diameter of a 3 mm vessel. The measurements are repeatable and comprise a sensitive and accurate method of assessing changes in coronary artery diameter under a variety of interventions in the conscious animal (67).

Telemetry of Pressures, Flows, and Dimensions

Extension of the measurement techniques described above to include radiotelemetry of the biological signals has obvious utility in situations in which the experimental design precludes the use of cables, tethers, and the laboratory environment. Examples include activities such as free-ranging exercise, the recording of data from intractable animals such as large primates (69) (Fig. 9), as well as studies of animals in their natural habitat. Because our laboratory has been interested in this area (31–33,35,42–47, 70–72), the design of the instruments previously described has been planned to include the parameters of low power requirements, battery operation, small size, and minimum parts to facilitate the telemetry of these parameters.

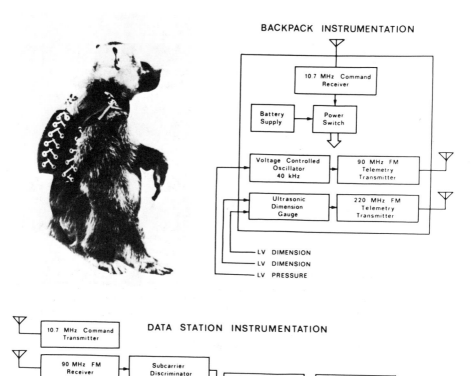

FIG. 9. Radiotelemetry of physiological measurements in conscious, unrestrained baboons. The instrumentation carried by the baboon in a backpack is shown schematically. The backpack contained the dual dimension/pressure telemetry apparatus plus batteries, which were used to power the system. An RF controlled interrogator was used to activate a motor-driven pump to infuse 1000 ml saline. The electronic instrumentation in the remote data station, used to receive and process the electronic signals, is schematically depicted at the bottom. From ref. 69, with permission of the American Society for Clinical Investigation.

The telemetry systems we have developed fall into two categories: flow–pressure systems and pressure–dimension systems. The uniqueness of both the cw ultrasonic Doppler flowmeter and the pulsed transit-time dimension gauge generally preclude their simultaneous use, owing to the generation of mutual interference. However, the electromagnetic flow system can be compatible with the ultrasonic dimension system.

FM–FM modulation techniques have been used for many years and are well understood. The development of integrated microcircuit amplifiers has allowed the design of small, low-power voltage controlled oscillators (VCO) with millivolt sensitivity, which are used to frequency-multiplex several physiologic signals onto a common RF carrier. Our design results in a VCO with 20 mV sensitivity for a frequency deviation of $\pm 7.5\%$, power consumption of 30 mW including pressure transducer excitation, and a size of 1 in. $\times$ 1/2 in. $\times$ 3 in. These VCO designs are used with center frequencies of 14.5, 22, 30, and 40 kHz to telemeter four low-frequency (DC to 100-Hz) signals on a common carrier. The VCOs are supplied power from battery-operated voltage regulators, and temperature-induced drift is approximately 50 parts per million per degree centigrade. Miniature 100-MHz FM transmitters of approximately the same size are used to complete the transmitting system.

The mobile receiving station consists of an FM receiver that is a slightly modified stereo high-fidelity unit, coupled with a bank of commercially available subcarrier frequency discriminators (Airpax FDS-30). This system receives and detects the RF signal from the transmitter and separates the individual subcarrier signals for conversion to individual analog voltages proportional to the physiologic data. These signals are then recorded on analog magnetic tape recorders for later playback on a strip chart oscillograph. Because the ultrasonic Doppler flow signal prior to demodulation consists of a spectrum of signals from 200 Hz to 20 kHz, this signal is telemetered directly on the RF carrier, while one of the 40-kHz VCOs is used to telemeter pressure. The receiving station for this flow–pressure system consists of an adjustable bandpass filter, which excludes the VCO signal from the flow detection process, and a subcarrier discriminator that has a built-in filter to exclude the flow data.

It is important to note that these telemetry systems are neither the smallest, lightest, nor most novel approaches yet attempted. However, these systems have the advantage of utility. The size and power consumption of the electronics are reasonable where the size of the experimental animals is somewhat dictated by the degree of surgery and the size of the transducers implanted.

Externalization of the transducer leads and the use of these systems in a backpack arrangement have several advantages over totally implanted systems. The externalized system can easily be shared among a number of animals. It can be calibrated and repaired easily, and its expense is appreciably less than an implanted system. The possibility for electronic failure in the hostile environment of an implanted system requires extreme attention to the problem of long-term insulation. Moreover, if problems do occur in the electronics, the experimental preparation is usually not recoverable.

Instrumentation for Smaller Animals

Most of the instrumentation described in this chapter is too large for use in smaller animals such as the rabbit or rat. Developments in smaller transducer design, along with improvements in tether systems, which can couple fluid catheters to external transducers as well as accommodate the wiring from flow and dimension transducers, now make it feasible to adapt some of these measurement techniques for these smaller animals. In our laboratory, as well as others, small tether systems containing two to three fluid couplings and as many as 10 electrical circuits allow chronic continuous measurements from conscious rats, instrumented with an indwelling catheter for infusion of fluids, a catheter in the left ventricle for the measurement

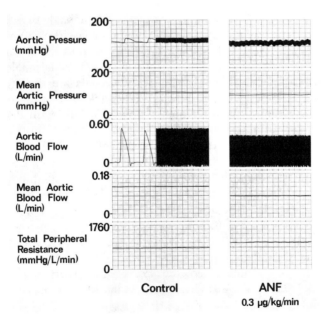

FIG. 10. The effect of 0.3µg/kg/min infusion of atrial natriuretic factor (ANF) on phasic and mean measurements of aortic pressure and aortic blood flow and on computed total peripheral resistance in a conscious rat before (*left panel*) and 30 min after (*right panel*) infusion. Note that ANF reduced mean aortic blood flow (cardiac output) more than arterial pressure, indicating a rise in peripheral resistance. From ref. 74, with permission of the American Heart Association, Inc.

of left ventricular pressure and dP/dt, and either an electromagnetic or transit-time flow probe around the ascending aorta to measure cardiac output (73,74). Figure 10 depicts signals from such an instrumented conscious rat, demonstrating that the economies of size and scale can be taken advantage of, in this case, in a study of the effects of atrial natriuretic factor on total peripheral resistance.

The catheters must be maintained through the tether system, by slow infusion of a small amount of heparin, to maintain long-term patency of the catheters. The small size of tubing necessary for implant (0.96 mm, o.d.), restricts the nominal use of the catheters to measurement and infusion, since withdrawal of blood is difficult and avoidance of clotting is a problem, both in the catheter and in the fluid swivel.

The transit-time flowmeter seems to be more stable on the aorta of these chronically instrumented animals than the electromagnetic probe, since the fit of the electromagnetic probe is extremely critical for success with such a small artery (3 mm). The relaxed constraint on fit associated with the transit-time probe ensures a better chance of success in this application although the *in vitro* calibration may require adjustment, due to the curved section of artery on which the flow probe is implanted.

SUMMARY

The chronically instrumented conscious animal model can be used to provide an important tool for the assessment of the effects of putative toxic substances on cardiovascular function (75). This chapter updates techniques that have been used routinely in our laboratory for the measurement of arterial, atrial, and ventricular pressures, blood flows to the heart, brain, kidney, intestine, and skeletal muscle, and ventricular and vascular dimensions, in animals ranging in size from calves, baboons, dogs, and rhesus monkeys to the rat (75). The application of radiotelemetry techniques to the measurement of these physiological variables has also been described. These techniques permit the continuous high-fidelity assessment of cardiovascular dynamics in conscious, unrestrained animals without the confounding influence of anesthesia and acute surgical trauma. Thus direct and reflex effects of toxic substances on cardiovascular function can be continuously monitored. Finally, the effect of these environmental agents can be reevaluated in these chronically instrumented, conscious animal models following the experimental induction of a disease state.

ACKNOWLEDGMENTS

This work was supported by U.S. Public Health Service Grants HL38070, HL33107, and HL33065 and NASA Grant NAG 2 451.

REFERENCES

1. Harlan WR, Sharrett AR, Weill H, Turino GM, Borhani NO, and Resnekov L. Impact of environment on cardiovascular disease. Report of the American Heart Association Task Force on Cardiovascular Disease. *Circulation* 1981;63:242A–250A.

2. Rosenman KD. Cardiovascular disease and environmental exposure. *Br J Ind Med* 1979;36:85–97.

3. Manders WT, Vatner SF. Effects of sodium pentobarbital anesthesia on left ventricular function and distribution of cardiac output, with particular reference to the mechanism for tachycardia. *Circ Res* 1976;39:512–517.

4. Vatner SF, Smith NT. Effects of halothane on left ventricular function and distribution of regional blood flow in dogs and primates. *Circ Res* 1974;34:155–167.

5. Vatner SF. Effects of anesthesia on cardiovascular control mechanisms. *Environ Health Perspect* 1978;26:193–206.

6. Vatner SF, Franklin D, Braunwald E. Effects of anesthesia and sleep on circulatory response to carotid sinus nerve stimulation. *Am J Physiol* 1971;220:1249–1255.

7. Vatner SF, Higgins CB, Braunwald E. Sympathetic and parasympathetic components of reflex tachycardia induced by hypotension in conscious dogs with and without heart failure. *Cardiovasc Res* 1974;8:153–161.

8. Vatner SF, Franklin D, Van Citters RL, and Braunwald E. Effects of carotid sinus nerve stimulation on the coronary circulation of the conscious dog. *Circ Res* 1970;17:11–21.

9. Vatner SF, Franklin D, Van Citters RL, Braunwald E. Effects of carotid sinus nerve stimulation on blood-flow distribution in conscious dogs at rest and during exercise. *Circ Res* 1970;27:495–503.

10. Vatner SF, Higgins CB, Franklin D, Braunwald E. Extent of carotid sinus regulation of the myocardial contractile state in conscious dogs. *J Clin Invest* 1972;51:995–1008.

11. Vatner SF, McRitchie RJ. Interaction of chemoreflex and pulmonary inflation reflexes in regulation of coronary circulation in conscious dogs. *Circ Res* 1975;37:664–673.

12. Vatner SF, Priano LL, Rutherford JD, Manders WT. Sympathetic regulation of the cerebral circulation by the carotid chemoreceptor reflex. *Am J Physiol* 1980;238:H594–H598.

13. Zimpfer M, Sit SP, Vatner SF. Effects of anesthesia on the carotid chemoreceptor reflex. *Circ Res* 1981;44:400–406.

14. Higgins CB, Vatner SF, Franklin D, Braunwald E. Extent of regulation of the heart's contractile state in the conscious dog by alteration in the frequency of contraction. *J Clin Invest* 1973;52:1187–1194.

15. Vatner SF, Monroe RG, McRitchie RJ. Effects of anesthesia, tachycardia, and autonomic blockade on the Anrep effect in intact dogs. *Am J Physiol* 1975;226:1450–1456.

16. Boettcher DH, Vatner SF, Heyndrickx GR, Braunwald E. Extent of the utilization of the Frank–Starling mechanism in conscious dogs. *Am J Physiol* 1978;3:H338–H345.

17. Vatner SF, Boettcher DH. Regulation of cardiac output by stroke volume and heart rate in conscious dogs. *Circ Res* 1978;42:557–561.

18. Vatner SF, Boettcher DH, Heyndrickx GR, McRitchie RJ. Reduced baroreflex sensitivity with volume loading in conscious dogs. *Circ Res* 1975;37:236–242.

19. Vatner SF. Effects of hemorrhage on regional blood flow distribution in dogs and primates. *J Clin Invest* 1974;54:225–235.

20. Zimpfer M, Manders WT, Barger AC, Vatner SF. Pentobarbital alters compensatory neural and hormonal mechanisms in response to hemorrhage. *Am J Physiol* 1981;243:H713–H721.

21. Higgins CB, Millard RW, Braunwald E, Vatner SF. Effects and mechanisms of action of dopamine on regional hemodynamics in the conscious dog. *Am J Physiol* 1973;225:432–437.

22. Vatner SF, Higgins CB, Braunwald E. Effects of norepinephrine on coronary circulation and left ventricular dynamics in the conscious dog. *Circ Res* 1974;34:812–823.

23. Vatner SF, Millard RW, Higgins CB. Coronary and myocardial effects of dopamine in the conscious dog: parasympatholytic augmentation of pressor and inotropic actions. *J Pharmacol Exp Ther* 1973;187:280–295.

24. Higgins CB, Vatner SF, Braunwald E. Regional hemodynamic effects of a digitalis glycoside in the conscious dog with and without experimental heart failure. *Circ Res* 1972;30:406–417.

25. Vatner SF, Higgins CB, Franklin D, Braunwald E. Effects of digitalis glycoside on coronary and systemic dynamics in conscious dogs. *Circ Res* 1971;28:470–479.

26. Vatner SF, Higgins CB, Patrick T, Franklin D, Braunwald E. Effects of cardiac depression and of anesthesia on the myocardial action of a cardiac glycoside. *J Clin Invest* 1971;50:2585–2595.
27. Vatner SF, Marsh JD, Swain JA. Effects of morphine on coronary and left ventricular dynamics in conscious dogs. *J Clin Invest* 1975;55:207–217.
28. Vatner SF, Baig H, (Introduced by Dexter L). The effects of inotropic stimulation on ischemic myocardium in conscious dogs. *Trans Assoc Am Physicians* 1979;91:282–293.
29. Vatner SF, Braunwald E. Effects of chronic heart failure on the inotropic response of the right ventricle of the conscious dog to a cardiac glycoside and to tachycardia. *Circulation* 1974;50:728–734.
30. Van Citters RL, Franklin D. Telemetry of blood pressure in free-ranging animals via an intravascular gauge. *J Appl Physiol* 1966;21:1633–1636.
31. Baig H, Patrick TA, Vatner SF. Implantable pressure gauges for use in chronic animals. In: Fleming DG, Ko WH, Neuman MR, eds. *Indwelling and implantable pressure transducers.* Cleveland, OH: CRC Press; 1977:35–43.
32. Franklin D, Vatner SF, Higgins CB, Patrick T, Kemper WS, Van Citters RL. Measurement and radiotelemetry of cardiovascular variables in conscious animals: techniques and applications. In: Harmison LT, ed. *Research animals in medicine.* Washington, DC: US Government Printing Office; 1973:1119–1133.
33. Patrick TA, Vatner SF, Kemper WS, Franklin D. Telemetry of left ventricular diameter and pressure measurements from unrestrained animals. *J Appl Physiol* 1974;37:276–281.
34. Vatner SF, Franklin D, Higgins CB, Van Citters RL. Backpack telemetry. In: McCutcheon EP, ed. *Chronically implanted cardiovascular instrumentation.* New York: Academic Press; 1973:357–364.
35. Vatner SF, Franklin D, Higgins CB, Patrick T, Braunwald E. Left ventricular response to severe exertion in untethered dogs. *J Clin Invest* 1972;51:3052–3060.
36. Pagani M, Mirsky I, Baig H, Manders WT, Kerkhof P, Vatner SF. Effects of age on aortic pressure–diameter and elastic stiffness–stress relationship in the unanesthetized sheep. *Circ Res* 1979;44:420–429.
37. Barber BJ, Quillen EW, Cowley AW Jr. An inexpensive pressure telemetry system. *Am J Physiol* 1980;239:H570–H572.
38. Vatner SF, Franklin D, Higgins CB, White S, Van Citters RL. Calibration of the ultrasonic Doppler flowmeter in situ. In: McCutcheon EP, ed. *Chronically implanted cardiovascular instrumentation.* New York: Academic Press; 1973:63–70.
39. Vatner SF, Franklin D, Van Citters RL. Simultaneous comparison and calibration of the Doppler and electromagnetic flowmeters. *J Appl Physiol* 1970;29:907–910.
40. Vatner SF, Young M, Patrick TA. Measurement of coronary blood flow in conscious animals. In: Altobelli SA, Voyles WF, Greene ER, eds. *Cardiovascular ultrasonic flowmetry.* New York: Elsevier/North-Holland; 1985:81–99.
41. Franklin D, Watson NW, Pierson KE, Van Citters RL. Technique for radiotelemetry of blood flow from unrestrained animals. *Am J Med Electron* 1966;5:24–28.
42. Vatner SF, Franklin D, Higgins CB, Patrick T, White S, Van Citters RL. Coronary dynamics in unrestrained conscious baboons. *Am J Physiol* 1971;221:1396–1401.
43. Franklin D, Vatner SF, Van Citters RL. Studies on peripheral vascular dynamics using animal models. In: *Animal models for biomedical research IV.* Washington, DC: National Academy of Sciences; 1971:74–84.
44. Higgins CB, Vatner SF, Franklin D, Braunwald E. Effects of experimentally produced heart failure on the peripheral vascular response to severe exercise in conscious dogs. *Circ Res* 1972;31:186–194.
45. Millard RW, Higgins CB, Franklin D, Vatner SF. Regulation of the renal circulation during severe exercise in normal dogs and dogs with experimental heart failure. *Circ Res* 1972;31:881–888.
46. Vatner SF. Effects of exercise and excitement on mesenteric and renal dynamics in conscious, unrestrained baboons. *Am J Physiol* 1978;3:H210–H214.
47. Vatner SF, Higgins CB, White S, Patrick T, Franklin D. The peripheral vascular response to severe exercise in untethered dogs before and after complete heart block. *J Clin Invest* 1971;50:1950–1960.
48. McLeod FD Jr. Directional Doppler demodulation. *20th ACEMB,* 1967; p 27.1 (abstract).
49. Baker DW. Pulsed ultrasonic Doppler flow-sensing. *IEEE Trans SU* 1970;17:170–185.
50. Hartley CJ, Hanley HG, Lewis RM, Cole JS. A multi-channel directional pulsed Doppler flowmeter. *Proc ACEMB,* 1974; p 339 (abstract).

51. Shen Y-T, Graham RM, Vatner SF. Effect of atrial natriuretic factor on blood flow distribution and vascular resistance in conscious dogs. *Am J Physiol* 1991;260:H1893–H1902.
52. Franklin D, Ellis R, Rushmer R. A pulsed ultrasonic flowmeter. *IRE Trans Med Electron* 1959;6:204–206.
53. Drost C. Vessel diameter-independent volume flow measurements using ultrasound. *Proceedings of the San Diego Biomedical Symposium* 1978;17:299–302.
54. Kolin A. Electromagnetic flowmeter: principle of method and its application to blood flow measurements. *Proc Soc Exp Biol Med* 1936;35:53–56.
55. Wetterer E. New methods of registering rate of blood circulation in unopened vessels. *Z Biol* 1937;98:26–36.
56. Ruterford JD, Vatner SF. Integrated carotid chemoreceptor and pulmonary inflation reflex control of peripheral vasoactivity in conscious dogs.*Circ Res* 1978;43:200–208.
57. Fryer T, Sandler H. Miniature battery operated electromagnetic flowmeter. *J Appl Physiol* 1971;31:622–628.
58. Rushmer RF, Franklin D, Ellis RM. Left ventricular dimensions recorded by sonocardiometry. *Circ Res* 1956;4:684–688.
59. Pagani M, Vatner SF, Baig H, et al. Measurement of multiple simultaneous small dimensions and study of arterial pressure–dimension relations in conscious animals. *Am J Physiol* 1978;4:H610–H617.
60. Heyndrickx GR, Millard RW, McRitchie RJ, Maroko PR, Vatner SF. Regional myocardial functional and electrophysiological alterations after brief coronary artery occlusion in conscious dogs. *J Clin Invest* 1975;56:978–985.
61. Hittinger L, Shannon R, Kohin S, Manders W, Kelly P, Vatner S. Exercise-induced subendocardial dysfunction in dogs with left ventricular hypertrophy. *Circ Res* 1990;66:329–343.
62. Theroux P, Ross J Jr., Franklin D, Kemper WS, Sasayama S. Regional myocardial function in the conscious dog during acute coronary occlusion and responses to morphine, propranolol, nitroglycerin, and lidocaine. *Circulation* 1976;53:302–314.
63. Vatner SF. Correlation between reductions in myocardial blood flow and function in conscious dogs. *Circ Res* 1980;47:201–207.
64. Prinzmetal M, Kennamer R, Merliss R, Wada T, Bor N. Angina pectoris. I. A variance form of angina pectoris. *Am J Med* 1959;27:375–388.
65. Hillis LD, Braunwald E. Medical progress: coronary artery spasm. *N Engl J Med* 1978;299:696–702.
66. Maseri A, L'Abbate A, Baroldi G, et al. Coronary vasospasm as a possible cause of myocardial infarction. A conclusion derived from a study of "pre-infarction" angina. *N Engl J Med* 1978;299:1271–1277.
67. Vatner SF, Pagani M, Manders WT, Pasipoularides AD. Alpha-adrenergic vasoconstriction and nitroglycerin vasodilation of large coronary arteries in the conscious dog. *J Clin Invest* 1980;65:5–14.
68. Vatner SF, Pagani M, Manders WT. Alpha adrenergic constriction of coronary arteries in conscious dogs. *Trans Assoc Am Physicians* 1979:229–238.
69. Zimpfer M, Vatner SF. Effects of acute increases in left ventricle preload on indices of myocardial function in conscious, unrestrained and intact, tranquilized baboons. *J Clin Invest* 1981;67:430–438.
70. Franklin D, Patrick T, Kemper S, Vatner SF. A system for radiotelemetry of blood pressure, blood flow, and ventricular dimensions from animals: a summary report. *Proceedings of International Telemetry Conference,* Washington, DC, September 1971, pp 244–250.
71. Van Citters RL, Franklin D, Vatner SF, Patrick T, Warren JV. Cerebral hemodynamics in the giraffe. *Trans Assoc Am Physicians* 1969;82:293–303.
72. Vatner SF, Patrick TA. Radio telemetry of blood flow and pressure measurements of untethered conscious animals. *Bibl Cardiol* 1974;34:1–11.
73. Shen Y-T, Vatner D, Gagnon H, Vatner S. Species differences in regulation of α-adrenergic receptor function. *Am J Physiol* 1989;257:R1110–R1116.
74. Shen Y-T, Young M, Ohanian J, Graham R, Vatner S. Atrial natriuretic factor-induced systemic vasoconstriction in conscious dogs, rats, and monkeys. *Circ Res* 1990;66:647–661.
75. Vatner SF, Patrick TA, Murray PA. Monitoring of cardiovascular dynamics in conscious animals. In: Van Stee EW, ed. *Cardiovascular toxicology.* New York: Raven Press, 1982; 35–55.

SECTION III

Ischemic Myocardial Cell Injury

Cardiovascular Toxicology, Second Edition,
edited by Daniel Acosta, Jr.
Raven Press, Ltd., New York © 1992.

4

Cellular and Molecular Basis of Toxic Cell Injury

Benjamin F. Trump and Irene K. Berezesky

*Department of Pathology, University of Maryland School of Medicine,
and Maryland Institute for Emergency Medical Services Systems,
Baltimore, Maryland 21201*

The purpose of this chapter is to review current knowledge concerning the cellular and molecular basis of toxic cell injury. Knowledge in this area has progressed rapidly during the past 20 years with most studies currently involving elucidation of the mechanisms involved in both lethal and sublethal injury, as well as in acute and chronic cell injury. This chapter focuses, in particular, on the morphologic, metabolic, and genetic events involved and also on the effects of altered ion homeostasis. A number of reviews are available on the pathophysiology of cell injury in general and the heart in particular, including Trump and Ginn, 1969 (1); Trump and Arstila, 1971 (2); Trump and Mergner, 1974 (3); Bowen and Lockshin, 1981 (4); Trump et al., 1982 (5); Mergner et al., 1990 (6); and Combs and Acosta, 1990 (7).

CHARACTERISTICS OF CELL INJURY

General

A cell injury may be defined as a stimulus or event that results in altering cellular homeostasis beyond the normal range (1–3). These alterations may be transient or prolonged and can therefore represent acute or chronic states. The injuries may also be lethal (i.e., injuries that result in cell death) or sublethal (i.e., injuries that even if prolonged may be compatible with continued survival of the cell through an altered homeostatic condition). Examples of lethal injury in the myocardium include the effects of total inhibition of ATP synthesis (e.g., anoxia, ischemia, or inhibitors of respiration and glycolysis). Examples of chronic sublethal injury include myocardial hypertrophy due to ventricular overload, fatty metamorphosis following exposure to a variety of toxic agents, or chronic mitochondrial abnormalities.

Following an acute lethal injury, two principal phases can be established following the application of the injurious stimulus. These are a phase prior to the point of cell death or "point of no return," the reversible phase, and a phase following cell death consisting of degradative changes, usually referred to as necrosis (1). The length of the prelethal or reversible interval varies with temperature, type of injury, and cell type. In the case of the myocardium, total ischemia at 37°C yields a reversible phase of approximately 30 min (8).

Classification of Cell Death

A number of classifications of cell death have been proposed. For purposes of the present chapter, we use the following classifications.

Instantaneous

Instantaneous cell death is usually within less than a second, occasioned by such treatments as ultra-rapid freezing or immersion in or perfusion with fixatives, such as glutaraldehyde or osmium tetroxide. This type of death is rare in living animals but is important because it distinguishes between the concepts of cell death and necrosis. With these types of instantaneous cell death, necrosis never occurs as the enzymes and factors responsible for degradation of cellular macromolecules are also rapidly inactivated.

Necrosis

The term "necrosis" is used to refer to the phase of degradation of cell components following irreversible injury *in vivo* (2,9). It is characterized by breakdown of cell macromolecules, including membranes, nucleic acids, and proteins, and, over a period of time, converts the cell to debris that eventually reaches equilibrium with the environment. At the light microscopic (LM) level, the characteristic changes of necrosis include: increasing eosinophilia of the cytoplasm, presumed to be due to denaturation of cytoplasmic proteins; nuclear chromatin clumping and shrinkage; and finally, karyolysis where the chromosomes are totally digested and the nucleus is only visible as a faint shadow. Gradually, the cellular debris is liquefied and/or removed by mononuclear phagocytes. *In vivo*, a zone of acute intense inflammation often surrounds the necrotic cells, which activates complement and other pathways, leading to the inflammatory response. In many cases, it is believed that the inflammatory response also contributes to further damage of cells at the margin of necrotic zones through release of injurious mediators, such as active oxygen species.

Autophagocytosis

Autophagocytosis is a process whereby organelles such as mitochondria, endoplasmic reticulum (ER), and peroxisomes are turned over by sequestration into the lysosomal system where extensive digestion and conversion to debris and residual bodies develops (10,11). Autophagy is seen in virtually all cells and, in most cases, consists of budding of portions of cytoplasm-containing organelles into the lumina of the cisternae of the ER. The subsequent double-membrane limited bodies, thus formed, ultimately fuse with primary and/or secondary lysosomes, resulting in the digestion of the sequestered organelles and the formation of a secondary lysosome. Autophagy is a common phenomenon under sublethal states of stress, including starvation, hormonal stimulation, and hypoxia and represents a normal mechanism for organelle turnover. The residual bodies formed by autophagocytosis accumulate in the cytoplasm and become auto-oxidized, forming lipofuscin pigment. Such accumulations are commonly observed in myocardial cells where they increase as a function of age. By LM, they can be observed as yellowish-brown autofluorescence cytoplasmic inclusions.

Autophagy thus represents a type of cell death and necrosis of organelles occurring within the lysosomal system, where they mix with other debris taken into the cell by endocytosis or phagocytosis. During the process of apoptosis, discussed later, cell fragments are commonly detached from apoptotic cells, undergo phagocytosis by adjacent parenchymal or mesenchymal cells, and then add heterophagic granules to the portfolio of the secondary lysosome. As these fragments may also contain organelles, including mitochondria, ER, and microbodies, it can be confusing to distinguish apoptosis from the process of autophagocytosis.

Extensive autophagocytosis has been described in cells to the point where the cytoplasm becomes virtually filled with engorged secondary lysosomes. It is still difficult to be certain whether or not this event is capable of leading the cell in question to death, although unquestionably the organelles within the autophagic vacuole are themselves dying and undergo necrosis.

Programmed Cell Death

The term "programmed cell death" is now used to refer to cells that die in a more or less predictable manner, following some type of scheduled agent, such as hormonal changes, alterations in growth factors, and alterations in nutrition, among others (12). Usually, the precise stimulus is not known. Since, however, this occurs in otherwise disease-free animals and plants, the term has thus been used to distinguish between a natural or "programmed" cell death that permits normal turnover of cells (as in maturation of the epidermal cells in the skin) as contrasted with "accidental" cell death that refers to cell death occurring from environmental or other factors including trauma, ischemia, anoxia, or xenobiotic chemicals. On the other hand, there is no doubt that overlap between these categories does occur and that while certain types of biologic cell responses typify programmed cell death, such as terminal differentiation and apoptosis, necrosis is typical of accidentally and environmentally induced cell death. However, it is also apparent that the two types may overlap in a particular case as more is learned. The thus far described examples of the types of programmed cell death are discussed next.

Apoptosis

The term "apoptosis" is derived from two Greek words, *apo,* meaning away from, and *ptosis,* meaning to fall. Apoptosis is therefore literally a falling away. This term thus refers to the blebbing and fragmentation of the cells undergoing this phenomenon. In a sense, the phenomenon is similar to apocrine secretion, which is a type of secretion in which part of the cytoplasm is budded away and enters the extracellular space (4,12,13).

The phenomenon of apoptosis occurs in a variety of physiologic and pathologic conditions, including normal development, hormone withdrawal as in the prostate gland following castration, turnover of lymphocytes, development of the nervous system including the eye, and many other examples that have been well reviewed by Wyllie and colleagues (13).

The phenomenon of apoptosis begins with striking changes in both the cytoplasm and the nucleus. The cytoplasm undergoes marked blebbing at the cell periphery, undoubtedly due to mediated changes in cytoskeletal–membrane interactions. Such interactions result in constriction of the blebs, pinching off and ultimately phagocytosis of the budded portions of cytoplasm by adjacent parenchymal or connective tissue cells. These buds then enter the phagolysosomal system of the phagocytizing cell and initially form large eosinophilic cytoplasmic inclusions of which the Councilman body in the liver is a classic example. Also, very early in the process, there is clumping of nuclear chromatin along the nuclear envelope and beginning fragmentation of the nucleus. This morphologic change in chromatin is accompanied by double-stranded DNA breaks that typically occur at internucleosomal regions, giving a characteristic "ladder" pattern on gels. This pattern is maintained and is particularly prominent in certain cells, such as lymphocytes.

As the process continues, the cytoplasm condenses and the nuclei become pyknotic, leading to the formation of "apoptotic" bodies, readily visible in H&E sections. These bodies are typical of hormone withdrawal in hormone-dependent organs and also occur prominently during development in several systems. Ultimately, the death of the fragments occurs by necrosis either in the extracellular space or within the phagolysosomes of the phagocytizing cell.

Terminal Differentiation

The phrase "terminal differentiation" has been commonly used to apply to a type of cell death often induced by growth factors, hormones, or other environmental changes by which cells in the mitotic cycle leave the cycle, usually from G1, and, instead of remaining available for recruitment back into the cycle, as in the case of renal tubular epithelium or hepatic parenchymal cells, undergo an irreversible program of commitment to a new phenotype. This new phenotype contains a variety of new expressed genes, which lead the cell to one that cannot divide and therefore that undergoes atrophy and death. A classic example is the keratin layer of the epidermis. During maturation from the basal layer, the epidermal cells undergo a terminal differentiation program and develop new cytoskeletal keratin proteins and active RNA and DNA synthesis, and then atrophy and form a keratinized cornified layer. A similar type of differentiation also occurs following injury in the bronchial epithelium, forming areas of "squamous metaplasia" (14). A variety of stimuli, including phorbol esters and growth factors such as TGF-β_1 (15) and serum (16), induce this in bronchial epithelia. Ionized cytosolic calcium ($[Ca^{2+}]_i$) seems to be involved in one type of signaling leading to this terminal differentiation program (17) and, in the case of keratinocytes, varying the extracellular ionized calcium (Ca^{2+}_e) is sufficient to induce such differentiation (18). It is of interest that many compounds and inflammatory agents that may be tumor promoters differentially induce this phenomenon in normal as compared to initiated cells, thus giving the initiated cells a growth advantage, one current hypothesis of tumor promotion (19).

Programmed Cell Death in Insects

Still another pattern of programmed cell death occurs in insect development. Bowen and Bowen (12) have carefully characterized this process and, again, it appears to involve lysosomal acid hydrolases, which in these cases may escape into the intracellular space, resulting in these types of programmed death.

Stages of Cell Injury

Some years ago, we investigated the reversible and irreversible changes in a variety of cell systems following lethal and sublethal injury (1,2,9,20–23). Based on these studies, we later characterized and classified these changes into stages of cell injury (Fig. 1) so as to permit the correlation of structure and function and to then codify the changes so as to be able to

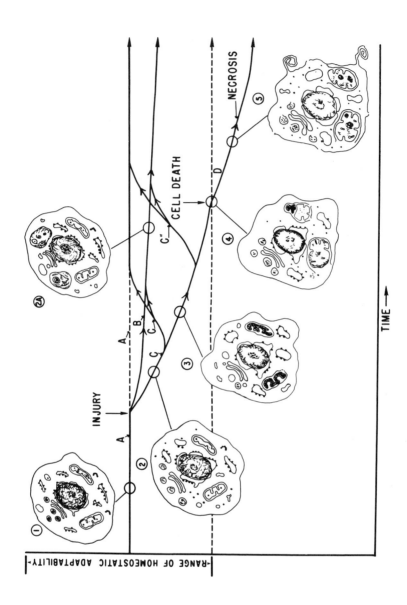

RANGE OF HOMEOSTATIC ADAPTABILITY

TIME →

INJURY

CELL DEATH

NECROSIS

A
B
C
C'
C"

A₁

①
②
②₁
③
④
⑤

compare differing injuries (for recent review, see ref. 24). The structural and functional characteristics of each stage are briefly discussed next.

Stage 1

Structure

Stage 1 is the normal cell (Fig. 2A). The mitochondria are in orthodox conformation and have well-defined granules. The nuclear chromatin is dispersed and numerous polysomes are located on the rough ER and in the cytosol.

Stage 2

Structure

The earliest changes are seen in this stage, often occurring within seconds after initiation of the injury. Cytoplasmic blebs form along cell surfaces, most prominently along free cell surfaces, such as lumina or capillary surfaces. These blebs have a low refractive index and are of low density, as observed by transmission electron microscopy (TEM). They usually contain free polysomes and other cytosolic components, but few organelles (25). Actin and tubulin fibers are detached from the plasma membrane and do not appear in the bleb itself; actin bundles do, however, appear at the bases of the blebs (25,26). Elsewhere in the cytosol, there is disorganization of the F-actin bundles. As the blebs grow, some constrict at the base and then detach, floating into the extracellular space. If the injury is removed prior to this point, the blebs are resorbed into the cytoplasm. At this phase, the ER becomes dilated and the lumen contains sparse flocculent filamentous material. This correlates with the changes in cellular volume and ion regulation. In the cytoplasm, the mitochondria often show loss of the normal matrical granules. There is clumping of the nuclear chromatin along the nuclear envelope and around the nucleolus (9).

FIG. 1. Diagrammatic conceptualization of the stages of cell injury. As described in the text. Stage 1 depicts a cell in a normal steady state (curve A). At the *arrow*, an injury is applied that may be acutely lethal or sublethal. In the case of a lethal injury, the cell loses homeostatic ability along curve C. Prior to the point of cell death, however, recovery can occur if the injurious stimulus is removed. Such recovery may then proceed along curve C' or curve". Note that incomplete recovery during the reversible phases after lethal injury might also result in a new steady state depicted by the right-hand limb of curves C' and C". From ref. 2, with permission.

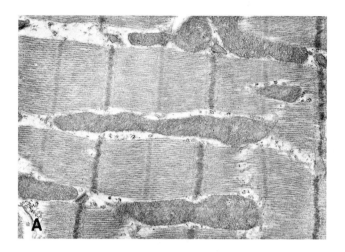

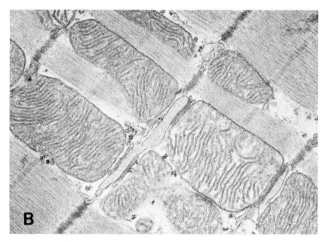

FIG. 2. Transmission electron micrographs (TEM) of dog myocardium. **A:** Control. Bands of myofilaments comprising the A and Z bands can be seen with mitochondria arranged in rows between the myofibrils. Stage 1. × 14,000. **B:** Following 15 min of·in vivo ischemia, note marked mitochondrial swelling of inner compartments. Stage 4a. × 20,000. From ref. 8, with permission. **C:** Following 60 min of in vivo ischemia, all mitochondria are markedly swollen and contain large flocculent densities, the hallmark of irreversibility. Stage 5. × 20,000. From ref. 8, with permission. **D:** Following 120 min of in vivo ischemia plus 24 hr reflow, mitochondria are swollen and contain large flocculent densities and occasional calcifications (*arrows*). Stage 5c. × 24,000. From ref. 42, with permission.

Function

In this stage, cellular ion shifts have begun. Depending on the type of injury, $[Ca^{2+}]_i$ may increase within a few seconds and $[Na^+]_i$, $[Cl^-]_i$, and H_2O_2 content also begin to increase, while $[K^+]_i$ decreases. In the case of anoxic injury, $[ATP]_i$ decreases rapidly, while $[ADP]_i$ increases (27). Coin-

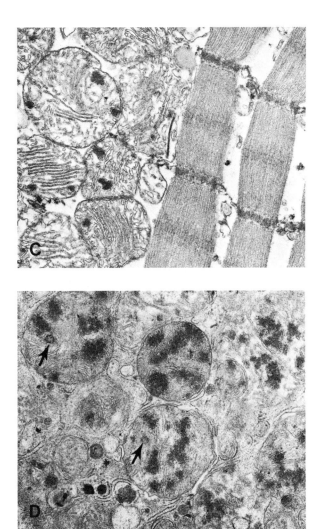

FIG. 2. *Continued.*

cident in time with the chromatin clumping, immediate early genes (e.g., *c-fos* and *c-jun*) begin to be expressed at higher levels (28–31).

Stage 3

Structure

The principal additional change in this stage is condensation of the inner mitochondrial compartments, which become reduced in volume and electron-dense, while, at the same time, the intracristal spaces become correspondingly enlarged (1). The ER continues to dilate, sometimes markedly so, creating large light microscopically visible cytoplasmic vacuoles termed "hydropic degeneration." As the dilatation is usually shared by the nuclear envelope, which is continuous with the ER, large perinuclear vacuoles often represent both dilated rough ER and dilated nuclear envelope.

Function

Condensed mitochondria typically occur under conditions where respiration and/or oxidative phosphorylation are inhibited. Thus in Stage 3, there are markedly reduced levels of ATP (27). As long as the mitochondria remain condensed, however, they seem to be reversibly altered, and, if reoxygenated or isolated at this stage and put into a phosphorylating medium, they will synthesize ATP and generate a normal membrane potential. This condensed appearance of the mitochondria is similar to that seen in mitochondria isolated in 0.25 M sucrose (3). The condensed conformation cannot apparently be maintained if significant damage to the inner membrane takes place, a change that also probably correlates with loss of the mitochondrial membrane potential.

Stages 4 and 4a

Structure

In these transitional stages toward irreversibility, the mitochondria show marked swelling of the inner compartment (Fig. 2B). This can be correlated with increased inner membrane permeability, as measured in isolated mitochondria, and with a decreasing ability to maintain a proton gradient. As the inner compartment swells, mitochondrial matrical enzymes have more access to and also probably leak into the surrounding cytosol.

Function

Functionally, the mitochondria have lost permeability control of the inner compartment, though if ATP–Mg^{2+} is added, permeability control can be restored (32). Respiratory control has been largely lost but if cells are restored to a normal environment or mitochondria are isolated and placed in a phosphorylating medium, recovery will occur. The changes in inner membrane permeability are related to modification of inner membrane phospholipids, which are modified and decrease in parallel with an increase of free fatty acids. If the injurious stimulus can be removed at this point, repair of the inner membranes takes place.

Stage 5

Structure

This stage represents the irreversibly altered cell (Fig. 2C) (1,2). The markedly swollen mitochondria have enlarged and now contain dense intramatrical inclusions known as "flocculent densities" and which represent precipitates of mitochondrial matrix protein (33). In addition, following certain types of injury, mitochondria exhibit calcium phosphate precipitates (Fig. 2D). These begin as small amorphous deposits, often near the cristae, which sometimes form annular aggregates; one mitochondrial profile often can have several such aggregates. If this process continues, the precipitates grow and become confluent. Also, the precipitates may become crystalline, forming aggregates of hydroxyapatite (Fig. 3) in the mitochondria (34,35).

Mitochondrial calcification in Stage 5 occurs only following certain types of injury. It has been observed that such calcification, even in dead cells, is an active process requiring electron transport. Accordingly, cells following injuries such as total ischemia (Fig. 4) or anoxia or injury from metabolic inhibitors such as CN or 2,4-DNP do not exhibit this calcification. Occasionally, intramitochondrial calcifications can be observed within myocardial infarcts *in vivo* or at the edges of ischemic areas. These calcifications

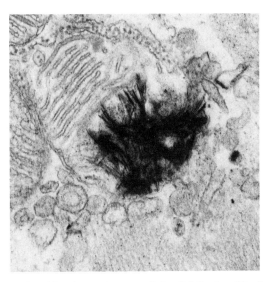

FIG. 3. A single mitochondrion in a rat myocardial cell following 60 min *in vivo* ischemia. Needle-shaped crystalline inclusions are seen, which reveal calcium and phosphate peaks when analyzed by energy dispersive x-ray microanalysis. × 55,000. From ref. 42, with permission.

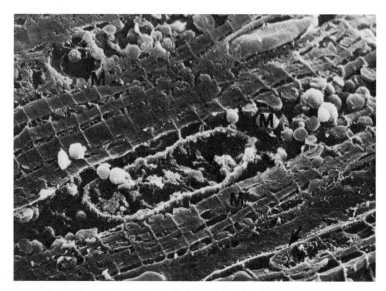

FIG. 4. Scanning electron micrograph (SEM) of dog myocardium following 60 min *in vivo* ischemia. Specimen was frozen following processing and then fractured so as to observe internal structures. Note the parallel rows of myofibrils and mitochondria (M) arranged in rows in the interfibrillar spaces and in the perinuclear region, as well as the ellipsoidal nucleus and chromatin clumping within. Also note the fractured mitochondrion (*arrow*) with its cristae. ×3500. From ref. 5, with permission.

are within cells near collaterals or at the border zone of the infarct where oxygen and substrates are available even to dying cells. As can be noted from the above morphological descriptions, mitochondrial changes are important in stage classification; these changes are illustrated diagrammatically in Fig. 5.

Function

In this stage, cells are beginning to reach equilibrium. $[Na^+]_i$, $[Cl^-]_i$, $[Ca^{2+}]_i$, and water content are high; $[K^+]_i$ and $[Mg^{2+}]_i$ are low. Most enzyme activities are reduced; an exception is the lysosomal acid hydrolases that typically maintain full activity in this stage. Mitochondrial phosphorylating

FIG. 5. A diagrammatic representation of mitochondrial profiles following cell injury: A, orthodox mitochondria (Stage 1); B, condensed (Stage 3); B_1, transitional form of condensed; B_2 and B_3, condensed mitochondria with flocculent densities or calcifications (Stage 3c); C and C_1, ring-formed condensed mitochondria; D, slightly swollen (Stage 4a); E, E_1, E_2, E_3, and E_4, various forms of highly swollen mitochondria with flocculent densities (Stage 5) or calcifications (Stage 5c). From ref. 3, with permission.

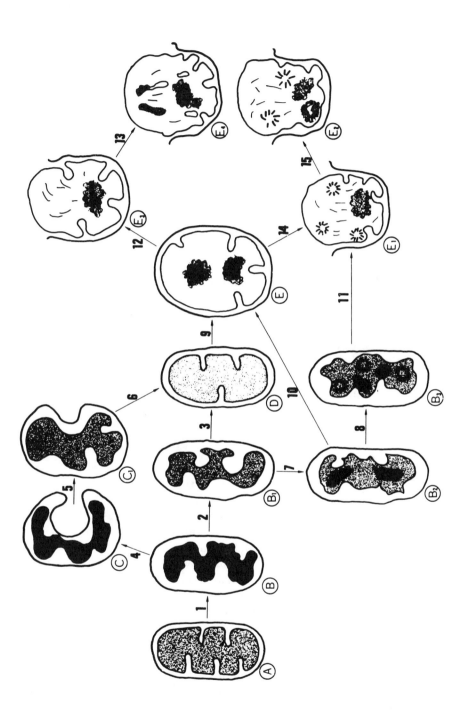

ability is irreversibly lost and mitochondrial matrix enzymes are in equilibrium with the cytosol. As the integrity of the cell membrane is violated, soluble enzymes (e.g., lactic dehydrogenase) escape from the cytosol into the extracellular space. Plasmalemmal membrane functions are lost, including Na^+/K^+–ATPase.

Stages 6 and 7

Structure

These stages occur during the necrotic phase with cell morphology now significantly altered by chromatin breakdown, marked membrane shape changes, myelin figure formation, and so on.

Function

Lysosomal hydrolases, although active long after cell death, have, at these stages, escaped from their compartments and catalyzed macromolecules in the cytoplasm, the organelles, and the nucleus. As time progresses, these cells find large amounts of Ca^{2+} and calcifications occur. The other cations reach equilibrium in the extracellular space. Finally, the cells also return to total equilibrium, though *in vivo*, necrotic debris is phagocytized by adjacent cells and digested within the phagolysosomal system of epithelium and macrophages.

PRINCIPAL MECHANISMS OF ACUTE LETHAL INJURY

Acute lethal injury can result from a variety of injurious stimuli, including toxic agents. Studies of many such conditions have made it clear that two mechanisms account for virtually all acute lethal injuries (1–3). These mechanisms are (a) interference with the integrity and/or function of the plasma membrane and (b) interference with cellular energy production.

Direct interference with cell membrane function is a common initial injurious action from a variety of toxic and injurious agents. Such include activation of the C5–9 complement sequence (36,37), oxidant stress (38), and a variety of SH-reactive compounds (39), including mercurials (34).

Interference with cellular energy metabolism commonly results from conditions that inhibit mitochondrial and/or glycolytic generation of ATP. Such conditions include anoxia or ischemia and inhibitors of respiration such as CN; uncouplers, such as 2,4-DNP; inhibitors of glycolysis, such as iodoacetic acid (IAA); and inhibitors of ATPases, such as oligomycin.

Changes in cellular metabolism constitute the fabric of the cellular reactions to acute and chronic injury. Previous studies from our laboratory have characterized many changes and, at the present time, we are engaged in determining the precise critical mechanisms involved in cell killing, cell recovery, and cell proliferation.

ION HOMEOSTASIS

Ion homeostasis and its role in the mechanism of subcellular events that follow acute and chronic cell injury have become widely recognized and studied over the years both by our own laboratory (24,40–48) and those of others (49–52). There is now no doubt that a variety of cellular events in cell injury are initiated by intracellular ion deregulation, particularly that of Ca^{2+}, Na^+, and H^+. Cell alterations involving changes in the metabolism and regulation of intracellular ions are extremely important as they form the basis of signaling, volume control, and energy metabolism control and also have an increasingly evident role in division and differentiation (53,54).

With the development of technologies such as energy dispersive x-ray microanalysis, total bound elements can be measured in unfixed, freeze-dried tissues and cells (Figs. 6 and 7). With the advent of even newer methodolo-

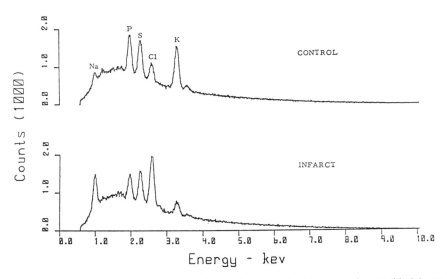

FIG. 6. Typical energy dispersive x-ray microanalysis spectra taken over freeze-dried 4-μm cryosections of myocardium from a patient who presented with a myocardial infarction. Note the increases in Na and Cl and the decrease in K in the infarct sample. Ca also is increased, but its small peak is obscured by the K beta peak.

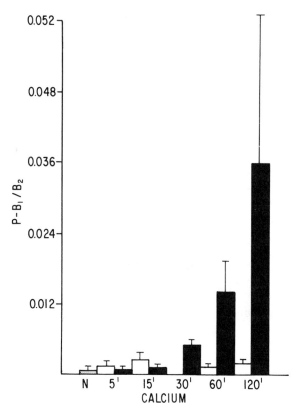

FIG. 7. Bar graph illustrating peak to background ratios (P-B_1/B_2) for calcium from energy dispersive x-ray microanalysis measurements obtained over 4-μm freeze-dried cryosections of rat myocardium following 5, 15, 30, 60, and 120 min occlusion of the coronary artery. N, normal unoperated animals; *white bars,* control right ventricle; *black bars,* ischemic left ventricle. From ref. 35, with permission.

gies such as image analysis paired with photon counting (Figs. 8 and 9), digital imaging fluorescence microscopy, and confocal laser scanning microscopy plus the development of new fluoroprobes, such as Fura-2, Fluo-3, Indo-1, Calcium green for Ca^{2+}; SBFI for Na^+; BCECF, SNARF for pH; Mag-Fura-5 for Mg^{2+}; and Rhodamine 123 for membrane potential, considerable progress has been made toward the understanding of ion homeostasis and the effects on it when deregulation occurs following cell injury. These last two techniques have allowed the investigator to image living cells and to not only measure concentration levels of these various cations but also to observe the exact location of their fluctuations (see Color Plates 1 and 2 on the following pages (47,48,50,54,59,71,89–91,99).

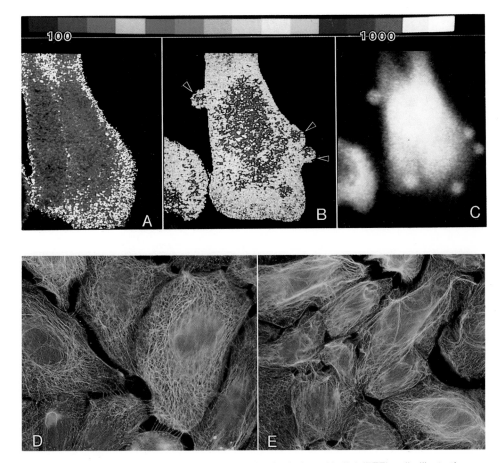

COLOR PLATE 1. Light micrographs of proximal tubule epithelial (PTE) cells illustrating various fluorescent procedures currently available for specialized studies. **A,B,C:** Digital imaging fluorescence microscopy of ratioed images of Fura-2-loaded cells at zero time (A) and at 14.75 min after treatment with 50 μM HgCl$_2$ plus 1.37 μM Ca^{2+} (B). Images are displayed in pseudocolor to indicate [Ca^{2+}]$_i$ levels (expressed in nM) as indicated on the color scale (blue ~60 nM; white > 2 μM). The fluorescein image (C) demonstrates Fura distribution at the same time as in (B). Blebs appeared at approximately 14 min after [Ca^{2+}]$_i$ was greater than 300 nM (B, *arrowheads*) (UV filter set). From ref. 89, with permission. **D,E:** Cells stained by indirect immunofluorescence procedures using monoclonal actin antibody (courtesy of Dr. R. Anthony). (D) Control cells showing a dense population of irregular thin filaments that intertwine and crisscross to form a compact meshlike arrangement. (E) Cells exposed to 3 mM KCN for 15 min at 37°C. The actin pattern is altered. Filaments show a haphazard arrangement and extend for long distances with only minor areas of overlap (FITC filter set). **F,G:** Cells exposed to 50 μM HgCl$_2$ plus 1.37 μM Ca^{2+}.

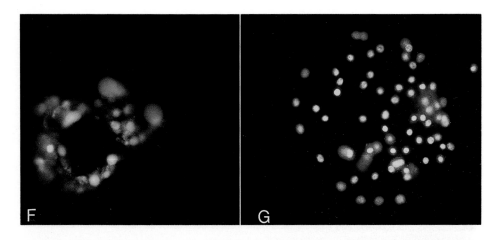

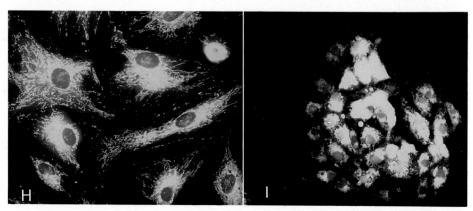

COLOR PLATE 1. *Continued.* (F) Cells preloaded with Fura-2 and in the presence of pro-pidium iodide (1 μM) at 40 min after treatment. The orange staining represents dead cells that have taken up propidium iodide. Most of the blue staining represents Fura-2 present in blebs. (G) Cells at 12 min after treatment in the presence of propidium iodide only. Many cells show loss of viability (UV filter set). **H,I:** Cells preloaded with Rhodamine 123. (H) Con-trol cells showing strandlike mitochondria. (I) Cells treated with 50 μM HgCl$_2$ plus 1.37 μM Ca^{2+} for 15 min. Mitochondria still retain Rhodamine 123, indicating maintenance of mem-brane potential; however, their shape has become globular (FITC filter set). From ref. 47, with permission.

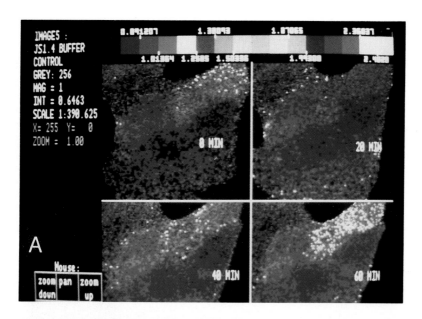

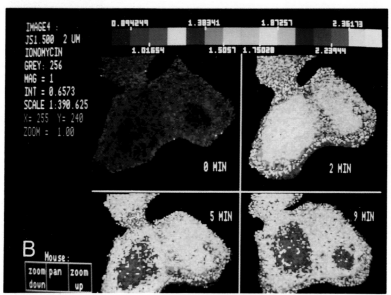

COLOR PLATE 2. Light micrographs of PTE cells treated with 25 mU/ml X/XOD. Cells were loaded with the fluorescent probe Fura-2, and $[Ca^{2+}]_i$ levels were measured using digital imaging fluorescence microscopy. **A:** Control cell. **B:** Treatment with 2 μM ionomycin (positive control) for 2, 5, and 9 min.

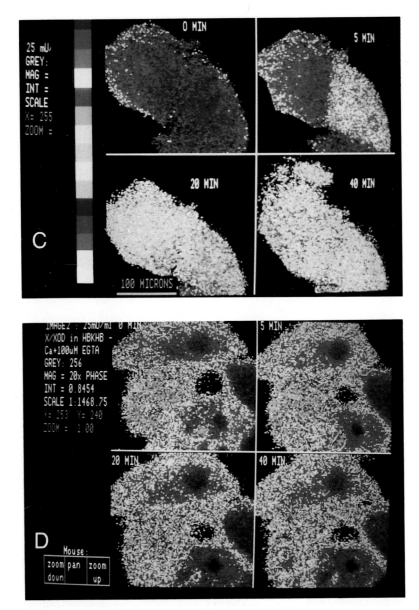

COLOR PLATE 2. *Continued.* **C:** Treatment with X/XOD for 5, 20, and 40 min in a medium with Ca^{2+}. **D:** Treatment with X/XOD for 5, 20, and 40 min in a medium containing no added Ca^{2+} and 100 μM EGTA. Note that X/XOD treatment in a "no" calcium medium did not increase [Ca^{2+}]$_i$ as compared to treatment with calcium in the medium. Images are shown in pseudocolor to indicate [Ca^{2+}]$_i$ levels (expressed in nM) as indicated on the color bars (blue ~60 nM; white > 2 μM). From ref. 59, with permission.

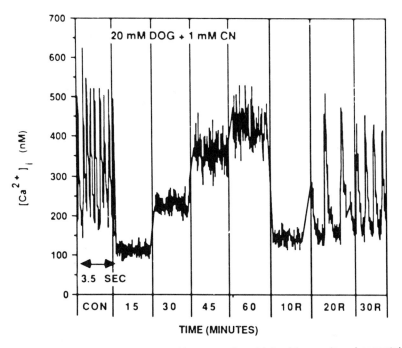

FIG. 8. $[Ca^{2+}]_i$ measurements, calibrated in nanomolar, obtained from cultured neonatal rat ventricular myocytes loaded with Fura-2 and treated with 20 mM 2-deoxy-D-glucose and 1 mM KCN for 60 min before return to control medium for 30 min. Measurements were obtained using 340/380 nm excitation produced by a microspectrofluorometer coupled by a quartz fiber optic to a microscope epi-illuminator. Emission (510 nm) was measured by photon counting. Note cessation of $[Ca^{2+}]_i$ upon exposure to DOG + CN, initial decrease of $[Ca^{2+}]_i$, and then its increase to peak systolic levels. Upon return to control medium, normal $[Ca^{2+}]_i$ transients are restored. From ref. 99, with permission.

Calcium

Normal Regulation

Normally, $[Ca^{2+}]_i$ is regulated at levels of about 100 nm by a combination of transport systems at the plasma membrane, the mitochondria, the ER, and subsets thereof (55,56). Each of these systems is energy dependent and also contains specific ion channels to control membrane permeation.

Plasma Membrane

The plasmalemma constitutes a major pathway for $[Ca^{2+}]_i$ regulation. Ca^{2+} entry may occur through gated or ungated channels and efflux through

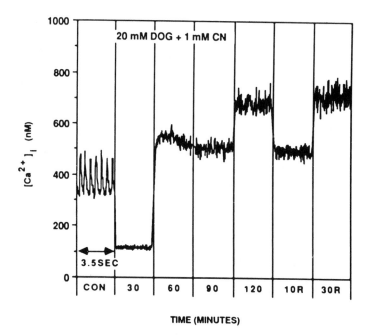

FIG. 9. Same conditions as in Fig. 8 except treatment was for 120 min before return to the control medium. DOG–CN results in an initial decrease followed by a sustained increase in $[Ca^{2+}]_i$. Upon return to the control medium, there is a slight decrease in $[Ca^{2+}]_i$ followed by a then persistent increase. From ref. 99, with permission.

Ca^{2+}–ATPase-dependent pathways. In several cell types, particularly excitable cells including the myocardium, Na^+/Ca^{2+} exchange represents a major participant in $[Ca^{2+}]_i$ regulation (57), and therefore toxins that interfere with the Na^+/K^+–ATPase or that otherwise modify Na^+ will have rapid secondary effects on $[Ca^{2+}]_i$. Modification of the plasmalemmal Ca^{2+} regulation therefore constitutes a major site of toxic effects on cell injury. Examples include complement (37), natural killer (NK) cell-induced cytotoxicity (58), and oxidative stress (59).

Mitochondria

The mitochondrial calcium uptake and release systems have been well characterized and, in many cells, including the myocardium, represent a large capacity system. Uptake is energy dependent and coupled with the generation of the proton gradient. Release occurs after cellular energy depletion or increase of NADPH. Cellular $[Ca^{2+}]_i$ increases after inhibition of ATP synthesis (49,51).

Endoplasmic Reticulum (ER)

The ER uptake and release pathways have also been well characterized, especially in muscle. The uptake system consists of a Ca^{2+} ATPase(s) that is sensitive to the compound thapsigargin and that causes immediate release of Ca^{2+} from the lumen. The related species of Ca^{2+}–ATPases in the sarcoplasmic reticulum (SR) or endoplasmic reticulum (ER) are now referred to as the (SERCA) gene family and have at least five different protein products (60). Thapsigargin inhibits all the SERCA enzymes with equal potency. This compartment also is sensitive to metabolites of the PI pathway, especially IP_3, which stimulates rapid release of Ca^{2+} and appears to represent a major link in transmembrane signaling (61,62). This particular Ca^{2+} interaction appears to represent an important link between the effects of acute injury and toxicity and those of chronic injury, including control of growth and differentiation (63).

Release of Ca^{2+}

The release of Ca^{2+} from the ER through channels occurs by two pathways including the IP_3-gated channel and a calcium-gated, ryanodine-sensitive receptor (64). Release of Ca^{2+} from the ER following IP_3 stimulation is followed by a sustained Ca^{2+} entry from the extracellular space. Thapsigargin has a similar effect, though it bypasses the IP_3 step and inhibits a Ca^{2+}–ATPase (60). Ca^{2+} release can also be regulated by SH groups.

Deregulation Following Injury

Because of its central role in the mediation of a number of intracellular events, acute or chronic deregulation of $[Ca^{2+}]_i$ by a cell injury (Fig. 10) would be expected to result in a variety of events. These events include activation of enzymes such as proteases, nucleases, and lipases; interaction with calmodulin; modulation of a variety of protein kinases; and alterations in cytoskeletal proteins. Some of these events may lead to terminal differentiation (19). Following injury, $[Ca^{2+}]_i$ deregulation can occur by any combination of the following: (a) influx from the extracellular space, (b) redistribution from the mitochondria, and (c) redistribution from the ER or parts thereof.

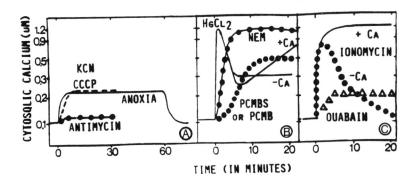

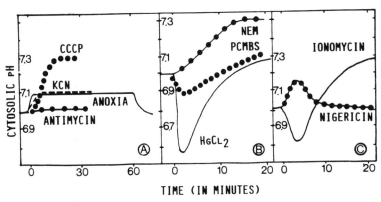

FIG. 10. The effect of different types of injury on cytosolic calcium of rabbit proximal tubule epithelial cells (PTE). Cells were cultured 8–12 days, loaded with Fura-2 (5 μM Fura-2-AM, 60 min, 25°C), and suspended by trypsinization. Spectrofluorometric measurements were made in HBSS + 10 mM Hepes, 1.37 mM CaCl$_2$, and 1 mg/ml glucose at 25°C. **A:** The effect of mitochondrial inhibitors on [Ca^{2+}]$_i$: anoxia, 5 mM KCN, 4 μM CCCP, and 5 μM antimycin. The increase in [Ca^{2+}]$_i$ seen with each is independent of [Ca^{2+}]$_e$ and is presumably due to release from mitochondria. Reoxygenation of anoxic cells leads to recovery of [Ca^{2+}]$_i$ to control levels. **B:** The effect of sulfhydryl inhibition with 250 μM NEM, 1 mM PCMBS, and 50 μM HgCl$_2$. The increased [Ca^{2+}]$_i$ seen with NEM and PCMBS is independent of [Ca^{2+}]$_e$ and is attributed mostly to release from the ER. HgCl$_2$ initially triggers release by CA^{2+} from the ER followed by activation of a plasma membrane Ca^{2+}/H$^+$ pump and then by influx of [Ca^{2+}]$_e$ when [Ca^{2+}]$_e$ is present. **C:** The effect of 5 μM ionomycin with 1.37 mM Ca^{2+} or less than 5 μM Ca^{2+} and 500 μM ouabain. Ionomycin causes redistribution of Ca^{2+} from ER and mitochondria as well as influx of [Ca^{2+}]$_e$. In the absence of [Ca^{2+}]$_e$, [Ca^{2+}]$_i$ recovers in part by means of a plasma membrane Ca^{2+}/H$^+$–ATPase. The elevation of [Ca^{2+}]$_i$ following inhibition of Na$^+$/K$^+$–ATPase with ouabain is due to increased Na$^+$/Ca^{2+} activity in response to elevated [Na$^+$]$_i$. From ref. 100, with permission.

Sodium

Normal Regulation

Na^+ entry into the cell is balanced by active extrusion via the ouabain-sensitive Na^+/K^+–ATPase, which is sensitive to cardiac glycosides (e.g., ouabain).

Deregulation

$[Na^+]_i$ regulation is intimately related to cell volume regulation. Cell volume regulation can be achieved in many cells if the Na^+/K^+–ATPase remains active. Following injury, however, when this is directly or indirectly inhibited, cells commonly swell and $[Na^+]_i$ increases, sometimes markedly. Any condition that lowers extracellular Na^{2+} or raises $[Na^{2+}]_i$ will favor the accumulation of $[Ca^{2+}]_i$.

pH

Normal Regulation

Normal intracellular pH (pH_i) appears to be significantly lower than plasma or tissue culture fluid, being about 7.2 (65). However, the actual pH of the interstitial fluid bathing most cells is considerably more difficult to measure and probably approximates pH_i.

Cellular pH is regulated by three principal mechanisms: cation (Na^+/Ca^{2+}) exchange, anion (HCO_3^-) exchange, and H^+–ATPases (65). The Na^+/H^+ exchanger is activated by low pH_i and by $[Na^+]_i$ increase. The activity of this exchanger can be stimulated by growth factors, probably involving phosphorylation and, under basal conditions, works to regulate pH at about 7.0. Following stimulation, the set point changes to 7.25, and therefore growth factors will result in alkalinization if the medium is below 7.2. However, this increase is minimized in the presence of normal amounts of HCO_3^-, which in most proliferating cells raises pH_i by Na^+-dependent Cl^-/HCO_3^- exchange.

Deregulation

Considerable current interest is attached to the regulation of pH_i in relation to transmembrane signaling, effects of growth factors, and regulation of viability following toxic injury.

The relation to cell division is striking, following fertilization of marine eggs, where division is preceded by an influx of Ca^{2+} and a rise in pH_i that is apparently related to the Na^+/H^+ antiport and can be inhibited by the diuretic amiloride (66). Under appropriate conditions (HCO_3^--free media), amiloride or weak acids will inhibit proliferation and alkalinization of the medium will promote it. Recently, Perona and Serrano (67) observed that chronically raising pH_i, by transfecting NIH–3T3 cells with yeast P-type H^+–ATPase, induced growth in soft agar, growth-factor independent proliferation, and tumorigenicity. Studies by Gillies et al. (68) indicate that at least some human tumor cells possess enough V-type H^+–ATPases to chronically raise pH_i.

Acidification of cells, on the other hand, appears to exert protective effects against a variety of toxic injuries. Penttila and Trump (69), for example, found that reduction of extracellular pH (pH_e) from 7.4 to 6.9 could double the life span of cells subjected to complete anoxia (see also ref. 70). Protection is also conferred against lethal injury by thermal injury as well as chemical toxins including $HgCl_2$. More recently, Lemasters' group reported that reducing the pH_e of the perfusion medium ameliorated the reperfusion injury in ischemic myocardium (71). This observation led these investigators to term this phenomenon the "pH paradox." The explanation for these effects is incomplete. Suggestions have included reduction of cell $[Na^+]_i$ and secondarily $[Ca^{2+}]_i$ through the Na^+/H^+ and Na^+/Ca^{2+} exchange mechanisms, respectively, prevention of Ca^{2+} entry, and competition between H^+ and Ca^{2+} for effects, resulting in inhibition of Ca^{2+}-mediated harmful events (e.g., phospholipase or protease activation).

Potassium

Normal Regulation

$[K^+]_i$ is regulated by a process similar to that for $[Na^+]_i$, using the Na^+/K^+–ATPase; however, different channels exist for this cation. A variety of K^+ channels participate in a variety of cellular functions and participate in signaling, at least in excitable cells. Current research is exploring the mechanism of this genetic diversity (72). A number of genes encoding K^+ channel polypeptides have been cloned on the basis of their similarity to the *Drosophila* shaker locus.

Deregulation

$[K^+]_i$ regulation is lost early and rapidly following a variety of acute injuries due to decreased cellular ATP and/or inhibition of the Na^+/K^+–ATPase at the plasmalemma.

Magnesium

Normal Regulation

Mg^{2+} is an essential element in cell function, participating in cellular energy metabolism in both photosynthesis and oxidative phosphorylation (73). In the case of oxidative phosphorylation, all ATP- or pH_i-requiring reactions are catalyzed by Mg^{2+}, which associates with ATP and other related compounds. Mg^{2+} does not form highly stable chelates with organic complexes and can be dissociated from ATP.

Mg^{2+} is essential for oxidative phosphorylation and changes in $[Mg^{2+}]_i$ are probably involved in its regulation. $[Mg^{2+}]_i$ participates in many other aspects of normal cell metabolism, including ribosomal structure and function and in $[Ca^{2+}]_i$ regulation, where $[Mg^{2+}]_i$ is a cofactor and participates in the mediation or regulation. In the nucleus, Mg^{2+} exhibits strong binding to DNA and it appears that sections of chromosomes are maintained structurally by Mg^{2+} and Ca^{2+}. The mitochondrial matrix contains about 41% of the Mg^{2+}, the inner membrane base 50%, the outer membrane 4%, and the inner membrane 5%.

Deregulation

Changes in $[Mg^{2+}]_i$ in relation to altered cell structure and function have not, thus far, been thoroughly characterized—principally because, until recently, methods for its measurement have not been available. More recently, however, with the development of the fluorescent probe, Mag Fura-2, insights are beginning to accrue concerning its role in altered cell metabolism.

It is known that Mg^{2+} is essential for mitochondrial contraction following swelling and it is often added *in vitro* as Mg^{2+}–ATP complex. Similarly, the effects of Mg^{2+}–ATP on resuscitation of patients and animals following hemorrhagic shock have been established (74). Rats maintained on magnesium-deficient diets developed mitochondrial swelling within 10 days. Changes in total cellular Mg^{2+} have not been observed in our experience until very late following cell injury, probably during the necrotic phase in contrast to changes in total sodium, potassium, and chloride (35). Thus significant loss of total $[Mg^{2+}]_i$ probably represents a manifestation of rather later effects of lethal injury. On the other hand, we and others have noted rapid increases of $[Mg^{2+}]_i$ within seconds or minutes following models of anoxic or ischemic injury or treatment of cells with uncouplers of mitochondrial oxidative phosphorylation. Increases of $[Mg^{2+}]_i$ therefore probably represent a loss from the mitochondrial compartment coupled with dissociation of Mg^{2+}–ATP complexes and, as such, increases of $[Mg^{2+}]_i$ probably can be used to reflect mitochondrial energy production. In addition to the effects of $[Mg^{2+}]_i$ on mitochondrial function and structure, protein synthesis, and DNA transcription, alterations of $[Mg^{2+}]_i$ may also play a role in cytoskeletal organization.

ENERGY METABOLISM

There are many types of important cell injuries that exert a primary effect on energy metabolism, predominantly on mitochondrial ATP synthesis, though some affect primarily anaerobic glycolysis, while other injuries, such as ischemia, affect both eventually (75). Effects on mitochondrial ATP synthesis can be classified into: (a) inhibitors of electron transport, including anoxia or ischemia, and chemical inhibitors of electron transport, including KCN, CO, antimycin, and rotenone; (b) primary uncouplers of mitochondrial oxidative phosphorylation, including halogenated phenols such as 2,4-DNP and phenachlorophenol and hydralzines such as FCCP. These compounds disperse the mitochondrial potential and proton gradient, some acting as proton ionophores. Mitochondrial uncoupling can also occur secondary to other injuries resulting, for example, from increased $[Ca^{2+}]_i$ or primary damage to the mitochondrial inner membrane (e.g., phospholipase attack); and (c) inhibitors of oxidative phosphorylation (e.g., oligomycin), which inhibit the H^+–ATPase of the inner membrane. Treatment of cells or tissues *in vivo* or *in vitro* with any of these conditions results in rapid arrest of ATP synthesis within the cell and, in the case of agents that change plasma membrane permeability, acute loss of ATP from the cells. The rate of ATP decline can be extremely rapid, requiring, for example, only a few seconds or minutes in the case of kidney cortex following clamping of the renal artery (76). This results in transient increases in the ADP/ATP ratio within cells, followed by continued conversion of ATP to ADP and of AMP to xanthine, ultimately reducing total adenine nucleotides. The rate of ATP decline is related to the rate of utilization of ATP by the cell, which is dependent on ATPases. Therefore reduction of temperature or inhibition of ATPases can retard the decline of ATP and prolong cell survival. Chaudry (74) has reported that addition of Mg^{2+}–ATP can reverse some aspects of cell injury.

ALTERED GENE EXPRESSION

Immediate Early Genes

c-fos

The oncogene *c-fos* is an example of an immediate gene that is activated by a number of acute cell injuries or stimuli including oxidant stress (Figs. 11–13), calcium ionophores (30,31,77–80), growth factors, and reflow after ischemic injury (81,82). All the functions of *c-fos* are not known. It appears

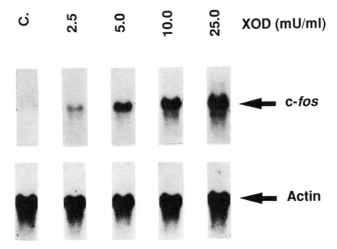

FIG. 11. Northern analysis showing the dose response of c-*fos* expression by X/XOD in primary cultures of rat PTE. Cultures were treated with 500 μM xanthine (X) and 2.5 – 25 mU/ml XOD for 30 min. The same membrane was rehybridized with an actin probe to ensure that the same amount of mRNA was loaded to each lane. From ref. 31, with permission.

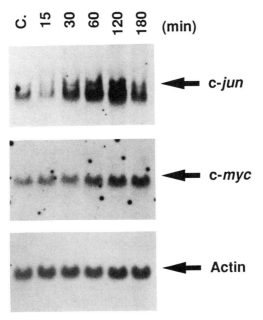

FIG. 12. Kinetics of the expression of c-*myc* and c-*jun* in rat PTE primary cultures following X/XOD (500 μM/25 mU/ml) treatment for 15, 30, 60, 120, and 180 min. From ref. 31, with permission.

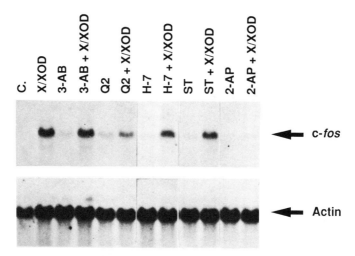

FIG. 13. Modification of c-*fos* expression by X/XOD in rat primary PTE cultures. X/XOD is the sample treated with 500μM X and 25 mU/ml XOD for 30 min. The following samples were incubated in 3-aminobenzimide (3-AB) (10 mM), Quin 2/AM (Q2) (30 μM), H-7 (25nM), staurosporine (ST) (50 nM), and 2-aminopurine (2-AP) (10 mM) alone or with X/XOD. C. represents the control from an untreated culture. From ref. 31, with permission.

to relate to the early events in cell division, although it is reported to also increase in terminally differentiated cells, such as neurons, following appropriate stimulation.

The mechanism of activation is currently under study in many laboratories. Since the calcium ionophore A23187 and thapsigargin (63) readily activate c-*fos*, a role for $[Ca^{2+}]_i$ seems likely. Furthermore, the cell injuries thus far studied (e.g., oxidant stress) also induce early increases in $[Ca^{2+}]_i$ (59), which precede the stimulation of c-*fos* (30,31). Such increases in $[Ca^{2+}]_i$ may also be associated with calcium endonuclease-induced breaks in DNA, which in turn induce poly-ADP ribosylation. Cerutti et al. (28) have proposed a role for poly-ADP ribosylation of proteins in c-*fos* induction. Pretreatment of cells with Quin 2 to buffer $[Ca^{2+}]_i$ increase has been found to be preventive against DNA strand breaks (83).

Stress Genes

Much of the work on stress genes has involved the "heat shock proteins" (HSP), originally described in *Drosophila*. These proteins, which have now been extensively subdivided into families (see reviews in refs. 84 and 85), are evoked in virtually all prokaryotic and eukaryotic forms and various classes are induced by a variety of stressors including heat, ATP depletion, heavy metal intoxication, ischemia (86), and oxidant stress (87).

Typically, the shock response is characterized by specific and transient induction of heat shock gene expression, blockade of normal translation with preferential translation of heat shock proteins, and induction of thermotolerance or, in some cases, protection against other forms of cell injury. HSP70 and HSP90 have been investigated the most extensively. HSP90 represents the non-DNA-binding component of the steroid receptor and appears to be involved in complexes with several oncogenic tyrosine-specific kinases including v-*src*. HSP70 is associated with a variety of cell phenomena involving binding to unfolded proteins in an ATP-dependent manner. Such unfolding may occur during normal turnover or during exposure to denaturing conditions as often occurs after lethal cell injury.

HYPOTHESIS

Through the years, based on our experiments and those in the literature, we have continued to develop a working hypothesis of the response of cells to acute, lethal, and sublethal injury as ideas are proposed and data are confirmed (Fig. 14). This hypothesis has and continues to focus on the role of ion deregulation, especially that of $[Ca^{2+}]_i$ (40–48,88).

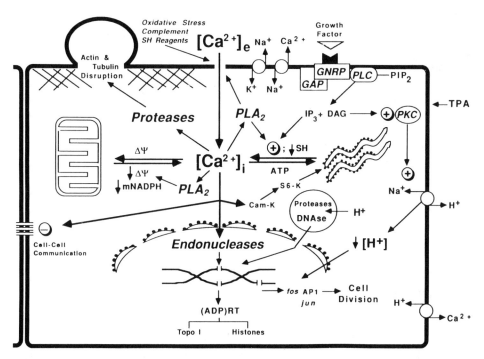

FIG. 14. A diagrammatic representation of a cell illustrating our current working hypothesis concerning the role of $[Ca^{2+}]_i$ in cell injury. From ref. 48, with permission.

Regulation of [Ca^{2+}]$_i$

Regulation of [Ca^{2+}]$_i$ at normal levels approximates 100 nM. In Fig. 14, note the ATP-dependent regulation by the plasma membrane, the mitochondria, and the ER. Several of the Ca^{2+}-activated systems are shown, including Ca^{2+}-activated proteases, phospholipases, and nucleases; integrity of gap junctions; and effects on calmodulin and calmodulin-dependent processes, including modulation of the cytoskeleton.

Relationship to Signaling

Relationship to signaling is shown on the right-hand side of the diagram. Note that signaling, involving ion deregulation, can be initiated by either growth factors or other extracellular stimuli binding to receptors and activating pathways involving cyclic GMP or cyclic AMP at the cell membrane. In the case of G protein signaling, calcium-dependent phospholipase C appears to be involved with the liberation of membrane phosphoinositide metabolites, such as IP$_3$ and diacylglycerol (DAG) (92). IP$_3$ results in rapid loss of Ca^{2+} from the ER, increasing [Ca^{2+}]$_i$, which may in turn induce further signal transmission. Furthermore, increases of [Ca^{2+}]$_i$ in many cells open calcium channels at the cell membrane, causing an influx of Ca^{2+}$_e$. DAG is capable of activating protein kinase C (PKC), which is also directly activated by phorbol esters, such as TPA (93). Actually, it is a growing family of PKC whose total function is not currently understood. Several of these are calcium dependent and increases of [Ca^{2+}]$_i$ may act synergistically with direct stimulation (e.g., by TPA). Other protein kinases are activated by cyclic AMP kinases, some of which stimulate phosphorylation of calcium-reactive sites on the SR, such as phospholamban, and on the troponin–tropomyosin complex.

Regulation of the membrane G proteins in the active versus the inactive state is accomplished through regulator proteins, including GAP, which interacts with the protein to downregulate it to the inactive state, thus stopping a signal. It has been observed that mutations in G proteins, such as those induced by mutations of the oncogene *ras,* interfere with this regulation and that the modified protein can remain in the active state, thus perpetuating the signaling process (94).

Other activities of PKC include activation of the Na$^+$/H$^+$ antiport, which is involved in regulation of [pH]$_i$ and, under appropriate conditions, can result in alkalinization of the cytoplasm.

The action of the signaling pathway on the ER through IP$_3$ can be simulated by compounds, such as thapsigargin, which induce release of Ca^{2+} from the ER by inhibition of uptake. This can result in activation of many of the processes, including gene expression, that are triggered by growth factor or hormone stimulation. This area thus provides an important link between xenobiotic treatment of cells or other types of cell injury and normal stimulation. The normal control mechanisms can return calcium homeostasis to normal through the normal calcium translocation systems described above; however, if these are modified, for example, with *ras* mutations or with continued increase of $[Ca^{2+}]_i$ by changes of membrane permeability, continued and inappropriate signaling will occur.

Cytoskeleton

Alterations of the cytoskeleton appear to play an active and possibly fundamental role in many sublethal and lethal reactions to injury. These can involve actin and associated proteins, tubulin, and intermediate filaments, including keratin. Regulation of $[Ca^{2+}]_i$ can be involved in the modification of all components of the cytoskeleton. Some of these interactions involve phosphorylation, for example, phosphorylation of tubulin may be a controlling factor in mitosis, and formation of the spindle and interactions with troponin C permits actin and myosin interactions.

Some of the early changes following sublethal injury include bleb formation (Fig. 15), which clearly results from increased $[Ca^{2+}]_i$ (25,50,91,95) and

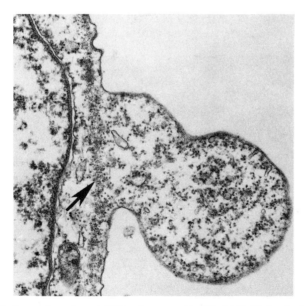

FIG. 15. TEM of a portion of a rat PTE cell exposed to 50 μM HgCl$_2$ for 4 min at 37°C with low Ca^{2+}$_e$. Note the bands of fine filaments, probably representing actin, at the base of the blebs (*arrow*). × 25,000. From ref. 25, with permission.

modification of actin and tubulin (Figs. 16–18) (26). The detachment of actin from the membrane in the region of the bleb and possibly contraction, forming a band of actin at the base of the bleb, seem to be common to many types of bleb formation. In ruffles, phospholipase A_2 has been localized in blebs (96). At least some of this appears to involve calcium-activated proteases, as inhibitors such as leupeptin and antipain can markedly modify bleb for-

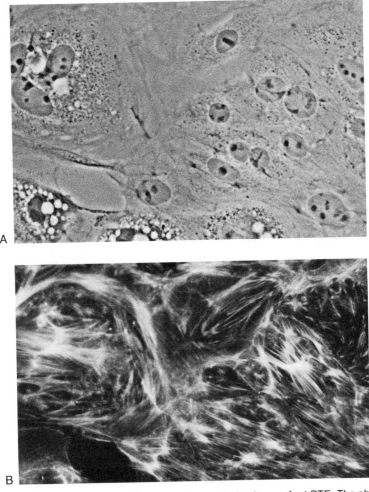

A

B

FIG. 16. Photomicrographs of untreated, 4-day, control cultures of rat PTE. The phase contrast photomicrograph (**A**) shows the spread-out, flat appearance typical of these cultured cells. Fluorescein phalloidin staining (**B**, the same field as A) shows abundant stress fibers as long, fluorescent cables spanning the long axis of control cells. In (B), heavy staining (*arrowheads*) is identified with the nuclear area in (A). ×260. From ref. 26, with permission.

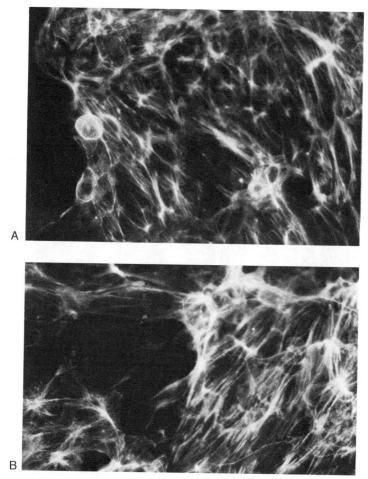

FIG. 17. Photomicrographs of PTE stained with fluorescein phalloidin after exposure to 10 μM HgCl₂ for 2 min (**A**) and 10 min (**B**). ×260. From ref. 26, with permission.

mation. Kolber et al. (97) have observed that modification and actin with cytochalasin results in DNA strand breaks.

In terminal differentiation in the skin, epithelium, and bronchial epithelium, increased $[Ca^{2+}]_i$ seems to modify expression of keratin intermediate filaments and formation of cross-linked bundles of keratin (17,18).

Gene Activation

As shown in Fig. 14, modification of cell ions can modify gene expression. Increases of $[Ca^{2+}]_i$ result in activation of several immediate early and stress

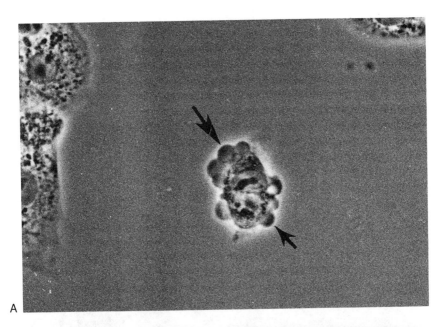

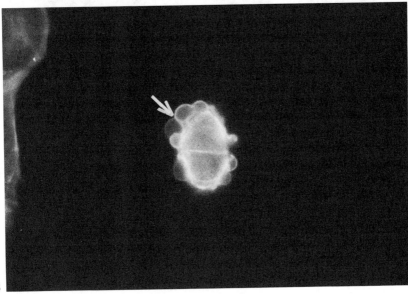

FIG. 18. Phase contrast (**A**) and fluorescent (**B**) photomicrographs of PTE after 6-min exposure to 100 μM HgCl$_2$. Actin filaments are absent in the cytoplasm and interior of blebs (*arrows*), but there is a clear band of fluorescent staining around each cell and four of the blebs (B). ×260. From ref. 26, with permission.

genes, including c-*fos,* c-*jun,* c-*myc* (97,98), and hsp70 (85). Some of this activation appears to result from phosphorylation of regulatory proteins. In some cases, poly-ADP ribosylation seems to represent a control mechanism. Poly-ADP ribosylation is stimulated by DNA strand breaks, which in turn can result from calcium activation of endonucleases (e.g., following oxidant injury). The role of altered $[pH]_i$ in this process is currently being investigated; however, regulation in the physiologic range is essential for DNA replication and transcription to occur.

Changes in Cell Junctions

Increases of $[Ca^{2+}]_i$ result in decreased cell–cell communications or changes in GAP junction proteins. It has been proposed that decreased cell–cell communication is an early change in tumor promotion and can, in fact, be used as a screening test for putative tumor promotors. Decreased concentrations of $[Ca^{2+}]_e$ also affect cell–cell communication and, if prolonged, can result in detachment of desmosomes, intermediate junctions, and tight junctions.

Changes in Cell Membranes

During the progression from sublethal to lethal injury, marked alterations in membrane integrity occur involving all membranes within the cell. In mitochondria, for example, change from the condensed to the swollen conformation is a result of mitochondrial swelling and modification of inner membrane phospholipids. The cell undergoes swelling due largely to the Donnan effect in the absence of ion regulation, especially $[Na^+]_i$. The cytoplasmic blebs become more numerous and, ultimately, marked increases of plasmalemmal permeability occur, permitting escape of cytosolic enzymes and ultimately leading to cell death. These membrane effects appear to be the direct result of activation of calcium-dependent phospholipases and proteases. Although initially these are apparently repairable (e.g., mitochondrial swelling even of the high amplitude variety can reverse), they ultimately become irreversible, an event that appears to correlate with the point of cell death.

CONCLUSIONS

For many years, the study of toxic cell injury has been one in which the understanding of the relationship between basic cellular structure and function to the disease process has been of paramount importance. As these studies have evolved, relating molecular mechanisms to aid in our understanding of these phenomena has also become important. Cell injury as well as cell death play important roles, not only in disease but also in the normal process of cell development and embryonic maturation. From the above discussion, it can be seen that we now know that a variety of cellular events in both acute and chronic cell injury, including neoplasia, are closely related if not initiated by intracellular ion deregulation. This conclusion has been made possible through the recent development of new methodologies, such as digital imaging fluorescence microscopy. It is through the use of this technique that investigators can now image living cells and, using appropriate fluorescent probes such as Fura-2 for $[Ca^{2+}]_i$, locate and measure concentration levels. Although $[Ca^{2+}]_i$ appears to be of particular importance, other ions are important as well, especially $[Na^+]_i$ and $[H^+]_i$. Examples include the fact that Ca^{2+}-activated endonucleases may well play a role in DNA damage following an acute nonmutagenic toxic injury, such as that induced by oxidative stress, and that $[Ca^{2+}]_i$ deregulation and alkalinization of the cytoplasm may ultimately lead to prolonged states of disordered cell division and cell differentiation. Although much more needs to be clarified before any conclusions can be made, it is quite clear that toxic cell injury is a fundamental biologic process and that further understanding of the cellular and molecular mechanisms involved could well lead to modification of the cell to toxic insults. It is our hypothesis, based on many years of experimentation, that a wide variety of phenomena that occur following cell injury are due to ion deregulation.

ACKNOWLEDGMENTS

This work was supported by NIH Grant DK15440 and Navy N00014-88-K-0427. This is contribution No. UM#3021 from the Cellular Pathobiology Laboratory.

REFERENCES

1. Trump BF, Ginn FL. The pathogenesis of subcellular reaction to lethal injury. In: Bajusz E, Jasmin G, eds. *Methods and achievements in experimental pathology,* vol IV. Basel: Karger; 1969:1–29.
2. Trump BF, Arstila AU. Cell injury and cell death. In: LaVia MF, Hill RB Jr, eds. *Principles of pathobiology.* New York: Oxford University Press; 1971:9–95.
3. Trump BF, Mergner WJ. Cell injury. In: Zweifach BW, Grant L, McClusky RT, eds. *The inflammatory process,* vol 1. New York: Academic Press, 1974:115–257.
4. Bowen ID, Lockshin RA. *Cell death in biology and pathology.* London: Chapman and Hall; 1981.
5. Trump BF, Berezesky IK, Cowley RA. The cellular and subcellular characteristics of acute and chronic injury with emphasis on the role of calcium. In: Cowley RA, Trump BF, eds. *Pathophysiology of shock, anoxia, and ischemia.* Baltimore: Williams & Wilkins; 1982:6–46.
6. Mergner WJ, Jones RT, Trump BF. *Cell death. Mechanisms of acute and lethal injury,* vol 1. New York: Field & Wood Medical Publishers; 1990.
7. Combs AB, Acosta D. Toxic mechanisms of the heart: a review. *Toxicol Pathol* 1990;18:583–596.

8. Trump BF, Mergner WJ, Kahng MW, Saladino AJ. Studies on the subcellular pathophysiology of ischemia. *Circulation [Suppl. I]* 1976;53:17–26.

9. Trump BF, Goldblatt PJ, Stowell RE. Studies of mouse liver necrosis *in vitro*. Ultrastructural and cytochemical alterations in hepatic parenchymal cell nuclei. *Lab Invest* 1965;14:1969–1999.

10. Marzella L, Glaumann H. Autophagy, Microautophagy and crinophagy as mechanisms for protein degradation. In: Glaumann H, Ballard J, eds. *Lysosomes: their role in protein breakdown*. London: Academic Press; 1987:319–367.

11. Lee HK, Marzella L. Transport of macromolecules to lysosomes. In: Thoene JG, ed. *Pathophysiology of lysosomal transport*. Boca Raton, FL: CRC Press; 1992 (in press).

12. Bowen ID, Bowen SM. *Programmed cell death in tumours and tissues*. London: Chapman and Hall; 1990.

13. Wyllie AH. Cell death: a new classification separating apoptosis from necrosis. In: Bowen ID, Lockshin RA, eds. *Cell death in biology and pathology*. London: Chapman and Hall; 1981:9–34.

14. McDowell EM, Trump BF. Histogenesis of preneoplastic and neoplastic lesions in tracheobronchial epithelium. *Surv Synth Pathol Res* 1983;2:235–279.

15. Pfeifer AM, Lechner JF, Masui T, Reddel RR, Mark GE, Harris CC. Control of growth and squamous differentiation in normal human bronchial epithelial cells by chemical and biological modifiers and transferred genes. *Environ Health Perspect* 1989;80:209–220.

16. Lechner JF, Haugen A, McClendon IA, Shamsuddin AKM. Induction of squamous differentiation of normal bronchial epithelial cells by small amounts of serum. *Differentiation* 1984;25:229–237.

17. Miyashita M, Smith MW, Willey JC, Lechner JF, Trump BF, Harris CC. Effects of serum, transforming growth factor type β, or 12-*O*-tetradecanol-phorbol-13-acetate on ionized cytosolic calcium concentration in normal and transformed human bronchial epithelial cells. *Cancer Res* 1989;49:63–67.

18. Yuspa S, Hennings H, Tucker R, Jaken S, Kilkenny A, Roop D. (1988). Signal transduction for proliferation and differentiation in keratinocytes. *Ann NY Acad Sci* 1988;548:191–196.

19. Hennings H, Kruszewski FH, Yuspa SH, Tucker RW. Intracellular calcium alterations in response to increased external calcium in normal and neoplastic keratinocytes. *Carcinogenesis* 1989;10:777–780.

20. Trump BF, Benditt EP. Electron microscopic studies of human renal disease. Observations of normal visceral glomerular epithelium and its modification in disease. *Am J Pathol* 1962;11:753–781.

21. Goldblatt PJ, Trump BF, Stowell RE. Studies on necrosis of mouse liver *in vitro*. Alterations in some histochemistry demonstrable hepatocellular enzymes. *Am J Pathol* 1965;47:183–208.

22. Trump BF, Bulger RE. Studies of cellular injury in isolated flounder tubules. III. Light microscopic and functional changes due to cyanide. *Lab Invest* 1968;18:721–730.

23. Glaumann B, Trump BF. Studies on the pathogenesis of ischemic cell injury. III. Morphological changes of the proximal pars recta tubules (P3) of the rat kidney made ischemic *in vivo*. *Virchows Arch [B]* 1975;19:303–323.

24. Trump BF, Berezesky IK. The role of sodium and calcium regulation in toxic cell injury. In: Mitchell JR, Horning MG, eds. *Drug metabolism and drug toxicity*. New York: Raven Press; 1984:261–300.

25. Phelps PC, Smith MW, Trump BF. Cytosolic ionized calcium and bleb formation after acute cell injury of cultured rabbit renal tubule cells. *Lab Invest* 1989;60:630–642.

26. Elliget KA, Phelps PC, Trump BF. HgCl$_2$-induced alteration of actin filaments in cultured primary rat proximal tubule epithelial cells labelled with fluorescein phalloidin. *Cell Biol Toxicol* 1991;7:263–280.

27. Mergner WJ, Chang SH, Marzella L, Kahng MW, Trump BF. Studies on the pathogenesis of ischemic cell injury. VII. ATPase of rat kidney mitochondria. *Lab Invest* 1979;40:686–694.

28. Cerutti P, Larsson R, Krupitza G, Muehlematter D, Crawford D, Amstad P. Pathophysiological mechanisms of oxidants. In: Cerutti PA, Fridovich I, McCord JM, eds.

Oxy-radicals in molecular biology and pathology. New York: Alan R Liss; 1988:493–507.

29. Cerutti PA, Trump BF. Inflammation and oxidative stress in carcinogenesis. *Cancer Cells* 1991;3:1–7.

30. Maki A, Swann J, Berezesky I, Trump B. Oxidative stress induces c-*fos* expression in primary cultures of rat proximal tubular epithelium (PTE)—abstract. *Circ Shock* 1990;31:38.

31. Maki A, Berezesky IK, Fargnoli J, Holbrook NJ, Trump BF. The role of [Ca^{2+}]$_i$ in induction of c-*fos*, c-*jun*, and c-*myc* mRNA in rat PTE following oxidative stress. *FASEB J* 1992; 919–924.

32. Mergner WJ, Smith MA, Trump BF. Studies on the pathogenesis of ischemic cell injury. IV. Alteration of ionic permeability of mitochondria from ischemic rat kidney. *Exp Mol Pathol* 1977;26:1–12.

33. Collan Y, McDowell EM, Trump BF. Studies on the pathogenesis of ischemic cell injury. VI. Mitochondrial flocculent densities in autolysis. *Virchows Arch [B]* 1981; 35:189–199.

34. Gritzka TL, Trump BF. Renal tubular lesions caused by mercuric chloride. Electron microscopic observations: degeneration of the pars recta. *Am J Pathol* 1968;52:1225–1277.

35. Osornio-Vargas AR, Berezesky IK, Trump BF. Progression of ion movements during acute myocardial infarction in the rat. An x-ray microanalysis study. *Scan Electron Microsc* 1981;2:463–472.

36. Shin ML, Carney DF. Cytotoxic action and other metabolic consequences of terminal complement proteins. In: Shin ML, ed. *Progress allergy,* vol 40. Karger: Basel; 1988:40–51.

37. Papadimitriou JC, Ramm LE, Drachenberg CB, Trump BF, Shin ML. Quantitative analysis of adenine nucleotides during the prelytic phase of cell death mediated by C5b-9. *J Immunol* 1991;147:212–217.

38. Fridovich I. The biology of oxygen radicals. *Science* 1978;201:875–880.

39. Sahaphong S, Trump BF. Studies of cellular injury in isolated kidney tubules of the flounder. V. Effects of inhibiting sulfhydryl groups of plasma membrane with the organic mercurials PCMB (parachloromercuribenzoate) and PCMBS (parachloromercuribenzenesulfonate). *Am J Pathol* 1971;63:277–297.

40. Trump BF, Berezesky IK, Phelps PC. Sodium and calcium regulation and the role of the cytoskeleton in the pathogenesis of disease: a review and hypothesis. *Scan Electron Microsc* 1981;2:434–454.

41. Trump BF, Berezesky IK. The role of calcium in cell injury and repair. A hypothesis. *Surv Synth Pathol Res* 1985;4:248–256.

42. Trump BF, Berezesky IK, Osornio-Vargas A. Cell death and the disease process. The role of cell calcium. In: Bowen ID, Lockshin RA, eds. *Cell death in biology and pathology.* London: Chapman and Hall; 1981:209–242.

43. Trump BF, Berezesky IK. Cellular ion regulation and disease: a hypothesis. In: Shamoo AE, ed. *Current topics in membranes and transport,* vol 25: *Regulation of calcium transport across muscle membranes.* New York: Academic Press; 1985:279–319.

44. Trump BF, Berezesky IK. Mechanisms of cell injury in the kidney: the role of calcium. In: Fowler BA, ed. *Mechanisms of cell injury: implications for human health.* Chichester: Wiley; 1987:135–151.

45. Trump BF, Berezesky IK. Cell injury and cell death. The role of ion deregulation. *Comments Toxicol* 1989;3:47–67.

46. Trump BF, Berezesky IK. Ion deregulation in injured proximal tubule epithelial cells. In: Bach PH, Lock EA, eds. *Nephrotoxicity. In vitro to in vivo animals to man.* New York: Plenum Press; 1989:731–741.

47. Trump BF, Berezesky IK, Smith MW, Phelps PC, Elliget KA. The relationship between cellular ion deregulation and acute and chronic toxicity. *Toxicol Appl Pharmacol* 1989;97:6–22.

48. Trump BF, Berezesky IK. The importance of calcium regulation in toxic cell injury. Studies utilizing the technology of digital imaging fluorescence microscopy. *Clin Lab Med* 1990;10:531–547.

49. Nicotera P, Hartzell P, Baldi C, Svensson S, Bellomo G, Orrenius S. Cystamine induces toxicity in hepatocytes though the elevation of cytosolic Ca^{2+} and the stimulation of a nonlysosomal proteolytic system. *J Biol Chem* 1986;261:14628–14635.

50. Lemasters J, DiGuiseppi J, Nieminen A, Herman B. Blebbing, free Ca^{2+} and mitochondrial membrane potential preceding cell death in hepatocytes. *Nature* 1987; 325:78–81.

51. Orrenius S, McConkey DJ, Bellomo G, Nicortera P. Role of Ca^{2+} in toxic cell killing. *Trends Pharmacol Sci* 1989;10:281–285.

52. Van Rooijen N. High and low cytosolic Ca^{2+} induced macrophage death? Hypothesis. *Cell Calcium* 1991;12:381–384.

53. Trump BF, Berezesky IK. Ion regulation, cell injury and carcinogenesis. *Carcinogenesis* 1987;8:1027–1031.

54. Trump BF, Berezesky IK, Smith MW, Phelps PC, Elliget KA. The role of ion deregulation in cell injury and carcinogenesis. *Methodological surveys in biochemistry and analysis: biochemical approaches to cellular calcium.* 1989:19:439–452.

55. Carafoli E. Intracellular calcium homeostasis. *Annu Rev Biochem* 1987;56:395–433.

56. Rasmussen H. The cycling of calcium as an intracellular messenger. *Sci Am* 1989;108:66–73.

57. Pritchard K, Ashley CC. Na^+/Ca^{2+} exchange in isolated smooth muscle cells demonstrated by the fluorescent calcium indicator fura-2. *FEBS Lett* 1986;195:23–27.

58. McConkey DJ, Chow SC, Orrenius S, Jondal M. NK cell-induced cytotoxicity is dependent on a Ca^{2+} increase in the target. *FASEB J* 1990;4:2661–2664.

59. Swann JD, Smith MW, Phelps PC, Maki A, Berezesky IK, Trump BF. Oxidative injury induces influx-dependent changes in intracellular calcium homeostasis. *Toxicol Pathol* 1991;19:128–137.

60. Lytton J, Westlin M, Hanley MR. Thapsigargin inhibits the sarcoplasmic or endoplasmic reticulum Ca–ATPase family of calcium pumps. *J Biol Chem* 1991;266:17967–17071.

61. Berridge MJ, Galione A. Cytosolic calcium oscillators. *FASEB J* 1988;2:3074–3082.

62. Gill D, Ghosh T, Mullaney J. Calcium signaling mechanisms in endoplasmic reticulum activated by inositol 1,4,5-triphosphate and GTP. *Cell Calcium* 1989;10:363–374.

63. Schontal A, Sugarman J, Brown JH, Hanley MR, Feramisco JR. Regulation of c-*fos* and c-*jun* protooncogene expression by the Ca^{2+}–ATPase inhibitor thapsigargin. *Proc Natl Acad Sci USA* 1991;88:7096–7100.

64. Iino M, Kobayashi T, Endo M. Use of ryanodine for functional removal of the calcium store in smooth muscle cells of the guinea-pig. *Biochem Biophys Res Commun* 1988;152:417–422.

65. Chen LK, Boron WF. Intracellular pH regulation in epithelial cells. *Kidney Int [Supp]* 1991;40:S11–S17.

66. Epel D. The cascade of events initiated by rises in cytosolic Ca^{2+} and pH following fertilization in sea urchin eggs. In: Boynton AL, McKeehan WL, Whitfield JF, eds. *Ions, cell proliferation and cancer.* New York: Academic Press; 1982:327–340.

67. Perona R, Serrano R. Increased pH and tumorigenicity of fibroblasts expressing a yeast proton pump. *Nature* 1988;334:438–440.

68. Gillies RJ, Martinez-Zaguilan R, Martinez GM, Serrano R, Perona R. Tumorigenic 3T3 cells maintain an alkaline intracellular pH under physiological conditions. *Proc Natl Acad Sci USA* 1990;87:7414–7418.

69. Penttila A, Trump BF. Extracellular acidosis protects Ehrlich ascites tumor cells and rat renal cortex against anoxic injury. *Science* 1974;185:277–278.

70. Shanley PF, Johnson GC. Calcium and acidosis in renal hypoxia. *Lab Invest* 1991;65:298–305.

71. Bond JM, Herman B, Lemasters JJ. Protection by acidotic pH against anoxia/reoxygenation injury to rat neonatal cardiac myocytes. *Biochem Biophys Res Commun* 1991;179:798–803.

72. Chung S, Reinhart PH, Martin BL, Brautigan D, Levitan IB. Protein kinase activity closely associated with a reconstituted calcium-activated potassium channel. *Science* 1991;253:560–562.

73. Aikawa JK. *Magnesium: its biological significance.* Boca Raton, FL: CRC Press; 1981.
74. Chaudry IH. Use of ATP following shock and ischemia. *Ann NY Acad Sci* 1990;603:130–141.
75. Weinberg JM. The cell biology of ischemic renal injury. *Kidney Int* 1991;39:476–500.
76. Mergner WJ, Marzella LL, Mergner G, Kahng MW, Smith MW, Trump BF. Studies on the pathogenesis of ischemic cell injury. VII. Proton gradient and respiration of renal tissue cubes, renal mitochondria and submitochondrial particles following ischemic injury. *Beitr Pathol* 1977;161:260–271.
77. Crawford D, Zbinden I, Amstrad P, Cerutti P. Oxidant stress induces the proto-oncogenes c-*fos* and c-*myc* in mouse epidermal cells. *Oncogene* 1988;3:27–32.
78. Cowley BD Jr, Chadwick LJ, Grantham JJ, Calvet JP. Sequential protooncogene expression in regenerating kidney following acute renal injury. *J Biol Chem* 1989;264:8389–8393.
79. Curran T, Franza BR. *Fos* and *jun:* the AP-1 connection. *Cell* 1988;55:395–397.
80. Herbst H, Milani S, Schuppan D, Stein H. Temporal and spatial patterns of proto-oncogene expression at early stages of toxic liver injury in the rat. *Lab Invest* 1991;65:324–333.
81. Rosenberg ME, Paller MS. Differential gene expression in the recovery from ischemic renal injury. *Kidney Int* 1991;39:1156–1161.
82. Schiaffonati L, Rappocciolo E, Tacchini L, Cairo G, Bernelli-Zazzera A. Reprogramming of gene expression in postischemic rat liver: induction of proto-oncogenes and hsp 70 gene family. *J Cell Physiol* 1990;143:79–87.
83. Cantoni O, Sestili P, Cattabeni F, et al. Calcium chelator quin 2 prevents hydrogen-peroxide-induced DNA breakage and cytotoxicity. *Eur J Biochem* 1989;182:209–212.
84. Lindquist S. The heat shock protein. *Annu Rev Genet* 1988;22:631–677.
85. Welch WJ. The mammalian stress response: cell physiology and biochemistry of stress proteins. In: Morimoto Tissieres R, Georgopoulos C, eds. *Stress proteins in biology and medicine.* Cold Spring Harbor, NY: Cold Spring Harbor Laboratory Press; 1990:223–278.
86. Cairo G, Bardella L, Schiaffonati L, Bernelli-Zazzera A. Synthesis of heat shock proteins in rat liver after ischemia and hyperthermia. *Hepatology* 1985;5:357–361.
87. Blake MJ, Gershon D, Fargnoli J, Holbook NJ. Discordant expression of heat shock protein mRNAs in tissues of heat-stressed rats. *J Biol Chem* 1990;265:15275–15279.
88. Trump BF, Jones TW, Elliget KA, et al. Relation between toxicity and carcinogenesis in the kidney: an heuristic hypothesis. *Renal Failure* 1990;12:183–191.
89. Smith MW, Phelps PC, Trump BF. Cytosolic Ca^{2+} deregulation and blebbing after $HgCl_2$ injury to cultured rabbit proximal tubule cells as studied by digital imaging microscopy. *Proc Natl Acad Sci USA* 1991;88:4926–4930.
90. Smith MW, Phelps PC, Trump BF. Injury-induced changes in cytosolic Ca^{2+} in individual rabbit proximal tubule cells. *Am J Physiol* 1992; F647–F655.
91. Nieminen A, Gores G, Dawson T, Herman B, Lemasters J. Toxic injury from mercuric chloride in rat hepatocytes. *J Biol Chem* 1990;265:2399–2408.
92. Berridge MJ, Irvine RF. Inositol triphosphate, a novel second messenger in cellular signal transduction. *Nature* 1984;312:315–321.
93. Nishizuka Y. The role of protein kinase C in cell surface signal transduction and tumour promotion. *Nature* 1984;308:693–698.
94. Freissmuth M, Casey PJ, Gilman AG. G proteins control diverse pathways of transmembrane signaling. *FASEB J* 1989;3:2125–2131.
95. Nicotera P, Hartzell P, Davis G, Orrenius S. The formation of plasma membrane blebs in heptocytes exposed to agents that increase cytosolic Ca^{2+} is mediated by activation of a non-lysosomal proteolytic system. *FEBS Lett* 1986;209:139–144.
96. Bar-Sagi D, Suhan JP, McCormick F, Feramisco JR. Localization of phospholipase A_2 in normal and *ras*-transformed cells. *J Cell Biol* 1988;106:1649–1658.
97. Kolber MA, Broschat KO, Landa-Gonzalez B. Cytochalasin B induces cellular DNA fragmentation. *FASEB J* 1990;4:3021–3027.
98. Morgan JI, Curran T. Regulation of c-*fos* expression by voltage-dependent calcium channels. In: Fiskum G, ed. *Cell calcium metabolism. Physiology, biochemistry, pharmacology, and clinical implications.* New York: Plenum Press; 1989:305–312.

99. Morris AC, Hagler HK, Willerson JT. Relationship between calcium loading and impaired energy metabolism during Na^+,K^+ pump inhibition and metabolic inhibition in cultured neonatal cardiac myocytes. *J Clin Invest* 1989;83:1876.

100. Trump BF, Smith MW, Phelps PC, Regec AL, Berezesky IK. The role of ionized cytosolic calcium ($[Ca^{2+}]_i$) in acute and chronic cell injury. In: Lemasters JJ, Hackenbrook CR, Thurman RG, Westerhoff HV, eds. *Integration of mitochondrial function*. New York: Plenum Press; 1988:437–444.

Cardiovascular Toxicology, Second Edition,
edited by Daniel Acosta, Jr.
Raven Press, Ltd., New York © 1992.

5

Pathobiology of Myocardial Ischemic Injury

L. Maximilian Buja

Department of Pathology and Laboratory Medicine, The University of Texas
Medical School at Houston, and Texas Heart Institute, Houston, Texas 77225

Myocardial ischemia is a state of myocardial impairment that results from inadequate coronary perfusion of oxygenated blood relative to the metabolic demands of the myocardium (1,2). Thus ischemic heart disease involves an imbalance in the normal integrated function of the coronary vasculature and the myocardium. The major consequences of myocardial ischemia are depressed myocardial contractile function, arrhythmias, and myocardial necrosis (infarction).

ROLE OF CORONARY ALTERATIONS IN MYOCARDIAL ISCHEMIA

Observations in Humans

Atherosclerosis leads to progressive narrowing of the coronary arteries and predisposes to the development of ischemic heart disease (3). However, the pathogenesis of acute ischemic heart disease involves the occurrence of an acute pathophysiological alteration in the presence of coronary atherosclerosis of variable severity (4–11). The acute pathophysiological event may involve a stress-induced increase in myocardial oxygen demand or an impairment in the oxygen-carrying capacity of the blood. However, many cases of acute ischemic heart disease results from a primary alteration in the coronary vasculature leading to decreased delivery of blood to the myocardium. These alterations involve platelet aggregation, vasoconstriction (coronary spasm), and thrombosis superimposed on atherosclerotic lesions (Fig. 1).

An acute alteration of an atherosclerotic plaque often initiates acute narrowing or occlusion of the coronary artery. Acute changes in plaques consist of fissures, ulceration, and rupture, with injury to the endothelium and surface cap of the plaque as the initiating event. Precipitation of these changes

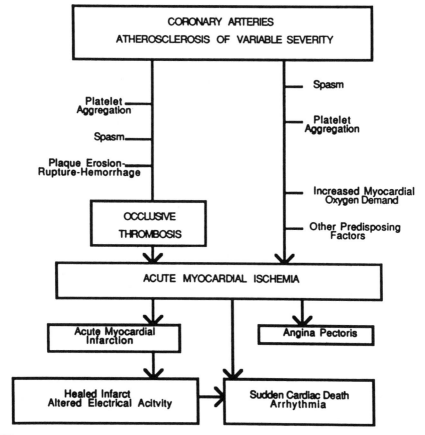

FIG. 1. Pathogenetic mechanisms of acute ischemic heart disease and potential clinical outcomes. Adapted from ref. 4.

likely requires chronic or recurrent injury, which may result from hemodynamic trauma as well as from toxic effects of products produced by degeneration of the plaque constituents. Occlusive coronary thrombi overlying fissured, ulcerated, or ruptured plaques are found in over 90% of cases of acute transmural myocardial infarction. This finding is the basis for the successful application of thrombolytic therapy for the treatment of acute myocardial infarction by coronary reperfusion. In syndromes of ischemic heart disease other than acute myocardial infarction, including unstable angina pectoris and sudden cardiac death, acute alterations of the coronary arteries also are frequently observed. These include endothelial disruption, plaque fissuring, platelet aggregation, and nonocclusive or occlusive thrombi.

Observations in Experimental Models

Insights into the role of coronary factors in the pathogenesis of acute myocardial ischemia have been provided by a canine model in which coronary stenosis with endothelial injury has been produced by placement of a plastic constrictor on a roughened area of the left anterior descending coronary artery (10,11). Coronary injury in the model results in the development of cyclic blood flow alterations, which are characterized by periods of progressive reduction to a nadir of blood flow followed by abrupt restoration of blood flow. These cyclic blood flow alterations are due to recurrent platelet aggregation at the site of coronary stenosis. There also is evidence that the process is driven by several platelet-derived mediators, including thromboxane A_2 (TxA$_2$) and serotonin (10,11). The cyclic blood flow alterations are mediated both by anatomic obstruction of the coronary artery by aggregated platelets as well as by excessive vasoconstriction produced by TxA$_2$, serotonin, and possibly other products released from the platelets (Fig. 2). Endothelial damage, leading to loss of prostacyclin and endothelium-derived relaxing factor, also contributes to the process. The cyclic blood flow alterations can be inhibited by treatment with TxA$_2$ synthesis inhibitors, TxA$_2$ receptor antagonists, and serotonin receptor antagonists (10,11). In a chronic model with cyclic blood flow alterations for several days, the animals develop intimal proliferation at the site of coronary stenosis with further nar-

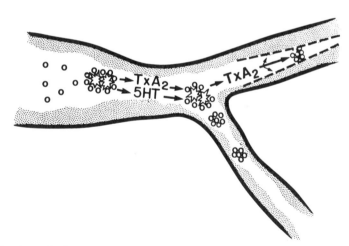

FIG. 2. A schematic diagram indicating the role of platelet-mediated mechanisms of induction of acute myocardial ischemia. Platelet aggregation develops in atherosclerotic coronary arteries at sites of endothelial injury. Aggregating platelets release mediators, including thromboxane A_2 (TxA$_2$) and serotonin (5HT), which cause further platelet aggregation downstream and vasoconstriction. From ref. 10, with permission.

rowing of the lumen (12). This process is likely mediated by multiple growth factors, including platelet-derived growth factor (PDGF) released from platelets.

Clinical Correlates

The observations derived from the canine cyclic blood flow model have implications for the pathogenesis of acute ischemic heart disease (8–12). Endothelial injury developing at a site of coronary stenosis can initiate changes leading to impaired coronary perfusion and myocardial ischemia. Endothelial injury predisposes to recurrent platelet aggregation, which produces anatomic obstruction compounded by vasoconstriction. TxA_2 and serotonin are important mediators of the process. Recurrent episodes of platelet aggregation may lead to further coronary stenosis as a result of intimal proliferation (12). A clinical counterpart of the latter phenomena may be the intimal proliferation that frequently occurs following percutaneous transluminal coronary angioplasty (PTCA) in humans. The process of recurrent platelet aggregation may result at any stage in the development of occlusive coronary thrombosis, although spontaneous resolution is also possible. Studies in humans have also provided evidence of platelet aggregation as well as release of TxA_2 and serotonin in patients with unstable angina pectoris (7,10,11). Thus there is strong evidence that endothelial injury and platelet aggregation are key factors in the mediation of acute ischemic heart disease.

MECHANISMS OF MYOCARDIAL ISCHEMIC INJURY

Metabolic Alterations

The major metabolic alterations induced by myocardial ischemia involve impaired energy and substrate metabolism (1,2). Oxygen deprivation results in a rapid inhibition of mitochondrial oxidative phosphorylation, the major source of cellular ATP synthesis. Initially, there is compensatory stimulation of anaerobic glycolysis for ATP production from glucose. However, glycolysis leads to the accumulation of hydrogen ions and lactate with resultant intracellular acidosis and inhibition of glycolysis (13,14). Fatty acid metabolism as well as glucose metabolism is impaired (15). Free fatty acids in the ischemic myocardium are derived from endogenous as well as exogenous sources, the magnitude of the latter depending on the degree of collateral perfusion. Inhibition of mitochondrial β-oxidation leads to the accumulation of long-chain acylcarnitine, long-chain acyl CoA, and free fatty acids. Initially, the free fatty acids are esterified into triglycerides, giving rise to fatty change in the myocardium. However, as esterification becomes blunted, free fatty acids increase (Fig. 3).

Myocardial ischemia is initially manifested by impaired excitation contraction coupling with resultant reduction in contractile activity of the ischemic myocardium (16). The associated early metabolic changes include a declining ATP level, leakage of potassium from myocytes, intracellular aci-

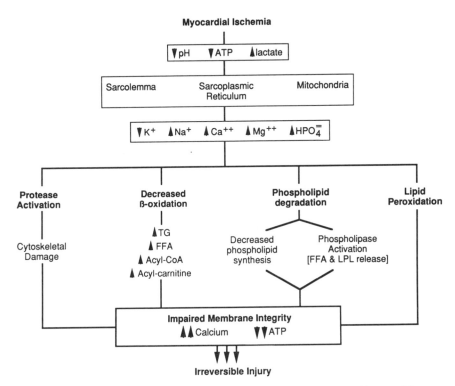

FIG. 3. Postulated sequence of alterations involved in the pathogenesis of irreversible myocardial ischemic injury. Oxygen deficiency induces metabolic changes, including decreased ATP, decreased pH, and lactate accumulation, in ischemic myocytes. The altered metabolic milieu leads to impaired membrane transport with resultant derangements in intracellular electrolytes. An increase in cytosolic Ca^{2+} may trigger the activation of proteases and phospholipases with resultant cytoskeletal damage and impaired membrane phospholipid balance. Lipid alterations include increased phospholipid (PL) degradation with release of free fatty acids (FFA) and lysophospholipids (LPL) and decreased phospholipid synthesis. Lipid peroxidation occurs as a result of attack by free radicals produced at least in part by the generation of excess electrons (e^-) in oxygen-deprived mitochondria. Free radicals also may be derived from metabolism of arachidonic acid and catecholamines, metabolism of adenine nucleotides by xanthine oxidase in endothelium (species dependent), and activation of neutrophils and macrophages. The irreversible phase of injury appears to be mediated by severe membrane damage produced by phospholipid loss, lipid peroxidation, and cytoskeletal damage. From ref. 15, with permission.

dosis, and accumulation of inorganic phosphate. However, the precise mechanism responsible for the excitation–contraction uncoupling and contractile depression of the ischemic myocardium has not been resolved and is the subject of continuing investigation. Nevertheless, the loss of contractile activity probably has a beneficial secondary effect by prolonging myocardial viability as a result of a major reduction in the demand for ATP.

Altered Ionic Homeostasis

The metabolic derangements discussed above lead to dysfunction of membrane pumps and channels with resultant derangements in intracellular electrolyte homeostasis. The earliest manifestation of membrane dysfunction is a net loss of potassium due to accelerated efflux of the ion from ischemic myocardial cells (2,16,18). The mechanism is currently uncertain, since the potassium efflux occurs before a severe reduction in ATP (17). Once ATP reduction is of sufficient magnitude, impaired function of the sodium/potassium–ATPase occurs. This is accompanied by an accumulation of sodium, chloride, and water in the cells; further loss of potassium; loss of cell volume regulation; and cell swelling (19). Another early change involves an initial increase in free intracellular magnesium level followed by progressive loss of magnesium (18). This is related in part to release of magnesium–ATP complexes as ATP depletion occurs. Finally, progressive changes in intracellular calcium homeostasis occur that may be of particular importance in the development of lethal cell injury.

Role of Calcium

The intracellular calcium level regulates normal cardiac function, and deranged calcium balance contributes significantly to the pathogenesis of myocardial cell injury (20–22). The intracellular calcium level is regulated by several processes (20). At the level of the sarcolemma, the voltage-dependent calcium channel is responsible for the slow inward current of the normal action potential; the sodium–calcium exchanger modulates intracellular calcium levels; and the calcium–ATPase mediates a calcium efflux pathway. At the level of the sarcoplasmic reticulum, the calcium/magnesium–ATPase and phospholamban mediate calcium uptake and release on a beat-to-beat basis. Intracellular calcium levels also are modulated by uptake and storage of calcium in the mitochondria and binding of calcium to calcium-binding proteins.

The total intracellular calcium concentration is on the order of 1–2 mM, with most of this calcium bound to cellular proteins (20–22). The free cytosolic ionized calcium concentration is approximately 100–300 nM during diastole and approximately 1 μM during systole. Beat-to-beat regulation of the cell calcium level involves voltage-dependent calcium influx across the sarcolemma followed by calcium-induced calcium release from the sarcoplasmic reticulum, with the latter providing the major source of the calcium that binds to the myofilaments and activates cardiac contraction. Diastole is mediated by a reuptake of calcium into the sarcoplasmic reticulum, thereby lowering the cytosolic free-calcium level.

Recent studies have confirmed that, at an early stage of myocardial hypoxic and ischemic injury, normal calcium transients are lost and the cytosolic free-calcium concentration increases into the micromolar range (23–26). Multiple mechanisms may be involved, including a net influx of calcium across the sarcolemma as well as loss of calcium from intracellular storage sites in the sarcoplasmic reticulum and mitochondria (20–26). These changes reflect membrane dysfunction, which is induced by ATP depletion and intracellular acidosis. The postulated consequences of an increase in cytosolic calcium include activation of phospholipases, proteinases, and calcium-dependent ATPases.

Progressive Membrane Damage

The conversion from reversible to irreversible myocardial injury is mediated by progressive membrane damage (Fig. 3). A number of factors may contribute to the more advanced stages of membrane injury. Cellular and organellar membranes consist of a phospholipid bilayer containing cholesterol and glycoproteins. The phospholipid bilayer is maintained by a balance between phospholipid degradation and synthesis. In myocardial ischemia, progressive phospholipid degradation occurs, probably as a result of the activation of one or more phospholipases secondary to an increase of cytosolic calcium or possibly other metabolic derangements (16). Phospholipase A- and phospholipase C-mediated pathways may be involved. Phospholipid degradation results in a transient increase in lysophospholipids, which are subsequently degraded by other lipases, as well as the release of free fatty acids. Thus phospholipid degradation contributes to the accumulation of various lipid species in ischemic myocardium. These lipids include free fatty acids, lysophospholipids, long-chain acyl CoA, and long-chain acylcarnitines (27,28). These molecules are amphiphiles (molecules with hydrophilic and hydrophobic portions). As a result of their amphiphatic property, these molecules accumulate in the phospholipid bilayers, thereby altering the fluidity and permeability of the membranes (29).

Initially, phospholipid degradation appears to be balanced by energy-dependent phospholipid synthesis. However, degradation eventually becomes predominant, with the result that net phospholipid depletion on the order of approximately 10% of total phospholipid content occurs after 3 hr of coronary occlusion. Although this net change in total phospholipid content is relatively small, it is associated with the development of significant permeability and structural defects, which are inhibited by agents that inhibit phospholipid degradation (30).

Myocardial ischemia also induces the generation of free radicals and toxic oxygen species derived from several sources (31–34). As a result of impaired oxidative metabolism, ischemic mitochondria generate an excess number of reducing equivalents that may initiate the generation of free radicals. Free radicals also can be produced by the enzymatic and nonenzymatic metabolism of arachidonic acid derived from phospholipid degradation and of catecholamines released from nerve terminals (see below). Endothelium of several species contains xanthine dehydrogenase, which may be converted to xanthine oxidase during ischemia. The xanthine oxidase can then metabolize adenine nucleotides derived from the metabolism of ATP. Neutrophils and macrophages invading ischemic tissue represent another source of free radicals. The major free-radical cascade involves a generation of superoxide anions followed by the production of toxic oxygen species, including the hydroxyl radical. A major target of free radicals is cell membranes, where the free radicals act on unsaturated fatty acids in membrane phospholipids leading to their peroxidation. Thus free radicals can be generated during myocardial ischemia and this process can be accelerated by reoxygenation.

Another potential factor in membrane injury involves disruption of the cytoskeleton, thereby affecting the anchoring of the sarcolemma to the interior of the myocyte (35–37). Vinculin has been identified as a cytoskeletal protein involved in this process. It is postulated that ischemia leads to disruption of cytoskeletal filaments connecting the sarcolemma to the myofibrils as a result of activation of proteases by increased cytosolic calcium or other mechanisms. After such disruption, the ischemic myocyte becomes more susceptible to the effects of cell swelling following accumulation of sodium and water. This process leads to the formation of subsarcolemmal blebs followed by rupture of the membrane. Such injury is likely accelerated by the effects of reperfusion, which allows for increased sodium, chloride, water, and calcium accumulation in the injured cells. Marked reactivation of contraction occurs as a result of increased calcium influx coupled with regeneration of ATP by mitochondria resupplied with oxygen. The resultant hypercontracture will accelerate membrane rupture following cytoskeletal disruption. The process just described may represent an important mechanism of reperfusion injury (38,39).

Thus the transition from reversible to irreversible myocardial damage appears to be mediated by membrane injury secondary to progressive phospholipid degradation, free-radical effects, and damage to the cytoskeletal anchoring of the sarcolemma. The consequences of this vicious cycle are loss of membrane integrity and further calcium accumulation with secondary ATP depletion (Fig. 3).

Autonomic Alterations and Arrhythmogenesis

Myocardial ischemia is accompanied by significant alterations in the autonomic nervous system. A major acute ischemic episode generates a stress reaction leading to elevation of circulating catecholamines. Within the ischemic myocardium, norepinephrine is released from injured nerve terminals, resulting initially in a redistribution of catecholamines followed by their eventual depletion (40). Alterations in adrenergic receptors develop, such as increases in the numbers of β- and α-adrenergic receptors on the sarcolemmal membrane (41,42). Initially, excess catecholamine stimulation is coupled to increased intracellular metabolism, mediated in part through the adenylate cyclase system. Eventually, uncoupling occurs between intracellular metabolism and receptor stimulation. However, this coupling can be restored and heightened upon reperfusion. Excess catecholamine stimulation can have a number of untoward consequences, including enhanced intracellular calcium influx as well as arrhythmogenesis.

Arrhythmias and conduction disturbances occur commonly in association with myocardial ischemia and may range from mild alterations to ventricular fibrillation. Arrhythmias are particularly common during the early phase of an ischemic episode as well as at the onset of reperfusion (2). It is likely that different mechanisms operate in different phases of ischemic arrhythmias (2). The arrhythmias may be mediated by metabolic alterations including a high concentration of potassium in the extracellular space adjacent to cardiac myocytes and nerve terminals (2); accumulation of lysophospholipids, long-chain acyl compounds, and free fatty acids in myocardial membranes (28); the alterations in the adrenergic system described above (40–42); and intracellular electrolyte alterations, including accumulation of intracellular calcium (43).

EVOLUTION OF MYOCARDIAL INFARCTION

Progression of Myocardial Ischemic Injury

In humans, the left ventricular subendocardium is the region most susceptible to myocardial ischemic injury. This is also true for the dog, which is the most common species used for experimental studies of myocardial ischemia. The susceptibility of the subendocardium relates to a more tenuous oxygen supply–demand balance in this region versus the subepicardium. This in turn is related to the pattern of distribution of the collateral circulation as well as local metabolic differences in subendocardial versus subepicardial myocytes.

Following coronary occlusion, the myocardium can withstand up to about

20 min of severe ischemia without developing irreversible injury. However, after about 20–30 min of severe ischemia, irreversible myocardial injury develops. The subsequent degradative changes give rise to recognizable myocardial necrosis. In the human and dog, myocardial necrosis first appears in the ischemic subendocardium, because this area generally has a more severe reduction in perfusion compared to the subepicardium. Over the ensuing 3–6 hr, irreversible myocardial injury progresses in a wavefront pattern from the subendocardium into the subepicardium (2,44). In the experimental animal and probably in humans as well, most myocardial infarcts are completed within approximately 6–8 hr after the onset of coronary occlusion. A slower pattern of evolution of myocardial infarction, however, can occur when the coronary collateral circulation is particularly prominent and/or when the stimulus for myocardial ischemia is intermittent, for example, in the case of episodes of intermittent platelet aggregation before occlusive thrombosis.

Histologic and Ultrastructural Changes

Established myocardial infarcts have distinct central and peripheral regions (Fig. 4) (2,22,44,45). In the central zone of severe ischemia, the necrotic myocytes exhibit clumped nuclear chromatin; stretched myofibrils with widened I bands; mitochondria containing amorphous matrix (flocculent) densities composed of denatured lipid and protein and linear densities representing fused cristae; and defects (holes) in the sarcolemma. In the peripheral region of an infarct, which has some degree of collateral perfusion, many necrotic myocytes exhibit disruption of the myofibrils with the formation of dense transverse (contraction) bands; mitochondria containing calcium phosphate deposits as well as the amorphous matrix densities; variable amounts of lipid droplets; and clumped nuclear chromatin. A third population of cells at the outermost periphery of infarcts contain excess numbers of lipid droplets but do not exhibit the features of irreversible injury just described. The pattern of injury seen in the infarcted periphery is also characteristic of myocardial injury produced by temporary coronary occlusion followed by reperfusion. In general, the most reliable ultrastructural features of irreversible injury are the amorphous matrix densities in the mitochondria and the sarcolemmal defects.

Determinants of Myocardial Infarct Size

The myocardial bed-at-risk, or risk zone, refers to the mass of myocardium that receives its blood supply from a major coronary artery that develops occlusion (44). Following occlusion, the severity of the ischemia is determined by the amount of preexisting collateral circulation into the myocardial bed-at-risk. The collateral blood flow is derived from collateral chan-

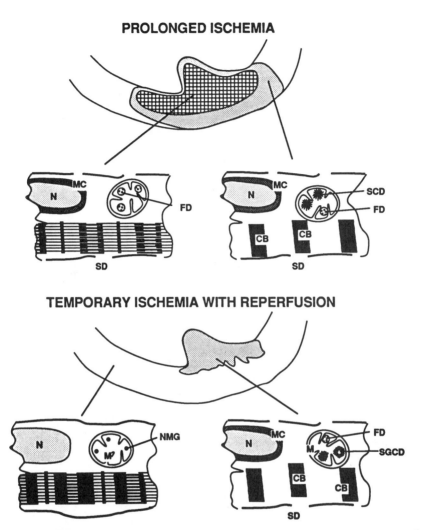

FIG. 4. Schematic diagram of morphological features of myocardial cell injury present in different regions of transmural infarcts produced by permanent coronary occlusion (*upper panel*) and subepicardial infarcts produced by temporary ischemia followed by reperfusion (*lower panel*). With prolonged coronary occlusion, myocardial necrosis is established in the subendocardium within 40–60 min, progresses in a wavefront pattern into the subendocardium of the region at risk (risk zone), and is completed by 3–6 hrs. With prolonged coronary occlusion, the myofibrils of myocytes in the central infarct region are hyperrelaxed as compared to those in the normal tissue depicted in the lower panel, and the mitochondria contain flocculent densities composed of denatured lipid and protein. The myofibrils of myocytes in the peripheral infarct region are formed into contraction bands and the mitochondria show calcium deposits as well as flocculent densities. With temporary ischemia and reperfusion, injury is limited to the subendocardium and is characterized by myofibrillar contraction bands and early mitochondrial calcification. N, nucleus; MC, marginated chromatin; SD, sarcolemmal defect; M, mitochrondia; FD, flocculent (amorphous) density; NMG, normal matrix granule; CD, contraction band; SCD, spicular calcium deposit; SGCD, small (granular) calcium deposit. From ref. 22, with permission.

nels connecting the occluded and nonoccluded coronary systems. With time, there is progressive increase in coronary collateral blood flow. However, much of this increase in flow may be too late to salvage significant amounts of myocardium.

The size of the infarct is determined by the mass of necrotic myocardium within the bed-at-risk. The bed-at-risk will also contain viable but injured myocardium. The border zone refers to the nonnecrotic but dysfunctional myocardium within the ischemic bed-at-risk. The size of the border zone varies inversely with the relative amount of necrotic myocardium, which increases with time as the wavefront of necrosis progresses. The border zone exists primarily in the subepicardial half of the bed-at-risk and has very little lateral dimension, owing to a sharp demarcation between vascular beds supplied by the occluded and patent major coronary arteries.

Thus the major determinants of ultimate infarct size are the duration and severity of ischemia, the size of the myocardial bed-at-risk, and the amount of collateral blood flow available shortly after coronary occlusion. Infarct size also can be influenced by the major determinants of myocardial metabolic demand, which are heart rate, wall tension (determined by blood pressure), and myocardial contractility.

Modulating Influences of Preconditioning, Stunning, and Reperfusion

The rate of progression of myocardial necrosis can be influenced by prior short intervals of coronary occlusion. Jennings and colleagues showed that the extent of myocardial necrosis following 60–90 min of coronary occlusion was significantly less in animals that had been pretreated with one or more 5-min intervals of coronary occlusion prior to the induction of permanent occlusion (46,47). However, after 120 min of coronary occlusion, the effect on infarct size is lost. This phenomenon is known as preconditioning (46–50). Recent evidence has indicated that a reduced rate of ATP depletion correlates with the beneficial effects of preconditioning (47). Further studies have suggested that activation of adenosine receptors may mediate the process of preconditioning (50). This interesting phenomenon is currently a subject of active investigation.

The progression of myocardial ischemia can be influenced profoundly by reperfusion. However, the effects of reperfusion are complex (38,39). Reperfusion clearly can limit the extent of myocardial necrosis if instituted early enough after the onset of coronary occlusion. However, reperfusion also changes the pattern of myocardial injury by causing hemorrhage within the severely damaged myocardium and by producing a pattern of myocardial injury characterized by contraction bands and calcification. Reperfusion also accelerates the release of intracellular enzymes from damaged myocardium. This may lead to a marked elevation of serum levels of these enzymes without necessarily implying further myocardial necrosis. The timing of reperfusion is critical to the outcome, with the potential for myocardial salvage being greater the earlier the intervention. Although reperfusion can clearly salvage myocardium, it may also induce additional injury. The concept of reperfusion injury implies the development of further damage, as a result of the reperfusion, to myocytes that were injured but that remained viable during a previous ischemic episode. Such injury may involve functional impairment, arrhythmia, and/or progression to cell death.

Persistent functional depression, requiring up to 24 hr or more for recovery, develops on reperfusion, even after relatively brief periods of coronary occlusion, on the order of 15 min, which are insufficient to cause myocardial necrosis. This phenomenon has been referred to as myocardial stunning (38,39). Free-radical effects and calcium loading have been implicated in its pathogenesis (51,52). After longer intervals of coronary occlusion on the order of 2–4 hr, there is actual necrosis involving the subendocardium and even more severe and persistent functional depression occurs. In our studies, after 2 hr of coronary occlusion, left ventricular regional sites of moderate dysfunction during ischemia recovered normal or near normal regional contractile function after 1–4 weeks of reperfusion, whereas after 4 hr of coronary occlusion, contractile dysfunction persisted after 4 weeks of reperfusion (53,54). Thus, depending on the interval of coronary occlusion before reperfusion, variable degrees of either contractile dysfunction, necrosis, or both are seen with reperfusion. The mechanisms of reperfusion injury are under active investigation. Further information regarding reperfusion injury is discussed in another chapter of this volume.

Measurement of Myocardial Infarct Size

Pathologic analysis of infarct size has provided a "goal standard" in assessing the accuracy of various noninvasive diagnostic tests for myocardial infarction. Although extensive investigation in this area has been conducted, noninvasive determination of infarct size remains a challenge (55). Techniques that have been used have included various electrocardiographic methods, quantitation of serum enzyme release, and various scintigraphic approaches. Our group has extensively evaluated the use of technetium stannous pyrophosphate scintigraphy for detection and sizing of myocardial infarcts, while other groups have evaluated the other approaches. Further work is needed to perfect methods for noninvasive detection and quantification of the myocardial bed-at-risk. This then will allow an analysis of absolute infarct size as well as infarct size as a percentage of the bed-at-risk.

Therapeutic Interventions

Continuing efforts have been made to develop therapeutic approaches to limiting infarct size since the extent of myocardial necrosis is a major determinant of prognosis following myocardial infarction. Experimental studies have shown that evaluation of a therapeutic agent should take into account both the influence of the size of the myocardial bed-at-risk and the amount of collateral perfusion over a given time interval of coronary occlusion. If an intervention produces a smaller infarct as a percentage of the bed-at-risk at any given level of residual perfusion, then it can be concluded that the intervention has an independent effect on myocardial ischemic cell injury. Various pharmacological approaches have been aimed at improving myocardial metabolism, increasing myocardial blood flow, reducing cellular calcium overload, and preventing free-radical-mediated effects. The most important advance in recent years has been the advent of thrombolytic therapy to provide reperfusion of the ischemic myocardium. This approach has initiated a new era of treatment of acute myocardial infarction (56). Ongoing investigations are aimed at developing pharmacological interventions that can be coupled with thrombolytic therapy to provide optimal protection and salvage of the ischemic myocardium.

REFERENCES

1. Hillis LD, Braunwald E. Myocardial ischemia. *N Engl J Med* 1977;296:971–978,1034–1041,1093–1096.
2. Reimer KA, Ideker RE. Myocardial ischemia and infarction: anatomic and biochemical substrates for ischemic cell death and ventricular arrhythmias. *Hum Pathol* 1987; 18:462–475.
3. Buja LM, Clubb FJ Jr, Bilheimer DW, Willerson JT. Pathobiology of human familial hypercholesterolemia and a related animal model, the Watanabe heritable hyperlipidemic rabbit. *Eur Heart J* 1990;11(Suppl E):41–52.
4. Buja LM, Hillis LD, Petty CS, Willerson JT. The role of coronary arterial spasm in ischemic heart disease. *Arch Pathol Lab Med* 1981;105:221–226.
5. Hirsh PD, Campbell WB, Willerson JT, Hillis LD. Prostaglandins and ischemic heart disease. *Am J Med* 1981;71:1009–1026.
6. Davies MJ, Thomas AC, Knapman PA, Hangartner JR. Intramyocardial platelet aggregation in patients with unstable angina pectoris suffering sudden ischemic cardiac death. *Circulation* 1986;73:418–427.
7. Fitzgerald DJ, Roy L, Catella F, Fitzgerald GA. Platelet activation in unstable coronary disease. *N Engl J Med* 1986;315:983–989.
8. Buja LM, Willerson JT. The role of coronary artery lesions in ischemic heart disease: insights from recent clinicopathologic, coronary arteriographic, and experimental studies. *Hum Pathol* 1987;18:451–461.
9. Buja LM, Willerson JT. Relationship of ischemic heart disease to sudden cardiac death. *J Forensic Sci* 1991;36:25–33.
10. Willerson JT, Hillis LD, Winniford M, Buja LM. Speculation regarding mechanisms responsible for acute ischemic heart disease syndromes. *J Am Coll Cardiol* 1986;8:245–250.
11. Willerson JT, Golino P, Eidt J, Campbell WB, Buja LM. Specific platelet mediators and unstable coronary artery lesions: experimental evidence and potential clinical implications. *Circulation* 1989;80:198–205.
12. Willerson JT, Yao S-K, McNatt J, et al. Frequency and severity of cyclic flow alteration and platelet aggregation predict the severity of neointimal proliferation following experimental coronary stenosis and endothelial injury. *Proc Natl Acad Sci USA* 1991; 88:10624–10628.

13. Neely JR, Morgan HE. Relationship between carbohydrate and lipid metabolism and the energy balance of heart muscle. *Annu Rev Physiol* 1974;36:413–459.
14. Neely JR, Grotoyohann LW. Role of glycolytic products in damage to ischemic myocardium: dissociation of adenosine triphosphate levels and recovery of function of reperfusion ischemic hearts. *Circ Res* 1984;55:816–824.
15. Buja LM. Lipid abnormalities in myocardial cell injury. *Trends Cardiovasc Med* 1991;1:40–45.
16. Carmeliet E. Myocardial ischemia: reversible and irreversible changes. *Circulation* 1984;70:149–151.
17. Venkatesh N, Lamp ST, Weiss JN. Sulfonylureas, ATP-sensitive K^+ channels, and cellular K^+ loss during hypoxia, ischemia, and metabolic inhibition in mammalian ventricle. *Circ Res* 1991;69:623–637.
18. Thandroyen FT, Bellotto D, Katayama A, Hagler HK, Miller J, Willerson JT, Buja LM. Subcellular electrolyte alterations during hypoxia and following reoxygenation in isolated rat ventricular myocytes. *Circ Res* 1992; in press.
19. Buja LM, Willerson JT. Abnormalities of volume regulation and membrane integrity in myocardial tissue slices after early ischemic injury in the dog: effects of mannitol, polyethylene glycol, and propranolol. *Am J Pathol* 1981;103:79–95.
20. Braunwald E. Mechanism of action of calcium-channel-blocking agents. *N Engl J Med* 1982;307:1618–1627.
21. Buja LM, Hagler HK, Willerson JT. Altered calcium homeostasis in the pathogenesis of myocardial ischemic and hypoxic injury. *Cell Calcium* 1988;9:205–217.
22. Hagler HK, Buja LM. Subcellular calcium shifts in ischemia and reperfusion. In: Piper HM, ed. *Pathophysiology of severe ischemic myocardial injury*. Boston: Kluwer Academic Publishers; 1990:283–296.
23. Morris AC, Hagler HK, Willerson JT, Buja LM. Relationship between calcium loading and impaired energy metabolism during Na^+,K^+ pump inhibition and metabolic inhibition in cultured neonatal rat cardiac myocytes. *J Clin Invest* 1989;83:1876–1887.
24. Lee H-C, Smith N, Mohabir R, Clusin WT. Cytosolic calcium transients from the beating mammalian heart. *Proc Natl Acad Sci USA* 1987;84:7793–7797.
25. Marban E, Kitakaze M, Kusuoka H, Porterfield JK, Yue DT, Chacko VP. Intracellular free calcium concentrations measured with ^{19}F NMR spectroscopy in intact ferret hearts. *Proc Natl Acad Sci USA* 1987;84:6005–6009.
26. Steenbergen C, Murphy E, Levy L, London RE. Elevation in cytosolic free calcium concentration early in myocardial ischemia in perfused rat heart. *Circ Res* 1987;60:700–707.
27. Katz AM, Messineo FC. Lipid–membrane interactions and the pathogenesis of ischemic damage in the myocardium. *Circ Res* 1981;481:1–16.
28. Corr PB, Gross RW, Sobel BE. Amphipathic metabolites and membrane dysfunction in ischemic myocardium. *Circ Res* 1984;55:135–154.
29. Buja LM, Miller JC, Krueger GRF. Altered membrane fluidity occurs during metabolic impairment of cardiac myocytes. *In Vivo* 1991;5:239–243.
30. Jones RL, Miller JC, Hagler HK, Chien KR, Willerson JT, Buja LM. Association between inhibition of arachidonic acid release and prevention of calcium loading during ATP depletion in cultured neonatal rat cardiac myocytes. *Am J Pathol* 1989;135:541–556.
31. Burton KP. Superoxide dismutase enhances recovery following myocardial ischemia. *Am J Physiol* 1985;248:H637–H643.
32. Burton KP. Evidence of direct toxic effects of free radicals on the myocardium. *Free Radical Biol Med* 1988;4:15–24.
33. McCord JM. Oxygen-derived free radicals in postischemic tissue injury. *N Engl J Med* 1985;312:159–163.
34. Burton KP, Morris AC, Massey KD, Buja LM, Hagler HL. Free radicals alter ionic calcium levels and membrane phospholipids in cultured rat ventricular myocytes. *J Mol Cell Cardiol* 1990;22:1035–1047.
35. Steenbergen C, Hill ML, Jennings RB. Volume regulation and plasma membrane injury in aerobic, anaerobic, and ischemic myocardium in vitro: effects of osmotic cell swelling on plasma membrane integrity. *Circ Res* 1985;57:864–875.
36. Steenbergen C, Hill ML, Jennings RB. Cytoskeletal damage during myocardial isch-

emia: changes in vinculin immunofluorescence staining during total in vitro ischemia in canine heart. *Circ Res* 1987;60:478–486.

37. Ganote CE, VanderHeide RS. Cytoskeletal lesions in anoxic myocardial injury: a conventional and high-voltage electron-microscopic and immunofluorescence study. *Am J Pathol* 1987;129:327–334.
38. Weisfeldt ML. Reperfusion and reperfusion injury. *Clin Res* 1987;35:13–20.
39. Hearse DJ, Bolli R. Reperfusion-induced injury: manifestations, mechanisms and clinical relevance. *Trends Cardiovasc Med* 1992; In press.
40. Muntz KH, Hagler HK, Boulas JH, Willerson JT, Buja LM. Redistribution of catecholamines in the ischemic zone of dog heart. *Am J Pathol* 1984;114:64–78.
41. Sharma AD, Saffitz JE, Lee BI, Sobel RE, Corr PB. Alpha adrenergic-mediated accumulation of calcium in reperfused myocardium. *J Clin Invest* 1983;72:802–818.
42. Thandroyen FT, Muntz KH, Buja LM, Willerson JT. Alterations in beta-adrenergic receptors, adenylate cyclase, and cyclic AMP concentrations during acute myocardial ischemia and reperfusion. *Circulation* 1990; 82(Suppl II):HH30–HH37.
43. Thandroyen FT, Morris AC, Hagler HK, Ziman B, Pai L, Willerson JT, Buja LM. Intracellular calcium transients and arrhythmia in isolated heart cells. *Circ Res* 1991;69:810–819.
44. Reimer KA, Jennings RB. The "wavefront phenomenon" of myocardial ischemic cell death. II. Transmural progression of necrosis within the framework of ischemic bed size (myocardium at risk) and collateral flow. *Lab Invest* 1979;40:633–644.
45. Buja LM, Tofe AJ, Kulkarni PV, et al. Sites and mechanisms of localization of technetium-99m phosphorous radiopharmaceuticals in acute myocardial infarcts and other tissues. *J Clin Invest* 1977;60:724–740.
46. Murry CE, Jennings RB, Reimer KA. Preconditioning with ischemia: a delay of lethal cell injury in ischemic myocardium. *Circulation* 1986;74:1124–1136.
47. Murry CE, Richard VJ, Reimer KA, Jennings RB. Ischemic preconditioning slows energy metabolism and delays ultrastructural damage during a sustained ischemic episode. *Circ Res* 1990;66:913–931.
48. Cohen MV, Liu GS, Downey JM. Preconditioning causes improved wall motion as well as smaller infarcts after transient coronary occlusion in rabbits. *Circulation* 1991; 84:341–349.
49. Iwamoto T, Miura T, Adachi T, Noto T, Ogawa T, Tsuchida A, Iimura O. Myocardial infarct size-limiting effect of ischemic preconditioning was not attenuated by oxygen free-radical scavengers in the rabbit. *Circulation* 1991;83:1015–1022.
50. Liu GS, Thronton J, Van Winkle DM, Stanley AWH, Olsson RA, Downey JM. Protection against infarction afforded by preconditioning is mediated by A_1 adenosine receptors in rabbit heart. *Circulation* 1991;84:350–356.
51. Bolli R, Patel BS, Jeroudi MO, Lai EK, McCay PB. Demonstration of free radical generation in "stunned" myocardium of intact dogs with the use of the spin trap alpha-phenyl N-tert-butyl nitrone. *J Clin Invest* 1988;82:476–485.
52. Kusuoka H, Porterfield JK, Weisman HF, Weisfeldt ML, Marban E. Pathophysiology and pathogenesis of stunned myocardium: depressed Ca^{2+} activation of contraction as a consequence of reperfusion-induced cellular calcium overload in ferret hearts. *J Clin Invest* 1987;79:950–961.
53. Bush LR, Buja LM, Samowitz W, Rude RE, Watham M, Tilton GD, Willerson JT. Recovery of left ventricular segmental function after long-term reperfusion following temporary coronary occlusion in conscious dogs: comparison of 2 and 4 hour occlusions. *Circ Res* 1983;53:248–263.
54. Bush LR, Buja LM, Tilton G, Wathen M, Apprill P, Ashton J, Willerson JT. Effects of propranolol and diltiazem alone and in combination on the recovery of left ventricular segmental function after temporary coronary occlusion and long term reperfusion in conscious dogs. *Circulation* 1985;72:413–430.
55. Buja LM, Willerson JT. Infarct size—can it be measured or modified in humans? *Prog Cardiovasc Dis* 1987;29:271–289.
56. Gunnar RM, Passamani ER, Bourdillon PD, et al. Guidelines for the early management of patients with acute myocardial infarction. *J Am Coll Cardiol* 1990;16:249–292.

Cardiovascular Toxicology, Second Edition,
edited by Daniel Acosta, Jr.
Raven Press, Ltd., New York © 1992.

6

Reperfusion Injury to the Heart

Is It a Phenomenon?

Robert A. Kloner and Karin Przyklenk

The Heart Institute Research Department, Hospital of the Good Samaritan, and Department of Medicine, Section of Cardiology, University of Southern California, Los Angeles, California 90017

The 1980s marked a revolution in the treatment of patients with acute myocardial infarction. While in the 1960s and 1970s only the complications of acute myocardial infarction (such as heart failure or arrhythmias) were treated, in the 1980s the infarct itself was treated by limiting its development with thrombolysis. Thrombolytic therapy with agents such as tissue plasminogen activator, streptokinase, and anisoylated plasminogen streptokinase activator complex can successfully lyse obstructing coronary artery thrombi in the setting of acute myocardial infarction. These agents, by reperfusing ischemic tissue, limit the size of myocardial infarction, enhance recovery of left ventricular function, and improve survival.

There is no doubt that timely reperfusion for the treatment of evolving myocardial infarction has beneficial effects. However, there is considerable debate as to whether additional benefit may be obtained by treating the phenomenon of reperfusion injury. Reperfusion injury has been broadly defined as cellular damage induced by the act of reperfusion *per se* (1–3). More specifically, it has been suggested that restoration of blood flow may lethally injure or kill a population of cells that were viable at the time of reflow (4).

Whether lethal reperfusion injury truly exists remains controversial. In the discussion that follows we review the evidence both in favor of and against this phenomenon. Potential mechanisms for reperfusion injury are also discussed. In addition, we review the concept that other forms of reperfusion injury, besides lethal reperfusion injury, may occur.

WHAT IS LETHAL REPERFUSION INJURY?

Several experimental studies have clarified the development of myocardial infarction during proximal coronary artery occlusion and the salvage of

131

tissue that occurs with early reperfusion. For example, a 15-min episode of proximal coronary artery occlusion followed by reperfusion in the canine preparation results in reversible ischemic injury: that is, myocardial cells do not die due to the ischemic insult (5). If the duration of ischemia is extended to 40–60 min, myocytes in the most ischemic subendocardial layers of the heart become necrotic, but tissue in the midmyocardial and subepicardial layers of the ischemic zone are salvaged by reperfusion. As the duration of coronary occlusion is extended to 3 hr, more tissue in the midmyocardial and subepicardial layers undergoes necrosis. Finally, with a permanent coronary artery occlusion (i.e., no reperfusion) the location of necrosis extends from subendocardial to subepicardial layers, resulting in a transmural or nearly transmural myocardial infarction (6–8).

This progression of myocyte death from subendocardium to subepicardium, first described by Reimer and Jennings (6,7), has been termed the "wavefront phenomenon" of necrosis. Their results and those of other researchers (8) have confirmed that the earlier one reperfuses an evolving myocardial infarction, the greater the amount of tissue that will be salvaged. In most experimental models, reperfusion beyond 3–6 hr of coronary occlusion will not salvage significant amounts of tissue. If, however, some myocardium dies due to reperfusion *per se* (i.e., lethal reperfusion injury), it might be possible to further enhance myocardial salvage by blunting this so-called reperfusion injury.

The concept of lethal reperfusion injury holds that there are a group of cells (presumably located in the midmyocardium) that are "hovering between life and death" at the end of the period of ischemia. Restoration of blood flow to these cells, resulting in an influx of fluid and electrolytes and the generation of toxic oxygen radicals, then precipitates cell death (2). Therapy designed to attenuate lethal reperfusion injury should salvage these cells and thereby result in myocardial infarcts that are smaller than those observed with reperfusion alone. That is, limiting reperfusion injury may extend the "window in time" following coronary occlusion in which reperfusion can salvage tissue.

DOES LETHAL REPERFUSION INJURY EXIST?

Reperfusion Injury Due to Oxygen Free Radicals

Many of the studies that support the hypothesis that lethal reperfusion injury is a real phenomenon have used pharmacologic therapy at the time of reperfusion to attempt to reduce infarct size above and beyond that achieved by reperfusion alone. The difference in infarct size between the control and treated group would then represent necrosis due to lethal reperfusion injury.

One of the first studies to support the concept that lethal reperfusion injury exists—and that it is due to oxygen free-radical damage—was reported by Jolly and colleagues (9). Using an anesthetized canine preparation, a proximal coronary artery was occluded for 90 min followed by 24 hr of reperfusion. One group of dogs received the oxygen free-radical scavenging agents superoxide dismutase (SOD) plus catalase 15 min prior to reperfusion and for 45 min thereafter. This treated group demonstrated a significant reduction in infarct size when compared with untreated controls. A second study by Ambrosio and co-workers (10) assessed infarct size produced by 90 min of coronary artery occlusion and 24 hr of reflow. Area of necrosis in animals randomized to receive SOD at the moment of reperfusion was reduced to *half* the infarct size observed in the control group. These data suggest that significant amounts of tissue had died during reperfusion in the control group, and that this lethal form of reperfusion injury could be treated with oxygen radical scavenging agents.

These two studies stimulated tremendous excitement, as they revived the concept that reperfusion injury could be modified. Several negative studies, however, soon followed: other investigators failed to show that oxygen radical scavenging agents given prior to or at the time of reperfusion were capable of limiting infarct size in canine models (11–16). For example, Przyklenk and Kloner (16) examined the effect of administering SOD plus catalase at the time of reflow in canine myocardium subjected to 2 hr of ischemia and 4 hr of reflow. SOD + catalase did not produce on overall reduction in infarct size or enhance recovery of contractile function, suggesting that scavenging of oxygen radicals at the time of reperfusion did not significantly reduce myocyte death. However, further analysis of the cardiac ultrastructure revealed that SOD + catalase did reduce damage to the subendocardial microvasculature: small vessels, including capillaries, exhibited less endothelial swelling, blebs, gaps, and disruption in treated animals than in controls. In addition, regional myocardial blood flow following reperfusion was significantly higher in animals that received SOD + catalase at the time of reflow. Thus although SOD + catalase did not limit reperfusion injury *per se,* results of this study suggest that scavenging agents may have a protective effect on the vascular endothelium.

As might be expected, there is very little data available regarding the efficacy of SOD in clinical instances of ischemia/reperfusion. In a preliminary report by Werns et al. (17), either placebo or SOD was administered for the initial hour following reperfusion to patients who underwent angioplasty for the treatment of acute myocardial infarction. No improvement in either global or regional left ventricular function was observed in patients who received the scavenging agent.

The discrepancy between studies showing substantial reductions in cell necrosis with oxygen radical scavengers versus no reduction in infarct size with these agents remains unresolved. The failure of these agents to limit necrosis when infarct size was assessed more than 24 hr following reflow has been attributed to the theory that, in some studies, infusion of SOD was discontinued too early during the reperfusion phase. SOD has a short biological half-life of less than 10 min; thus stopping the infusion early after reperfusion would result in a rapid fall in plasma levels, and loss of any therapeutic effect. As oxygen radicals are thought to be generated both at the time of reflow (perhaps by the xanthine oxidase pathway) and during the acute inflammatory response (by activated neutrophils), the duration of treatment versus the duration of reperfusion may be an important factor. Using SOD conjugated to polyethylene glycol (thereby extending the half-life to more than 30 hr), Tamura and colleagues (18) documented a sustained reduction in infarct size in dogs that underwent 90 min of coronary occlusion and 4 days of reflow. However, a recent study by Tanaka and associates (19) did not confirm these positive effects with the SOD conjugate.

It has been suggested that SOD may not be the optimal agent to reduce free-radical-mediated damage. As the SOD molecules are too large to cross the cell membrane, this agent may not be able to scavenge intracellular sources of free radicals (such as those originating from the mitochondrial electron transport chain). Other more permeable antioxidants might be better choices for the treatment of free-radical-mediated lethal reperfusion injury.

These conflicting studies provide no consensus as to whether lethal free-radical-mediated reperfusion injury truly exists. In fact, the majority of recent reports have concluded that free-radical-mediated reperfusion injury does not contribute significantly to myocyte necrosis in the setting of ischemia/reflow. These disparate experimental data, combined with the disappointing preliminary clinical results obtained by Werns et al. (17), make it unlikely that oxygen radical scavengers will be administered to patients undergoing reperfusion for the treatment of acute myocardial infarction.

Reperfusion Injury Due to Calcium Overload

Another theory regarding "lethal reperfusion injury" is that cell death at the time of reflow is due to calcium overload upon reperfusion (1,4). In the mid-1970s Whalen and co-workers (20) observed that the subendocardium of canine hearts subjected to a 40-min episode of transient coronary artery occlusion demonstrated a marked increase in tissue calcium levels. More specifically, calcium phosphate appeared to be located in granular densities within the mitochondria. Subendocardial tissue subjected to 40 min of ischemia already exhibited evidence of irreversible cell injury, characterized by breaks in the sarcolemmal membrane, and amorphous (nongranular) densities within the mitochondria. However, within minutes of reperfusion, the myocytes developed explosive cellular swelling, contraction bands, and the granular-type (i.e., calcium phosphate) densities (21). This led Jennings and colleagues (20,21) to hypothesize that the increase in calcium content occurred in cells that had already been irreversibly damaged by the ischemic episode: the increased edema and calcium uptake associated with reperfusion were merely a consequence of the inability of the dead myocytes to regulate cell volume and electrolyte influx.

Whether preventing calcium influx into cells at the end of an ischemic episode can actually salvage cells and prevent so-called lethal reperfusion injury in an *in vivo* model of coronary occlusion/reperfusion is unknown. The experimental literature is replete with studies investigating the effects of calcium blockers in models of ischemia/reperfusion (22,23). Some calcium blockers such as verapamil, when administered both during ischemia and following reperfusion, have been shown to reduce or delay development of myocardial infarct size in experimental models (24,25). However, our laboratory has observed that when intracoronary verapamil is given only during the reperfusion phase, it has no effect on myocardial infarct size (26). In addition, limited data obtained from patients who have received nifedipine plus thrombolysis for acute myocardial infarction have not shown benefits on either global or regional left ventricular function (27).

Thus, similar to the oxygen radical scavenging hypothesis, there is no clear evidence that calcium blockers can prevent lethal reperfusion injury. The role of calcium in lethal reperfusion injury therefore remains uncertain. However, this does not rule out the possibility that other means of prevention of "leaky" sarcolemma membranes (with subsequent reduction of calcium flux into cells) might reduce cell damage.

STUNNED MYOCARDIUM: A FORM OF NONLETHAL REPERFUSION INJURY?

While the concept of lethal reperfusion injury remains controversial, there is no doubt that stunned myocardium is a real phenomenon. Stunned myocardium refers to prolonged postischemic dysfunction of viable myocardium salvaged by reperfusion (28). This phenomenon was first characterized in experimental animal studies: for example, a transient coronary artery occlusion of 15 min followed by reperfusion was associated with depressed regional function for hours to days following reflow, despite the fact that no myocardial infarct was present (29). Postischemic "stunning" has been documented by a host of laboratories, and there is now evidence that this phenomenon also occurs in patients (30).

Stunned myocardium may represent a functional and nonlethal form of reperfusion injury (2). This concept is supported by the observation that oxygen free radicals formed upon reperfusion lead to postischemic dysfunction (31). Both *in vitro* and *in vivo* evidence indicates that reperfusion of reversibly ischemic myocardium is associated with an accelerated "burst" of free-radical production within the initial seconds following reflow (32,33). Furthermore, low levels of oxygen radical generation have been detected for as long as 3 hr following a 15-min episode of transient ischemia (34). These oxygen-centered radicals can cause peroxidation of membrane lipids, resulting in defects in both sarcolemmal and sarcoplasmic reticular membrane structure and function. Injury to these membranes can lead to altered calcium handling and hence defective myocyte function.

The concept that oxygen radicals generated upon reperfusion contribute to postischemic dysfunction is further supported by the fact that superoxide dismutase and catalase have consistently been shown to enhance recovery of function in models of brief ischemia reperfusion (35–37). This is true whether these agents are administered prior to the ischemic episode or immediately before the onset of reperfusion. In addition, Bolli et al. (34) documented that the spin trapping agent α-phenyl-*N*-tert-butyl-nitrone improved function of the stunned myocardium while "trapping" (i.e., scavenging) oxygen and carbon-centered radicals.

Another observation that supports the hypothesis that stunned myocardium represents a functional form of reperfusion injury is that small doses of intracoronary nifedipine (which did not reduce blood pressure or increase regional myocardial blood flow) infused 30 min after reperfusion enhanced the return of function of myocardium stunned by brief episodes of ischemia (38). These data support the concept that ongoing postischemic dysfunction can be improved or reversed even when calcium blockers are administered after reperfusion.

ALTERATIONS IN MICROVASCULAR FUNCTION AS A FORM OF REPERFUSION INJURY

When severely ischemic myocardium develops necrosis and is then reperfused, areas within the infarct fail to reperfuse and remain deprived of blood flow. This observation has been termed the no-reflow phenomenon and has been documented in both animal and human studies (39,40).

The cause of no-reflow appears to be actual morphologic damage to the microvasculature, characterized by localized areas of endothelial edema that cause the cells to protrude or "bleb" and obstruct the lumen of the vessel, endothelial gaps, loss of pinocytotic vesicles within the endothelium, deposition of fibrin, red blood cell plugging (rouleaux formalin) (39), and neutrophil plugging. These irreversibly damaged blood vessels are located within areas where the myocytes are frankly necrotic.

Zones of no-reflow appear as perfusion defects when fluorescent dyes or carbon particles are injected post-reperfusion. They are also characterized by severely depressed regional myocardial blood flow, as measured by radioactive microspheres (39,41). Some studies have shown that the extent of the no-reflow zone increased as a function of time following reperfusion (42,43). In this regard, some investigations consider no-reflow as a form of lethal reperfusion injury to the microvasculature. As described earlier, it is interesting to note that the oxygen radical scavengers SOD + catalase administered at the time of reperfusion reduced vascular damage and blunted no-reflow following 2 hr of coronary occlusion (16). However, since no-reflow areas are always confined well within the area where myocytes are already dead, it is doubtful that no-reflow contributes to lethal myocyte injury.

In addition to the no-reflow phenomenon, there is also evidence for a "low-reflow" phenomenon (41). Low-reflow consists of a mild to moderate reduction in regional myocardial blood flow, which occurs in the subepicardial, peri-infarct zone of reperfused infarcts. In contrast to no-reflow, this mild depression in blood flow is associated with viable myocytes and nonnecrotic microvessels.

Low reflow may represent another form of functional reperfusion injury. The microvasculature, although nonnecrotic, may demonstrate altered function during reperfusion. For example, following brief periods of ischemia and reperfusion, the response of the microvasculature to vasodilators and reactive hyperemia is blunted ("vascular stunning") (44). This same phenomenon has recently been described in viable reperfused subepicardial myocardium following a 90-min coronary artery occlusion (45). Whether these microcirculatory abnormalities are due to damage that occurs during ischemia or damage that occurs only in the reperfusion phase remains to be determined.

SUMMARY

The concept of reperfusion injury is multifaceted and may manifest itself in multiple forms (Table 1). For example, reperfusion injury may be "functional," as in the postischemic contractile abnormalities of viable myocytes (stunned myocardium). This concept is supported by reports that agents administered following reperfusion enhance the recovery of stunned, postischemic tissue. In addition, there may be two forms of vascular reperfusion injury. One is seen as the "no-reflow" phenomenon and is associated with microvascular necrosis. The fact that the size of the no-reflow zone enlarges as reperfusion progresses may suggest a form of lethal microvascular reper-

TABLE 1. *Theoretical types of reperfusion injury*

  I. Injury to myocytes
    a. Lethal reperfusion injury
    b. Functional (nonlethal) reperfusion injury (stunned myocardium)
  II. Injury to vessels
    a. Lethal reperfusion injury? (i.e., the "no-reflow" phenomenon)
    b. Functional (nonlethal) reperfusion injury (i.e., the "low-reflow" phenomenon) or reduced coronary vasodilator reserve

---

fusion injury. In contrast, the "low-reflow" phenomenon may represent a form of nonlethal or functional vascular reperfusion injury in which nonnecrotic microvessels exhibit reduced vasodilator reserve.

The controversial form of damage induced by reflow is "lethal" reperfusion injury—the concept that reperfusion *per se* causes some myocytes to die. Experimental studies provide no consensus as to whether lethal reperfusion injury truly exists. Furthermore, it will be even more difficult to determine whether lethal reperfusion injury is of clinical importance: a large patient population would need to be studied, and some adjuvant pharmacologic therapy plus thrombolytic agent would need to reduce infarct size to a greater extent than that achieved by thrombolysis alone. Clinical documentation of lethal reperfusion injury is further confounded by the difficulties in measuring infarct size in humans (i.e., usually by indirect techniques such as QRS scoring on the electrocardiogram, or CK-MB enzyme analysis). Further study is clearly needed to conclusively prove or disprove the concept of lethal reperfusion injury and assess its importance in clinical instances of ischemia/reperfusion.

REFERENCES

1. Weisfeldt ML. Reperfusion and reperfusion injury. *Clin Res* 1987;35:13–20.
2. Kloner RA, Przyklenk K, Whittaker D. Deleterious effects of oxygen radicals in ischemia/reperfusion. Resolved and unresolved issues. *Circulation* 1989;80:1115–1127.
3. Simpson PJ, Lucchesi BR. Free radicals and myocardial ischemia and reperfusion injury. *J Lab Clin Med* 1987;110:13–30.
4. Braunwald E, Kloner RA. Myocardial reperfusion: a double-edge sword? *J Clin Invest* 1985;76:1713–1719.
5. Jennings RB, Schaper J, Hill ML, Steenberger C Jr, Reimer KA. Effect of reperfusion late in the phase of reversible ischemic injury: changes in cell volume, electrolytes, metabolites, and ultrastructure. *Circ Res* 1985;56:262–278.
6. Reimer KA, Lowe J, Rasmussen M, Jennings RB. The "wavefront phenomenon" of ischemic cell death I. Myocardial infarct size vs. duration of occlusion in dogs. *Circulation* 1977;56:786–794.
7. Reimer KA, Jennings RB. The "wavefront phenomenon" of myocardial ischemic cell death. II: Transmural progression of necrosis within the framework of ischemic bed size (myocardium at risk) and collateral flow. *Lab Invest* 1979;40:633–644.
8. Ellis SG, Henschke CI, Sandor T, Wynne J, Braunwald E, Kloner RA. Time course of functional and biochemical recovery of myocardium salvaged by reperfusion. *J Am Coll Cardiol* 1983;1:1047–1055.
9. Jolly SR, Kane WJ, Bailie MB, Abrams GD, Lucchesi BR. Canine myocardial reperfusion injury: its reduction by the combined administration of superoxide dismutase and catalase. *Circ Res* 1984;54:227–285.
10. Ambrosio G, Becker LC, Hutchins GM, Weisman HF, Weisfeldt ML. Reduction in experimental infarct size by recombinant human superoxide dismutase: insights into the pathophysiology of reperfusion injury. *Circulation* 1986;74:1424–1433.
11. Uraizee A, Reimer KA, Murry CE, Jennings RB. Failure of superoxide dismutase to limit size of myocardial infarction after 40 minutes of ischemia and 4 days of reperfusion in dogs. *Circulation* 1987;75:1237–1248.
12. Richard VJ, Murry CE, Jennings RB, Reimer KA. Therapy to reduce free radicals during early reperfusion does not limit the size of myocardial infarcts caused by 90 minute of ischemia in dogs. *Circulation* 1988;78:473–480.

13. Gallagher KP, Buda AJ, Pace D, Gerren RA, Shlafer M. Failure of superoxide dismutase and catalase to alter size of infarction in conscious dogs after 3 hours of occlusion followed by reperfusion. *Circulation* 1986;73:1065–1070.
14. Patel B, Jeroudi MO, O'Neill PG, Roberts R, Bolli R. Effect of human recombinant superoxide dismutase on canine myocardial infarction. *Am J Physiol* 1990; 258:H369–H380.
15. Nejima J, Knight DR, Fallon JT, et al. Superoxide dismutase reduces reperfusion arrhythmias but fails to salvage regional function or myocardium at risk in conscious dogs. *Circulation* 1989;79:143–153.
16. Przyklenk K, Kloner RA. "Reperfusion injury" by oxygen-derived free radicals? Effect of superoxide dismutase plus catalase given at the time of reperfusion, on myocardial infarct size, contractile function, coronary microvasculature, and regional myocardial blood flow. *Circ Res* 1989;64:86–96.
17. Werns S, Brinker J, Gruber J, et al. A randomized, double-blind trial of recombinant human superoxide dismutase (SOD) in patients undergoing PTCA for acute MI. *Circulation* 1989;80(Suppl II);II-113.
18. Tamura Y, Chi L, Driscoll EM, Hott PT, Freeman BA, Gallagher KP, Lucchesi BR. Superoxide dismutase conjugated to polyethylene glycol provides sustained protection against myocardial ischemia/reperfusion injury in canine heart. *Circ Res* 1988;63:944–959.
19. Tanaka M, Stober RC, Fitz Harris GP, Jennings RB, Reimer KA. Evidence against the "early protection-delayed death": hypothesis of superoxide dismutase therapy in experimental myocardial infarction. Polyethylene glycol–superoxide dismutase plus catalase does not limit myocardial infarct size in dogs. *Circ Res* 1990;67:636–644.
20. Whalen P, Hamilton D, Ganote CE, Jennings RB. Effect of a transient period of ischemia on myocardial cells. I. Effect on cell volume regulation. *Am J Pathol* 1974;24:381–398.
21. Kloner RA, Ganote CE, Whalen DA, Jennings RB. Effect of a transient period of ischemia on myocardial cells. II. Fine structure during the first few minutes of reflow. *Am J Pathol* 1974;74:399–422.
22. Kloner RA, Braunwald E. Effects of calcium channel antagonists on infarcting myocardium. *Am J Cardiol* 1987;59:84B–94B.
23. Kloner RA, Przyklenk R. Progress in cardioprotection: the role of calcium antagonists. *Am J Cardiol* 1990;66:2H–9H.
24. Reimer KA, Jennings RB. Verapamil in two reperfusion models of myocardial infarction. Temporary protection of severely ischemic myocardium without limitation of ultimate infarct size. *Lab Invest* 1984;51:655–660.
25. Hoff PT, Tamura Y, Lucchesi BR. Cardioprotective effects of amlodipine on ischemia and reperfusion in two experimental models. *Am J Cardiol* 1990;66:10H–16H.
26. Lo HM, Kloner RA, Braunwald E. Effect of intracoronary verapamil on infarct size in the ischemic; reperfused canine heart: critical importance of the timing of treatment. *Am J Cardiol* 1985;56:672–677.
27. Erbel R, Pop T, Meinertz T, et al. Combination of calcium channel blocker and thrombolytic therapy in acute myocardial infarction. *Am Heart J* 1988;115:529–538.
28. Braunwald E, Kloner RA. The stunned myocardium-prolonged post-ischemic ventricular dysfunction. *Circulation* 1982;66:1146–1149.
29. Heyndrickx GR, Millard RW, McRitchie RJ, Maroko PR, Vatner SF. Regional myocardial function and electrophysiological alterations after brief coronary artery occlusion in conscious dogs. *J Clin Invest* 1975;56:978–985.
30. Kloner RA, Przyklenk K, Rahimtoola SH, Braunwald E. Myocardial stunning and hibernation: mechanisms and clinical implications. In: Braunwald E, ed. *Heart disease update*. Philadelphia: Saunders; 1990:241–256.
31. Bolli R. Mechanisms of myocardial "stunning." *Circulation* 1990;82:723–738.
32. Garlick PB, Davies MJ, Hearse DJ, Slater TF. Direct detection of free radicals in the reperfused rat heart using electron spin resonance spectroscopy. *Circ Res* 1987;61:757–760.
33. Zweier JL. Measurement of superoxide derived free radicals in the reperfused heart: evidence for a free radical mechanism of reperfusion injury. *J Biol Chem* 1988;263:1353–1357.

34. Bolli R, Patel BS, Jeroudi MO, Lai EK, McCay PB. Demonstration of free radical generation in "stunned" myocardium of intact dogs with the use of the spin trap α-phenyl-*N*-tert-butyl nitrone. *J Clin Invest* 1988;82:476–485.
35. Myers ML, Bolli R, Lekich RF, Hartley CJ, Roberts R. Enhancement of recovery of myocardial function by oxygen free radical scavengers after reversible regional ischemia. *Circulation* 1985;72:912–921.
36. Przyklenk K, Kloner RA. Superoxide dismutase plus catalase improve contractile function in the canine model of "stunned myocardium." *Circ Res* 1986;58:148–156.
37. Gross GJ, Farber NE, Hardman HF, Warltier DC. Beneficial actions of superoxide dismutase and catalase in stunned myocardium of dogs. *Am J Physiol* 1986;250:H372–H377.
38. Przyklenk K, Ghafari GB, Eitzman DT, Kloner RA. Nifedipine administered after reperfusion ablates systolic contractile dysfunction of postischemic "stunned" myocardium. *J Am Coll Cardiol* 1989;13:1176–1183.
39. Kloner R, Ganote CE, Jennings RB. The "no-reflow" phenomenon following temporary coronary occlusion in the dog. *J Clin Invest* 1974;54:1496–1508.
40. Schafer T, Montz R, Mathey DG. Scintographic evidence of the "no-reflow" phenomenon in human beings after coronary thrombolysis. *J Am Coll Cardiol* 1985;5:593–598.
41. Kloner RA, Alker KJ. The effect of streptokinase on intramyocardial hemorrhage, infarct size, and the no-reflow phenomenon during coronary reperfusion. *Circulation* 1984;70:513–521.
42. Jeremy RW, Links JM, Becker LC. Progressive failure of coronary flow during reperfusion of myocardial infarction: documentation of the no reflow phenomenon with positron emission tomography. *J Am Coll Cardiol* 1990;16:695–704.
43. Ambrosio G, Weisman HF, Mannisi JA, Becker LC. Progressive impairment of regional myocardial perfusion after initial restoration of postischemic blood flow. *Circulation* 1989;80:1846–1861.
44. Nicklas JM, Gips ST. Decreased coronary flow reserve after transient myocardial ischemia in dogs. *J Am Coll Cardiol* 1989;13:195–199.
45. Vanhaecke J, Flameng W, Borgers M, Jang IK, Van de Werf F, DeGeest H. Evidence for decreased coronary flow reserve in viable postischemic myocardium. *Circ Res* 1990;67:1201–1210.

SECTION IV

Cardiac Toxicology

Cardiovascular Toxicology, Second Edition,
edited by Daniel Acosta, Jr.
Raven Press, Ltd., New York © 1992.

7

Cardiotoxicity of Anthracyclines and Other Antineoplastic Agents

Kathleen A. Havlin

Department of Medicine, Temple University Comprehensive Cancer Center, Philadelphia, Pennsylvania 19140

The treatment of malignant disease with antitumor agents has become more widespread with the availability of more active drugs and treatment regimens. Adjuvant treatment programs attempting to eradicate microscopic disease are commonplace for breast, colon, osteosarcoma, and testicular tumors, and investigational in a number of other solid tumors. Neoadjuvant chemotherapy programs preceding definitive local treatment are now employed in the therapy of osteosarcomas, head and neck tumors, and, in some cases, non-small-cell lung cancer. Patients with advanced testicular tumors, small cell lung cancer, lymphomas, myeloma, and leukemias enjoy prolonged survival and, in some cases, are cured, with chemotherapy as primary treatment. Many patients with metastatic and/or advanced disease will receive successful palliative treatment with antineoplastics. The gains of these treatment programs are not without risks of complications due to the toxic agents employed. This chapter is a review of the cardiotoxic effects of the commonly used anthracyclines, a discussion of possible mechanisms of action and prevention, as well as additional discussion of other antineoplastics with cardiotoxic effects.

ANTHRACYCLINES

Doxorubicin and Duanorubicin

The anthracyclines, doxorubicin and daunorubicin, are among the most widely used antineoplastics having established response rates in leukemias as well as a variety of solid tumors (1,2). Danuorubicin has the more limited spectrum of activity primarily in acute leukemias. The clinical manifestations of cardiotoxicity from anthracyclines can be divided into two categories: (a) acute effects manifested by electrocardiographic changes and (b) a cumulative dose-dependent cardiomyopathy.

Electrocardiographic changes noted in association with the administration of the anthracyclines include ST–T wave changes, sinus tachycardia, ventricular and atrial ectopy, atrial tachyarrhythmia, and low voltage QRS complex (3–5). The most common EKG finding noted in studies using continuous electrographic recording devices is ventricular ectopy (6,7). In general, EKG changes are reversible and of little clinical consequence; however, cardiac arrest, presumably due to a dysrhythmia, has been reported (8).

The more serious toxicity of the anthracyclines and their dose-limiting effect is a dose-dependent cardiomyopathy. The overall incidence of cardiomyopathy has ranged from 0.4 to 10% with an associated mortality rate of 28–61% (3,9–11). Based on a number of studies, the onset of symptoms of congestive heart failure (CHF) following the last dose of anthracycline ranged from 2 days to 10.3 years (11–13). One study (3) reported a shorter median time (25 days) to CHF in fatal cases than in nonfatal cases (56 days).

Risk factors for the development of anthracycline cardiomyopathy have been identified. For both doxorubicin and daunorubicin, a dose–response relationship exists between the total dose of anthracycline and the development of CHF. Initial studies reporting doxorubicin cardiotoxicity identified a dose of 600 mg/m^2 as the cardiotoxic threshold above which CHF was more likely to occur (14,15). In large retrospective reviews of over 4000 patients, Von Hoff and colleagues identified an increasing probability of developing congestive heart failure as the dose of the anthracycline was increased. The cumulative probability of developing CHF with doxorubicin was 3% at 400 mg/m^2 and 7% at 550 mg/m^2. The greatest increase in the slope of the curve was noted at the 550-mg/m^2 total dose level (11) (Fig. 1). For daunorubicin, the incidence of CHF at 600 mg/m^2 was 1.5% with an increase to 12% at a total dose of 1000 mg/m^2 (5). More recently, a study of escalating doses of doxorubicin in patients with advanced breast cancer noted significant decreases in left ventricular function by radionuclide multigated blood pool scans (MUGA) at a mean dose of 459 mg/m^2 (SD ± 165 mg/^{2}) (16). These data continue to support an approximate dose of 550 mg/m^2 as a threshold for increased risk for the development of cardiotoxicity as identified by Von Hoff and colleagues.

The schedule of doxorubicin administration has been shown to influence the incidence of both drug-induced noncardiac as well as cardiac toxicity. Multiple studies have shown that weekly administration or prolonged infusions of doxorubicin decrease the incidence of drug-induced cardiomyopathy without sacrificing efficacy (17–21). Other risk factors frequently mentioned for the development of anthracycline-induced CHF include advanced age of the patient (11,22), preexisting cardiac disease (3,15), prior mediastinal radiation (3,15,23), and concomitant administration of other cytotoxic agents (3,4,24–27).

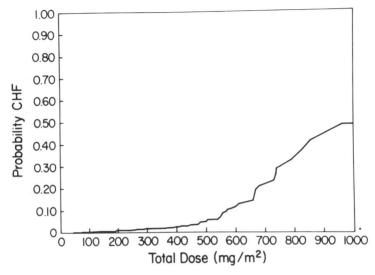

FIG. 1. Cumulative probability of developing doxorubicin-induced congestive heart failure (CHF) versus total cumulative dose of doxorubicin in 3941 patients receiving doxorubicin. From ref. 11, with permission.

Prospective evaluation of cardiac function during treatment with anthracyclines has become standard practice. Noninvasive methods in use include serial EKGs for change in QRS voltage (28), rest and exercise radionuclide angiography for measurement of left ventricular ejection fraction (29–31), exercise and Doppler echocardiographic analysis of left ventricular function (32–34), and QRS–Korotkoff interval (35). The gold standard for measurement of cardiac damage due to anthracyclines is endomyocardial biopsy with the designated pathological changes, rated 0–3, correlating with the degree of toxicity. A pathological score of 0 denotes no changes; 1 notes early myofibrillar dropout and/or swelling of the sarcoplasmic reticulum; 2 reveals progressive myofibrillar dropout, cells with cytoplasmic vacuolization, or both; 3 reveals diffuse myocyte damage with marked cellular changes in mitochondria, nuclei, and sarcoplasmic reticulum, and cell necrosis (36). Despite some evidence of lack of correlation between cardiac biopsy scores and radionuclide measurement of left ventricular ejection fraction, of the noninvasive methods, radionuclide angiography appears to be the most practical and reliable method of serial assessment of cardiac function (37,38). Recommendations for discontinuation of anthracycline therapy include ejection fractions (EFs) less than 45% at rest, failure to increase the EF with exercise, or greater than 10% decrease from a normal pretreatment level (31,39,40).

The actual mechanism of anthracycline cardiotoxicity remains elusive. No single theory adequately explains or integrates our current understanding of the clinical, biochemical, and molecular effects of these agents on cardiac structure and function. Similarly, the cytotoxicity of the anthracyclines has undergone extensive scrutiny over the years. A variety of biochemical effects are known including inhibition of nucleic acid metabolism due to intercalation with DNA, chelation of transition metal ions, participation in oxidation–reduction reactions, and binding to cell membranes (41–43). Unfortunately, the precise mechanism of the cytotoxic action of anthracyclines has yet to be defined. There is emerging evidence, however, that the cytotoxic/antitumor effect may be related to the activation of topoisomerase-II-mediated DNA cleavage rather than the DNA intercalation itself (44).

The ultrastructural changes seen with anthracycline therapy are well documented and reproducible in a variety of laboratory animals as well as humans (45–48). As mentioned earlier, these changes reveal several cellular abnormalities including myofibrillar loss and cytoplasmic vacuolization due to swelling of the sarcotubular system, structural abnormalities in the mitochondria with deposits of electron-dense bodies, and increased numbers of lysosomes (49,50).

Multiple researchers have attempted to explain the ultrastructural changes seen in myocardial cells after treatment with anthracyclines in terms of a unifying theory of action. There are several leading hypotheses of anthracycline cardiotoxicity. These include (a) free-radical formation with subsequent membrane damage and interference with energy metabolism, (b) interference with calcium metabolism, (c) the effect of histamine and other catecholamines, and (d) toxicity due to a cardiotoxic metabolite.

Free-radical formation by doxorubicin and the resulting cardiac DNA and membrane damage have been extensively studied and considered critical in the evolution of anthracycline-induced cardiotoxicity (46,51,52). The quinone-containing anthracyclines (doxorubicin, daunorubicin, epirubicin) were first noted to produce free radicals in the mid-1970s. Under aerobic conditions such as those in the myocardium, the quinone can be reduced to a free radical (semiquinone) by several electron-donating enzyme systems, such as NADPH and cytochrome P-450 reductase, and NADH dehydrogenase. The semiquinone free radicals subsequently react with molecular oxygen to form superoxide, hydrogen peroxide, and hydroxyl radical and, in turn, result in lipid peroxidation of cell membranes with continued generation of additional free radicals. Interaction with and damage to the cell membrane then influences cell permeability and function. The generation of these free radicals with accumulation of lipid peroxides is well documented (46,53). In addition, it is clear that free-radical formation occurs at a variety of sites including the cytosol, mitochondria, and sarcoplasmic reticulum and possibly explains the ultrastructural lesions commonly seen (54). Free radicals also impair sequestration of calcium by the sarcoplasmic reticulum and ultimately may result in decreased calcium stores, resulting in impaired contractility and relaxation of cardiac muscle (55,56). Increased calcium influx and myocardial calcium content have also been described with treatment with doxorubicin (57,58).

Free radicals may also be generated by nonenzymatic reactions of iron with doxorubicin with similar consequences. Although little free iron is present within the myocardium, there is evidence that doxorubicin can abstract iron from ferritin (59).

Interference with calcium metabolism may be a direct result of effects on cellular membranes rather than on the inciting event in anthracycline-induced cardiotoxicity. Early on it was thought that increased levels of intracellular calcium were responsible for mitochondrial dysfunction with resultant depletion of high-energy phosphate stores and contractile dysfunction. The electron-dense bodies seen in mitochondria were found to contain calcium (60). Accumulation of calcium was well documented *in vivo* in mitochondria in a variety of organs in the rabbit treated with chronic administration of doxorubicin (57,61). Recent data, however, point more toward an initial deficiency of intracellular calcium and its resultant effects on calcium flux and muscle contraction (62). Studies with combinations of calcium-channel blocking drugs thought to prevent calcium accumulation with anthracycline treatment have provided conflicting data regarding their influence on cardiotoxic effects (63–65).

Another theory of anthracycline cardiotoxicity revolves around the involvement of histamine and other vasoactive substances as causative agents. Support for this theory comes from experiments examining histopathologic lesions produced in rabbits after histamine infusions, which were found to be similar to doxorubicin-induced lesions (66). These same authors were able to show that histamine release was stimulated *in vitro* by doxorubicin. Additional studies by others have supported these findings as well as documented prevention of histamine release with the use of inhibitors such as theophylline and disodium cromoglycate and the free-radical scavenger *N*-acetylcysteine, which was also found to inhibit the release of histamine (67). Klugman and colleagues also noted the absence of typical histopathologic cardiac lesions in the animals treated with the inhibitors.

The possibility of a metabolite of doxorubicin as the offending cardiotoxic agent has also been suggested (68–70). Olson and colleagues compared the *in vitro* cardiotoxic effects of doxorubicin and doxorubicinol, the carbon-13 alcohol metabolite of doxorubicin. In their study, doxorubicinol was found to be a more potent inhibitor of contractile function, membrane-associated ion pumps, and greatly decreased calcium loading within the sarcoplasmic reticulum vesicles. In addition, the authors noted intracardiac conversion of doxorubicin to doxorubicinol, further supporting previous evidence of accumulation in cardiac tissue in a time-dependent fashion (68,71). Of interest, the authors found that doxorubicin maintained greater cytotoxicity in three pancreatic adenocarcinoma cell lines over the metabolite, suggesting separation of cytotoxic and cardiotoxic effects.

Perhaps one of the more enlightening aspects providing some insight into mechanisms of cardiotoxicity has been the various agents tested to prevent cardiac toxicity. These agents include coenzyme Q (72), N-acetylcysteine (NAC) (73), prenylamine (74), and the bispiperazinedione ICRF-187 (75). Inhibition of coenzyme Q (CoQ_{10}), a mitochondrial enzyme involved in oxidative phosphorylation, results in cardiac lesions in the rat similar to those seen with doxorubicin cardiotoxicity (76). Investigators described the prevention of experimental cardiotoxicity by doxorubicin with the addition of CoQ_{10} (ubiquinone) in the isolated rabbit heart model (77). These same investigators administered ubiquinone to rabbits and were able to demonstrate prevention of doxorubicin cardiotoxicity *in vivo* (78). More recently, CoQ_{10} has been studied for its therapeutic effect in dilated cardiomyopathy with evidence of efficacy (79).

Prenylamine is a calcium-channel blocking agent that has undergone investigation in Argentina. After obtaining laboratory evidence of cardioprotection in animals, investigators proceeded with a small randomized trial in patients (80,81). Cardiotoxicity as evidenced by congestive cardiomyopathy and supraventricular dysrhythmia was seen in the untreated patients. There were no cardiac events in the group treated with prenylamine. As mentioned earlier, other studies have not revealed a benefit with the use of other calcium-channel blockers.

N-acetylcysteine (NAC) is a sulfhydryl compound shown in mice to confer cardiac protection from doxorubicin treatment theoretically through increased sulfhydryl content in the heart (73). However, when a randomized trial with the oral form was conducted in cancer patients, treatment with NAC did not confer significant cardioprotection (82).

ICRF-187 is an iron chelating agent whose chelating properties were first noted during Phase I testing of the compound as an antineoplastic agent (83). Prevention of anthracycline cardiotoxicity is thought to be prevented by the binding of ICRF-187 to ferrous at intracellular sites that would normally complex with doxorubicin. It is the iron–doxorubicin complex that is thought to be responsible for the generation of free radicals with the subsequent cascade of events leading to cardiac damage (46,84).

More recently, doxorubicin has been administered to patients in a liposome-encapsulated form with a suggestion of less cardiac toxicity as determined by radionuclide ejection fraction and, in a few patients, Billingham score on endomyocardial biopsy (85,86). Of all these agents, only ICRF-187 has been studied in a randomized, prospective fashion and has shown consistent evidence of modulating cardiotoxicity due to anthracyclines (75).

In summary, there are several theories of the mechanism of anthracycline cardiotoxicity without an all-encompassing theory to explain the myriad properties and effects of this class of antineoplastic agent. Further investigation and elucidation are required and ongoing. ICRF-187 continues to show promise as a clinically useful agent in the prevention of doxorubicin cardiotoxicity.

Anthracycline Analogs

Over 1000 anthracycline derivatives have been synthesized with the hope of retaining therapeutic efficacy with less toxicity of both myelosuppression and cardiotoxicity (87). Only compounds with cytotoxicity preclinically at least equal to doxorubicin are then tested further to ascertain their toxicity profile. Determining whether these analogs are beneficial and less toxic than doxorubicin continues to be an active area of investigation. The following briefly reviews the cardiotoxicity seen with several of the compounds in clinical use or undergoing clinical evaluation (Fig. 2).

Esorubicin (4'-Deoxydoxorubicin)

Esorubicin is an anthracycline analog synthesized by the removal of the hydroxyl group from the 4' carbon of the sugar moiety of the parent compound, doxorubicin. Recent follow-up of 136 patients treated with esorubicin on 1 of 2 CALGB Phase II protocols was reported (88). Serial MUGA scans were obtained in 36 of 44 patients who received more than four cycles of therapy. Decreases in left ventricular ejection fraction of more than 5% were noted at doses of 240 mg/m^2 and more than 10% at doses of 480 mg/m^2. Overall, cardiotoxicity was observed in 11 patients (8%) without previous anthracycline or history of cardiovascular disease. Cardiotoxicity described included overt congestive heart failure, asymptomatic decreases in left ventricular ejection fraction, sinus tachycardia, and one myocardial infarction.

4'-Epidoxorubicin

Epirubicin is a stereoisomer of doxorubicin with a different configuration of the hydroxyl group in the 4' position of the sugar moeity. Cardiotoxicity similar in scope to that reported for doxorubicin has been reported with epirubicin. In two studies of patients with advanced breast cancer without prior treatment with an anthracycline, congestive heart failure was reported in four patients who received cumulative doses of epirubicin greater than 1000 mg/m^2 (89) and in one patient who received a total dose of 797 mg/m^2 (90). There have been several studies recently reported, which have included endomyocardial biopsies as part of the evaluation documenting cardiotoxicity due to epirubicin (91–93). In all these studies, the type and severity of

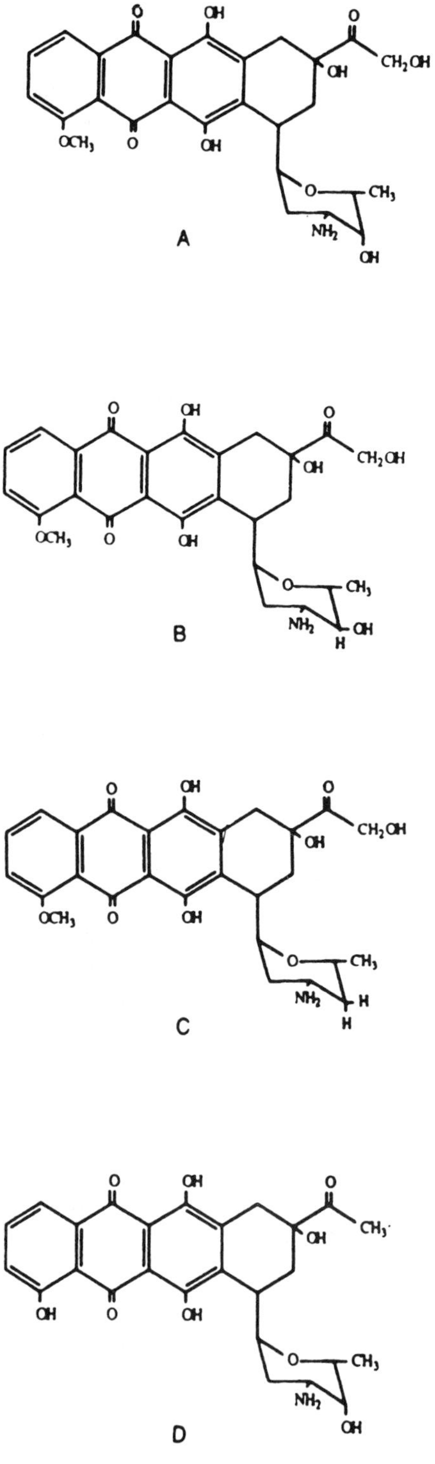

FIG. 2. Anthracyclines. **A:** Doxorubicin. **B:** Epirubicin. **C:** Esorubicin. **D:** Idarubicin.

histologic abnormalities were similar to those seen with doxorubicin and correlated with increasing doses of epirubicin. Dardir and colleagues noted a statistically significant correlation (p = .0006) between the total dose of epirubicin and pathologic changes quantified by the use of the Billingham scale (82). In one study, doses smaller than 500 mg/m^2 were not associated with cardiotoxicity. However, at doses of 500–1000 mg/m^2, 2% of the patients developed congestive heart failure with an increase to 35% of the patients developing congestive heart failure at cumulative doses greater than 1000 mg/m^2 (83).

Idarubicin (4-Demethoxydaunorubicin)

Idarubicin differs from the parent compound, doxorubicin, in substitution of the C-4 methoxyl group with a hydrogen atom. During Phase I testing with the agent, the significant cardiotoxicity described was limited to patients who had received previous treatment with anthracyclines. Therefore postulating a direct cause and effect was not possible (94–96). The cardiotoxicity described ranged from asymptomatic EKG changes to overt congestive heart failure requiring therapy and discontinuation of the idarubicin. In Phase II studies, decreases in left ventricular ejection fraction without clinical signs of cardiac failure were seen infrequently and were limited to patients who had received prior anthracyclines (97–101). In these studies, cumulative doses of 800 mg/m^2 orally and 169 mg/m^2 intravenously were tolerated without signs of clinical congestive heart failure.

Mitoxantrone (Novantrone)

Mitoxantrone, a substituted anthraquinone, was developed in an attempt to achieve similar antitumor activity of the anthracyclines but with less toxicity. Despite modifications, mitoxantrone has been reported to have cardiac effects although on a lesser scale than the anthracyclines. Described cardiac toxicity includes decreases in left ventricular ejection fraction (LVEF) and congestive heart failure (102). Dysrhythmias have been noted infrequently (103). In large series including a randomized study comparing cytoxan, doxorubicin, and 5-flourouracil to cytoxan, mitoxantrone, and 5-fluorouracil in patients with metastatic breast cancer, the incidence of congestive heart failure was less than 2% (94,104,105). The majority of patients experiencing congestive heart failure have received more than 120 mg/m^2 of mitoxantrone but similar toxicity has been reported at lower doses both in patients with and without prior exposure to an anthracycline (95,106,107). Treatment of CHF related to mitoxantrone therapy usually responds to management with digoxin, diuretics, and discontinuation of mitoxantrone with the possibility of eventual return to a baseline cardiac status (98). A small number of endomyocardial biopsies have been done and reveal changes consistent with anthracycline-induced cardiomyopathy (108,109). Predisposing factors to mitoxantrone cardiotoxicity include prior anthracycline therapy, mediastinal irradiation, and prior cardiovascular disease, with prior anthracycline therapy the most important factor (110). In patients previously treated with anthracyclines, the incidence of CHF is negligible up to doses of 100 mg/m². In patients without previous treatment with anthracyclines, doses up to 160 mg/m² appear to be tolerated without significant cardiotoxicity (111). Careful monitoring of cardiac ejection fraction at cumulative doses greater than 100 mg/m² is recommended especially in those at risk for development of cardiac toxicity. Toxicology studies performed in beagle dogs did not reveal clinical manifestations of CHF or EKG changes (112). Abnormalities on endomyocardial biopsies in dogs were limited to dilatation of the sarcoplasmic reticulum (113). In one study, mitoxantrone was shown to be an antioxidant inhibiting both basal and drug-induced peroxidation of lipids (114). It follows that if lipid peroxidation is important in the development of cardiotoxicity of anthracyclines and anthracycline-like drugs, mitoxantrone theoretically has the potential for causing less cardiotoxicity. To date this has been shown to be the case clinically as well.

OTHER ANTITUMOR AGENTS

Cyclophosphamide

Severe hemorrhagic cardiac necrosis has been reported in the transplant setting at doses of 120–240 mg/kg given over 1–4 days (115–117). The presenting symptoms are tachycardia and refractory congestive heart failure. EKG changes reveal sinus tachycardia, low voltage QRS complex, ST segment elevation, and nonspecific ST–T wave changes. Left ventricular systolic function as assessed by echocardiographic fractional shortening have been shown to be significantly decreased from baseline in patients with and without clinical symptoms of heart failure (118). Significant increases in LDH and CPK suggesting myocardial damage are seen in approximately one-half of the patients. Symptoms of cardiac necrosis may not become evident until 2 weeks after dosing but are rapidly fatal when present (119). Pathological findings at autopsy include dilated heart, patchy transmural hemorrhages, focal areas of fibrinous pericarditis and myocardial necrosis, and interstitial lesions consisting of hemorrhage, edema, and fibrin deposition (109,110). There is emerging data that the intracellular thiol, glutathione, may play a role in the protection against cardiac injury due to cyclophosphamide (120).

There is some evidence that cyclophosphamide in combination with other agents, particularly BCNU, 6-thioguanine, cytosine arabinoside, and total body irradiation, may be more cardiotoxic than cyclophosphamide alone (121). In one study, 4 of 15 patients died of acute myopericarditis using the combination of BCNU, cyclophosphamide, 6-thioguanine, and cytosine arabinoside (107). Another study reported a 9% incidence of fatal cardiomyopathy and/or pericarditis with this same combination or high-dose cyclophosphamide and total body irradiation (122). An additional 22% of patients experienced nonfatal congestive heart failure. The majority of patients in each of these studies had received prior anthracyclines possibly compounding their risk of developing cardiotoxicity from these regimens.

A more recent study has evaluated the cardiotoxicity of cyclophosphamide in twice-daily higher dose compared to a lower daily dose schedule (123). Left ventricular ejection fractions did not change significantly in either group; however, four of the five patients who developed clinical cardiotoxicity (four pericarditis; one congestive heart failure) were in the higher dose group. The conclusion of the authors was that the twice-daily dosing schedule although not completely without cardiotoxicity resulted in less ventricular dysfunction. As more experience is gained in bone marrow transplantation, it will be important to identify regimens and dosing schedules that allow for efficacy without excessive toxicity.

5-Fluorouracil (5-FU)

The reported incidence of cardiac side effects with 5-fluorouracil (5-FU), a widely used antimetabolite, is low, at approximately 1.6% (124). Angina with ischemic EKG changes is the most frequent cardiac toxicity noted. The first reports of chest pain associated with ischemic EKG changes in patients receiving 5-FU occurred in 1975. All three patients failed to have subsequent evidence of a myocardial infarction; EKG abnormalities resolved with discontinuation of the drug (125). Ischemic EKG changes, left ventricular dysfunction, and hypotension with dyspnea associated with infusions of 5-FU alone and in combination with cisplatin have been reported (126,127). Severe but reversible heart failure with global hypokinesis and cardiogenic shock has been reported in association with continuous infusions of 5-FU (128–130). Extensive cardiac evaluations have been performed in a small number of these patients without documentation of significant coronary artery disease or clear evidence of vasospasm (119–121, 131–133). The episodes of severe heart failure and cardiogenic shock resolved with aggressive support following discontinuation of the 5-FU infusion in most reported cases. Conflicting evidence exists regarding the efficacy of nitrates and/or calcium-channel blocking agents in preventing anginal episodes, which suggests that mechanisms other than coronary vasospasm may be involved in the cardiac effects of 5-fluorouracil (134–136). Myocardial infarctions have been reported in a small number of patients as well as deaths in patients refractory to supportive therapy (121–124).

The mechanism by which 5-FU causes cardiotoxicity is unknown. Possible etiologies include vasospasm, a direct cardiotoxic effect either from 5-FU or one of its metabolites, or some other metabolic derangement lead ing to either an increase in metabolic demands or a decrease in the available energy to meet those demands. Comparisons have been made to the "stunned myocardium," a syndrome of reversible postischemic ventricular dysfunction (137). Little animal data exist to support any particular theory at the present time. There is laboratory evidence of persistent radioactivity in the myocardium of mice injected with ^{14}c-labeled 5-FU 96 hr after injection, suggesting delayed metabolism in the heart (138). In addition, both the pharmacokinetics and the toxicity profiles of oral, bolus intravenous, and prolonged intravenous administration of 5-FU are known to differ. Lower but sustained plasma levels and less myelosuppression and greater mucositis noted with the prolonged infusion (139). These differences may ultimately provide insight into the mechanism of 5-FU cardiotoxicity.

Cisplatin

Cisplatin, a bifunctional alkylating agent with a broad spectrum of activity, is associated with rare reports of cardiotoxicity. Cisplatin-induced bradycardia (140) and paroxysmal supraventricular tachycardia have been reported (141,142). Ischemic vascular events with myocardial infarctions in young patients with and without mediastinal radiation who were treated with cisplatin-based combination chemotherapy are among the most serious toxicities reported with the agent (143,144). Coronary artery spasm was documented in one patient at cardiac catheterization in the absence of atherosclerotic disease. Two cases of severe coronary artery atherosclerosis and one case of fibrous intimal proliferation in young males with testicular cancer after cisplatin-based chemotherapy have been documented (145,146). None of the patients was considered to have had significant risk factors for coronary artery disease; only one patient had received thoracic irradiation.

Amsacrine (AMSA)

This drug is an acridine orange derivative with documented activity in acute leukemia and lymphoma. Reported cardiac toxicity with this agent has included dysrhythmias (147–149), ventricular dysfunction (150), and acute myocardial necrosis (151) although the latter occurred after administration of multiple drugs and in the setting of progressive disease. Significant QT prolongation may be the initial effect resulting in increased vulnerability to ventricular dysrhythmias as noted by some authors (152,153). The presence of hypokalemia may compound the risk of developing a dysrhythmia (139,140,154). One study of heavily pretreated patients concluded that an anthracycline dose greater than 400 mg/m^2 and administration of more than 200 mg/m^2 of AMSA over 48 hr were related to an increased risk of cardiac effects associated with the AMSA therapy (141). Four of the six patients who developed clinical congestive heart failure in that study were in this high-risk group. To date, a cumulative dose effect and its relationship to cardiotoxicity have not been demonstrated for this agent (145).

Studies in rabbits at high doses and dogs using toxic doses of high, lethal, and supralethal doses of AMSA revealed marked effects on atrioventricular and intraventricular conduction systems (155). First and second degree A-V block, prolongation of QRS and QT intervals, ventricular premature contractions, atrial flutter, and ventricular tachycardia were among the noted effects.

Cytosine Arabinoside (ARA-C)

Cytarabine, a nucleoside analog, effective in treating acute leukemia rarely causes cardiotoxicity. There are, however, case reports of a cardiac dysrhythmia (156) and acute pericarditis encountered during high-dose therapy (157). At the time of the pericarditis, the patient was in complete clinical remission from acute lymphocytic leukemia. Pericardial fluid analysis was negative for tumor or an infectious agent. No evidence of myocardial damage either clinically or by laboratory studies was noted during the episode of pericarditis.

BIOLOGICALS

Interferon

The incidence of cardiovascular toxicity associated with interferon therapy has been in the range of 5–12% (158,159). Increasing dose, increasing age, and a prior history of cardiovascular disease appear to be risk factors for the development of cardiotoxicity with the interferons (149).

The most frequently reported cardiac toxicities are primarily hypotension and tachycardia and may be related to the febrile reaction commonly seen rather than a direct cardiotoxic effect (160). Nonfatal dysrhythmias, predominantly supraventricular tachyarrhythmias, have been described in patients receiving interferon therapy (161). Early clinical trials in France were temporarily halted due to four deaths from myocardial infarctions in patients treated with interferon (162). Myocardial infarctions in patients with and without prior cardiac histories have been reported (151,163–165). Infrequent reports of congestive heart failure with short-term and prolonged administration of interferons have been described (151,166–168). The report of three patients with Kaposi's sarcoma and HIV-positive state suggests a possible synergism between interferon and the HIV virus. Postmortem findings in one case revealed four-chamber enlargement without evidence of coronary artery disease, fibrosis, amyloid, or inflammatory infiltrates, suggesting a drug-related etiology of the cardiomyopathy (169).

Although the reports of cardiovascular toxicities with interferon treatment overall are infrequent, older patients and those with a history of previous cardiac events may be at increased risk for the development of cardiac toxicity from interferons.

Interleukin-2 (IL-2)/Lymphokine-Activated Killer Cells (LAK)

Significant cardiotoxicity with interleukin-2 alone and in combination with lymphokine-activated killer cells has been documented by all centers involved in these investigations. The incidence of hypotension requiring pharmacologic support with vasopressors was 65% in 317 patients treated at the National Cancer Institute (NCI) (170). Dysrhythmias, primarily supraventricular tachyarrhythmias, occurred in 9.7% of courses. Angina or ischemic changes were noted in 2.6% of patients and myocardial infarction in 1.5%. Hemodynamic changes seen in patients receiving IL-2/LAK therapy consisted of a decrease in mean arterial pressure and systemic vascular resistance with an increase in heart rate and cardiac index (161,171). Cardiac dysfunction with significantly decreased stroke index and left ventricular stroke work associated with a reduction in left ventricular ejection fraction was also noted in the NCI study. Complete heart block has been documented in one patient (172). Severe myocarditis with lymphocytic and eosinophilic infiltrates with areas of myocardial necrosis on autopsy have been documented in one patient on high-dose IL-2 therapy (173). The hemodynamic changes seen are consistent with those seen in early septic shock (174). The etiology of the hypotension is thought to be due to an increase in vascular permeability (capillary leak phenomenon) leading to both a decrease in intravascular volume and a reduction in systemic vascular resistance (164, 175). The actual mechanism by which this high-output/low-resistance state occurs is currently unknown. Leading possibilities include a direct effect of IL-2 or an indirect effect mediated by another cytokine or substance released by IL-2. Investigational studies with IL-2 in various schedules and doses are ongoing.

SUMMARY

Cardiotoxicity primarily due to treatment with anthracyclines continues to provide a fertile area of research for scientists and physicians. Further research is required to unravel the precise mechanism of anthracycline cardiotoxicity. The search for a less cardiotoxic but equivalent cytotoxic anthracycline analog continues to be an active focus of preclinical and clinical research. With the increasing use of antineoplastics in the treatment of malignant disease, there has been increased recognition of varied cardiac effects with multiple agents. Undoubtedly, this body of knowledge will continue to grow and result in additional research questions over the coming years.

REFERENCES

1. Blum RH, Carter SK. Adriamycin: a new anticancer drug with significant clinical activity. *Ann Intern Med* 1974;80:249–259.
2. Young RC, Ozols RF, Myers CE. The anthracycline antineoplastic drugs. *N Engl J Med* 1981;305:139–153.
3. Minow RA, Benjamin RS, Gottleib JA. Adriamycin (NSC-123127) cardiomyopathy—an overview with determination of risk factors. *Cancer Chemother Rep* 1975;6:195–201.
4. Praga C, Beretta G, Vigo PL, et al. Adriamycin cardiotoxicity: a survey of 1273 patients. *Cancer Treat Rep* 1979;63:827–834.
5. Van Hoff DD, Rozenoweig M, Layard M, Slavik M, Muggia FM. Daunomycin-induced cardiotoxicity in children and adults. A review of 110 cases. *Am J Med* 1977;62:200–208.
6. Freiss GG, Boyd JF, Geer MR, Garcia JC. Effects of first-dose doxorubicin on cardiac rhythm as evaluated by continuous 24-hour monitoring. *Cancer* 1985;56:2762–2764.
7. Steinberg JS, Cohen AJ, Wasserman AG. Acute arrhythmogenicity of doxorubicin administration. *Cancer* 1987;60:1213–1218.
8. Wortman JE, Lucas JS, Schuster E, Thiele D, Logue GL. Sudden death during doxorubicin administration. *Cancer* 1979;44:1588–1591.
9. Halazun JF, Wagner HR, Gaeta JF, Sinks LF. Daunorubicin cardiac toxicity in children with acute lymphocytic leukemia. *Cancer* 1974;33:545–554.
10. LaFrak EA, Pitha J, Rosenheim S, O'Bryan RM, Burgess MA, Gottleib JA. Adriamycin (NSC 123127) cardiomyopathy. *Cancer Chemother Rep* 1975;6(3):203–208.
11. Von Hoff DD, Laylard MW, Basa P, Davis HL, Von Hoff AL, Rozenoweig M, Muggia FM. Risk factors for doxorubicin-induced congestive heart failure. *Ann Intern Med* 1979;91:710–717.
12. Freter CE, Lee TC, Billingham ME, Chak L, Bristow MR. Doxorubicin cardiac toxicity manifesting seven years after treatment. *Am J Med* 1986;80:483–485.
13. Lipshultz SE, Colan SD, Gelber RD, Perez-Atayde AR, Sallan SE, Sanders SP. Late cardiac effects of doxorubicin therapy for acute lymphoblastic leukemia in childhood. *N Engl J Med* 1991;324:808–815.
14. Bonadonna G, Beretta G, Tancini G, et al. Adriamycin (NSC-123127) studies at the Instituto Nazionale Tumori, Milan. *Cancer Chemother Rep* 1975;6(2):231–245.
15. Cortes EP, Lutman G, Wanka J, Wang JJ, Pickren J, Wallacae J, Holland JF. Adriamycin (NSC-123127) cardiotoxicity: a clinicopathologic correlation. *Cancer Chemother Rep* 1975;6((2):215–225.
16. Jones RB, Holland JF, Bhardwaj S, Norton L, Wilfinger C, Strashun A. A phase I–II study of intensive-dose adriamycin for advanced breast cancer. *J Clin Oncol* 1987;5:172–177.
17. Weiss AJ, Metter GE, Fletcher WS, Wilson WL, Grage TB, Ramirez G. Studies on adriamycin using a weekly regimen demonstrating its clinical effectiveness and lack of cardiac toxicity. *Cancer Chemother Rep* 1976;60:813–822.
18. Chlebowski R, Pugh R, Paroly W, Heuser J, Pajak T, Jacobs E, Bateman JR. Adriamycin on a weekly schedule: clinically effective with low incidence of cardiotoxicity. *Clin Res* 1979;27:53A.
19. Legha SS, Benjamin RS, Mackay B, et al. Reduction of doxorubicin cardiotoxicity by prolonged continuous intravenous infusion. *Ann Intern Med* 1982;96:133–139.

20. Lum BL, Svee JM, Torti FM. Doxorubicin: alteration of dose scheduling as a means of reducing cardiotoxicity. *Drug Intell Clin Pharm* 1985;19:259–264.
21. Gundersen S, Kvinnsland S, Klepp O, Kvaloy S, Lund E, Host H. Weekly adriamycin versus VAC in advanced breast cancer. A randomized trial. *Eur J Cancer Clin Oncol* 1986;22(12):1431–1434.
22. Bristow MR, Mason JW, Billingham ME, Daniels JR. Doxorubicin cardiomyopathy: evaluation by phonocardiography, endomyocardial biopsy, and cardiac catheterization. *Ann Intern Med* 1978;88:168–175.
23. Merrill J, Greco FA, Zimbler H, et al. Adriamycin and radiation: synergistic cardiotoxicity. *Ann Intern Med* 1975;82:122–123.
24. Kushner JP, Hansen VL, Hammar SP. Cardiomyopathy after widely separated courses of adriamycin exacerbated by actinomycin-D and mithramycin. *Cancer* 1975;36:1577–1584.
25. Smith PJ, Ekert H, Waters KD, Matthews RN. High incidence of cardiomyopathy in children treated with adriamycin and DTIC in combination chemotherapy. *Cancer Treat Rep* 1977;61:1736–1738.
26. Buzdar AV, Legha SS, Tashima CK, et al. Adriamycin and mitomycin-C: possible synergistic cardiotoxicity. *Cancer Treat Rep* 1978;62:1005–1008.
27. Watts RG. Severe and fatal anthracycline cardiotoxicity at cumulative doses below 400 mg/m^2: evidence for enhanced toxicity with multiagent chemotherapy. *Am J Hematol* 1991;36:217–218.
28. Minow RA, Benjamin RS, Leo ET, Gottlieb JA. Adriamycin cardiomyopathy—risk factors. *Cancer* 1977;39:1397–1402.
29. Alexander J, Dainiak N, Berger HJ, et al. Serial assessment of doxorubicin cardiotoxicity with quantitative radionuclide angiocardiography. *N Engl J Med* 1979;300:278–283.
30. Singer JW, Narahara KA, Ritchie JL, Hamilton GW, Kennedy JW. Time and dose-dependent changes in ejection fraction determined by radionuclide angiography after anthracycline therapy. *Cancer Treat Rep* 1978;62:945.
31. Palmeri ST, Bonow RO, Myers CE, et al. Prospective evaluation of doxorubicin cardiotoxicity by rest and exercise radionuclide angiography. *Am J Cardiol* 1986;58:607–613.
32. Bloom KR, Bini RM, Williams CM, Sonley MJ, Gribbin MA. Echocardiography in adriamycin cardiotoxicity. *Cancer* 1978;41:1265–1269.
33. Marchandise B, Schroeder E, Boslv A, Doyen C, Weynants P, Kremer R, Pouleur H. Early detection of doxorubicin cardiotoxicity: interest of Doppler echocardiographic analysis of the left ventricular filling dynamics. *Am Heart J* 1989;118:92–98.
34. Weesner KM, Bledsoe M, Chauvenet A, Wofford M. Exercise echocardiography in the detection of anthracycline cardiotoxicity. *Cancer* 1991;68:435–438.
35. Greco FA. Subclinical adriamycin cardiotoxicity: detection by timing the arterial sounds. *Cancer Treat Rep* 1978;62:901–905.
36. Billingham ME, Bristow MR, Glatstein E, Mason JW, Masek MA, Daniels JR. Adriamycin cardiotoxicity: endomyocardial biopsy evidence of enhancement by irradiation. *Am J Surg Pathol* 1977;1:17–23.
37. Marshall RC, Berger HJ, Reduto LA, Gottschalk A, Zaret BL. Variability in sequential measures of left ventricular performance assessed with radionuclide angiocardiography. *Am J Cardiol* 1978;41:531–536.
38. Ewer MS, Ali MK, Mackay B, et al. A comparison of cardiac biopsy grades and ejection fraction estimations in patients receiving adriamycin. *J Clin Oncol* 1984;2:112–117.
39. Steinberg JS, Wasserman AG. Radionuclide ventriculography for evaluation and prevention of doxorubicin cardiotoxicity. *Clin Ther* 1985;7:660–667.
40. Piver MS, Marchetti DL, Parthasarathy KL, Bakshi S, Reese P. Doxorubicin hydrochloride (adriamycin) cardiotoxicity evaluated by sequential radionuclide angiocardiography. *Cancer* 1985;56:76–80.
41. Pigram WJ, Fuller W, Amilton LDH. Stereochemistry of intercalation: interaction of daunomycin with DNA. *Nature* 1972;235:17–19.
42. Murphree SA, Cunningham LS, Hwang KM, et al. Effects of adriamycin on surface properties of sarcoma 180 ascites cells. *Biochem Pharmacol* 1976;25:1227–1231.

43. Sinha BK. Binding specificity of chemically and enzymatically activated anthracycline anticancer agents to nucleic acids. *Chem Biol Interact* 1980;30:67–77.

44. Tewey KM, Chen GI, Nelson EM, Lui LF. Intercalative antitumor drugs interfere with the breakage–reunion reaction of mammalian DNA topoisomerase II. *J Biol Chem* 1984;259:9182–9187.

45. Janke RA. An anthracycline antibiotic-induced cardiomyopathy in rabbits. *Lab Invest* 1974;30:292–303.

46. Meyers CE, McGuire WP, Liss RH, Ifrim I, Grotzinger K, Young RC. Adriamycin: the role of lipid peroxidation in cardiac toxicity and tumor response. *Science* 1977;197:165–167.

47. Billingham ME. Some recent advances in cardiac pathology. *Hum Pathol* 1979;10:367–386.

48. Singal PK, Segstro RJ, Singh RP, Kutryk MJ. Changes in lysosomal morphology and enzyme activities during the development of adriamycin-induced cardiomyopathy. *Can J Cardiol* 1985;1:139–147.

49. Olson HM, Young DM, Prieur DJ, LeRoy AF, Reagan RL. Electrolyte and morphologic alterations of myocardium in adriamycin-treated rabbits. *Am J Pathol* 1974; 77:439–454.

50. Ferrans VJ. Overview of cardiac pathology in relation to anthracycline cardiotoxicity. *Cancer Treat Rep* 1978;62:955–961.

51. Doroshow JH. Effect of anthracycline antibiotics on oxygen radical formation in rat heart. *Cancer Res* 1983;43:460–472.

52. Rajagopalan S, Politi PM, Sinha BK, Myers CE. Adriamycin-induced free radical formation in the perfused rat heart: implications for cardiotoxicity. *Cancer Res* 1988; 48:4766–4769.

53. Singal PK, Pierce GN. Adriamycin stimulates low-affinity Ca^{++} binding and lipid peroxidation but depresses myocardial function. *Am J Physiol* 1986;250:H419–H425.

54. Doroshow JH. Role of reactive oxygen production in doxorubicin cardiac toxicity. In: Hacker MP, Lazo JS, Tritton TR, eds. *Organ directed toxicities of anticancer drugs.* The Hague: Martinus Nijhoff; 1988:31–40.

55. Abramson JJ, Salama G. Sulfhydryl oxidation and calcium release from sarcoplasmic reticulum. *Mol Cell Biochem* 1988;82:81–84.

56. Olson RD, Mushlin PS. Doxorubicin cardiotoxicity: analysis of prevailing hypotheses. *FASEB J* 1990;4:3076–3086.

57. Olson HM, Young DM, Prieur DJ, LeRoy AF, Reagan RL. Electrolyte and morphologic alterations of myocardium in adriamycin-treated rabbits. *Am J Pathol* 1974; 77:439–454.

58. Azuma J, Sperelakis N, Hasegawa H, et al. Adriamycin cardiotoxicity: possible pathogenic mechanisms. *J Mol Cell Cardiol* 1981;13:381–397.

59. Zweier JL, Gianni L, Muindi J, Myers CE. Differences in O_2 reduction by the iron complexes of adriamycin and daunomycin: the importance of side chain hydroxyl group. *Biochim Biophys Acta* 1986;884:326–336.

60. Singal PK, Forbes MS, Sperelakis N. Occurrence of intramitochondrial Ca^{++} granules in a hypertrophied heart exposed to adriamycin. *Can J Physiol Pharmacol* 1983; 62:1239–1244.

61. Revis N, Marusic N. Effects of doxorubicin and its aglycone metabolite on calcium sequestration by rabbit heart, liver, and kidney mitochondria. *Life Sci* 1979;25:1055–1064.

62. Jensen RA. Doxorubicin cardiotoxicity: contractile changes after long term treatment in the rat. *J Pharmacol Exp Ther* 1986;236:197–203.

63. Maisch B, Gregor O, Zuess M, Kocksiek K. Acute effect of calcium channel blockers on adriamycin exposed adult cardiocytes. *Basic Res Cardiol* 1985;80:626–635.

64. Rabkin SW. Interaction of external calcium concentrations and verapamil on the effects of doxorubicin (adriamycin) in the isolated heart preparation. *J Cardiovasc Pharmacol* 1983;5:848–855.

65. Suzuki T, Kanda H, Kawai Y, Tominaga K, Murata K. Cardiotoxicity of anthracycline antineoplastic drugs—clinicopathological and experimental studies. *Jpn Circ J* 1979;43: 1000–1008.

66. Bristow MR, Kantrowitz NE, Harrison WD, Minobe WA, Sageman WS, Billingham

ME. Mediation of subacute anthracycline cardiotoxicity in rabbits by cardiac histamine release. *J Cardiovasc Pharmacol* 1983;5:913.

67. Klugman FB, Decorti G, Candussio L, Grill V, Mallardi F, Baldini L. Inhibitors of adriamycin-induced histamine release *in vitro* limit adriamycin cardiotoxicity *in vivo*. *Br J Cancer* 1986;54:743–748.

68. Del Tacca M, Danesi R, Ducci M, Bernardini C, Romanini A. Might adriamycinol contribute to adriamycin-induced cardiotoxicity? *Pharmacol Res Commun* 1985;17:1073–1084.

69. Boucek RJ, Olson RD, Brenner DE, Ogunbumni EM, Inui M, Fleischer S. The major metabolite of doxorubicin is a potent inhibitor of membrane-associated ion pumps: a correlative study of cardiac muscle with isolated membrane fractions. *J Biol Chem* 1987;262:15851–15856.

70. Olson RD, Mushlin PS, Brenner DE, et al. Doxorubicin cardiotoxicity may be due to its metabolite, doxorubicinol. *Proc Natl Acad Sci USA* 1988;85:3585–3589.

71. Peters JH, Gordon GR, Kashiwase D, Acton EM. Tissue distribution of doxorubicin and doxorubicinol in rats receiving multiple doses of doxorubicin. *Cancer Chemother Pharmacol* 1981;7:65–70.

72. Cortes EP. Adriamycin cardiotoxicity: early detection by systolic time interval and possible prevention by coenzyme Q10. *Cancer Treat Rep* 1978;62:887.

73. Doroshow JH, Locker GY, Ifrim I, Myers CE. Prevention of doxorubicin cardiotoxicity in the mouse by *N*-acetylcysteine. *J Clin Invest* 1981;68:1053–1064.

74. Milei J, Marantz A, Ale J, Vazquez A, Buceta JE. Prevention of adriamycin-induced cardiotoxicity by prenylamine: a pilot double blind study. *Cancer Drug Delivery* 1987;4:129–136.

75. Speyer JL, Green MD, Jacquotte AZ, et al. ICRF-187 permits longer treatment with doxorubicin in women with breast cancer. *J Clin Oncol* 1992;10:117–127.

76. Combs AB, Kishi T, Poter TH, Folkers K. Models for clinical disease. I. Biochemical cardiotoxicity of coenzyme Q_{10} inhibitor in rats. *Res Commun Chem Pathol Pharmacol* 1976;13:333–339.

77. Bertazzoli C, Sala L, Tosano MG. Antagonistic action of ubiquinone on experimental cardiotoxicity of adriamycin in isolated rabbit heart. *Int Res Commun Sys Med Sci* 1975;3:367.

78. Bertazzoli C, Sala L, Socia E, Ghione M. Experimental adriamycin cardiotoxicity prevented by ubiquinone *in vivo*. *Int Res Commun Sys Med Sci* 1975;3:468.

79. Langsjoen PH, Langsjoen PH, Folkers K. A six-year clinical study of therapy of cardiomyopathy with coenzyme Q_{10}. *Int J Tissue Reactions* 1990;12(3):169–171.

80. Milei J, Vazquez A, Boveris A, et al. The role of prenylamine in the prevention of adriamycin-induced cardiotoxicity. A review of experimental and clinical findings. *J Int Med Res* 1988;16:19–30.

81. Milei J, Marantz A, Ale J, Vazquez A, Buceta JE. Prevention of adriamycin-induced cardiotoxicity by prenylamine: a pilot double blind study. *Cancer Drug Delivery* 1987;4:129–136.

82. Myers CE, Bonow R, Palmeri S, et al. A randomized controlled trial assessing the prevention of doxorubicin cardiomyopathy by *N*-acetylcysteine. *Semin Oncol* 1983;10(1 suppl 1):53–55.

83. Von Hoff DD, Howser D, Lewis B, Holcenberg J, Weiss R, Young RC. Phase I study of ICRF-187 using a daily for 3 days schedule. *Cancer Treat Rep* 1981;65:249–252.

84. Hasinoff BB. The interaction of the cardioprotective agent ICRF-187 ((+);-1,2-bis(3,5-dioxopiperazinyl-1-yl)propane); its hydrolysis product (ICRF-198); and other chelating agents with the Fe(III) and Cu(II) complexes of adriamycin. *Agents Actions* 1990;29:374–381.

85. Balazsovits JAE, Mayer LD, Bally MB, Cullis PR, McDonnell M, Ginsberg RS, Falk RE. Analysis of the effect of liposome encapsulation on the vesicant properties, acute and cardiac toxicities, and antitumor efficacy of doxorubicin. *Cancer Chemother Pharmacol* 1989;23:81–86.

86. Treat J, Greenspan A, Forst D, et al. Anti-tumor activity of liposome-encapsulated doxorubicin in advanced breast cancer: Phase II study. *J Natl Cancer Inst* 1990;82:1706–1710.

87. Weiss RB, Sarosy G, Clagett-Carl K, Russo M, Leyland-Jones B. Anthracycline

analogs: the past, present, and future. *Cancer Chemother Pharmacol* 1986;18:185–197.

88. Ringenberg QS, Propert KJ, Muss HB, et al. Clinical cardiotoxicity of esorubicin (4'-deoxydoxorubicin,DxDx): prospective studies with serial gated heart scans and reports of selected cases. *Invest New Drugs* 1990;8:221–226.

89. Jain KK, Casper ES, Geller NL, et al. A prospective randomized comparison of epirubicin and doxorubicin in patients with advanced breast cancer. *J Clin Oncol* 1985;3:818–826.

90. Havsteen H, Brynjolf I, Svahn T, Dombernowsky P, Godtfredsen J, Munck O. Prospective evaluation of chronic cardiotoxicity due to high-dose epirubicin of combination chemotherapy with cyclophosphamide, methotrexate, and 5-fluorouracil. *Cancer Chemother Pharmacol* 1989;23:101–104.

91. Dardir MD, Ferrans VJ, Mikhael YS, et al. Cardiac morphologic and functional changes induced by epirubicin chemotherapy. *J Clin Oncol* 1989;7:947–958.

92. Nielsen D, Jensen JB, Dombernowsky O, et al. Epirubicin cardiotoxicity: a study of 135 patients with advanced breast cancer. *J Clin Oncol* 1990;8:1806–1810.

93. Macchiarini P, Danesi R, Mariotti R, et al. Phase II study of high-dose epirubicin in untreated patients with small-cell lung cancer. *Am J Clin Oncol* 1990;13(4):302–307.

94. Berman E, Wittes RE, Leyland-Jones B, et al. Phase I and clinical pharmacology studies of intravenous and oral administration of 4-demethoxydaunorubicin in patients with advanced cancer. *Cancer Res* 1983;43:6096–6101.

95. Daghestani AN, Arlin ZA, Leyland-Jones B, et al. Phase I and II clinical and pharmacological study of 4-demethoxydaunorubicin (idarubicin) in adult patients with acute leukemia. *Cancer Res* 1985;45:1408–1412.

96. Tan CTC, Hancock C, Steinherz P, et al. Phase I clinical pharmacological study of 4-demethoxydaunorubicin (idarubicin) in children with advanced cancer. *Cancer Res* 1987;47:2990–2995.

97. Kris MG, Gralla RJ, Kelsen DP, et al. Phase II trial of oral 4-demethoxydaunorubicin in patients with non-small cell lung cancer. *Am J Clin Oncol* 1985;8:377–379.

98. Martoni A, Pacciarini MA, Pannuti F. Activity of 4-demethoxydaunorubicin by the oral route in advanced breast cancer. *Eur J Cancer Clin Oncol* 1985;21:803–806.

99. Gillies H, Liang R, Rogers H, et al. Phase II trial of idarubicin in patients with advanced lymphoma. *Cancer Chemother Pharmacol* 1988;21:261–264.

100. Chisesi T, Capnist G, De Dominicis E, Dini E. A phase II study of idarubicin (4-demethoxydaunorubicin) in advanced myeloma. *Eur J Cancer Clin Oncol* 1988;24:681–684.

101. Villani F, Galimberti M, Comazzi R, Crippa F. Evaluation of cardiac toxicity of idarubicin (4-demethoxydaunorubicin). *Eur J Cancer Clin Oncol* 1989;25:13–18.

102. Shenkenberg TD, Von Hoff DD. Mitoxantrone: a new anticancer drug with significant clinical activity. *Ann Intern Med* 1986;105:67–81.

103. Gams RA, Wesler MJ. Mitoxantrone cardiotoxicity: results from Southeastern Cancer Study Group. *Cancer Treat Symp* 1984;3:31–33.

104. Clark GM, Tokaz LK, Von Hoff DD, Thoi LL, Coltman CA Jr. Cardiotoxicity in patients treated with mitoxantrone on Southwest Oncology Group phase II protocols. *Cancer Treat Symp* 1984;3:25–30.

105. Bennett JM, Muss HD, Doroshow JH, et al. A randomized multicenter trial comparing mitoxantrone, cyclophosphamide, and fluorouracil in the therapy of metastatic breast carcinoma. *J Clin Oncol* 1988;6:1611–1620.

106. Schell FC, Yap H-Y, Blumenschein G, Valdivieso M, Bidey M. Potential cardiotoxicity with mitoxantrone. *Cancer Treat Rep* 1982;66:1641–1643.

107. Coleman RE, Maisey MN, Khight RK, Rubens RD. Mitoxantrone in advanced breast cancer—a phase II study with special attention to cardiotoxicity. *Eur J Cancer Clin Oncol* 1982;20:771–776.

108. Aapro MS, Alberts DS, Woolfenden JM, Mackel C. Prospective study of left ventricular function using radionuclide scans in patients receiving mitoxantrone. *Invest New Drugs* 1983;1:341–347.

109. Unverferth DV, Bashore TM, Magrien RD, Fetters JK, Neidhart JA. Histologic and functional characteristics of human heart after mitoxantrone therapy. *Cancer Treat Symp* 1984;3:47–53.

110. Crossley RJ. Clinical safety and tolerance of mitoxantrone. *Semin Oncol* 1984;11(3 suppl 1):54–58.

111. Posner LE, Dukart G, Goldberg J, Bernstein T, Cartwright K. Mitoxantrone: an overview of safety and toxicity. *Invest New Drugs* 1985;3:123–132.
112. Henderson BM, Dougherty WJ, James VC, Tilley LP, Noble JF. Safety assessment of a new anticancer compound, mitoxantrone, in beagle dogs: comparison with doxorubicin. I. Clinical observations. *Cancer Treat Rep* 1982;66:1139–1143.
113. Sparano BM, Gordon G, Hall C, Iatropoulos MJ, Noble JF. Safety assessment of a new anticancer compound, mitoxantrone, in beagle dogs: comparison with doxorubicin. II. Histologic and ultrastructural pathology. *Cancer Treat Rep* 1982;66:1145–1158.
114. Kharasch ED, Novak RF. Inhibition of adriamycin-stimulated microsomal lipid peroxidation by mitoxantrone and ametantrone, two new anthracenedione antineoplastic agents. *Biochem Biophys Res Commun* 1982;108:1346–1352.
115. O'Connell TX, Berenbaum MC. Cardiac and pulmonary effects of high doses of cyclophosphamide and isophosphamide. *Cancer Res* 1974;34:1586–1591.
116. Applebaum FR, Strauchen JA, Graw GR Jr, Savage DD, Kent KM, Ferrans VJ, Herzig CP. Acute lethal carditis caused by high dose combination chemotherapy. *Lancet* 1976;1:58–62.
117. Goldberg MA, Antin JH, Guinan EC, Rappeport JM. Cyclophosphamide cardiotoxicity: an analysis of dosing as a risk factor. *Blood* 1986;68:1114–1118.
118. Gottdiener JS, Applebaum FR, Ferrans VJ, Deisseroth A, Zeigler J. Cardiotoxicity associated with high-dose cyclophosphamide therapy. *Arch Intern Med* 1981;141:758–763.
119. Slavin RE, Millan JC, Mullins CM. Pathology of high dose intermittent cyclophosphamide therapy. *Hum Pathol* 1975;6:693–709.
120. Friedman HS, Colvin OM, Aisaka K, et al. Glutathione protects cardiac and skeletal muscle from cyclophosphamide-induced toxicity. *Cancer Res* 1990;50(8):2455–2462.
121. Trigg ME, Finlay JL, Bozdech M, Gilnbert E. Fatal cardiac toxicity in bone marrow transplant patients receiving cytosine arabinoside, cyclophosphamide, and total body irradiation. *Cancer* 1987;59:38–42.
122. Cazin B, Gorin NC, Laporte JP, et al. Cardiac complications after bone marrow transplantation. *Cancer* 1986;57:2061–2069.
123. Braverman AC, Antin JH, Plappert MT, Cook EF, Lee RT. Cyclophosphamide cardiotoxicity in bone marrow transplantation: a prospective evaluation of new dosing regimens. *J Clin Oncol* 1991;9:1215–1223.
124. La Bianca R, Beretta G, Clerici M, et al. Cardiac toxicity of 5-fluorouracil: a study of 1083 patients. *Tumori* 1982;68:505–510.
125. Dent RG, McCall I. 5-Fluorouracil and angina. *Lancet* 1975;1:347–348.
126. Jakubowski AA, Kemeny N. Hypotension as a manifestation of cardiotoxicity in three patients receiving cisplatin and 5-fluorouracil. *Cancer* 1988;62:266–269.
127. Rezkalla S, Kloner RA, Enslev J, et al. Continuous ambulatory ECG monitoring during fluorouracil therapy: a prospective study. *J Clin Oncol* 1989;7:509–514.
128. Chaudary S, Song SYT, Jaski BE. Profound yet reversible heart failure secondary to 5-fluorouracil. *Am J Med* 1988;85:454–456.
129. McKendall GR, Shurman A, Anamur M, Most AS. Toxic cardiogenic shock associated with infusion of 5-fluorouracil. *Am Heart J* 1988;118:184–186.
130. Martin M, Diaz-Rubio E, Furio V, Blazquez J, Almenarez J, Farina J. Lethal cardiac toxicity after cisplatin and 5-fluorouracil chemotherapy. *Am J Clin Oncol* 1989;12(3):229–234.
131. Collins C, Weiden PL. Cardiotoxicity of 5-fluorouracil. *Cancer Treat Rep* 1987;71:733–736.
132. Freeman NJ, Costanza ME. 5-Fluorouracil-associated cardiotoxicity. *Cancer* 1988;61:36–45.
133. Ensley JF, Patel B, Kloner R, Kish JA, Wynne J, Al-Surraf M. The clinical syndrome of 5-fluorouracil cardiotoxicity. *Invest New Drugs* 1989;7:101–109.
134. Oleksowicz L, Bruckner HW. Prophylaxis of 5-fluorouracil induces coronary vasospasm with calcium channel blockers. *Am J Med* 1988;85:750–751.
135. Kleiman NS, Lehane DE, Geyer CE, Pratt CM, Young JB. Prinzmetal's angina during 5-fluorouracil chemotherapy. *Am J Med* 1987;82:566–568.
136. Patel B, Kloner RA, Ensley J, Al-Surraf M, Kish J, Wynne J. 5-Fluorouracil cardiotoxicity: left ventricular dysfunction and effect of coronary vasodilators. *Am J Med Sci* 1987;294:238–243.

Cardiovascular Toxicology, Second Edition,
edited by Daniel Acosta, Jr.
Raven Press, Ltd., New York © 1992.

8

Cardiovascular Toxicity of Antibacterial Antibiotics

*Rebecca S. Keller, †‡Janet L. Parker, and
*‡H. Richard Adams

*Departments of *Veterinary Biomedical Sciences and †Physiology, and ‡the Dalton
Research Center, University of Missouri–Columbia, Columbia, Missouri 65211*

Toxic side effects of clinically important antibacterial antibiotics usually can be explained either by hypersensitivity (allergic reactions) or by cytotoxic lesions in susceptible tissues after repeated treatment. Occasionally, however, untoward patient responses to antibiotics are encountered that can be explained neither by immunologic mechanisms nor by overt cytotoxicity damage. Rather, the chemical structures of some antibiotic molecules allow them to pose as native ligands and to therefore be recognized by specific binding domains on excitable membranes of eukaryotic cells. The resulting interaction between the antibiotic-ligand and the receptive membrane binding site modulates or even prevents the normal membrane functions associated with these sites, thereby leading to dysfunction of homeostatic regulatory activities of the affected host cell.

Indeed, there is considerable evidence that the pharmacodynamic profiles of certain antibiotic agents encompass direct actions on peripheral cardiorespiratory control mechanisms that can be explained best by antibiotic interaction with membrane binding sites of host cells. Antibiotics chemically related to neomycin and streptomycin (i.e., the aminoglycosides) are exemplary in this respect [1–15]. These drugs retard somatic neuromuscular function via an inhibitory action at the prejunctional terminal of motor axons [16]; they also disrupt excitation–contraction coupling across the sarcolemmal membrane of vascular smooth muscle and myocardium [1,5,7,15]. These actions share a common basic mechanism in that aminoglycoside antibiotics reversibly interact with Ca^{2+} binding domains on excitable membranes of neurons, vascular smooth muscle, and cardiac myocyte [6,14,16]. Much less is known about the mechanisms whereby other types of antibiotics disrupt cardiovascular functions.

The clinical significance of the direct cardiovascular depressant actions of antibiotics remains conjectural, but several case reports can be interpreted as support for this contention. Cardiac asystole (17,18), circulatory collapse (19), cardiopulmonary arrest (20), cardiac dysrhythmias (21), cardiac decompensation in congestive heart failure (22), and hypotensive episodes (19,23–25) have been linked to antibiotic administration. However, little definitive information is available about either the clinical importance of antibiotic-related cardiovascular problems or the precise mechanisms responsible for such activities. The present chapter is an overview of this problem area with primary emphasis on the direct cardiovascular actions of the aminoglycoside antibiotics. The authors reviewed this field a decade ago (1,7), and the current chapter comprises a condensation of this earlier information along with an update on more recent publications focusing on cardiovascular toxicity and related membrane actions of antibiotics. Neither an exhaustive examination of all antibiotics nor a review of all related publications was attempted. Rather, our goal was to consider selected key reports that best typify the types of cardiovascular toxicities that can be associated with direct membrane actions of antibacterial antibiotics. Circulatory disturbances associated with anaphylactic reactions to antibiotics or cytotoxicity of antineoplastic antibiotics were not considered in this discussion.

CLINICAL REPORTS

Direct cardiovascular toxicity of antibiotics is encountered infrequently during the therapy of bacterial infections, thus leading to the general understanding that antibacterial antibiotics are innocuous to the heart and vasculature. Certainly this assumption is valid relative to the management of uncomplicated infections in otherwise uncompromised patients. However, appropriate antimicrobial therapy and its unquestionable beneficial results have led to the frequent use of these drugs without reconsideration by the clinician of potential cardiovascular toxicities. Although antibiotics are rarely considered when untoward hemodynamic responses are examined for etiologic or iatrogenic factors, episodes of circulatory dysfunction related to antibiotics occasionally have been detected in individuals with primary circulatory disease or serious systemic illness.

In an early report over 30 years ago, Swain et al. (26) referred to "peripheral circulatory disturbances" and anginal syndrome in tubercular patients treated with large doses of streptomycin; circulatory collapse was seen with chloramphenicol. Hypotensive episodes occurred during therapy with gentamicin (24,25,87), streptomycin (19,23,62), neomycin (19), lincomycin (17), and kanamycin (18). Such hemodynamic responses usually were not attributed to direct cardiovascular depressant effects of the involved antibiotics, but were unexplained or assumed to be secondary to bacteremia or respiratory depression. For instance, cardiorespiratory arrest occurred shortly after intravenous administration of a kanamycin overdosage in a patient seriously ill with abdominal abscessation, and Ream (18) assumed that this episode of cardiac standstill was secondary to apnea and hypoxemia. However, the immediate onset of cardiac asystole suggests that direct myocardial depression was involved.

More than 250 case reports of acute adverse patient responses to antibiotic therapy were reviewed by Pittinger et al. (19) in 1970. The majority of these problems were associated with the concurrent administration of anesthetics, muscle relaxants, or other antibiotics. Most attention was directed toward the respiratory depressant effects of the antibiotics as responsible mechanisms. Several cases of circulatory collapse, some terminating in death, were reported (19).

Hypotension was detected by Cohen et al. (23) in a patient treated with streptomycin during the postoperative period after heart surgery. These investigators believed that a myocardial depressant action of streptomycin was responsible, owing to an accumulation of the antibiotic in the serum secondary to renal dysfunction (23); they did not consider the related possibility that myocardial depression associated with surgery could have predisposed the heart to the deleterious action of streptomycin.

In 1990, Nattel et al. (21) reported on several clinical episodes of a bizarre type of cardiac dysrhythmia produced by erythromycin. This antibiotic can induce a long QT syndrome with accompanying ventricular tachycardia characterized as a form of "torsades de pointes." Nattel et al. (21) cautioned that ECG monitoring may be wise when intravenous erythromycin is used in patients with predisposing factors for long QT syndrome, such as hypokalemia and hypomagnesemia or pretreatment with antiarrhythmic drugs.

Although controlled studies in humans are not available, the nature of antibiotic-induced cardiovascular effects is no doubt dependent on the rate and route of administration, as well as on the total amount of the drug. With lincomycin, for example, Novak et al. (27) found that intravenous infusion of up to 1.5 g over 60 min produced no significant cardiovascular changes. However, Waisbren (20) reported on four cases of cardiopulmonary arrest after rapid intravenous administration of large doses of this antibiotic. Daubeck et al. (17) successfully resuscitated a lincomycin-treated patient after 90 min of cardiac arrest; arrest was attributed to massive intravenous overdosage of the antibiotic.

Daynes (22) associated streptomycin administration with an exacerbation of heart failure in patients with advanced pulmonary tuberculosis. A considerable number of the tuberculous patients with chronic congestive heart failure died soon after beginning therapy with streptomycin, isoniazid, and ethionamide. Daynes (22) suggested that the myocardial depressant action of streptomycin was involved, and he reported a decreased mortality rate when kanamycin was substituted for streptomycin. However, since kanamycin can also depress cardiac function (12,23,28), the causal relationship between streptomycin and heart failure in these cases is tenuous.

Indeed, it should be emphasized that a direct causal relationship between antibiotics and cardiovascular depression was rarely established in the above-mentioned reports. Evaluation of adverse patient responses was retrospective and evidence for antibiotic participation usually was circumstantial at best. However, because of the serious outcome of some of the clinical episodes, investigators have attempted to identify and characterize cardiovascular depressant actions of antibiotics using laboratory animals as test subjects. Based on such studies, the circulatory effects of certain antibiotics reflect a net response dependent on changes in several different physiologic systems. Some antibiotics, for instance, can (a) directly depress the heart and vasculature, (b) indirectly affect these tissues secondarily to respiratory insufficiency, and even (c) disrupt autonomic control of the circulation.

RESPIRATORY DEPRESSANT ACTIONS

Clinical recognition of respiratory depressant actions of antibiotics can be traced to Pridgen in 1956 (29). He reported that two infants developed apnea and later died subsequent to intraperitoneal lavage with neomycin. Pridgen (29) suggested that the antibiotic exerted a neuromuscular blocking effect that led to respiratory paralysis. Numerous clinical and research studies have validated that neomycin and other aminoglycosides do indeed possess neuromuscular blocking properties (16,19,30–33). Considerably less information is available about the neuromuscular effects of other antibiotics that also exert this action, such as the tetracyclines, lincomycin, and polymyxins (16,31,34–52).

The actions of antibiotics at the somatic neuromuscular junction are important to the present discussion for two major reasons. First, and obviously, if the respiratory depressant effects are sufficient to impede pulmonary exchange of oxygen and carbon dioxide, then the cardiovascular system will be affected by hypoxemia, acidemia, and autonomic reflex adjustments. Second, the mechanism of the inhibitory action of the aminoglycosides at the motor end plate has provided important information about the basic interaction of these agents with excitable membranes.

The neuromuscular blocking effect of aminoglycoside antibiotics involves two separate mechanisms. First, they exert a prejunctional effect by decreasing the release of the neurotransmitter acetylcholine from the motor neuron (35,36). Second, they also exert a "curare-like" postjunctional blocking effect either by altering the sensitivity of the nicotinic receptor of the skeletal myofiber to acetylcholine or by modulating receptor-coupled ion channel conductance. The prejunctional inhibitory action is generally viewed as the dominant mechanism, but species and even muscle differences may exist (11,16,37).

To delineate prejunctional from postjunctional actions of gentamicin, Torda (38) measured the quantal content of end-plate potential (EPP) along with miniature end-plate potentials (MEPP) and miniature end-plate currents

(MEPC) in a toad sartorius nerve–muscle preparation. Torda (38) observed a marked reduction in the quantal content of the EPP, confirming that gentamicin inhibited neuromuscular transmission by preventing transmitter release from the cholinergic axon terminal. The effects of gentamicin on postjunctional events were not evident until the concentration of gentamicin was increased to an order of magnitude above that necessary for neuromuscular blockade (38).

Caputy and co-workers (39) studied the effects of 14 antibiotics on neuromuscular transmission in a rat nerve–muscle preparation; conclusions from this study were that neomycin has both pre- and postjunctional effects, while tobramycin acts predominantly prejunctionally and netilmicin acts postjunctionally. Fiekers (42) concurred with previous workers and concluded that the major mechanism of neuromuscular blockade by aminoglycosides is a competitive antagonism with Ca^{2+} at a prejunctional site. Fiekers (43) also reported that neomycin and streptomycin have different postjunctional mechanisms. Neomycin interacts with the open configuration of the ionic channels associated with the acetylcholine receptor; whereas streptomycin seemingly blocks the receptor (43).

To more clearly describe the mechanism of antibiotic action at the prejunctional site, Talbot (45) studied the effects of pH on transmitter release and Ca^{2+} antagonism by aminoglycosides in a frog nerve–muscle preparation. Talbot (45) found that a decrease in pH caused potentiation of the inhibitory aminoglycoside actions, due to a possible pH-dependent regulation of the voltage-dependent Ca^{2+}-mediated release of acetylcholine. Atchison and colleagues (47) examined the effects of antibiotics on calcium uptake into isolated nerve terminals; they studied aminoglycosides, lincosamides, tetracyclines, and polymyxins. The results of their experiments confirmed other studies, indicating that the prejunctional mechanism by which aminoglycoside antibiotics induce neuromuscular blockade is by antagonism of Ca^{2+} entry through voltage-gated calcium channels across the axon terminal membrane. In another study of isolated neurons, Nation and Roth (48) proposed that neomycin's prejunctional inhibitory activity is dependent on binding of the antibiotic to axonal membrane phospholipids.

In summary, numerous types of antibiotics can disrupt somatic neuromuscular function, but the responsible mechanisms are varied and often poorly delineated. The neuromuscular actions of the aminoglycoside antibiotics have been relatively well defined. Although aminoglycosides disrupt postjunctional receptor events, their dominant neuromuscular blocking action depends on a decrease in the release of acetylcholine from cholinergic neurons; these agents interfere with the participation of Ca^{2+} in the excitation–secretion coupling process of the axon terminal membrane (16,35,36). This action is reversed by Ca^{2+} in a competitive-like manner (33); in certain details it simulates the inhibitory effects of magnesium; and it depends on a binding of the antibiotic to plasma membrane phospholipids where Ca^{2+} is normally distributed. Studies with other tissues have shown clearly that the

Ca^{2+} antagonistic activity of the aminoglycosides is not restricted to somatic nerve terminals. Indeed, it is manifested in excitable membranes of different tissues in which Ca^{2+} serves as a coupling agent between membrane depolarization and cellular events such as muscle contraction and exocytotic release of neurotransmitters.

AUTONOMIC EFFECTS

In view of basic similarities at all peripheral cholinergic neuroeffector junctions, it is not surprising that antibiotics that inhibit motor end-plate function also interfere with neurotransmission in autonomic ganglia (53–55). The ganglionic blocking effect of the aminoglycosides seems to be due principally to a Ca^{2+}-related decrease in the discharge of acetylcholine from the presynaptic neuron (56). Wright and Collier (56) reported that aminoglycosides similarly decrease the release of the sympathetic neurotransmitter, norepinephrine, from adrenergic axons. Thus the bradycardia and hypotensive responses to the aminoglycosides in intact animals (2,3,13) could be due partly to blockade of sympathetic ganglia and adrenergic neuroeffector junctions of the heart and blood vessels.

Indeed, the fact that bradycardia rather than tachycardia occurs in conjunction with the hypotensive response suggests that these agents either directly suppress the sinoatrial node, inhibit sympathetic reflex drive to the heart, or both. On the other hand, aminoglycosides depress both cardiac and arterial muscles even when these tissues are isolated *in vitro* from autonomic and humoral control factors (7,12,14). The relative importance of autonomic effects in the intact subject remains questionable. The direct influence of these agents on the circulatory system is likely to be more important than effects secondary to autonomic changes but, admittedly, more comparative information is needed in this area.

CARDIOVASCULAR EFFECTS

Background

Relatively few systematic investigations of cardiovascular actions of therapeutically useful antibiotics have been reported. In an early study, Swain et al. (26) found that the canine heart–lung preparation was depressed by several chemically unrelated antibiotics such as chloramphenicol, streptomycin, and tetracycline. Mechanisms were not identified, but potential interactions with digitalis-sensitive functions were suggested. Leaders et al. (57) reported that tetracycline, chloramphenicol, oleandomycin, streptomycin, and dihydrostreptomycin decreased contractile strength of perfused rabbit hearts. Mechanisms were not identified, but streptomycin also decreased coronary flow (57). Since streptomycin decreased myocardial contractile force and thereby reduced myocardial oxygen demand, Leaders et al. (57) did not determine if the decrease in coronary flow produced by this antibiotic was caused by a direct vasoconstrictor action or was secondary to an autoregulated increase in coronary vascular resistance due to the fall in myocardial oxygen demand.

In an interesting study of the canine microcirculation, Stallworth et al. (58) concluded that vascular reactivity and blood pressure could be influenced by commonly used anti-infectious drugs such as penicillin-G-potassium, tetracycline hydrochloride, chloramphenicol sodium succinate, nitrofurantoin sodium, and sodium cephalothin. These investigators reported that three of nine dogs treated with large doses of penicillin-G-potassium developed acute circulatory shock and died. Stallworth et al. (58) attributed these responses to allergic reactions to the penicillin. However, such a high incidence of pencillin sensitivity in a random population of mongrel dogs is exceedingly unlikely, if not impossible. Stallworth et al. (58) did not consider the more obvious explanation of direct cardiac toxicity owing to the large amounts of potassium these dogs received. Bolus injections of potassium salts can evoke cardiac arrest owing to depolarization of excitable membranes and thus electromechanical quiescence of the heart. Penicillin-G-sodium was found to have no discernible cardiovascular effects either in control dogs or in dogs subjected to an experimental form of circulatory shock (13). Ingredients of commercial preparations of antibiotics should be considered by investigators when responsibilities for adverse responses are assigned.

For another example, Gross et al. (59) reported that intravenous injection of a preparation of oxytetracycline in propylene glycol provoked transient sinoatrial arrest and circulatory collapse in unanesthetized calves. This adverse reponse could be reproduced by injection of propylene glycol vehicle but not by aqueous preparations of oxytetracycline (59).

Oxytetracycline in ascorbic acid vehicle was reported by McCullough and Wallace (60) to inhibit vasoconstrictor responses to norepinephrine and histamine in rabbit ear arteries, but mechanisms were not identified. The vascular and sympathetic nervous system activity of oxytetracycline was studied in more detail by Kalsner (61) using rabbit aortic strips and perfused rabbit ear arteries. Kalsner (61) found no evidence for an *in vitro* effect of 0.1 mM oxytetracycline on sympathetic nerve stimulation or contractile responses to norepinephrine. However, a limitation of that study is that only one concentration of oxytetracycline, 0.1 mM, was tested; larger concentrations may well have influenced sympathetic neuroeffector function or vascular reactivity.

Intravenous administration of the macrolide antibotics erythromciyn, oleandomycin, spiramycin, and leucomycin reduced blood pressure in pentobarbital anesthetized dogs (62). The response to erythromycin was not abolished by bilateral cervical sympathectomy, bilateral cervical vagotomy, spinal cord transections, or atropine. The hypotensive action of these anti-biotics was not a direct effect, however, but was apparently secondary to histamine release (62).

Cohen et al. (23) reported on a rather detailed hemodynamic study of several antibiotics in dogs. Intravenous infusions of streptomycin, tetracycline, kanamycin, vancomycin, erythromycin, and colymycin reduced cardiovascular function in a dose-dependent manner. Streptomycin decreased left ventricular pressure and its rate of development ($+dP/dt_{max}$) in Langendorff cat heart preparations, as did tetracycline, kanamycin, vancomycin, and chloramphenicol. Cohen et al. (23) proposed that electrolyte disturbances were probably involved in the cardiac depressant effect of streptomycin; however, they neither suggested nor studied Ca^{2+} as claimed later by De Morais et al. (63) and Sohn and Katz (64).

Aminoglycoside Antibiotics

Taken in concert, the preceding series of experimental studies with various antibiotics provided little information about responsible cellular mechanisms, but yielded convincing evidence that several clinically useful antibiotics could directly affect vascular smooth muscle and cardiac function. Subsequently, studies in different laboratories were directed toward identification of hemodynamic mechanisms of different antibiotics, with much emphasis on the aminoglycosides.

In Vivo Studies

Cardiovascular manifestations of acute toxicity of several antibiotics were studied in nonhuman primates and dogs anesthetized with pentobarbital (2,3,13). These animals were maintained on artificial respiration, thereby avoiding circulatory effects secondary to neuromuscular blockade and respiratory insufficiency. Intravenous administration of penicillin G and cephalothin in doses from 10 to 40 mg per kg body weight produced no discernible circulatory effects (13). In contrast, bolus intravenous injections of large amounts of neomycin, tobramycin, or gentamicin consistently depressed cardiovascular function expressed as dose-dependent reductions of systemic blood pressure, cardiac output, left ventricular contractile force (LVCF), the first derivative of LVCF ($+dP/dt_{max}$), peak systolic left ventricular pressure (LVP), $+dP/dt_{max}$, and heart rate (2,3,13).

As outlined earlier, Vital Brazil and Prado-Franceschi (35,36) suggested that aminoglycosides compete with Ca^{2+} for membrane receptive areas on the somatic nerve terminal, thereby preventing the participation of Ca^{2+} in the excitation–secretion coupling process [see Pittinger and Adamson (16) for review]. Indirect evidence for Ca^{2+}–aminoglycoside antagonism in other tissues can be interpreted from early hemodynamic experiments. For example, Swain et al. (26) observed that Ca^{2+} exerted some antagonistic activity toward the *in vitro* cardiodepressant effects of streptomycin and dihydrostreptomycin. Similarly, Corrado (53), Wolf and Wigton (65), and Pandey et al. (66) reported that circulatory responses to streptomycin were "reversed" or "restored" by Ca^{2+}. The site or specificity of such interactions was not known. Wolf and Wigton (65) speculated that vascular tissue was affected directly; whereas Corrado (53) and Pandey et al. (66) assumed autonomic ganglia were involved.

The specificity of Ca^{2+}–aminoglycoside interaction was tested *in vivo* in a comparative study of the circulatory effects of Ca^{2+} and two other cardiovascular stimulants, isoproterenol and norepinephrine, in primates treated with neomycin (2). The catecholamines rapidly antagonized the hemodynamic depressant effects of the antibiotic, but the positive actions of the amines were only transient. Conversely, cardiovascular functions depressed by neomycin were rapidly restored to, and maintained at, control levels by a single injection of an amount of calcium chloride "equipotent" to the catecholamines. The differing responsiveness to Ca^{2+} and the catecholamines in antibiotic-treated monkeys was interpreted as evidence for a reversible inhibitory action of aminoglycosides on Ca^{2+}-dependent functions in the heart, the vasculature, or both (2).

In Vivo *Studies in Compromised Subjects*

Although direct *in situ* cardiovascular actions of antibiotics are unlikely to be clinically relevant under usual conditions, we were concerned that such actions could be manifested in those individuals already experiencing circulatory instability. We tested this hypothesis by administering different antibiotics to control dogs and to dogs subjected to an experimental form of gram-negative endotoxemia (13). During the circulatory shock model induced by *E. coli* endotoxemia, the cardiovascular depressant actions of aminoglycoside antibiotics were indeed relatively enhanced compared to effects in control dogs, as illustrated with gentamicin in Fig. 1. We advised that rapid intravenous injection of such antibiotics should be approached cautiously in patients with preexisting hemodynamic dysfunctions, and we suggested that the myocardium and the vasculature could be involved in adverse cardiovascular responses of aminoglycoside antibiotics in endotoxemic subjects (13).

Vascular Smooth Muscle

Streptomycin was reported to produce vasodilation in the perfused hindlimb preparation of the dog (23). Wolf and Wigton (65) later confirmed the

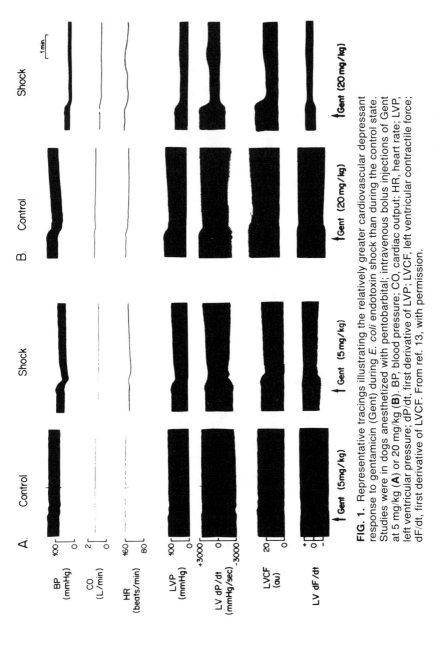

FIG. 1. Representative tracings illustrating the relatively greater cardiovascular depressant response to gentamicin (Gent) during *E. coli* endotoxin shock than during the control state. Studies were in dogs anesthetized with pentobarbital; intravenous bolus injections of Gent at 5 mg/kg (**A**) or 20 mg/kg (**B**). BP, blood pressure; CO, cardiac output; HR, heart rate; LVP, left ventricular pressure; dP/dt, first derivative of LVP; LVCF, left ventricular contractile force; dF/dt, first derivative of LVCF. From ref. 13, with permission.

vasodilator properties of streptomycin using perfused kidneys of dogs. Importantly, Ca^{2+} antagonized the vasodilator activity of streptomycin in this study (65). It was not clear, however, if perfusion pressure changes in the hindlimb and kidney represented direct effects of the antibiotics on contractile function of vascular smooth muscle or if vascular resistance changes were indirect and reflected autoregulatory adjustments to metabolic changes in the skeletal muscle or renal parenchymal tissues.

Direct evidence for a Ca^{2+}-antagonistic action of aminoglycosides was obtained initially from experiments with ^{45}Ca and rabbit aorta (9). Arterial tissue was selected for use in this study for two reasons. First, the direct vascular effects of the aminoglycosides were believed to be important to the net hemodynamic response of mammals to these drugs. Second, vascular smooth muscle represented an excellent model system for elucidating effects of aminoglycosides that perhaps could be extrapolated to excitable membranes of other tissues. In brief, streptomycin, neomycin, gentamicin, and kanamycin characteristically decreased ^{45}Ca uptake and increased ^{45}Ca efflux in a sustained manner in vascular smooth muscle (8–10,67,68). Reciprocally, Ca^{2+} inhibited the uptake and increased the efflux of ^{14}C-gentamicin (69). Thus there seemed to be some type of competition between aminoglycosides and Ca^{2+} for membrane binding sites in the vascular smooth muscle cells.

Effects of aminoglycosides on Ca^{2+} movement were demonstrated not only in rabbit aorta but also in different vascular beds of dogs and nonhuman primates. Vessels studied included the aorta and the renal, superior mesenteric, femoral, coronary, carotid, and terminal mesenteric arteries (8,67,70). The disruptive effect of aminoglycosides on Ca^{2+} homeostasis was manifested at cellular membrane sites important to contractile reactivity of the vessels; these antibiotics inhibited arterial contractions induced by norepinephrine, angiotensin II, serotonin, histamine, Ca^{2+}, and depolarizing concentrations of K^+ (8,10,67,68).

Based on differing inhibitory effects of the antibiotics on contractile responses and ^{45}Ca movement, it was proposed that these drugs exert their Ca^{2+} antagonistic activity by inhibiting the uptake, reuptake, and/or binding of Ca^{2+} at superficial membrane sites (for details, see refs. 7, 9, 71, and 72). We suggested that anionic binding sites of membrane phospholipids interacted with, or were in some way affected by, the polycationic aminoglycosides. The phospholipid-membrane perturbation resulting from such aminoglycoside–membrane interaction would decrease the capacity of the cell membrane to bind and store Ca^{2+}. Such action(s) would in turn decrease the availability of membrane-bound Ca^{2+} for intracellular movement to the contractile proteins of the vascular smooth muscle cell, thereby inhibiting contractile responses to vasostimulatory interventions that act through mobilization of Ca^{2+} from superficial membrane stores (9,67).

The Ca^{2+}-inhibiting activity of the aminoglycosides was more pronounced in small resistance arteries than in large conduit vessels (e.g., effects on coronary arteries and terminal mesenteric arteries > carotid arteries > aorta) (8,67). It was concluded that small, highly reactive vessels such as terminal mesenteric arteries and also coronary arteries depend more on a superficial membrane source of Ca^{2+} than do large conduit vessels (8,67). The dependence of coronary arteries on a superficial source of Ca^{2+} for norepinephrine responses was reported later by van Breeman et al. (73). Thus it seemed that the aminoglycosides might be useful as model drugs for probing Ca^{2+}-dependent events in excitable tissues that rely on mobilization of superficial Ca^{2+} for intracellular functions.

In addition, it was postulated that the disruptive effect of aminoglycosides on Ca^{2+} homeostasis at superficial membrane sites could explain the inhibitory activity of these agents in excitable tissues other than vascular smooth muscle alone (9). Direct evidence for Ca^{2+}–aminoglycoside antagonism has been obtained in several different tissues, including sarcoplasmic reticulum of skeletal muscle (74), inner ear tissues (75), intestinal smooth muscle (63), and cholinergic neurons (56). Based on studies with renal and inner ear isolates, Schacht and co-workers (75,76) suggested that neomycin inhibits the turnover of membrane polyphosphoinositides and their ability to bind Ca^{2+}. It now seems clear that the renal and ototoxicity of the aminoglycosides is associated with the interaction of these agents with membrane phospholipids that are directly or indirectly involved in Ca^{2+} movements.

Myocardium

In view of the participation of superficially localized Ca^{2+} in activation of myocardial contractions, and in view of previous studies pointing toward cardiodepressant actions of aminoglycosides (2,23,26), it seemed likely that these antibiotics affected Ca^{2+} metabolism in the heart. Gentamicin, a representative aminoglycoside, depressed isometric contractions of atrial myocardium from rats and guinea pigs in a concentration-dependent manner (4,6,12). Similar negative inotropic effects were seen with kanamycin, amikacin, and sisomicin in guinea pig atria (12). Using rat ventricular muscle, Sohn and Katz (64,77) subsequently verified the direct myocardial depressant effects of kanamycin and streptomycin.

The negative inotropic action of large concentrations of gentamicin was antagonized by excess Ca^{2+} in a competitive manner (4,12). In contrast, effects of the antibiotic were only partially antagonized by norepinephrine, isoproterenol, digoxin, or increased frequency of beating (4,12). These data showed that the negative inotropic action of an aminoglycoside could be completely antagonized by an increase in the concentration of interstitial Ca^{2+}, but not by interventions that mobilized available membrane-bound pools of Ca^{2+}.

The Ca^{2+}-related myocardial depressant action of aminoglycosides was supported by data presented in abstract form, which showed that gentamicin decreased ^{45}Ca tissue spaces in beating, but not in quiescent, atrial muscle of the guinea pig (78). This inhibitory action was demonstrable if the Ca^{2+} concentration of the bathing medium was low (1.0 mM) rather than high (2.5 or 10.0 mM). These data were later published in a comprehensive review of aminoglycoside effects in vascular tissue (71). Lullman and Schwarz (79) subsequently reported similar inhibition of Ca^{2+} binding to atrial myocardium by gentamicin and also by sisomicin and dibekacin.

Further study showed that the cardiac depressant action of gentamicin (6) and other aminoglycosides was augmented considerably when myocardial contractions were dependent on an increased influx of Ca^{2+} through slow cation channels of the sarcolemma. These channels are responsible for the influx of Ca^{2+} during the plateau phase of the cardiac action potential; Ca^{2+} influx through slow channels couples membrane excitation to activation of the contractile proteins (80,81). The inhibitory effect of gentamicin on slow Ca^{2+} contractile responses provided evidence that aminoglycosides in some way affect either the transport system responsible for Ca^{2+} influx through the slow channels of the cell membrane, the availability of Ca^{2+} for translocation to these sites, or both. Myographic tracings illustrating the enhanced negative inotropic action of gentamicin in heart muscle contracting under Ca^{2+} channel-activated conditions are presented in Fig. 2. We proposed that aminoglycosides decrease the systolic influx of Ca^{2+} in contracting myocardial cells by inhibiting the uptake or binding of Ca^{2+} at superficial binding sites of the sarcolemma, thereby reducing the quantity of membrane-bound Ca^{2+} available for movement into the myoplasm during depolarization of the cell membrane (4,6).

The inhibitory influence of gentamicin on slow inward Ca^{2+} channels in heart muscle (6) was later confirmed by different investigators. Hino et al. (82) reported that gentamicin remarkably diminished the slow inward current measured in guinea pig papillary muscle by a single sucrose-gap voltage-clamp technique. Hino et al. (82) also demonstrated depression of the slow inward Ca^{2+} current at low concentrations of gentamicin and depression of the time-dependent outward current only at high concentrations of gentamicin. The inhibitory action of gentamicin was expressed rather selectively on the peak amplitude of the slow inward current, since the antibiotic did not affect the time course, voltage dependency of steady-state inactivation or activation, or reversal potential of the current. Addition of exogenous Ca^{2+} reversed the inhibitory effects of gentamicin on the slow inward current. Concurring with previous reports (6), Hino et al. (82) proposed that the depressant action of gentamicin on slow inward current in myocardial cells was due to a blockade of slow channels, with the antibiotic dislocating Ca^{2+} from slow channel binding sites on the external surface of the sarcolemma. In agreement with this theory, numerous studies have shown aminoglycoside

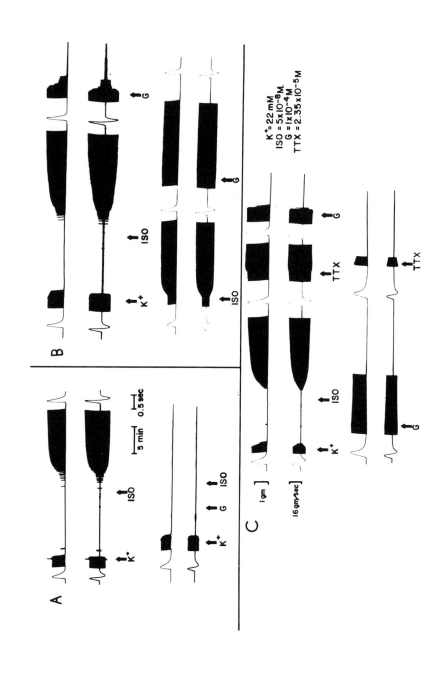

K⁺ = 22 mM
ISO = 5×10⁻⁸ M.
G = 1×10⁻⁴ M
TTX = 2.35×10⁻⁵ M

A

ISO

G   ISO

K⁺

K⁺

5 min   0.5 sec

B

G

ISO

K⁺

G

ISO

C

1 gm

16 gm/sec

K⁺

ISO

TTX

G

TTX

G

inhibition of Ca^{2+} binding using isolated membrane preparations (83,84). Lullmann and Schwarz (79) demonstrated Ca^{2+} binding abnormalities induced by gentamicin in intact cardiac muscle. They too concluded that the functional depression caused by gentamicin is not due to a decrease in extracellular Ca^{2+}, but rather a decrease in the amount of Ca^{2+} bound to the sarcolemmal membrane of the cardiac tissue.

De la Chapelle-Groz and Athias (85) studied the effect of gentamicin on cultured cardiac myocytes; they obtained results consistent with the above studies in that gentamicin antagonized the inotropic actions of Ca^{2+}. One of the main objectives in their study was to compare the actions of gentamicin with other known Ca^{2+} antagonists to ascertain the binding site on the cardiac myocyte where gentamicin acts as a ligand. The actions of La^{3+} and EDTA most closely resembled the actions of gentamicin on cardiac myocytes. This indicates that since gentamicin has been shown not to chelate Ca^{2+} ions, the action of gentamicin is more like that of La^{3+}, as also suggested by earlier studies (88). Therefore it was concluded that gentamicin binds to an extracellular site of the cardiac membrane, which normally binds Ca^{2+}. Hashimoto and colleagues (86) demonstrated the close resemblance of gentamicin–Ca^{2+} antagonism with Co^{2+}–Ca^{2+} antagonism. Their data suggested that gentamicin may be binding to the same site as Co^{2+} and Ca^{2+}; however, they provided no direct evidence for this proposal. Co^{2+} has been shown to compete with Ca^{2+} for binding sites in the membrane at the site of Ca^{2+} channels (87). These investigators also demonstrated that prolongation of the open state of the Ca^{2+} channel by the Ca^{2+} channel agonist Bay k 8644 had little effect on the action of gentamicin or Co^{2+}. This is consistent with the theory that gentamicin dislocates Ca^{2+} from the cardiac sarcolemmal membrane (6), and that with less membrane-bound Ca^{2+}, there is less Ca^{2+} available for entry through the opened channel irrespective of how long the channel may be open.

Calcium flow through the slow cation channels of the cardiac cell membrane is inhibited by several chemical agents referred to commonly as "Ca^{2+} antagonists" or "slow channel blockers." Included in this group are the organic compounds such as verapamil and D600 and the cationic or inorganic

----

FIG. 2. Effects of gentamicin (G) in guinea pig left atria contracting under normal (5.4 mMK⁺) or "slow channel activated" (22 mM K⁺–isoproterenol) conditions. **A:** Contractions (CT) ceased after 22 mM K⁺ but were restored by isoproterenol (ISO) (*upper tracings*). Pretreatment with G (0.1 mM) prevented restoration of contractions by ISO (*lower tracings*). **B:** G abolished contractions of muscle beating under high K⁺–ISO conditions (*upper tracings*); however, G had no effect in the ISO-treated atria beating under normal K⁺ (5.4 mM) conditions (*lower tracings*). **C:** Tetrodotoxin (TTX) did not stop contractions of atria beating under high K⁺–ISO conditions; whereas G blocked contractions (*upper tracings*). Conversely, under control conditions (5.4 mM K⁺; no ISO), G has little effect whereas TTX stopped contractions (*lower tracings*). The time markers in (A) and the calibration markers and drug concentrations in (C) apply to all tracings. Stimulation frequency is 0.2 Hz. From ref. 6, with permission.

Ca^{2+} antagonists such as lanthanum (La^{3+}) and manganese (Mn^{2+}) (6,88). Based on the selective inhibitory action of small amounts of gentamicin on slow Ca^{2+} contractile responses, we proposed the aminoglycosides as putative members of the list of slow Ca^{2+} channel blockers in heart muscle (6).

Comparative cardiac studies were done with La^{3+}, D600, and gentamicin using the inotropic response to changes in heart rate as a test inotropic intervention (88). The positive inotropic response of heart muscle to increased frequency of stimulation is thought to involve increased Ca^{2+} influx and/or increased releasability of membrane Ca^{2+} (88). The negative inotropic effect of D600 was more pronounced at high rates of stimulation (>1.4 Hz) than at low rates (<0.8 Hz). On the other hand, La^{3+} and gentamicin decreased the positive inotropic response to increased beating rates throughout the frequency range that was examined (0.1–2.2 Hz). Further study showed that the pharmacodynamics of the myocardial effects of gentamicin were less complex than those exhibited by either La^{3+} or D600 (88).

For example, contractile strength of gentamicin-depressed heart muscle consistently recovered to near control values within 10 min after the muscle was placed in a drug-free control medium. Muscle treated with an equipotent concentration of La^{3+} or D600 failed to regain 50% of basal inotropy even after recovery in normal bathing medium for 1 hr. Furthermore, D600-treated muscle still displayed an inversion of the amplitude–frequency curve after the recovery period. In La^{3+}-treated muscle, contractile responses to high rates of stimulation were attenuated, and responses to low frequencies were actually enhanced after the recovery period. In contrast, the inhibitory activity of a comparable concentration of gentamicin seemed completely reversible since inotropic responses to changes in heart rate were quite normal after recovery from this antibiotic (88), as compared with La^{3+} and D600 in Fig. 3.

Rapid recovery of mechanical function strongly suggested the recovery of an active physiologic process rather than cytotoxic damage inflicted on the myocytes by the antibiotic. Thus although gentamicin inhibits slow Ca^{2+} responses (6), the inotropic effects of this agent could be differentiated from the poorly reversible and more complex actions of the well-known Ca^{2+} antagonists D600 and La^{3+} (88) (Fig. 3). We suggested that these characteristics enhance the utility of gentamicin as a model Ca^{2+} channel blocking drug for those types of studies requiring recovery of contractile function, and warrant further study for potential application in cardiologic investigations (88). The negative inotropic potency of the aminoglycosides is less than that of the organic Ca^{2+} antagonists D600 and verapamil but is of a similar order of magnitude as the cationic Ca^{2+} antagonists such as La^{3+} and Mn^{2+} (88).

Cation channel blockade by aminoglycosides has now been reported not only in vascular muscle (8–10) and myocardium (6), but also in other tissues, for example, neomycin block of slowly inactivating Ca^{2+} channels in clonal GH3 pituitary cells (89), aminoglycoside block of N-type Ca^{2+} channel of

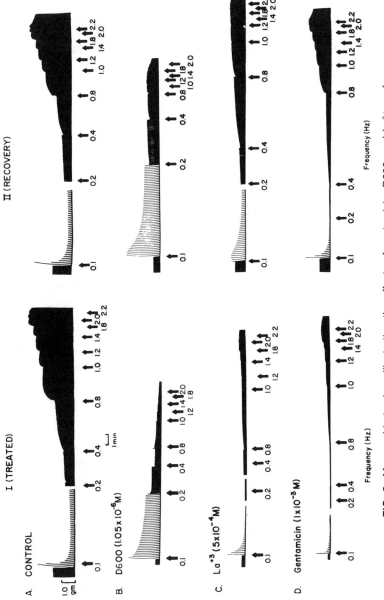

FIG. 3. Myographic tracings illustrating the effects of gentamicin, D600, and La³⁺ on frequency–force relationships of isolated heart muscle while the drug was present in the bathing medium (I, Treated) and again 1.5–2 hr after recovery in control bathing medium (II, Recovery). Tension and time scales in I (A) apply to all tracings. From ref. 88, with permission.

rat brain synaptosomes (90), neomycin block of inward Ca^{2+} current in paramecium (91), gentamicin block of voltage-gated Ca^{2+} channels in cochlear outer hair cells (92), and aminoglycoside block of Ca^{2+}-activated K^+ channels from rat brain synaptosomal membranes incorporated into planer lipid bilayers (93). These types of studies have substantiated clearly that toxicities of aminoglycoside antibiotics in different types of host cells depend on a common type of molecular mechanism involving disruption of Ca^{2+}-dependent signaling across excitable membranes.

Other Antibiotic Agents

In addition to the aminoglycosides, several other antimicrobial as well as non-antimicrobial antibiotics have been reported to affect myocardial activity. In most cases, however, little is known about the mechanism(s) of their cardiac depressant actions, and interactions with cellular functions have not been intensely investigated.

Cardiac depressant effects have been described for several of the macrolide antibiotics including erythromycin and oleandomycin (94). Leaders et al. (57) reported hypotension and slowed heart rate in anesthetized rabbits treated with oleandomycin, as well as decrease in the beating rate and contractile amplitude of isolated rabbit hearts. Intravenous injection of erythromycin was shown to produce dose-dependent decreases in both blood pressure and myocardial contractile force in anesthetized dogs (23). Regan et al. (95) reported that erythromycin may cause arrhythmias and ventricular tachycardia in the ischemic ventricle or in the digitalis-treated animal, possibly by enhancing intracellular potassium loss. Clinically, erythromycin has been associated with cardiac dysrhythmias characterized by the long QT syndrome and accompanying ventricular tachycardia waveform known as "torsades de pointes" (21). Cardiac transmembrane potential experiments showed that erythromycin prolonged action potential duration and reduced phase zero depolarization rate, effects consistent with the fast Na^+ channel blocking properties of quinidine and other Class IA antiarrhythmic drugs (21). Alteration of ion fluxes by erythromycin is a likely factor responsible for the cardiac effects of this type of antibiotic.

Lincomycin has been shown to produce adverse effects on myocardial impulse transmission. Daubeck et al. (17) observed cardiac arrest and ventricular fibrillation in a patient following an inadvertent overdose of lincomycin. Spurred by the clinical incident, these investigators examined lincomycin-induced hypotension, arrhythmias, cardiac slowing, and ventricular fibrillation in subsequent canine studies. These abnormalities were dependent on rate of administration of lincomycin as well as on the amount of drug given. The arrhythmias appeared to result from decreased excitability and conduction velocity; arrhythmias caused by lincomycin may be potentiated by digitalis (17).

Chloramphenicol, in addition to its well-known toxic effects on bone marrow, has also been shown to produce negative inotropic and chronotropic effects in a number of cardiac preparations (23,26,57). The myocardial depressant effects of chloramphenicol were incompletely antagonized by Ca^{2+} or ouabain (26) and seem additive to the depression produced by halothane (77). Isometric contractions of isolated rat heart muscle were depressed by chloramphenicol, but the degree of depression was considerably less than that obtained with kanamycin or streptomycin (64,77). Propranolol or atropine had no effect on the response to chloramphenicol in the isolated toad heart, suggesting that the negative inotropic and chronotropic effects of this agent resulted from a myocardial cell interaction rather than an alteration in the release or response to endogenous autonomic mediators (96). Inhibition of protein synthesis has been implicated in the altered heart beat response to chloramphenicol in explanted chick embryos (97).

Vancomycin reduced pressure development and $+ dP/dt_{max}$ in both the left and right ventricles of anesthetized dogs (23). The cardiac depressant action of vancomycin was confirmed in isolated cat hearts (23).

Several of the polyene group of antifungal agents have been shown to depress myocardial contractility and induce electrical disturbances in isolated cardiac preparations. Arora and Arora (98,99) demonstrated that eurocidine, pentamycin, fungichromin, and amphotericin B diminished the amplitude of contraction in perfused Langendorff preparations of several species. The accompanying disturbances in electrical activity in response to candicidin and amphotericin B appeared to result from changes in myocardial ion transport similar to those induced by toxic concentrations of ouabain (100). Ruiz-Ceretti et al. (101) examined the effects of amphotericin B on electrical activity in isolated rabbit hearts and found a decrease in both amplitude and rate of depolarization of the cardiac action potential within 15 min after exposure to the drug. The authors concluded that the subsequent disappearance of the plateau phase of the action potential was due to inhibition of slow inward current by the antibiotic. This proposal is further supported by the observation that one of the first changes observed in the electrocardiogram following administration of amphotericin B is prolongation of the P–R interval (101). Since the slow current is thought to contribute as much as 30% to the depolarizing current in the nodal cells, inhibition of the slow current by amphotericin B could be the mechanism underlying the decrease in atrioventricular conduction seen with this drug. Using voltage clamp techniques, Schanne et al. (102) showed that this antibiotic blocked the ionic channels involved in activation of the slow inward current and suggested this mechanism for explaining the depression of contractility observed in rabbit hearts (102). It should be emphasized, however, that amphotericin B is not typical of a "Ca^{2+} antagonist, slow channel blocker" since it affects action potential parameters other than the plateau alone. Indeed, it may also exert a blocking effect on sodium channels responsible for rapid depolarization of the transmembrane potential (102).

To further complicate the amphotericin B story, studies reported in 1988 indicated that this drug provokes *in vivo* renal arterial vasoconstriction (103). This response was inhibited by the Ca^{2+} channel blocking agent verapamil, but not by angiotensin II receptor blockade or renal sympathectomy (103). Verapamil is a vasodilator agent, and its inhibition of amphotericin B-induced renal vasoconstriction may reflect simple physiologic antagonism between a vasodilator and a vasoconstrictor. On the other hand, since amphotericin B can act as a Ca^{2+} ionophore in liposomes (104), perhaps it may also enhance Ca^{2+} influx in some intact cells such as renal vascular smooth muscle.

Considering the well-known Ca^{2+}-chelating properties of the tetracyclines, it is not surprising that this group of antibiotics can produce toxic effects on the cardiovascular system. Cardiovascular depressant effects have been observed in intact animals and in isolated cardiac preparations from different laboratory animal species (23,26,57). Swain et al. (26) used an isolated dog heart–lung preparation and reported a complete reversal of tetracycline-induced myocardial depression by Ca^{2+}. The possibility that this interaction was due to a Ca^{2+}-chelating activity of tetracycline was tested by comparing tetracycline, Ca^{2+}, and disodium ethylenediaminetetracetate (EDTA). Calcium similarly reversed the effects of increasing doses of both EDTA and tetracycline. The comparison was limited, however, because of precipitate formation of the tetracycline–Ca^{2+} complex. These results indicate an important difference in the mechanism by which tetracyclines exert their cardiotoxic effects in comparison to that of other antibiotics. Whereas the aminoglycosides, polyenes, and macrolides are thought to have a direct action on some myocardial cellular process, it appears the tetracyclines may act simply by lowering Ca^{2+} levels in plasma or the extracellular space. Further studies are needed, however, to completely discount a direct cardiac action of tetracyclines independent of Ca^{2+} chelation.

Considerable information about the myocardial toxicity of valinomycin, a macrocyclic antibiotic, has been obtained by Sperelakis and co-workers (105,106). Valinomycin was found to block the Ca^{2+}-dependent, slowly rising electrical response (slow response) induced by isoproterenol in hearts whose fast Na^+ channels were voltage inactivated by partial depolarization with elevated K^+ solution. This agent also markedly shortened the ventricular action potential plateau, as well as lowered the ATP level. Other metabolic inhibitors, such as cyanide or dinitrophenol, also produced action potential shortening and slow response blockade concomitant with a lowering of the ATP level (106). Glucose elevation to 27 or 55 mM or treatment with insulin was found to reverse the effects of valinomycin and restore the Ca^{2+}-dependent slow responses of guinea pigs and chick embryo hearts. Vogel and Sperelakis (106) thus concluded that since elevated glucose uptake should lead to an increased availability of ATP, the electrophysiological effects of valinomycin are owed largely to metabolic poisoning rather than to a direct effect of the cardiac sarcolemma.

SUMMARY

Mechanisms

The spectrum of cardiovascular effects of antibiotics, as with other types of drugs, depends on the pharmacodynamic profiles of the individual agents. Circulatory dysfunction induced by certain antibiotics can be secondary to neuromuscular paralysis and respiratory insufficiency, primary to direct depressant actions on the heart and blood vessels, or caused by a combination of direct and indirect effects.

The inhibitory influence of the aminoglycosides on Ca^{2+} homeostasis in peripheral neurons, vascular smooth muscle, and the myocardium no doubt explains the capability of this particular group of antibiotics to disrupt hemodynamic control mechanisms. This characteristic of the aminoglycosides does not seem to be attributable to overt cytotoxic damage of cardiovascular tissues but is related to a reversible interaction of these agents with Ca^{2+} binding sites of excitable membranes. Many of the biologic actions of aminoglycosides in mammals, including cellular damage to the kidney and inner ear tissues, also are associated in some way with perturbation of membrane phospholipids where Ca^{2+} normally is distributed.

Indeed, no doubt prompted by early work from Schacht's group (75,76), recent studies have shown convincingly that aminoglycosides alter interactions between Ca^{2+} and polyphosphatidylinositol elements in membranes of various types of eukaryotic cells (107–110). The phosphoinositides are believed to represent the membrane receptors that misconstrue aminoglycosides as native ligands. Resulting interactions between the phosphoinositide and the aminoglycoside-ligand displace Ca^{2+} from its normal binding domain, and thereby disrupt cell membrane homeostasis and signal transduction mechanisms that depend on phosphoinositide–Ca^{2+} interactions (75,76,107–110). This paradigm is believed to account for many actions of aminoglycosides, for example, nephro- and ototoxicity (75,76,84,107), inhibition of platelet function (108), inhibition of platelet-derived growth factor actions (110), and perhaps even modulation of pertussis sensitivity of G-protein-regulated polyphosphoinositide phosphodiesterase activity in the promyelocytic HL60 cell (109). Future studies involving aminoglycoside antibiotics and phosphoinositides in membranes from myocardial and vascular tissues will add new critical information concerning the molecular mechanisms responsible for cardiovascular actions of this important group of antibiotics.

Relatively less is known about mechanisms of cardiovascular toxicities of other antibiotics that also can affect hemodynamics. Lincomycin can induce neuromuscular paralysis but also seems to exert direct effects on cardiac impulse conduction. Tetracyclines can influence respiratory and myocardial functions; these activities appear to be related, at least in part, to chelation of Ca^{2+} or other cations. Chloramphenicol spares the somatic neuromuscu-

TABLE 1. *Cardiovascular depressant effects of aminoglycoside antibiotics*

Antibiotic	Species	Preparation	Effect	Comments	References
Streptomycin	Dog	In vivo	Cardiovascular depression	During anesthesia	23
	Dog	Perfused kidney	Vasodilation	During anesthesia	65
	Cat, rabbit	In vitro (Langendorff)	Contractile depression		23, 57
	Human		Suspected cardiac depression	Tuberculous patients with congestive heart failure	22
	Dog	In vitro (heart–lung)	Cardiac depression		26
	Dog, cat, rhesus monkey	In vivo	Hypotension	During anesthesia	3, 66
	Rat	In vitro (ventricular muscle)	Contractile depression	Additive with halothane	64, 77
	Human	In vivo	Persistent hypotension	After cardiac surgery	23
	Rabbit	In vivo	Hypotension	During anesthesia; $ED_{50} = 40$ mg/kg	57
Dihydrostreptomycin	Rabbit	In vitro (Langendorff)	Contractile depression		57
	Rabbit	In vivo	Hypotension	During anesthesia; $ED_{50} = 40$ mg/kg	57
Kanamycin	Dog	Heart–lung	Contractile depression		26
	Human		Cardiac arrest	IV Overdose	18
	Rabbit	In vitro (Langendorff)	Contractile depression		28
	Dog	In vivo	Cardiovascular depression	During anesthesia	23
	Dog	In vivo	No effects	Unanesthetized, slow IV drip	106
	Guinea pig	In vitro (atrial muscle)	Contractile depression	30% Depression with 3.8 mM	12
	Rat	In vitro (ventricular muscle)	Contractile depression	Additive with halothane	64, 77

Drug	Species	Preparation	Effect	Comment	Ref.
Neomycin	Human		Cardiovascular depression	Review of case reports	19
	Rhesus monkey, baboons	In vivo	Cardiovascular depression	During anesthesia	2, 3
Gentamicin	Rat	In vitro (atrial muscle)	Contractile depression	Antagonized by Ca^{2+}	4
	Rhesus monkey	In vivo	Cardiovascular depression	During anesthesia; antagonized by Ca^{2+}	2
	Dog	In vivo	Cardiovascular depression	Potentiated in shock	13
	Guinea pig	In vitro (ventricular muscle)	Reduced slow inward Ca^{2+} current	Voltage clamp	82
	Guinea pig	In vitro (atrial muscle)	Inhibited ^{45}Ca binding	Other aminoglycosides	79
	Rat	Cultured ventricular myocytes	Negative inotrope and chronotrope	Antagonized by Ca^{2+}	85
	Guinea pig	In vitro (atrial muscle)	Contractile depression	Blocked slow Ca^{2+}-dependent contractions	6
	Dog	Papillary muscle	Reduced contractile force	During anesthesia	82
	Dog	SA-node	Slowed SA rate	During anesthesia	82
	Dog	AV-node	AV block (large doses)	During anesthesia	82
	Dog	In vitro (ventricular muscle)	Negative inotrope	Compared with Co^{2+} and Bay k 8644	86
	Guinea pig	In vitro (atrial muscle)	Contractile depression	Comparison with La^{3+} and D600	88
Amikacin	Guinea pig	In vitro (atrial muscle)	Contractile depression	34% Depression with 4 mM	12
	Dog	In vivo	No effects	Unanesthetized; slow IV drip	106
Sisomicin	Guinea pig	In vitro (atrial muscle)	Contractile depression	45% Depresion with 2 mM	12

TABLE 2. *Cardiovascular effects of several antibiotics*

Antibiotic	Species	Preparation	Effect	Comments	References
Tetracyclines	Dog	In vitro (heart–lung)	Contractile depression	Ca^{2+} chelation	26
	Dog	In vivo	Cardiovascular depression	During anesthesia	23
	Cat, rabbit	In vitro (Langendorff)	Contractile depression	During anesthesia;	23, 57
	Rabbit	In vivo	Hypotension	$ED_{50} = 120$ mg/kg	57
Chloramphenicol	Rabbit, cat	In vitro (Langendorff)	Contractile depression	During anesthesia;	23, 57
	Rabbit	In vivo	Hypotension	$ED_{50} = 120$ mg/kg	57
	Dog	In vitro (heart–lung)	Contractile depression		26
	Toad	In vitro	Contractile depression		96
	Chick	In vitro	Decreased pulsatile rate	Embryonic chick heart	97
	Rat	In vitro (ventricular muscle)	Contractile depression	Additive with halothane	64, 77
Erythromycin	Cat	In vitro (Langendorff)	Contractile depression		23
	Dog	In vivo	Cardiovascular depression	During anesthesia; histamine release	23, 62, 95
	Human		Cardiac dysrhythmia	Torsades de pointes	21
	Dog	Purkinje fiber	Prolonged action potential	Inhibit Na^+ channel	21
	Rat	In vitro (atrial muscle)	Negative inotrope	Other macrolides	94
Lincomycin	Dog	In vivo	Ventricular arrhythmias	After digitalis or ischemia	95

188

Drug	Species	Preparation	Effect	Condition	Ref.
Oleandomycin	Human		Cardiac arrest	Overdose IV	17
	Rabbit	In vitro (Langendorff)	Contractile depression		57
	Rabbit	In vivo	Hypotension	During anesthesia; $ED_{50} = 80$ mg/kg	57
Colymycin	Dog	In vivo	Hypotension	During anesthesia	62
	Dog	In vivo	Cardiovascular depression	During anesthesia	23
Vancomycin	Dog	In vivo	Cardiovascular depression	During anesthesia	23
	Cat	In vitro (Langendorff)	Contractile depression		23
Amphotericin B	Rabbit	In vitro (Langendorff)	Electromechanical depression	Decreased action potential plateau	101
	Guinea pig	In vitro (Langendorff)	Contractile depression; decreased coronary flow; decreased heart rate		99, 100
Candicidin	Guinea pig	In vitro (Langendorff)	Contractile depression; systolic arrest; decreased heart rate; decreased coronary flow		100
	Rat	In vitro (Langendorff)	Contractile depression; altered electrolyte balance		98
Valinomycin	Guinea pig, chick	In vitro	Contractile depression	Blocks slow Ca^{2+} responses by metabolic poisoning	104, 105

lar junction but, under some conditions, may affect inotropic and chrono-tropic responsiveness of cardiac tissue. The circulatory depressant actions of erythromycin and related antibiotics seem to depend on histamine release, but a disruption of potassium distribution in the heart may also be involved. More information is needed in this neglected field of antibiotic pharmacol-ogy–toxicology.

Clinical Aspects

Although experimental studies have established the potential for untoward cardiovascular effects of several clinically important antibiotics (Tables 1 and 2), most of the data cannot be extrapolated directly to clinical medicine. Greater-than-therapeutic doses of antibiotics administered by intravenous bolus injections were commonly studied in animals subjected to circulatory stress associated with surgical instrumentation and general anesthesia. Con-centrations of antibiotics many times greater than those that occur in plasma of patients generally are needed *in vitro* to directly depress myocardial or arterial contractility. Buyniski and Bierwagen (111) demonstrated that even large amounts of the aminoglycosides kanamycin and amikacin exert little or no detectable hemodynamic effects when administered by slow intrave-nous drip to unanesthetized dogs.

On the one hand, therefore, we must conclude that cardiovascular de-pressant effects of antibiotics are unlikely to be clinically relevant in the routine therapy of uncomplicated infections in otherwise normal patients. The beneficial results of appropriate antibiotic therapy are unquestionable, and the present discussion should not be considered reason to withhold antibiotic treatment when sensitivity tests and clinical experience dictate otherwise.

On the other hand, however, the serious and even disastrous outcome of some of the clinical incidents should not be disregarded. Inadvertent over-dosage of antibiotics undoubtedly was involved in several cases, and preex-isting circulatory dysfunction or systemic illness seemed contributory. Neu-romuscular effects may dominate if myoneural or pulmonary disease has decreased the margin of safety of impulse transmission in respiratory mus-cles. On the other hand, direct cardiovascular effects may become more important if congestive heart failure, circulatory shock, myocardial infarc-tion, or other circulatory ailments have diminished cardiac reserve. Thus, as a few investigative groups forewarned (1,5,13,19,23,64), the circulatory ef-fects of certain antibiotics may well become a relevant issue if the patient's cardiovascular system is compromised by disease, general anesthesia, drugs, or any other intervention that directly or indirectly depresses physi-ologic reactivity of the heart and the vasculature.

ACKNOWLEDGMENTS

This work was supported in part by National Heart, Lung, and Blood Institute Research Grant HL-36079 and National Heart, Lung, and Blood Institute Research Career Development Award K04-HL-01669 for J. L. Parker.

REFERENCES

1. Parker JL, Adams HR. Cardiovascular depressant effects of antibiotics. In: Van Stee EW, ed. *Cardiovascular toxicology.* New York: Raven Press; 1982:327–351.
2. Adams HR. Cardiovascular depressant effects of neomycin and gentamicin in rhesus monkeys. *Br J Pharmacol* 1975;54:453–462.
3. Adams HR. Cardiovascular depressant effects of the neomycin–streptomycin group of antibiotics. *Am J Vet Res* 1975;36:103–108.
4. Adams HR. Direct myocardial depressant effects of gentamicin. *Eur J Pharmacol* 1975;30:272–279.
5. Adams HR. Antibiotic-induced alterations of cardiovascular reactivity. *Fed Proc* 1976;35:1148–1150.
6. Adams HR, Durrett LR. Gentamicin blockade of slow Ca^{++} channels in atrial myocardium of guinea pigs. *J Clin Invest* 1978;62:241–247.
7. Adams HR, Durrett LR. Myocardial toxicity of antibiotics. In: T. Balaz, ed. *Cardiac toxicology,* vol 2. Boca Raton, FL: CRC Press; 1981:145–164.
8. Adams HR, Goodman FR. Differential inhibitory effects of neomycin on contractile responses of various canine arteries. *J Pharmacol Exp Ther* 1974;193:393–402.
9. Adams HR, Goodman FR, Lupean VA, Weiss GB. Effects of neomycin on tension and ^{45}Ca movements in rabbit aortic smooth muscle. *Life Sci* 1973;12:279–287.
10. Adams HR, Goodman FR, Weiss GB. Alteration of contractile function and calcium ion movements in vascular smooth muscle by gentamicin and other aminoglycoside antibiotics. *Antimicrob Agents Chemother* 1974;5:640–646.
11. Adams HR, Mathew BP, Teske RH, Mercer HD. Neuromuscular blocking effects of aminoglycoside antibiotics on fast- and slow-contracting muscles of the cat. *Anesth Analg* 1976;55:500–507.
12. Adams HR, Parker JL, Durrett LR. Cardiac toxicities of antibiotics. *Environ Health Perspect* 1979;26:217–223.
13. Adams HR, Parker JL, Mathew BP. Cardiovascular manifestations of acute antibiotic toxicity during *E. coli* endotoxin shock in anesthetized dogs. *Circ Shock* 1979;6:391–404.
14. Adams HR, Teske RH, Mercer HD. Anesthetic–antibiotic interrelationships. *J Am Vet Med Assoc* 1976;168:409–412.
15. Adams HR. Acute adverse effects of antibiotics. *J Am Vet Med Assoc* 1975;166:983–987.
16. Pittinger C, Adamson R. Antibiotic blockade of neuromuscular function. *Annu Rev Pharmacol* 1972;12:169–184.
17. Daubeck JL, Daughety MJ, Petty C. Lincomycin-induced cardiac arrest: a case report and experimental investigation. *Anesth Analg* 1974;53:563–567.
18. Ream CR. Respiratory and cardiac arrest after intravenous administration of kanamycin with reversal of toxic effects by neostigmine. *Ann Intern Med* 1963;59:384–387.
19. Pittinger CB, Eryasa Y, Adamson R. Antibiotic-induced paralysis. *Anesth Analg* 1970;49:487–501.
20. Waisbren BA. Lincomycin in larger doses (letter). *JAMA* 1968;206:2118.
21. Nattel S, Ranger S, Talajic M, Lemery R, Roy D. Erythromycin-induced long QT syndrome: concordance with quinidine and underlying cellular electrophysiologic mechanism. *Am J Med* 1990;89:235–238.

22. Daynes G. Drug-induced heart failure in advanced pulmonary tuberculosis. *S Afr Med J* 1974;48:2352–2353.
23. Cohen LS, Wechsler AS, Mitchell JH, Glick G. Depression of cardiac function by streptomycin and other antimicrobial agents. *Am J Cardiol* 1970;26:505–511.
24. Hall DA, McGibbon DH, Evans CC, Meadows GA. Gentamicin, tubocurarine, lignocaine, and neuromuscular blockade: a case report. *Br J Anaesth* 1972;44:1329.
25. Warner WA, Sanders E. Neuromuscular blockade associated with gentamicin therapy. *JAMA* 1971;215:1153.
26. Swain HH, Kiplinger GF, Brody TM. Actions of certain antibiotics on the isolated dog heart. *J Pharmacol Exp Ther* 1956;117:151–159.
27. Novak E, Vitti TG, Panzer JD. Antibiotic tolerance and serum levels after intravenous administration of multiple large doses of lincomycin. *Clin Pharmacol Ther* 1971; 12:793–797.
28. Ramos AO, Ramos L, de Luca AM. Acoes da Kanamicina nas musculaturas lisa e cardiaca. *Folia Clin Biol* 1961;21:156–162.
29. Pridgen JE. Respiratory arrest thought to be due to intraperitoneal neomycin. *Surgery* 1956;40:571–574.
30. Bruckner J, Thomas KC Jr, Bikhazi GB, Foldes FF. Neuromuscular drug interactions of clinical importance. *Anesth Analg* 1980;59:678–682.
31. Dretchen KL, Gergis SD, Sokoll MD, Long JP. Effect of various antibiotics on neuromuscular transmission. *Eur J Pharmacol* 1972;18:201–203.
32. Molgo J, Lemeignan M, Uchiyama T, Lechat P. Inhibitory effect of kanamycin on evoked transmitter release. Reversal by 3,4-diaminopyridine. *Eur J Pharmacol* 1979; 57:93–97.
33. Prado WA, Corrado AP, Marseillan RF. Competitive antagonism between calcium and antibiotics at the neuromuscular junction. *Arch Int Pharmacodyn* 1978;231:297–307.
34. Rubbo JT, Gergis SD, Sokoll MD. Comparative neuromuscular effects of lincomycin and clindamycin. *Anesth Analg* 1977;56(3):329–332.
35. Vital Brazil O, Prado-Franceschi J. The nature of the neuromuscular block produced by neomycin and gentamicin. *Arch Int Pharmacodyn* 1969;179:78–110.
36. Vital Brazil O, Prado-Franceschi J. The neuromuscular blocking action of gentamicin. *Arch Int Pharmacodyn* 1969;179:65–77.
37. Dretchen KL, Sokoll MD, Gergis SD, Long JP. Relative effects of streptomycin on motor nerve terminal and end-plate. *Eur J Pharmacol* 1973;22:10–16.
38. Torda T. The nature of gentamicin-induced neuromuscular block. *Br J Anaesth* 1980;52:325–329.
39. Caputy AJ, Kim YI, Sanders DB. The neuromuscular blocking effects of therapeutic concentrations of various antibiotics on normal rat skeletal muscle: a quantitative comparison. *J Pharmacol Exp Ther* 1981;217(2):369–378.
40. Farley JM, Wu CH, Narahashi T. Mechanism of neuromuscular block by streptomycin: a voltage clamp analysis. *J Pharmacol Exp Ther* 1982;222(2):488–493.
41. Paradelis AG, Tsouras JS, Latsoudes P, Demetriou T, Triantaphyllidis C. Neuromuscular blocking activity of dibekacin, a new semisynthetic aminoglycoside antibiotic. *Experientia* 1980;36:867–868.
42. Fiekers JF. Effects of the aminoglycoside antibiotics, streptomycin and neomycin, on neuromuscular transmission. I. Presynaptic considerations. *J Pharmacol Exp Ther* 1983;225(3):487–495.
43. Fiekers JF. Effects of the aminoglycoside antibiotics, streptomycin and neomycin, on neuromuscular transmission. II. Postsynaptic considerations. *J Pharmacol Exp Ther* 1983;225(3):496–502.
44. Del Pozo E, Baeyens JM. Effects of calcium channel blockers on neuromuscular blockade induced by aminoglycoside antibiotics. *Eur J Pharmacol* 1986;128:49–54.
45. Talbot PA. Potentiation of aminoglycoside-induced neuromuscular blockade by protons in vitro and in vivo. *J Pharmacol Exp Ther* 1987;241(2):686–694.
46. Baeyens JM, Del Pozo E. Comparison of the effects of calcium and the calcium channel stimulant Bay k 8644 on neomycin-induced neuromuscular blockade. *Pharmacol Toxicol* 1989;65:398–401.
47. Atchison WD, Adgate I, Beaman CM. Effects of antibiotics on uptake of calcium into isolated nerve terminals. *J Pharmacol Exp Ther* 1988;245(2):394–401.

48. Nation PN, Roth SH. The effects of neomycin on membrane properties and discharge activity of an isolated sensory neuron. *Can J Physiol Pharmacol* 1988;66:27–31.
49. Singh YN, Marshall IG, Harvey AL. Pre- and postjunctional blocking effects of aminoglycoside, polymyxin, tetracycline and lincosamide antibiotics. *Br J Anaesth* 1982; 54:1295–1305.
50. Fiekers JF, Henderson F, Marshall IG, Parsons RL. Comparative effects of clindamycin and lincomycin on end-plate currents and quantal content at the neuromuscular junction. *J Pharmacol Exp Ther* 1983;227(3):308–315.
51. Fiekers JF. Neuromuscular block produced by polymyxin B: interaction with end-plate channels. *Eur J Pharmacol* 1981;70:77–81.
52. Durant NN, Lambert JJ. The action of polymyxin B at the frog neuromuscular junction. *Br J Pharmacol* 1981;72:41–47.
53. Corrado AP. Ganglioplegic action of streptomycin. *Arch Int Pharmacodyn* 1958; 114:166–178.
54. Corrado AP, Ramos AO. Neomycin—its curariform and ganglioplegic actions. *Rev Brasil Biol* 1958;18:81–85.
55. Singh YN, Marshall IG, Harvey AL. Some effects of the aminoglycoside antibiotic amikacin on neuromuscular and autonomic transmission. *Br J Anaesth* 1978;50:109–117.
56. Wright JM, Collier B. The effects of neomycin upon transmitter release and action. *J Pharmacol Exp Ther* 1976;200:576–587.
57. Leaders F, Pittinger CB, Long JP. Some pharmacological properties of selected antibiotics. *Antibiotic Chemother* 1960;10:503–507.
58. Stallworth JM, Rodriguez O, Barrington BA. Microcirculatory responses to commonly used therapeutic drugs. *Am Surg* 1972;38:145–153.
59. Gross DR, Kitzman JV, Adams HR. Cardiovascular effects of intravenous administration of propylene glycol and of oxytetracycline in propylene glycol in calves. *Am J Vet Res* 1979;40:783–791.
60. McCullough DA, Wallace WFM. Inhibition of constrictor responses of the rabbit ear artery by a mixture of oxytetracycline and ascorbic acid. *Br J Pharmacol* 1975; 54:261.
61. Kalsner S. The lack of effect of oxytetracycline on response to sympathetic nerve stimulation and catecholamines in vascular tissue. *Br J Pharmacol* 1976;58:261–266.
62. Wakabayashi K, Yamada S. Effects of several macrolide antibiotics on blood pressure of dogs. *Jpn J Pharmacol* 1972;22:799–807.
63. De Morais IP, Corrado AP, Suarez-Kurtz G. Competitive antagonism between calcium and aminoglycoside antibiotics on guinea pig intestinal smooth muscle. *Arch Int Pharmacodyn* 1978;231:317–327.
64. Sohn YZ, Katz RL. Effects of certain antibiotics on isometric contractions of isolated heart muscle. *Can Anaesth Soc J* 1978;25:291–296.
65. Wolf GL, Wigton RS. Vasodilation induced by streptomycin in the perfused canine kidney. *Arch Int Pharmacodyn* 1971;194:285–289.
66. Pandey K, Kumar S, Badola RP. Neuromuscular blocking and hypotensive actions of streptomycin and their reversal. *Br J Anaesth* 1964;36:19–25.
67. Goodman FR, Adams HR, Weiss GB. Effects of neomycin on ^{45}Ca binding and distribution in canine arteries. *Blood Vessels* 1975;12:248–260.
68. Goodman FR, Weiss GB, Adams HR. Alterations by neomycin of ^{45}Ca movements and contractile responses in vascular smooth muscle. *J Pharmacol Exp Ther* 1974;188:472–480.
69. Goodman FR. Distribution of ^{14}C-gentamicin in vascular smooth muscle. *Pharmacology* 1978;16:17–25.
70. Goodman FR, Adams HR. Contractile function and ^{45}Ca movements in vascular smooth muscle of nonhuman primates: effects of aminoglycoside antibiotics. *Gen Pharmacol* 1976;7:227–232.
71. Goodman FR. Calcium related basis of action of vascular agents: cellular approaches. In: Weiss GB, ed. *Calcium in drug action.* New York: Plenum Press; 1978:331.
72. Weiss GB. Calcium and contractility in vascular smooth muscle. In: Narahashi T, Bianchi CP, eds. *Advances in general and cellular pharmacology II.* New York: Plenum Press; 1977:71–154.

73. van Breeman C, Siegel B, Hwang O. Differences in adrenergic activation of coronary and peripheral arteries. *Fed Proc* 1978;37:416(abstract).
74. Calviello G, Chiesi M. Rapid kinetic analysis of the calcium-release reticulum: the effect of inhibitors. *Biochemistry* 1989;28:1301–1306.
75. Orsulakova A, Stockhurst E, Schacht J. Effect of neomycin on phosphoinositide labeling and calcium binding in guinea pig inner ear tissues *in vivo* and *in vitro*. *J Neurochem* 1975;26:285–290.
76. Schibeci A, Schacht J. Action of neomycin on the metabolism of polyphosphoinositides in the guinea pig kidney. *Biochem Pharmacol* 1977;26:1769–1774.
77. Sohn YZ, Katz RL. Interaction of halothane and antibiotics on isometric contractions of rat heart muscle. *Anesth Analg* 1977;56:515–521.
78. Goodman FR, Adams HR. Negative inotropic effects of gentamicin in guinea pig left atria. *Fed Proc* 1976;35:613(abstract).
79. Lullmann H, Schwarz B. Effects of aminoglycoside antibiotics on bound calcium and contraction in guinea-pig atria. *Br J Pharmacol* 1985;86:799–803.
80. Pappano AJ. Calcium-dependent action potentials produced by catecholamines in guinea pig atrial muscle fiber depolarized by potassium. *Circ Res* 1970;27:379–389.
81. Thyrum PT. Inotropic stimuli and systolic transmembrane calcium flow in depolarized guinea pig atria. *J Pharmacol Exp Ther* 1974;188:166–179.
82. Hino N, Ochi R, Yanagisawa T. Inhibition of the slow inward current and the time-dependent outward current of mammalian ventricular muscle by gentamicin. *Pflugers Arch* 1982;394:243–249.
83. Gotanda K, Yanagisawa T, Satoh K, Taira N. Are the cardiovascular effects of gentamicin similar to those of calcium antagonists? *Jpn J Pharmacol* 1988;47:217–227.
84. Lohdi S, Weiner ND, Mechigian J, Schacht J. Ototoxicity of aminoglycosides correlated with their action on monomolecular films of polyphosphoinositides. *Biochem Pharmacol* 1980;29:597–601.
85. De la Chapella-Groz A, Athias P. Gentamicin causes the fast depression of action potential and contraction in cultured cardiocytes. *Eur J Pharmacol* 1988;152:111–120.
86. Hashimoto H, Yanagisawa T, Taira N. Differential antagonism of the negative inotropic effect of gentamicin by calcium ions, Bay k 8644 and isoprenaline in canine ventricular muscle: comparison with cobalt ions. *Br J Pharmacol* 1989;96:906–912.
87. Hagiwara S, Byerly L. Calcium channel. *Annu Rev Neurosci* 1981;4:69–125.
88. Durrett LR, Adams HR. A comparison of the influence of La^{3+}, D600, and gentamicin on frequency–force relationships in isolated myocardium. *Eur J Pharmacol* 1980;66:315–325.
89. Suarez-Kurtz G, Reuben JP. Effects of neomycin on calcium channel currents in clonal GH3 pituitary cells. *Pflugers Arch* 1987;410:517–523.
90. Wagner JA, Snowman AM, Olivera BM, Snyder SH. Aminoglycoside effects on voltage-sensitive calcium channels and neurotoxicity. *N Engl J Med* 1987;317:1669.
91. Gustin M, Hennessey TM. Neomycin inhibits the calcium current of paramecium. *Biochim Biophys Acta* 1988;940:99–104.
92. Dulon D, Zajic G, Aran JM, Schacht J. Aminoglycoside antibiotics impair calcium entry but not viability and motility in isolated cochlear hair cells. *J Neurosci Res* 1989;24:338–346.
93. Nomura K, Naruse K, Watanabe K, Sokabe M. Aminoglycoside blockade of Ca^{2+}-activated K^+ channel from rat brain synaptosomal membranes incorporated into planar bilayers. *J Membr Biol* 1990;115:241–251.
94. Tomargo J, De Miguel B, Tejerina MT. A comparison of josamycin with macrolides and related antibiotics on isolated rat atria. *Eur J Pharmacol* 1982;80:285–293.
95. Regan TJ, Khan MI, Oldewurtel HA, Passannante AJ. Antibiotic effect on myocardial K^+ transport and the production of ventricular tachycardia. *J Clin Invest* 1969;48:68A.
96. Banerjee S, Mitra C. Muscle relaxant properties of chloramphenicol. *J Pharm Sci* 1976;65:704–708.
97. Glanzer ML, Peaslee MH. Inhibition of heart beat development by chloramphenicol in intact and cardia bifida explanted chick embryos. *Experimenta* 1970;26:370–371.
98. Arora HRK. Effects of polyene antifungal antibiotics on the heart: a study with amphotericin B and endomycin. *Indian J Med Res* 1965;53:877–881.

99. Arora HRK, Arora V. A study on the cardiac actions of some polyene antibiotics. *Arch Int Pharmacodyn* 1970;185:234–245.
100. Arora V, Shah GF, Arora HRK. Effects of polyene-antifungal antibiotics on the perfused guinea pig heart. *Med Pharmacol Exp* 1967;17:391–396.
101. Ruiz-Ceretti E, Schanne OF, Bonnardeaux JL. Effects of amphotericin B on isolated rabbit hearts. *J Moll Cell Cardiol* 1976;8:77–88.
102. Schanne OF, Ruiz-Ceretti E, Deslauriers Y, Payet D, Soulier P, Demers JM. The effects of amphotericin B on the ionic currents of frog atrial trabeculae. *J Mol Cell Cardiol* 1977;9:909–920.
103. Tolins JP, Raij L. Adverse effect of amphotericin B administration on renal hemodynamics in the rat: neurohumoral mechanisms and influence of calcium channel blockade. *J Pharmacol Exp Ther* 1988;245:594–599.
104. Ramos H, de Murciano AA, Cohen BE, Bolard J. The polyene antibiotic amphotericin B acts as a Ca^{2+} ionophore in sterol-containing liposomes. *Biochim Biophys Acta* 1989;982:303–306.
105. Schneider JA, Sperelakis N. Valinomycin blockade of slow channels in guinea pig heart perfused with elevated K^+ and isoproterenol. *Eur J Pharmacol* 1974;27:349–354.
106. Vogel S, Sperelakis N. Valinomycin blockade of myocardial slow channels is reversed by high glucose. *Am J Physiol* 1978;235:H46–H51.
107. Marche P, Olier B, Girard A, Fillastre JP, Morin JP. Aminoglycoside-induced alterations of phosphoinositide metabolism. *Kidney Int* 1987;31:59–64.
108. Tysnes OB, Steen VM, Holmsen H. Neomycin inhibits platelet functions and inositol phospholipid metabolism upon stimulation with thrombin, but not with ionomycin or 12-O-tetradecanoyl-phorbol 13-acetate. *Eur J Biochem* 1988;177:219–223.
109. Cockcroft S, Stutchfield J. Effect of pertussis toxin and neomycin on G-protein-regulated polyphosphoinositide phosphodiesterase. *Biochem J* 1988;256:343–350.
110. Vassbotn FS, Langeland N, Holmsen H. Neomycin inhibits PDGF-induced IP_3 formation and DNA synthesis but not PDGF-stimulated uptake of inorganic phosphate in C3H/10T1/2 fibroblasts. *Biochim Biophys Acta* 1990;1054:207–212.
111. Buyniske JP, Bierwagen ME. Comparative effects of kanamycin and amikacin on aortic blood pressure, cardiac rate, and surface electrocardiogram in the conscious dog. *Res Commun Chem Pathol Pharmacol* 1975;11:327–330.

Cardiovascular Toxicology, Second Edition,
edited by Daniel Acosta, Jr.
Raven Press, Ltd., New York © 1992.

9

Bacterial Lipopolysaccharide (Endotoxin) and Myocardial Dysfunction

*‡Janet L. Parker and †‡H. Richard Adams

*Departments of *Physiology and †Veterinary Biomedical Sciences, and the ‡Dalton Research Center, University of Missouri–Columbia, Columbia, Missouri 65211*

> While it is generally conceded that peripheral vascular failure is the dominant factor concerned in the development of shock, from time to time suspicions have been voiced that the myocardium is also involved.—C. J. Wiggers, 1950 (1)

> There is now widespread recognition that most patients with sepsis and septic shock develop significant derangements of myocardial function.—J. E. Parrillo, 1990 (2)

Circulatory shock resulting from bacterial sepsis remains the most common cause of death in medical and surgical intensive care units in the United States (2–5). Mortality rates ascribed to septicemic shock remain as high as 30–60% despite aggressive clinical management with antibiotics, intravascular volume expansion, cardiovascular support drugs, and other interventions (4). The pathogenesis of shock is incompletely understood, but it unquestionably involves a highly complex and dynamic progression of hemodynamic and metabolic derangements eventually affecting virtually all organ systems. Profound cardiovascular dysfunction is believed to dominate as the ultimate cause of death in septicemic patients.

The lipopolysaccharide (LPS) constituent of the outer cell membrane of gram-negative bacteria, commonly referred to as endotoxin, is considered to be the primary bacterial-product toxin responsible for the development of host cell reactions to gram-negative sepsis and its subsequent cardiovascular manifestations (6–13). Upon entry into the host organism's circulation, LPS interacts with different types of cells including macrophages, polymorphonuclear leukocytes, platelets, and vascular endothelial cells. Cells activated by LPS are induced to release an impressive repertoire of endogenous compounds that normally serve immunomodulatory or inflammatory functions. These factors include immunopermissive cytokines such as tumor necrosis factor-α and interleukins, and fatty acid breakdown products such as the eicosanoids and platelet activating factor. In the septicemic patient these factors for some reason become pathophysiologic progenitors and mediators of LPS toxicity instead of physiologically containing the bacterial invaders. This complex cascade culminates in the severe cardiovascular dysfunction and multiorgan failure comprising septicemic shock.

Septic shock is characterized typically by low systemic vascular resistance, generalized maldistribution of tissue blood flows, and cardiac output inadequate relative to metabolic demands. The predominant historical viewpoint emphasized the role of peripheral vascular collapse, rather than myocardial failure, in the pathogenesis of circulatory shock. However, shock-related functional depression of the heart has now been documented in numerous clinical and experimental investigations using a wide variety of techniques and approaches (for reviews, see refs. 2–5 and 14–24). Current research efforts include not only validation of the presence of shock-induced myocardial depression in patients and intact animal models but also address: (a) cellular, subcellular, and biochemical mechanisms of disrupted excitation–contraction coupling of the heart in shock; (b) putative endogenous toxic mediators that could be involved in producing myocardial dysfunction in shock; and (c) potential chemotherapeutic interventions that may directly or indirectly improve myocardial contractile function in shock.

This chapter provides an overview of this area, with emphasis on: (a) the large body of clinical and experimental evidence indicating that impaired myocardial performance accompanies endotoxin and septic shock states; (b) cellular and biochemical mechanisms of disrupted excitation–contraction coupling processes of the cardiac myocyte in shock; and (c) potential *in vivo* mechanisms and mediators involved in the myocardial toxicity of endotoxicosis.

CARDIAC DYSFUNCTION IN CLINICAL LPS AND
SEPSIS SYNDROMES

Generally accepted concepts relative to the function of the heart in clinical shock states have undergone major transition and considerable controversy over the past several decades. Much of the discrepancies during this period relate to changes in (a) clinical recognition and characterization of the shock state itself, (b) criteria for identification of myocardial depression, and (c) major alterations in therapeutic management of shock, particularly relating to the more recent use of aggressive fluid resuscitation. The dynamic and precarious nature of shock and limited diagnostic capabilities have further increased the difficulty of studying intrinsic cardiodynamic function in shock patients. Despite these drawbacks, a large number of clinical studies have now provided convincing evidence for significant myocardial dysfunction in endotoxemic and septicemic patients.

Historically, septic shock was characterized by a hemodynamic pattern mainly of hypotension and low cardiac output (1,19,25). Aggressive administration of resuscitative fluids was not standard clinical practice during this period (prior to 1960), primarily because a convenient and accurate measure of LV end-diastolic filling volume or preload was unavailable (for reviews, see refs. 3, 18, and 19). The subsequent use of the pulmonary artery catheter to monitor pulmonary capillary wedge pressures provided information suggesting that the reduced cardiac output reported in previous studies resulted from reduced venous return and inadequate LV preload (19). Septic shock patients in more contemporary investigations generally receive large volumes of resuscitative fluids to achieve optimal preload. Under these conditions, most septic patients initially exhibit a "hyperdynamic" pattern of hemodynamic and cardiac function characterized by normal to high cardiac output and low systemic vascular resistance. Increased cardiac output in the majority of septic shock patients seemed inconsistent with the presence of heart failure, and renewed doubts and controversy about the involvement of myocardial dysfunction in the early hyperdynamic stages of shock.

Subsequent findings of Siegel et al. (26,27) indicated that septic shock patients may shift from a high cardiac output (hyperdynamic) to a low cardiac output (hypodynamic) state as circulatory shock progresses. Shoemaker (28) similarly reported a general pattern of normal to increased cardiac output early in patients in septic shock, followed by a precipitous fall in cardiac output and cardiac work in patients who subsequently died; indeed, cardiac output at the onset of therapeutic management has been closely proportional to survival following bacterial shock (29,30). Decreased LV stroke work in relation to right-sided filling pressure was observed by Siegel et al. (27) in 30 patients with bacterial shock of various causes. Those patients with hypodynamic (low output) septic shock states had poorer ventricular function relationships and tended to be the least responsive to therapy (31). Weisel et al. (32) measured the transient effects of fluid challenge on LV stroke work and pulmonary artery occlusive pressure and found evidence of impaired LV function in fatal cases of sepsis. The LV stroke work index in patients with low output septic shock was only 25% of normal values in the presence of a 200% increase in central venous pressure (CVP).

The premise that a hyperdynamic state of increased cardiac output is an indicator of a better prognosis during sepsis has not been accepted by all investigators. Several studies showed that most nonsurvivors maintained a normal or high cardiac index (CI), even within a few hours of death (33–36). In 1990, D'Orio et al. (35) reported an analysis of clinical, hemodynamic, and metabolic data from 26 consecutive septic shock patients before and during volume infusion. Mean CI was initially greater in survivors than nonsurvivors (4.5 versus 3.0 L/min/m^2), but none of the initial cardiovascular variables served as a reliable predictor for survival. During fluid loading, however, only survivors exhibited a normal cardiac response, as evidenced by the change in LV stroke work index (LVSWI) for a given increase in the pulmonary capillary wedge pressure as the index of LV preload. These investigators suggested that the LVSWI response to volume loading may be a better predictor of prognosis than total CI (35). Also in 1990, Jardin et al. (36) evaluated serial hemodynamic measurements and two-dimensional echo cardiographic studies in 21 patients with sepsis-related circulatory failure. Initial hemodynamic evaluation revealed severe ventricular systolic dysfunction in one-third of the patients, as evidenced by low CI and markedly reduced LV ejection fraction. The remaining patients exhibited an increased CI associated with tachycardia. Since LVEF remained normal despite low peripheral vascular resistance, they concluded the presence of moderate LV systolic dysfunction, even during the apparently hyperdynamic state of septic shock. Reinhart et al. (37) reported in 1990 that therapeutically induced increases in oxygen delivery (via inotropic support drugs) produced measurable but small increases in oxygen consumption (Vo_2) in septic shock patients; Vo_2 increases, however, were similar in survivors and nonsurvivors, suggesting that factors other than tissue oxygen deficit determined patient outcome. The use of pulmonary capillary wedge pressure as an index of LV end-diastolic pressure may be inaccurate in some conditions (38–41). Lefcoe and colleagues (39) reported wedge pressure to be 30 mm higher than LV end-diastolic pressure in five septic patients. Snyder (40) suggested that ventricular filling pressure may be consistently dissociated from wedge pressure in septic patients. If so, greater reliance may need to be placed on volume challenge, measurements of end-diastolic volume, or direct measures of left atrial or ventricular end-diastolic pressure to assure adequate ventricular filling.

Much insight has recently been provided by the work of Parrillo and co-workers (2–5,18,19), using simultaneous assessment of cardiac hemodynamics and measurements of radionuclide scan-determined LV end-systolic and end-diastolic volume indices in endotoxemic and septic shock patients. These investigators employed three different methods of quantifying serial ventricular performance in their subjects: ejection fractions, shifts in the Starling ventricular function curve based on LV end-diastolic volume index versus stroke work index, and the ventricular function curve response to intravascular volume expansion. In brief, their findings indicated that septic shock produced a profound decrease in systolic LV performance that was expressed as a substantial decrease in ejection fraction. Left ventricular dysfunction was most evident during the early course (1–3 days) of sepsis and was reversible by days 7–10 after the onset of sepsis. Intravascular volume expansion partially overcame the decrease in systolic performance early in shock but was less effective after progression of shock to the more severe stages (2–5,18,19). The impairment in LV systolic function was associated temporally with a dilatative increase in LV end-diastolic volume index. Dilation of the heart with increased end-diastolic volume tended to maintain the stroke volume index constant although ejection fraction remained low. However, the diastolic enlargement was dependent on the intravascular volume expansion. The end-diastolic volume index did not increase without volume expansion; instead, it seemingly decreased (18,19).

Vincent et al. (29) reported the presence of biventricular cardiac failure in the fatal progression of septic shock due to peritonitis. In contrast to the acute survivors, the fatal cases failed to respond to fluid repletion; instead, they demonstrated disproportionate increases in both right- and left-side filling pressures, increases in pulmonary vascular resistance, and decreased right and LV work capability. Recent studies documented right ventricular (RV) dysfunction in septic shock patients manifested as reduced RV ejection fraction with higher RV end-systolic volumes (42). Similar responses were observed by Bell and Thal (43) in another group of septic shock patients without preexisting heart disease. These patients responded to volume loading with a rapid rise in CVP without a concomitant increase in cardiac output. Early heart failure was suggested in some patients, although most showed evidence of cardiac failure after shock periods of longer than 24 hr. Right ventricular failure in shock has also been suggested by Clowes (44) and others (45) to be related to increased pulmonary vascular resistance and attendant elevation of impedance to RV ejection. Indeed, Schneider et al. (48) suggested that volume loading in some patients with septic shock does not result in increased forward flow because of RV failure associated with pulmonary hypertension (increased RV outflow pressure) and also coronary hypotension. Disparate changes in both preload and afterload may thus disorder biventricular working conditions and, ultimately, adversely affect output performance of both left and right ventricles in shock (42–50).

In summary, numerous clinical studies have now provided considerable evidence confirming the contention that septicemic circulatory shock is associated with reduced ventricular performance. Because of major changes in cardiac filling volumes and outflow resistance seen by both the RV and LV chambers, it has been difficult to distinguish intrinsic myocardial dysfunction from an otherwise normal heart that is forced to work-pump under abnormal preload and afterload conditions (17). The difficulty inherent to highly invasive monitoring in ill patients has prompted study of experimental shock models in laboratory animals.

CARDIAC DYSFUNCTION IN EXPERIMENTAL LPS AND SEPSIS MODELS: *IN VIVO* STUDIES

The complex issues involved in the experimental evaluation of cardiodynamic adjustments during shock were addressed previously by different groups (2–5,14,16–24). Much of the earlier investigations using experimental shock models followed a similar line of reasoning as that described in clinical reports. For instance, in 1956 Weil et al. (51) demonstrated that the heart appears to perform adequately in the early phase of endotoxin shock in the dog, but that the pooling of large volumes of blood in the liver and intestines elicits marked decreases in venous return and the heart is thus unable to maintain its output. Goodyer (52) reported no evidence of primary myocardial failure in early hemorrhagic or endotoxin shock in dogs and therefore concluded that peripheral mechanisms, rather than heart failure *per se*, were dominant in determining irreversibility in shock. Lefer (53) reported that LV performance (calculated as stroke output corrected for filling pressure) actually increased 2 hr after 0.75 mg/kg endotoxin administration in dogs; significant cardiodepression was not observed until 6–7 hr postendotoxin. Further evidence supportive of a lack of myocardial depression in the early phase of shock has been presented by other investigators on the basis of unaltered LV function curves (54–56), maximum velocity of contraction (V_{max}) (57), function of pumping heart preparations (58–61), and other *in vivo* indices of cardiac contractility (62–64). Indeed, Hess et al. (24) suggested that the early phase of experimental endotoxin or bacteremic shock may be analogous to the high-output/low-resistance stage of clinical septic shock, where cardiac output is relatively maintained without evidence of myocardial failure. Even in cases where decreases in LV pressure, LV maximal rate of pressure development ($+dP/dt_{max}$), or cardiac output were reported (65,66), investigators generally attributed these alterations to deficient venous return and LV preload and did not consider myocardial depression to be a major contributing factor.

On the other hand, Solis and Downing (67) reported initial evidence for reduced LV function curves in early endotoxemia in the cat. The initial resistance of the canine pumping heart preparation to the effects of endotoxin shock was initially shown by Hinshaw, Archer, and colleagues (68–71) and David and Rogel (72) to deteriorate after several hours. Notable cardiac dysfunction or failure was reported to occur as early as 4–7 hr following an LD_{70} endotoxin administration and was demonstrated by increased LV end-diastolic pressure, decreased cardiac power and myocardial efficiency, and depressed negative and positive dP/dt_{max} values. These authors suggested that abnormal ventricular diastolic filling and inadequate coronary perfusion result in progressively diminishing cardiac performance, often terminating in overt failure (69). Indeed, maintenance of coronary perfusion pressure and coronary blood flow has been shown to delay cardiac functional deterioration in both hemorrhagic (72) and endotoxin (69,73) shock.

As emphasized in previous reviews (16,17,22,74), the preponderance of early studies of shock cardiodynamics used indexes of myocardial inotropy that were sensitive to changes in preload and afterload. Such methods are limited because they cannot adequately sample intrinsic myocardial compartments independently of concurrent changes in peripheral vascular preconditions (14–17). More recent studies with improved technologies have reopened the issue of early cardiac participation in LPS-related shock syndromes.

The LV end-systolic pressure–volume relationship is believed to describe the inotropic state of the heart independently of changes in preload and afterload (22,74,75). Guntheroth et al. (76,77) used the LV end-systolic pressure–volume ratio technique in mongrel dogs and found that evidence for depressed myocardial contractility appeared early after endotoxin injection (2–6 hr) and persisted until death. Goldfarb et al. also used this ratio technique and consistently obtained similar evidence for an early and maintained reduction in myocardial contractility after endotoxin injection in both dogs (22,74,78,79) and pigs (80–82). Lee et al. (82) used an endotoxin-loaded osmotic pump to produce a state of "hyperdynamic" sepsis in pigs characterized by elevated cardiac output, heart rate, and LV systolic pressure. Hearts of surviving pigs (10 of 15) exhibited significantly depressed slope of the end-systolic pressure–diameter relationships (ESPDR) and percent shortening of short axis diameter, despite concomitant elevated rates of pressure development.

Other investigators have used basically similar end-systolic pressure–dimension relationships as an index of myocardial contractility in whole animal studies of shock but, in contrast, recorded no negative inotropism. That is, not only did endotoxemia not reduce myocardial contractility, it actually seemed to enhance myocardial contractility (83,84). This controversy was resolved recently when Law et al. (85) reported that β-adrenergic blockade with propranolol prevented the increase in end-systolic pressure–dimension ratio they normally observed in endotoxemic animals (83,84). Indeed, these investigators reported that after propranolol they now observed evidence of decreased myocardial contractility in their animal model of sepsis (85), consistent with other studies (78–82).

The preceding findings from different laboratories (76–85) emphasize two important caveats about *in situ* hemodynamic studies in shock research (17). First, compensatory release of epinephrine and norepinephrine acting on cardiac β-receptors can mask underlying myocardial depression, an often overlooked but fundamental characteristic of shock recognized years ago (86). Second, although the end-systolic pressure–volume relationship may describe the myocardial inotropic state independently of cardiac loading conditions, alterations in this relationship do not differentiate underlying abnormalities in intrinsic muscle mechanics from inotropic effects evoked by extrinsic factors such as catecholamines or other neurogenic or circulating cardioactive agents.

Papadakis and Abel (87) evaluated LV performance in canine endotoxin shock, using an intact open-chest experimental model wherein cardiac function curves were constructed at constant mean arterial pressure and heart rate (88). The $+dP/dt_{max}$ index of contractility was used along with LV end-diastolic pressure to assess directional changes in contractility under these controlled conditions. Interestingly, $+dP/dt_{max}$ was depressed early (60 min) during the 2-hr period after intravenous endotoxin, although coronary sinus flow was significantly elevated at 2 hr. These findings supported the view of an early and sustained depression of myocardial contractility in endotoxin shock unrelated to coronary hypoperfusion and its resulting detrimental effects on the myocardium. Abel and Beck (89) reported that with constant heart rate and preload, ventricular performance indicators tended to follow the afterload curve. The largest changes were observed in $-dP/dt_{max}$, perhaps suggesting an early disturbance in LV relaxation. These authors also appropriately cautioned about the difficulty of interpreting any *in vivo* parameter of cardiac performance under conditions of changing preload, heart rate, or afterload.

Findings from several studies using nonhuman primates also suggest strongly that the myocardium is adversely affected during shock, based primarily on abnormal relationships between ventricular filling pressure, cardiac output, and mean arterial pressure (58,90–93). Greenfield et al. (93) found that during fluid loading (colloid infusion) in monkeys, cardiac work in endotoxin-shocked animals was one-half that of control animals at equal end-diastolic ventricular pressures. Autopsy evaluation of these animals revealed evidence of myocardial edema and swelling of capillary endothelium in the endotoxin-treated group. Geocaris et al. (91) similarly demonstrated altered LV responses to fluid loading in an intact awake shock model in baboons. In 1990, the effects of endotoxemia on basic cardiovascular function were reported by Snow et al. (94) using *in situ* hearts of rhesus monkeys. These investigators reported an impairment of the heart's ability to maintain sufficient oxygen delivery, as measured by the reduction–oxidation state of cytochrome aa_3 during periods of increased work and oxygen delivery.

Evidence is emerging that in addition to the LV systolic contractile dysfunction in shock, the LV diastolic volume index and volume–pressure relationships are also altered. Parrillo and co-workers (95,96) recently conducted studies relevant to their clinical work (discussed above) using a canine model that simulates human septic shock. They documented that without intravascular volume loading, LV end-diastolic volume index fell while pulmonary capillary wedge pressure tended to increase (95,96); this set of findings suggested that septic shock *decreased* LV diastolic compliance and therefore increased its reciprocal, LV diastolic stiffness (97–99). This decrease in LV compliance was especially evident in nonsurvivors, where it was associated with greater decrements in stroke volume and stroke work indices (96). In contrast, intravascular volume loading resulted in an increase in LV end-diastolic volume index without a matching increase in pulmonary wedge pressure (95); this set of findings suggested that intravascular volume therapy *increased* LV diastolic compliance during sepsis (97–

99). This increase in LV compliance was associated with improved LV cardiodynamic indices and survival in both dogs (95,96) and humans (2,100).

The mechanism(s) responsible for the opposing interactive effects of septicemia and intravascular volume expansion on LV diastolic pressure–volume relationships is unknown. Nevertheless, as emphasized by Adams et al. (17), this series of studies by Parrillo and co-workers (2–5, 18,19,95,96,100) yielded three key findings. First, based on ejection fractions measured in conjunction with measurements of cardiac hemodynamics, the radionuclide scan technique provided substantial support for a reversible diminution of intrinsic LV contractile reserves in clinical and experimental sepsis. Second, septicemia also markedly altered LV diastolic function, first reducing end-diastolic compliance and then in some way setting the stage for ventricular dilation and an increase in LV compliance in response to intravascular volume expansion. Third, intravascular volume expansion substantially altered manifestation of the systolic and diastolic LV sequelae of septicemic shock. This third element clearly emphasized the difficulty of ascertaining changes in basal intrinsic myocardial function in patients or intact animals wherein the heart is influenced by the shock state and by numerous endogenously released factors as well as by therapeutic intervention.

Evidence for diastolic dysfunction in sepsis and endotoxin shock models has recently emerged from other laboratories as well. In 1990, Stahl et al. (101) evaluated cardiac responses to continuous high-volume fluid resuscitation in a chronic canine model of hyperdynamic sepsis. Septic animals demonstrated a significant reduction in systolic contractility, as evidenced by the use of a rate- and load-independent index of LV performance (E_{max} of the end-systolic pressure–volume relationship) confirming previous work by Goldfarb et al. (78–82). Abnormal diastolic function was indicated by significant progressive increases in unstressed and end-diastolic ventricular volumes, but significant decreases in myocardial compliance as quantitated by transmural pressure versus normalized volume–strain analysis. Thus intravascular volume expansion increased LV chamber compliance during sepsis by inducing LV chamber dilatation. However, stiffness of the myocardium itself actually increased (101). Evidence for increased LV stiffness was also observed early (2–4 hr) after endotoxemia in guinea pigs (102) and sepsis in rats (103). Thus fluid-induced increases in diastolic volume help maintain global cardiac performance during endotoxemia or sepsis. However, the intrinsic diastolic response of LV myocardium itself apparently entails an early increase in stiffness and a decrease in its reciprocal compliance (17,101–103), while the LV chamber size actually may be increasing owing to fluid-induced dilatation (101). Interestingly, in 1991, Walley and Cooper (104) concluded that impaired LV function during hypovolemic shock in a pig model is due entirely to increased diastolic stiffness.

CARDIAC DYSFUNCTION IN EXPERIMENTAL LPS AND SEPSIS MODELS: ISOLATED TISSUE STUDIES

Different investigative groups have evaluated different types of cardiac tissue preparations isolated from experimentally shocked animals (14–17,21,23,24,103). The approach of using isolated cardiac preparations was initiated in an attempt to circumvent the confounding influence of multiple extracardiac constraints operative in all previous studies with intact subjects. The shock models studied include acute endotoxemia, chronic endotoxemia, intraperitoneal sepsis, and bacteremia. Cardiac tissues include atrial muscle, ventricular muscle, sinoatrial tissue, isovolumetric LV preparations, and externally working LV preparations. The underlying rationale for these studies was to compare cardiodynamic responsiveness of hearts from animals in shock with appropriate sham-shock (control) hearts under equal conditions of preload, heart rate, temperature, and coronary perfusate composition. A tabulation of the results from some of these studies is provided (Table 1) and briefly summarized in this section.

Systolic Properties of the Heart After LPS and Sepsis

Cardiodynamic studies with hearts isolated from shocked animals yielded basically similar results; cardiac muscle removed from the complexity of the *in situ* LPS or septic shock environment consistently displayed a decrease in systolic contractile function irrespective of shock model or animal species (Table 1). This loss in contractile function was expressed as diminished length–tension curves in isolated atrial and ventricular muscles, diminished LV systolic pressure versus LV end-diastolic pressure curves in isovolumetric LV preparations, and diminished LV stroke volume versus left atrial filling pressure curves in externally working hearts. Hinshaw et al. (23,58–61,68–71), in a series of early reports, used blood-perfused pumping LV preparations isolated from dogs receiving LPS to document myocardial failure and decreased responsiveness to catecholamines. Similar effects on myocardial performance were obtained using a live *E. coli* bacteremia model (23,105). The concomitant presence of coronary hypotension was found to increase the incidence of endotoxin-induced myocardial failure in these preparations. These investigators suggested that myocardial edema and/or coronary hypoperfusion may contribute significantly to the endotoxin-induced reductions in myocardial function and responsiveness (71).

Examination of an isovolumetric LV model after 16–18 hr of *E. coli* endotoxemia in guinea pigs indicated that endotoxemia produced reductions in peak LV systolic pressure and also lowered the maximal rates for LV pressure increase ($+dP/dt_{max}$) and decrease ($-dP/dt_{max}$) (106). The contractile dysfunctions associated with this condition were not coupled to changes in heart rate, active state duration, or tissue water content; neither were they surmounted by pyruvate nor by maximally effective increments in coronary flow, end-diastolic stretch, or interstitial Ca^{2+} concentration (106). These findings led to the interpretation that the pathogenesis of endotoxemia and septicemia in some way entailed a decrease in intrinsic inotropic reserves of the left ventricle that was expressed as impaired isovolumic contraction and relaxation (106). The data from crystalloid-perfused hearts provided direct corroboration of cardiac contraction–relaxation disorders observed previously in more complex preparations of endotoxemia with blood-perfused dog hearts (68,69). Results obtained from crystalloid-perfused hearts also supported analogous findings obtained previously by Parker et al. (15,106–115) in isolated atrial and LV papillary muscle preparations harvested from guinea pig and rat endotoxin shock models.

The time course of intrinsic cardiac changes associated with shock were examined in the guinea pig endotoxemic model; based on isometric contractions of electrically paced atrial muscle, inotropic depression developed within 1–2 hr after intraperitoneal injection of *E. coli* endotoxin (113). Maximal loss of contractile function occurred between 6 and 16 hr after endotoxemia was initiated; the endotoxin-mediated inotropic changes were reversible with normal contractile function restored by 2 days after endotoxin injection (113). Similar temporal findings after LPS injection were obtained in preliminary studies with the isovolumetric LV preparation in guinea pig hearts (114). Thus it seems that intrinsic cardiac contractile dysfunction associated with endotoxemia is not simply terminal or agonal in onset but is present early (<4 hr) in the developmental phase of endotoxicosis. This early development of intrinsic cardiac dysfunction supports previous findings in intact dogs indicating that evidence of myocardial dysfunction in endotoxemia occurred within 2–4 hr after systemic exposure to endotoxin (76–79). Thus, owing to this timely appearance, it would seem that systolic myocardial dysfunction could contribute to the development of the hemodynamic instability characteristic of endotoxin and septic shock syndromes.

McDonough et al. (116–119) examined *in vitro* cardiac function of pumping hearts isolated from rat models of hyperdynamic sepsis. These studies confirmed a relatively early onset of myocardial dysfunction in these models. Hearts removed from septic rats during the hyperdynamic stage exhibited a downward and rightward shift in work–function curves, indicative of severe depression. These *in vitro* alterations were evident despite *in vivo* demonstration of significantly elevated cardiac output, tachycardia, elevated coronary blood flow, and unaltered blood pressure (116–119). No significant alterations in high-energy phosphate production or substrate utilization were observed, indicating that altered myocardial metabolism is not likely to be a significant contributor to the dysfunction (119). Furthermore, in these studies of early sepsis, the heart retained the ability to respond to β-adrenergic stimulation by catecholamines with increased inotropy and chronotropy

TABLE 1. *Studies of cardiac tissues isolated from endotoxic/septic animals*

Shock model	Species	Cardiac preparation	Key findings	References
Endotoxin	Guinea pig, rat	Atrial muscle, LV muscle	Decreased inotropy, decreased Ca^{2+} responses, early (<2 hr) onset	107–109, 111–113, 139, 140
Endotoxin	Guinea pig	Sinoatrial node–right atrium	Sick sinus syndrome	107
Endotoxin	Guinea pig	Isovolumetric LV	Decreased LV inotropy, impaired LV relaxation	102, 106, 107, 114
Hyperdynamic sepsis	Rat	Pumping LV	Decreased CO, decreased peak systolic pressure	116, 118, 119
Endotoxin	Rat	Pumping LV	Decreased CO, decreased peak systolic pressure, blunted adrenergic responsiveness	124, 125
Hyperdynamic sepsis	Rat	Pumping LV	Decreased CO, partially antagonized by verapamil and ouabain	117, 118
Endotoxin	Rat	Pumping LV	Decreased CO at 6 hr	123
Hyperdynamic sepsis	Rat	Perfused hearts	Unchanged myocardial concentrations of high-energy phosphates, total adenine nucleotides, and creatine	156
Endotoxin	Rat	Cardiac membranes	Altered β-adrenoreceptor–adenylate cyclase coupling	120, 121, 262, 263
Endotoxin	Rat	Pumping LV	Depressed function antagonized by dichloroacetate	128, 264
Endotoxin	Rat	Cardiac myocytes	Altered adrenergic responsiveness	126
Sepsis	Rat	Right atria	Chronotropic supersensitivity to β-agonists	122

Condition	Animal	Preparation	Finding	Ref.
Sepsis	Rat	Pumping LV	Streptozotocin-induced diabetes potentiated cardiac dysfunction	265
Sepsis	Rat	Isovolumetric LV	Cardiac depression antagonized by isoproterenol	121
Sepsis	Rat	SR membrane	Unaffected Ca–ATPase, increased Ca^{2+} uptake	153
Endotoxin	Dog	SR membranes	Reduced Ca^{2+}-induced Ca^{2+} release, decreased ryanodine binding	154
Endotoxin	Dog	LV myofibril	Depressed myofibrillar ATPase activity	24, 130–134
Endotoxin	Dog	SR membranes	Depressed Ca^{2+} uptake and ATPase activity	134–136
Endotoxin	Guinea pig	SR, SL membranes	Unaffected Ca^{2+} fluxes	151
Endotoxin	Dog	SL membranes	Altered phospholid composition, increased phospholipase A_2 activity	149, 266
Endotoxin	Dog	SL membranes	Altered Na–Ca exchange and stoichiometry	149
Endotoxin	Dog	SL membranes	Unaffected Na–Ca exchange and stoichiometry	150
Endotoxin	Dog	LV muscle strip	Impaired sodium pump activity (^{86}Rb uptake)	267
Endotoxin	Guinea pig	Isovolumetric LV	Reduced LV systolic pressure, increased diastolic chamber stiffness	102
Sepsis	Rat	Isovolumetric LV	Reduced LV systolic pressure, increased diastolic chamber stiffness	103
Endotoxin	Rat	Pumping LV	Exercise training improved LV function and responsiveness	129

Abbreviations: LV, left ventricular; CO, cardiac output; SR, sarcoplasmic reticulum; SL, sarcolemma.

(118,120,121). Smith and McDonough (121) reported that, with maximal iso-proterenol stimulation, isovolumically contracting hearts from septic animals were able to generate the same $+dP/dt_{max}$ as hearts from control animals exposed to lower levels of isoproterenol; there were no differences in inotropic indices between the two groups when expressed as a percent of the maximal $+dP/dt_{max}$ achieved. In addition, chronotropic supersensitivity of cardiac β-adrenoceptors was reported by this group to occur in this rat model of early sepsis (121,122). The chronotropic actions of isoproterenol and fenoterol appeared to be mediated by $β_2$-receptors in septic hearts and by $β_1$-receptors in control hearts (122). These studies (116–122) collectively suggest that in early sepsis the ability of the heart to modulate its inotropic state in response to β-adrenergic stimulation is operative despite intrinsic myocardial contractile dysfunction.

Chronic administration of endotoxin in rats by subcutaneous osmotic pump was shown by Fish et al. (123) to result in reduced *in vitro* cardiac work performance in the absence of *in vivo* evidence of cardiac dysfunction. These studies are consistent with the concept of the confounding influence of compensatory sympathoadrenal stimulation (absent in the *in vitro* heart preparations) in *in vivo* cardiovascular homeostasis during shock and sepsis (123).

In late sepsis or following acute intravenous endotoxin administration, myocardial adrenergic responsiveness may be altered (124–126). These findings may relate to alterations in both α- and β-adrenoceptors observed in other organs and cell types in endotoxemia and sepsis (127). Romanosky et al. (125) reported that isoproterenol increased mechanical work by hearts of endotoxin-treated rats (LD_{50}-6 hr), but not to the same level of performance as that of control hearts not given isoproterenol. Myocytes isolated from endotoxin-treated rats exhibited significantly blunted isoproterenol-stimulated accumulation of adenosine 3′,5′ cyclic monophosphate (cAMP) when compared to myocytes from control rats (126–129). Accumulation of cAMP in response to forskolin was similarly reduced (126,128). Binding studies using ($±$) [^{3}H]CGP 12177 suggested a 25% decrease in β-receptor density, with little effect on receptor affinity for the radiolabeled antagonist (126). Burns et al. (128) reported that amrinone augmented cAMP levels fivefold and increased contractility in endotoxin-shocked rats. Interestingly, DeBlieux et al. (129) recently reported that the reduced cAMP accumulation in response to isoproterenol and forskolin in endotoxin-treated rats may be prevented by exercise training. They proposed that training may maintain the integrity of the β-adrenergic receptor adenylate cyclase system during endotoxin challenge *in vivo* (129).

Diastolic Properties of the Heart After LPS and Sepsis

In contrast to the expanding database corroborating a dysfunction of LV *systolic* dynamics during endotoxemia and septicemia, less is known about the influence of these syndromes on intrinsic *diastolic* cardiodynamics, as introduced previously. Early studies using isovolumetric blood-perfused dog hearts indicated that global LV diastolic force increased after exposure to endotoxin, but this change was interpreted as a reflection of contractile failure rather than as a primary decrease in diastolic compliance (73). Hinshaw and co-workers (68) reported an increase in LV end-diastolic pressure and a decrease in LV $-dP/dt_{max}$ in pumping dog hearts exposed to endotoxemia. Numerous other studies have likewise indicated a reduction in LV $-dP/dt_{max}$ after LPS and sepsis (21,89,102,106), indicating slowed LV myocardial relaxation during early diastole.

Although an increase in LV end-diastolic pressure and a decrease in LV $-dP/dt_{max}$ have been interpreted as endotoxin-mediated changes in LV diastolic compliance or stiffness, interpretations about LV chamber compliance and stiffness cannot be derived from pressure measurements alone (97–99). Diastolic volume must be assessed along with diastolic pressure measurements before unique conclusions can be reached about diastolic pressure–volume relationships (i.e., compliance and stiffness) (97–99). Also, $-dP/dt_{max}$ is highly dependent on preload conditions, and it changes proportionately with changes in sarcomere length or other determinants that influence the magnitude of developed systolic pressure and $+dP/dt_{max}$ (97). Reductions in $-dP/dt_{max}$ can reflect nothing more than parallel changes in systolic function secondary to adjustments in cardiac loading conditions or inotropy. Thus end-diastolic compliance and the rate of ventricular relaxation can be independent variables (97), and changes in one of these variables does not necessarily indicate changes in the other (97).

Left ventricular end-diastolic pressure–volume (compliance) relationships were measured in beating hearts isolated from unresuscitated guinea pigs 16–18 hr after endotoxin (106). Results from this study suggested that intrinsic LV chamber stiffness was increased during endotoxemia, albeit these changes at 16–18 hr postendotoxin did not achieve statistical significance (106). However, recent studies by Parker et al. (102) with the guinea pig model indicated that LV chamber compliance was reduced significantly within 4 hr after induction of endotoxemia, with this reduced compliance partially waning during the next 48 hr *(unpublished observations)*. Thus in the absence of intravascular volume expansion, endotoxemia evoked an early reversible decrease in LV chamber compliance or distensibility.

Hearts isolated from a septic rat model likewise indicated an early reduction in LV diastolic compliance (103), consistent with findings from the guinea pig endotoxin model (102). Even when the LV chamber undergoes dilatation after intravascular volume expansion in experimental peritonitis in dogs, normalized LV volume–strain analyses indicated an increase in diastolic stiffness (decreased compliance) of LV myocardium itself (101). Parrillo and co-workers (2–5,18,19) found that intravascular volume expansion enhanced LV diastolic compliance in survivors of sepsis, while LV compli-

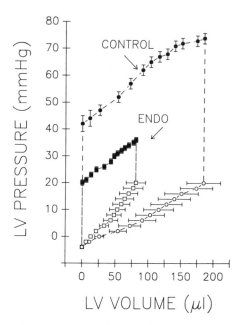

FIG. 1. Composite systolic and end-diastolic pressure–volume relationships in isovolumetric left ventricular preparations of coronary-perfused hearts isolated from control or endotoxemic guinea pigs 4 hr after intraperitoneal injection of either 1 mg/kg of *E. coli* endotoxin (Endo; n = 7) or saline (Control; n = 9). Values are means ± SE of developed systolic pressure (peak systolic pressure minus diastolic pressure; *filled symbols*) and end-diastolic pressure (*open symbols*). Note that systolic pressures are reduced and end-diastolic pressures are elevated in the endotoxin group; thus endotoxemia reduced LV contractility but also decreased LV chamber compliance or distensibility. Adapted from ref. 102.

ance was apparently reduced in nonsurvivors. Thus we would suggest that an early increase in LV diastolic stiffness may well signify a poor prognosis during sepsis, but that a subsequent decrease in LV stiffness (increase in compliance) owing to LV chamber dilatation signifies a beneficial response to intravascular volume resuscitation. Figure 1 illustrates impaired LV contractility concurrent with increased diastolic stiffness of the LV chamber in hearts isolated from guinea pigs 4 hr after the induction of *E. coli* endotoxemia (102).

CARDIAC SUBCELLULAR PREPARATIONS: DISRUPTED Ca^{2+} HANDLING AFTER LPS AND SEPSIS

A breakdown in the subcellular machinery of cardiac excitation–contraction coupling processes has been reported in several experimental shock states, including LPS, septic, and hemorrhagic shock. Evidence for Ca^{2+}-

related functional abnormalities has been obtained using isolated heart muscle preparations, as well as subcellular preparations of cardiac myofibrils, sarcoplasmic reticulum (SR), mitochondria, and sarcolemma. An understanding of these interrelating dysfunctional processes can provide greater insight into possible pathophysiologic and mechanical alterations associated with myocardial failure in shock syndromes.

Hess and colleagues (24,130–134), in an intensive series of studies, demonstrated depressed myofibrillar ATPase activity from ventricular tissue in global myocardial ischemia as well as in canine endotoxin shock. This group further reported that the canine endotoxin shock model was associated with depressed SR Ca^{2+} uptake and ATPase activity (134–136). This effect was greater in subendocardial SR and furthermore was correlated with a decrease in LV stroke work. Augmenting venous return was found to prevent endotoxin-induced decreases in Ca^{2+} uptake and ATPase activity, suggesting a synergistic effect of low venous return in producing these effects (135). In canine hemorrhagic shock, depressed myocardial contractility was associated with depression of myofibrillar ATPase activity characterized by decreased enzyme affinity for Ca^{2+}, as well as uncoupling of Ca^{2+} transport from ATPase hydrolysis in the SR (137). Hess and colleagues (134,135) postulated that a decreased amount of Ca^{2+} sequestered by the SR would decrease the rate of myocardial relaxation. Importantly, reduced SR Ca^{2+} accumulation would decrease the amount of this cation available for release by subsequent action potentials (134), thus contributing to the myocardial contractile depression observed in shock states.

Although loss of sarcolemmal (SL) integrity has been observed in ischemia and shock models using morphometric techniques (138,141–143), precise correlations between SL dysfunction and cardiac depression remain uncertain. Bhagat et al. (139,140) isolated cardiac fragments from guinea pigs subjected to *in vivo* endotoxin treatment; they reported reduced ^{45}Ca binding by a SL fraction but a lack of effect of this procedure on ^{45}Ca uptake by SR or mitochondrial fraction. Bhagat et al. (139) suggested that endotoxin shock may act at the cell membrane of the myocardial fiber to reduce the amount of Ca^{2+} released from superficial sites upon cellular depolarization. Parker and Adams (108) presented functional evidence suggesting that superficial Ca^{2+} stores of the cardiac sarcolemma may be an important target site in the endotoxin-shocked guinea pig. Atrial muscles from shocked animals demonstrated increased sensitivity and prolonged recovery from the negative inotropic actions of Mn^{2+} (thought to compete with Ca^{2+} at outer SL sites), gentamicin (a SL Ca^{2+} channel antagonist), and low Ca^{2+} medium. However, companion studies with D600, nifedipine, and slow Ca^{2+} channel-activation techniques (108) demonstrated that the slow Ca^{2+} channels remained operative in this shock model.

Increasing extracellular Ca^{2+} has been reported to reverse shock-induced cardiac depression in some shock models (108,109) but not in others

(106,112). The lack of complete reversal by Ca^{2+} may suggest permanent damage to the contractile machinery in those models (106). *In vitro* treatment of canine heart homogenates with *E. coli* endotoxin was reported by Liu and Spitzer (144) to result in decreased oxidation rates of palmitate, palmitoyl CoA, and lactate; the inhibitory effects of endotoxin were antagonized by EDTA and mimicked by exogenous Ca^{2+}. It was proposed that endotoxin released endogenous Ca^{2+} from the homogenates, perhaps by causing the membranes to "leak" Ca^{2+} (144). This free Ca^{2+} was thought to be the actual inhibitor of fatty acid and lactate oxidation. Although Mela et al. (145) could find no defect in cardiac mitochondrial oxidative metabolism and energy production in a canine endotoxin shock model, other studies have shown that mitochondria isolated from ischemic left ventricle exhibit reduced ATP production and a lower ATP/O ratio. This has been suggested by Hess (134) to relate to increased cytosolic free Ca^{2+} concentration (produced by failure of the SR pump), subsequent mitochondrial uptake of Ca^{2+}, and inhibition of phosphorylation and ultimately reduced energy available for contraction.

The SL Na–Ca exchanger facilitates the transmembrane movement of Ca^{2+} using the energy of an oppositely directed Na^+ gradient. The operation and direction of exchange can be affected by membrane potential and other interventions (146). Alterations in Na–Ca exchange of the cardiac myocyte could potentially affect Ca^{2+} regulation during both systole and diastole (147), and the exchanger system has been proposed as a target during certain pathophysiological insults such as ischemia, reperfusion injury, and endotoxin shock (148–150). Liu and Xuan (149) reported that Na–Ca exchange in cardiac SL vesicles from endotoxin-shocked dogs exhibited decreased activity and altered stoichiometry from 3 Na^+ per Ca^{2+} (146) to 2 Na^+ per Ca^{2+}. In contrast, Hale et al. (150) recently evaluated activity and stoichiometry of Na–Ca exchange using the thermodynamic approach of Reeves and Hale (146). These studies suggest that cardiac SL Na–Ca exchange activity was not altered in canine endotoxin shock and that the exchange process remained electrogenic with a stoichiometry of 3 Na^+ per Ca^{2+} (150). These studies were recently supported by those of Kutsky and Parker (151), with SL membrane vesicles prepared from a guinea pig endotoxin shock model. Calcium pump activity (energy-dependent Ca^{2+} uptake) was similar in sarcolemma from control and shock animals, and no intrinsic alteration in the rate or equilibrium Ca^{2+} concentration of Na–Ca exchange was observed. The electrogenic nature of the exchanger was maintained, suggesting that the stoichiometry was greater than 2 Na^+ per Ca^{2+} (151), results supporting the findings of Hale et al. (150). Since Na–Ca exchange and other Ca^{2+}-binding characteristics of the sarcolemma could be affected by changes in cardiac phospholipids, Hale et al. (152) evaluated cardiac sarcolemmal phospholipid profiles of hearts isolated from a guinea pig endotoxin shock model characterized by marked functional depression of the LV myocardium and altered responsiveness to Ca^{2+}-dependent inotropic interventions acting at SL sites (108,109). However, Hale et al. reported that cardiac SL phospholipid levels (measured by HPLC) of phosphatidyl ethanolamine, phosphatidyl choline, and sphingomylin were unaltered by endotoxemia when compared to sarcolemma from control subjects (152).

Several recent studies have evaluated Ca^{2+} fluxes of isolated SR vesicles prepared from septic or endotoxin rats (153), guinea pigs (151), and dogs (154). These studies used cardiac membrane preparations similar to those reported in the earlier studies by Hess and colleagues (24,134–136). McDonough (153) evaluated the capacity of the SR to take up Ca^{2+} as well as Ca^{2+}-stimulated ATPase activity in SR vesicles from a hyperdynamic sepsis model of decreased cardiac function. In contrast to the previous studies of endotoxemia in dogs (134–136) and rats (155), McDonough (153) reported that Ca^{2+} uptake in SR from septic rats was not depressed but in fact was increased compared to control SR. However, these results were consistent with those of Soulsby et al. (135) in which SR function was normal in endotoxic dogs when venous return was maintained (i.e., a hyperdynamic model). Recently, Kutsky and Parker (151) reported no significant alterations in active Ca^{2+} transport, Ca^{2+} ATPase activity, and passive Ca^{2+} efflux in SR membrane isolated from a guinea pig endotoxin shock model. Thus impaired SR Ca^{2+} pump activity or leak of Ca^{2+} from the SR does not appear to be a factor in the intrinsic myocardial dysfunction observed in this model (106–112). These data do not rule out the possibility that other influences (acidosis, toxins, ischemia, etc.) may be operative *in vivo* to indirectly alter Ca^{2+} fluxes and cardiac performance. In 1991 Liu and Wu (154) reported interesting data suggesting that Ca^{2+}-induced Ca^{2+} release from either passively or actively loaded SR vesicles was decreased in a canine endotoxin model. Furthermore, the binding of [^{3}H]ryanodine to cardiac SR was significantly reduced by 25%. Such derangements in the SR Ca^{2+} release channel may have potential significance in the shock-induced depression of myocardial contractility and diastolic function.

MEDIATORS OF MYOCARDIAL TOXICITY OF LPS AND SEPSIS

The etiologic mechanisms and pathways that couple complex systemic syndromes such as endotoxemia with intrinsic dysfunction of heart muscle remain questionable. Since the endotoxin molecule itself does not seem to possess direct cardiac inotropic actions (115), the endotoxemic syndrome apparently affects the heart through other more complex mechanistic pathways. Different abnormalities and mediators have been proposed as sole or adjunctive causes of endotoxin-induced cardiac changes, including circulating myocardial depressant peptides, activation of endogenous opiate systems, hematologic factors, release of various autacoids such as eicosanoids and cytokines, myocardial infiltration with leukocytes and generation of oxygen free radicals, and global or regional malperfusion of the heart (see refs. 2–4, 14–17, 24, and 74 for compilation). Many questions remain unanswered; however, recent studies have provided evidence that global myocardial ischemia is not a necessary prerequisite for the cardiodynamic complications of endotoxemia or sepsis (2–5,17,156–158).

Role of Myocardial Ischemia

Circulatory shock syndromes associated with endotoxemia and septicemia often are accompanied by systemic hypotension and therefore below-normal coronary perfusion pressures. These relationships have led to the idea that cardiac complications from these types of shock simply reflected inadequate coronary perfusion pressure and global myocardial ischemia. This hypothesis was supported by the fact that decreases in coronary blood flow were not uncommon observations after endotoxin injection (69,157, 159–164). However, the physiologic and pathophysiologic interactions between coronary blood flow and oxygen needs of cardiac tissue are exceedingly complex. An understanding of these relationships in shock requires a consideration not only of the quantity of coronary blood flow but also of cardiac workload dynamics and resulting autoregulation of coronary vascular resistance to match changing metabolic needs of the heart. In other words, the critical question is not whether coronary blood flow is reduced during shock; the critical question is whether myocardial blood flow is adequate to supply energy requirements of the heart during shock (16,17).

Coronary blood flow is determined by the interactions of vascular resistance, extravascular (compressive force) resistance, and perfusion pressure (165). The coronary circulation normally exhibits a tight relationship between cardiac metabolic rate and blood flow and near-ideal autoregulation of blood flow in response to changes in cardiac work. Endotoxin-induced myocardial hypoperfusion could result from increases in resistance (either vascular or extravascular), decreases in perfusion pressure, and/or malfunction in coronary blood flow autoregulation. Each of these mechanisms has been invoked as a cause for decreased or inadequate coronary blood flow leading to depressed cardiac function in endotoxin shock (17,69,159–164).

Elkins et al. (159) used cardiopulmonary bypass to separate the coronary and systemic circulations in dogs during endotoxic shock. Their data indicated intermediate levels of cardiac performance in dogs given endotoxin when normal coronary perfusion pressures were maintained. On the other hand, if the coronary circulation was perfused at pressures of 20–70 mm Hg during endotoxin, more substantial depression of cardiac function was observed. Similarly, Hinshaw et al. (69) used isolated hearts to investigate the relationship between coronary blood flow and cardiac function in endotoxin shock. Their results indicated that coronary hypotension plus endotoxin produced more cardiac depression than did endotoxin or coronary hypotension alone. Thus when endotoxin shock is accompanied by severe systemic hypotension (aortic pressure $\leq$ 50 mm Hg), myocardial hypoperfusion will be a likely adjunctive influence on cardiac function (69,159,160,162).

Bronsveld et al. (166,167) concluded that decreases in coronary blood flow recorded during endotoxic shock were not evidence of myocardial hypoperfusion because the blood flow was still matched to decreased cardiac metabolic demands (work of the heart). The regional distribution of coronary blood flow during endotoxin shock also generally supports the hypothesis that the heart can be adequately perfused even when total flow is decreased. The LV subendocardium is the cardiac tissue believed to be most vulnerable to hypoperfusion and/or ischemia. The subendocardium receives most or all of its blood flow during diastole, and the vasculature supplying the subendocardium is subjected to large intramyocardial compressive effects on resistance and capacitance (165). Therefore when myocardial perfusion is adequate, subendocardial blood flow is greater than or equal to subepicardial blood flow. When myocardial perfusion becomes compromised, subendocardial blood flow is less than subepicardial flow. Data from a recent study of acute endotoxemia in beagle dogs indicated that although total coronary blood flows were reduced substantially by endotoxin (157,168), the double product of heart rate X systolic aortic pressure also was correspondingly reduced (17). Since this double product index is believed to be directly proportional to myocardial oxygen demands, it would seem that the reduction in total coronary blood flow represented autoregulation of coronary vascular resistance brought about by the decreased need for cardiac energy requirements. This interpretation was supported by estimates of transmural blood flow distribution. Although coronary blood flows were decreased in this dog model of endotoxin shock, the subendocardial/subepicardial blood flow ratios of the left ventricle and septum were not significantly different from unity (157).

Somani and Saini (169) and Bronsveld et al. (166,167) likewise measured subendocardial/subepicardial ratios of 0.9–1 during endotoxic shock. Goldfarb et al. (80) also found normal transmural distribution of coronary blood flow in pigs given low doses of endotoxin (100 µg/kg), whereas pigs given high doses of endotoxin (250 µg/kg) had decreased coronary blood flow and decreased subendocardial/subepicardial ratios in combination with evidence of cardiac failure. The high-endotoxin-dose pigs also had mean arterial pressures of less than 60 mm Hg (80).

Coronary blood flows are not always decreased during endotoxemic and septicemic syndromes. In numerous studies, coronary flows have remained normal or even greater than necessary for supplying the metabolic needs of the heart (2,4,103,123). Cunnion et al. (158) reported that myocardial ischemia was not a cause of myocardial depression during septic shock in humans when mean arterial pressures remained at or above 60 mm Hg. Coronary blood flows in their patients were normal or even higher than those of control subjects. Goldfarb et al. (78) observed that low doses of endotoxin (100 μg/kg) in pigs did not decrease coronary blood flow although myocardial mechanical function seemed depressed. Lee et al. (82) found that coronary blood flow was not only maintained in chronic endotoxemic pigs with evidence of cardiac contractile dysfunction, but that coronary flow actually increased when cardiac workload was unchanged. Nishijima et al. (170) studied acute endotoxin injection in pigs and observed that coronary blood flow to the LV myocardium remained at control levels despite the presence of severe systemic hypotension. Fish et al. (123) similarly observed that coronary blood flows were well maintained even after 30 hr of endotoxin infusion in rats. Despite the adequacy of coronary blood flow, hearts isolated from the endotoxemic rats were dysfunctional with depressed left atrial filling pressure versus LV output curves (123). Thus some endotoxemic syndromes can be associated with relative overperfusion of the myocardium even in the presence of reduced contractile variables of the heart muscle. McDonough et al. (119) reached an analogous conclusion after reviewing coronary and cardiodynamic interrelationships developing during hyperdynamic sepsis.

The ultimate test of the adequacy of myocardial perfusion cannot be determined from measurements of coronary blood flow alone. Rather, as mentioned earlier, blood flow relative to the metabolic needs of the myocardium is the key element (17). We and others have measured myocardial energy stores and myocardial adenine nucleotide levels following endotoxin shock to evaluate the adequacy of coronary flow relative to metabolic demand of the heart (157). Although it appears that endotoxin altered myocardial metabolism and produced some subtle changes in various nucleotide concentrations in the heart, high-energy phosphate levels were maintained at control levels even in the presence of substantial reductions in coronary blood flows (157). The minimal changes seen in myocardial adenylates and in pyridine nucleotide coenzymes following endotoxin did not indicate that the hearts were in jeopardy from energy depletion as would be expected if coronary flows were inadequate. A similar maintenance of cardiac high-energy phosphate stores also was observed by McDonough et al. (156) in a hyperdynamic model of sepsis in rats that was characterized by myocardial contractile dysfunction in isolated hearts.

Circulating Cardiodepressant Toxins

The potential deleterious role of blood-borne substances that depress cardiac function in shock has been the basis of numerous publications for over two decades. One of the best known of these substances has been designated myocardial depressant factor (MDF). This term was first used in 1966 by Brand and Lefer (171) and Baxter et al. (172), working in independent laboratories, to describe the cardioinhibitory factors found in the plasma of cats in hemorrhagic shock and dogs in burn shock, respectively. Since then, extensive studies have attempted to characterize the chemical and biological properties of MDF, as well as other toxic factors now also purported to influence cardiac function in shock (14,173). Cardioinhibitory substances have now been reported to be present in endotoxin, hemorrhagic, cardiogenic, splanchnic ischemic, traumatic, and burn shock, and in many species including humans, baboons, dogs, rats, cats, and guinea pigs.

Plasma (or ultrafiltrates of plasma) obtained from animals in shock has been shown to markedly depress contractility of isolated heart muscle preparations (174). This cardiodepressant activity increased as the plasma was purified and it could not be attributed to acidemia, hyperosmolality, or altered ion contents of the plasma (171). Purified extracts of plasma obtained from cats in postoligemic shock reduced contractile force developed by isolated perfused cat hearts and isolated cat papillary muscle by over 50% within 5–10 min (174–176). Exogenously administered MDF (in concentrations thought to be present in the plasma of shocked animals) has been reported to impair cardiac contractility in the normal animal (177), as indicated by a 54% reduction in maximal LV power within 60 min, and the subsequent production of a state of shock. Contractile activity of cultured rat heart cells also has been shown by Carli et al. to be depressed by sera from endotoxin-shocked rats (178) or septic shock patients (179,180).

Neither the chemical structure nor the precise myocardial cellular action of MDF, or any of the other putative cardiotoxic factors of shock, have yet been identified. Several groups have recently reported evidence for partial or complete isolation of several substances and have published reports on their clinical and physical properties (181–184). The molecular weight (mol wt) of MDF in one study was reported to be about 500; it is water soluble and relatively insoluble in methylene chloride; the plasma concentration during shock is on the order of ng/ml (173,174). MDF can be inactivated by ashing or by the addition of trypsin or pronase, a nonspecific proteolytic enzyme (185,186). Greene et al. (187) reported the chromatographic isolation and purification of MDF from dogs in hemorrhagic shock. Biologic activity (bioassay of myocardial depression in feline papillary muscle) was found to reside in a peptide of three or four amino acid residues (glutamic acid, glycine, serine, and an unidentified amino substance). Low molecular weight substances (<1000 mol wt) have also been reported by Goldfarb and colleagues (181,183). Further work is needed to determine the exact identification and characterization of these compounds, as well as the precise cellular mechanisms whereby they may produce cardiac depression.

The formation and subsequent release into the circulation of cardiotoxic factors in shock have been postulated by many investigators to be intimately related to splanchnic ischemia (53,182,185,188–191). Indeed, intestinal venous plasma obtained from animals experiencing simulated intestinal shock (188,189) and splanchnic artery occlusion (190) has been shown to reduce contractility of isolated papillary muscles and perfused heart preparations. Systemic hypotension often develops as the shock state progresses and elicits hemodynamic processes that result in pancreatic and splanchnic hypoperfusion. Ischemia of the pancreas in shock has been reported to be more intense than that in other splanchnic organs (184) and resultant deleterious consequences of pancreatic hypoperfusion have been suggested to play a minor role in subsequent production of toxic factors (184). The prolonged deficit of blood flow causes local ischemia, hypoxia, and acidosis, which in turn is thought to set into motion certain cellular autolytic processes. The exocrine pancreas appears to be particularly susceptible to shock-induced ischemia and hypoxia, and considerable disruption of lysosomes and release of proteases from zymogen granules occur in the pancreatic cells (173, 184,191). Intracellular acidity may further increase the activity of lysosomal proteases and thereby promote their hydrolytic actions (173). In addition, zymogenic enzymes (such as trypsin, kallikrein, and phospholipase A) are activated and may act to lyse subcellular membranes to make cellular protein substances available for the hydrolytic action of the lysosomal proteases (184). A variety of biologically active peptides is formed as the separated and released proteases cleave the cellular protein substrates. MDF is thought to be one of the small peptides formed by this catalytic proteolysis and, after formation, is released through cell membranes and transported by the systemic circulation to the heart (184,191). In addition to its cardiotoxic effect, MDF is also thought to exert indirect positive feedback actions (coronary and splanchnic vasoconstriction, reticuloendothelial depression), which may further undermine circulatory dysfunction in shock.

Lefer (191) recently reviewed the pathophysiology and biological actions of MDF in shock, with particular relevance to direct and indirect interactions of MDF with other mediators. Foremost among the vasoconstrictor mediators that promote the formation or actions of MDF are believed to be eicosanoids and other lipids (thromboxane A_2, leukotriene D_2, and platelet activating factor). All of the eicosanoids proposed are essentially free of direct negative inotropic activity at concentrations comparable to those observed in shock (191); platelet activating factor, however, can exert direct depression of myocardial contractility (191,192). As MDF is produced, its pathophysiological effects may promote the continued production and actions of such lipid vasoactive mediators. A large variety of pharmacological agents have been reported to prevent MDF formation and exert beneficial actions during shock including angiotensin-converting enzyme inhibitors, angiotensin receptor antagonists, thromboxane antagonists, lipoxygenase inhibitors, leukotriene receptor antagonists, and calcium channel blockers (for review see ref. 191).

The findings described above are consistent with the hypothesis that circulating depressant factors are a common denominator producing cardiac depression in many forms of shock. However, none of these factors has been characterized in precise molecular terms, and it remains unknown whether they represent identical or unrelated substances (53,173). The presence and putative pathologic role of these substances in shock have been questioned by other investigators (14,23,24,58–61,68–71,193). Furthermore, acute pancreatectomy does not prevent myocardial dysfunction in shock (68,193), suggesting the lack of importance of humoral factors released from this organ. Certainly, the inability to isolate, purify, identify, and fully characterize a specific shock-induced cardiodepressant substance has played a principal role in the lack of general acceptance of the circulating cardiotoxic hypothesis in shock. Although a circulating myocardial depressant substance has been reported by Parrillo et al. (194) in human septic shock, the relationship between such factors and prognosis will require better understanding of both its structure and function.

Endogenous Opiates

The discovery of endogenous opiates has resulted in an exciting new era of research directed at uncovering physiologic and pathophysiologic roles subserved by this system. Holaday and Faden initially investigated the possibility that endogenous opiates (endorphins), released from the pituitary during stress, may contribute to the pathophysiology of shock states (195–200). These researchers reported that the specific opiate antagonist, naloxone, rapidly reversed hypotension in rat and canine models of hemorrhagic, endotoxin, and spinal shock (195,200). They subsequently provided evidence for a stereospecific action of naloxone at opiate receptors and suggested that naloxone competes by displacing endorphins and thus reversing their hypotensive effects (197,199). Naloxone improved LV contractility in hemorrhagic and endotoxemic dogs, based on findings of increased $+ dP/dt_{max}$, stroke volume, cardiac output, and MAP; total peripheral resistance and heart rate were unaffected (201,202). From these studies, it was suggested that the beneficial effects of naloxone in shock may be mediated by improvement of cardiac inotropic function. Curtis and Lefer (203) reported that naloxone treatment reduced circulating MDF concentrations and improved hemodynamic and metabolic variables in hemorrhagic shock. Other studies (204–210) have reported that naloxone, as well as certain other opiate antagonists, can improve cardiovascular variables in mice, rats, cats, rabbits, sheep, dogs, pigs, horses, monkeys, and human patients (for review, see ref. 197).

The precise mechanisms or sites of action whereby naloxone exerts these beneficial effects remain unresolved, but a preponderance of data indicate an important component of the CNS in the therapeutic effects of naloxone (197,198). Ventriculocisternal administration of naloxone was protective against severe hypotension in endotoxin (211) and hemorrhagic (198) shock. Naloxone had no effect after hypophysectomy, suggesting an important contribution of pituitary endorphins. Other data also suggest that the beneficial cardiovascular actions of naloxone may be mediated peripherally by sympathomedullary discharge. Koyama et al. (212) reported that both intracisternal and intravenously (iv) administered naloxone activates the efferent sympathetic nervous system, as measured by preganglionic splanchnic nerve activity.

Although opiate antagonism is a strategic tool with which to implicate endogenous endorphin involvement in shock, direct correlations between the studies described above and an endorphin-linked cardiac depression remain difficult to draw. Naloxone, in addition to being a broad-acting opiate antagonist at multiple opiate receptor types, also exerts a variety of peripheral effects that may not be related to its CNS effects (213,214), thus complicating the interpretation of studies using this agent to evaluate control mechanisms.

Several studies have been directed toward evaluating the direct myocardial effects of circulating endorphins and opiate antagonists in circulatory shock states. Increased serum β-endorphins have been reported in human patients in shock (215), but direct myocardial depression by endorphins has generally been discounted. However, Caffrey et al. (216) have demonstrated evidence for direct myocardial effects of opiates and opiate antagonists, utilizing local intracoronary injections of these agents in dogs. Intracoronary injection of the opiate receptor antagonist naloxone increased myocardial contractility; consistent with these results is the myocardial depression produced by local injections of opiates. Riggs et al. (217,218) and Vargish et al. (219,220) reported that high concentrations of an exogenous opioid, morphine sulfate, produced naloxone-sensitive decreases in heart rate and cardic output in isolated cardiac preparations. Lower concentrations of three opioid (δ) agonists (including leu-enkephalin) and an opioid μ agonist decreased cardiac output, but with a predominant action on heart rate (221).

In isolated heart muscle preparations, β-endorphins have been reported to exert cardiodepressant activity only at concentrations ($>10^{-8}$ mol) greatly exceeding those considered physiologic (10^{-11} mol) (215). Similarly, naloxone has been shown to lack inotropic activity in isolated heart muscles from control (215,222,223) as well as shocked animals (102,222,223) except at high concentrations (10–200 μg/ml) (214). Nonetheless, concentrations of endorphins measured in plasma or added *in vitro* may have little functional relevance to cardiac effects of endogenous opiates released in discrete areas where they then act on specific receptor populations.

Ruth and Eiden (224) recently demonstrated that 10^{-7} mol enkephalin (a dose that lacks direct inotropic activity) significantly antagonized the chronotropic effects of norepinephrine in isolated rat atria. These studies suggest a potential modulatory influence of endogenous opiates on autonomic control of cardiac function, an effect not unlike that previously observed at other noradrenergic prejunctional sites within the CNS. Caffrey et al. provided evidence that naloxone potentiates contractile responses to epinephrine in isolated arteries (225) and also that naloxone enhances the myocardial inotropic response to isoproterenol in the dog isolated heart–lung preparation (226). In the latter studies, naloxone increased the response to isoproterenol but had little effect alone (226). Importantly, the myocardial response to naloxone was dependent on β-adrenergic mechanisms and was eliminated by prior blockade with propranolol (226). In recent studies (227) this group further reported that the ability of naloxone to enhance the inotropic effect of epinephrine is not mediated through an increase in plasma epinephrine concentration secondary to a decrease in the disposal of circulating catecholamines. These data support the contention that naloxone's ability to improve cardiovascular indices may depend on circulating or neuronally released catecholamines. Caffrey and colleagues (227) proposed the interesting concept that endogenous opioids of myocardial origin may act as local "governors" or modulators of adrenergic responsiveness. However, the importance of this putative governing role of endogenous opioids to LPS-induced myocardial dysfunction remains unknown and questionable.

Free-Radical-Induced Myocardial Injury

Free-radical interactions have been implicated in a large number of disease states, including inflammation, radiation injury, ischemia, and, more recently, circulatory shock. Much evidence now indicates that irreversible cellular damage may be produced by the action of oxygen-derived radicals and intermediates such as superoxide anion, O_2^-; hydroxyl radical, OH; hydrogen peroxide, H_2O_2; and singlet oxygen (228). Free radicals have been shown in a variety of tissues to produce endothelial damage (229,230), vasodilation (231), intestinal mucosal epithelial lifting (232), lysosomal disruption (233), phospholipid membrane lysis (234,235), damaged mitochondria (228), increased vascular permeability (236), and disrupted Ca^{2+} transport of cardiac sarcoplasmic reticulum (237,238). The role of these highly reactive activated metabolites of oxygen in the pathogenesis of myocardial ischemia and shock has been investigated in a number of model systems and represents a distinctly new approach to the understanding of shock-induced myocardial injury.

Oxygen radicals can be generated by a variety of biological reactions. Most of these reactions result in the production of one (O_2^-), two (H_2O_2), or three (OH·) electron reduction of oxygen. A group of cellular enzymes involved in catalyzing oxidation reactions (e.g., xanthine oxidase, glycolate oxidase) result in univalent or divalent reduction of O_2 (228). Activation of polymorphonuclear leukocytes (PMNs) causes release of oxygen free radicals [via nicotinamide adenine dinucleotide phosphate (NADPH) oxidase], lysosomal enzymes, and arachidonic acid derivatives, which are capable of generating oxygen free radicals (228,239–241). Free radicals produced by such systems are highly energetic and reactive; cellular viability and protection crucially depend on their effective removal and control. Under normal conditions, various endogenous enzymatic mechanisms (e.g., superoxide dismutase, SOD; catalase; peroxidase) and other scavenging processes effectively operate to remove oxygen radicals (228). Imbalances in these interrelationships can produce profound biochemical alterations (228). Numerous studies have provided evidence suggesting that free-radical interactions may be involved in the damage observed in hypoxic and ischemic myocardium (228,237–244). Del Maestro (228) suggested that during partial ischemia and shock, free radicals are generated intracellularly, particularly in mitochondria. There is evidence that the heart mitochondrial electron-transfer system may function as a generator of superoxide radicals when all the components on the substrate side of cytochrome c are reduced; these may produce cellular damage when scavenging mechanisms are reduced, ineffective, or overwhelmed (228).

Specific alterations in cardiac sarcoplasmic reticulum produced by oxygen free radicals have been investigated by Hess et al. (237–239). Alterations in subcellular Ca^{2+} fluxes of sarcoplasmic reticulum have been described by this group in shock and myocardial ischemia and have been implicated in contributing to depressed cardiac contractility and irreversibility in shock. The addition of an oxygen free-radical generating system (xanthine–xanthine oxidase) to isolated sarcoplasmic reticulum produced severe depression of both Ca^{2+} uptake velocity and Ca^{2+}–adenosine triphosphatase (ATP) activity (237); the depressed Ca^{2+} uptake velocity remained depressed in the presence of acidosis (pH 6.4). Importantly, mannitol, a scavenger of the hydroxyl radical, and SOD restored the depressed Ca^{2+} uptake velocity. Manson and Hess (238) reported evidence that free radicals produced by activated leukocytes similarly depressed Ca^{2+} uptake rates; and furthermore, that this effect was reduced by catalase or SOD plus catalase. These authors have presented the concept that, since endotoxin is known to activate complement and lead to the production of complement components (C5a), the resulting C5a-activated leukocytes could release free radicals and potentially lead to the loss of contractility in cardiac muscle observed in septic shock. In this regard, Lefer et al. (243) have reported that the free-radical scavenger MK-447 improved myocardial contractility in myocardial ischemia and traumatic shock. Other studies have not provided support for beneficial actions of free-radical scavengers in endotoxin shock models, and this area remains a contentious issue relative to the putative role of reactive oxygen species in the cardiac toxicity of LPS (157,168,245,246).

Other Putative Mediators

A multitude of endogenously released vasoconstrictor and vasodilator agents has been implicated in the mediation of endotoxin and septic states, especially the vasoactive lipids such as leukotrienes, prostaglandins, thromboxanes, and PAF (for review, see refs. 245 and 247–251). The effects of many of these agents on the vasculature and other organ systems have been extensively documented and include active vasoconstriction, enhanced leakiness of capillary membranes, redistribution of blood flow, release of other shock mediators, bronchoconstriction, and platelet aggregation (191). Many of these mediators exert actions that may intensify or prolong the shock state.

Relative to the heart in shock, few of these vasoactive lipids have been demonstrated to produce direct negative inotropic effects. Stahl and Lefer (252) showed that PAF produces dose-dependent increases in coronary perfusion pressure and decreases in contractile force of isolated rat hearts perfused at constant flow. Interestingly, the LTD_4 antagonist LY-171,883 prevented the increase in perfusion pressure but did not antagonize the negative inotropic response. Thus the negative inotropic response to PAF is likely the result of both a direct negative inotropic action and an indirect vasoconstrictor effect via release of eicosanoid mediators (252). It has generally been reported that the other putative lipid mediators of shock decrease contractility secondary to their potent coronary constrictor effects (245,253,254), although certain aspects of this viewpoint remain controversial. Some studies (255–257) have provided evidence for negative inotropic effects of leukotrienes C_4 and D_4 independent of coronary flow reduction, perhaps due to inhibition of cardiac transsarcolemmal Ca^{2+} influx (256). In 1990, Karmazyn and Moffat (258) demonstrated a positive inotropic effect of low concentrations of LTC_4 and LTD_4 (0.01–0.50 ng/ml), concomitant with coronary artery constriction, and a negative inotropic effect at higher concentrations.

In addition to the potential direct effects, these vasoactive mediators have been proposed by Lefer (247) to interact with either the formation of MDF, its pathophysiological effects during shock, or both. Thus these agents, although lacking significant negative inotropic activity themselves, may exert biological effects that act in concert with MDF and amplify its cardiodepressant action. Specific interactions among the various vasoactive mediators, and their significance in the pathogenesis of cardiac dysfunction in shock, remain controversial and a current area of intensive research. Recently, new developments in the field of vascular endothelial cell pathophysiology have also suggested a vasoactive role of altered release of endothelial-derived relaxing factor (EDRF, possibly nitric oxide, NO) in endotoxin and shock states (246,259–261). This rapidly expanding area of research will likely provide significant new information during the next 5 years relative to a role of EDRF/NO and possible interactions with other mediators of LPS toxicity such as cytokines and PAF.

Finally, although macrophage-derived immunomodulatory cytokines such as tumor necrosis factor-α and the interleukins are now believed to play principal mediator roles in endotoxin and sepsis pathogenesis (9), the mechanistic pathways leading from cytokine induction to myocardial toxicity in these forms of circulatory shock currently are unknown.

CONCLUSION AND IMPLICATIONS

Sufficient clinical and experimental data are now available to assemble a consensus that LV contraction–relaxation mechanisms intrinsic to heart muscle itself are indeed disordered during endotoxemic and septicemic syndromes. Evidence from studies with isolated hearts indicate that endotoxin-induced cardiodynamic changes present as reduced myocardial contractility (lowered isovolumic LV $+dP/dt_{max}$), impaired relaxation during early diastole (reduced isovolumic LV $-dP/dt_{max}$), reduced chamber compliance or distensibility during late diastole, and reduced LV stroke volume and cardiac output. In the intact subject, these changes would result in impaired filling of the ventricles during diastole as well as reduced ejection during systole.

Intrinsic cardiac dysfunction in shock may be masked in intact subjects by compensatory activation of endogenous cardiostimulants such as catecholamines or, also importantly, by therapeutic interventions. Indeed, intravascular volume expansion markedly alters manifestation of intrinsic systolic and diastolic defects during shock. Shock-induced dysfunctional hearts can still respond to increases in end-diastolic sarcomere length; intravascular volume loading can thereby provide the depressed heart with adequate preload to maintain stroke volume at near normal values although ejection fraction can remain subnormal. Intravascular volume expansion evokes an apparent compensatory dilation of the heart during shock, thereby contributing to maintenance of stroke volume although reduced ejection fractions still identify the intrinsically dysfunctional heart. Thus in situ measurements either of stroke volume index or cardiac index alone may not accurately sample for altered heart function in septic shock patients.

Finally, clinical and experimental studies have indicated that inadequate myocardial blood flows are not necessary prerequisites for cardiac sequelae of endotoxemic and septicemic shock. Certainly, inadequate myocardial perfusion is likely to be an important confounding influence in those subsets of shock patients with preexisting ischemic (coronary artery) heart disease. Also, when the systemic hypotensive state becomes severe enough to halt or limit coronary vascular autoregulation, then myocardial malperfusion and ischemia may contribute to and exacerbate the cardiac changes already underway. Indeed, studies in 1991 suggested a maldistribution of heterogenous coronary blood flow in a hypotensive model of acute endotoxin shock in dogs (268); however, it was unclear if these changes were primary to LPS pathogenesis or simply a manifestation of the systemic hypotension and reduced coronary perfusion pressure. The fact remains that direct or indirect evidence of cardiac mechanical dysfunction can develop in LPS and sepsis syndromes while total coronary blood flow, myocardial subendocardial/subepicardial blood flow ratios, and LV concentrations of high-energy phosphates remain normal and adequate for the reduced workload imposed on the heart. The pathogenesis of intrinsic cardiac injury during endotoxemia and septicemia, although not requiring global myocardial ischemia as an obligatory etiologic factor, remains to be delineated.

ACKNOWLEDGMENTS

The authors wish to acknowledge Dr. C. E. Jones of the Department of Physiology of the Texas College of Osteopathic Medicine, Fort Worth, Texas, and Dr. M. H. Laughlin of the Department of Veterinary Biomedical Sciences of the University of Missouri, Columbia, Missouri, for their important contributions to refs. 16 and 17, which along with ref. 14 provided the background for this chapter.

This work was supported in part by Research Grant HL-36079 from the National Institutes of Health. J. L. Parker is the recipient of NIH Research Career Development Award HL-01169.

REFERENCES

1. Wiggers CJ. *Physiology of shock*. Cambridge, MA: The Commonwealth Fund/Harvard University Press; 1950.
2. Parrillo JE. Myocardial depression during septic shock in humans. *Crit Care Med* 1990;18:1183–1184.
3. Cunnion RE, Parrillo JE. Myocardial dysfunction in sepsis: recent insights. *Chest* 1989;95:941–945.
4. Parrillo JE. Cardiovascular pattern during septic shock. *Ann Intern Med* 1990;113:227–229.
5. Snell RJ, Parrillo JE. Cardiovascular dysfunction in septic shock. *Chest* 1991;99:1000–1009.
6. Danner RL, Elin RJ, Hosseini JM, Wesley RA, Reilly JM, Parrillo JE. Endotoxemia in human septic shock. *Chest* 1991;99:169–175.
7. Wolff SM, Bennett JV. Gram-negative rod bacteremia. *N Engl J Med* 1974;291:733–734.
8. Suffredini AF, Fromm RE, Parker MM, Brenner MB, Kovacs JA, Wesley RA. The cardiovascular response of normal humans to the administration of endotoxin. *N Engl J Med* 1989;321:280–287.
9. Raetz CR, Ulevitch RJ, Wright SD, Sibley CH, Ding A, Nathan CF. Gram-negative endotoxin: an extraordinary lipid with profound effects on eukaryotic signal transduction. *FASEB J* 1991;5:2652–2660.
10. Van Deventer SJH, Ten Cate JW, Ty Gat GNJ. Intestinal endotoxemia. *Gastroenterology* 1988;94:825–831.

11. Ravin HA, Rowley D, Jenkins C, Fine J. On the absorption of bacterial endotoxin from the gastrointestinal tract of the normal and shocked animal. *J Exp Med* 1960;112:783–792.
12. Fink MP. Gastrointestinal mucosal injury in experimental models of shock, trauma, and sepsis. *Crit Care Med* 1991;19:627–641.
13. Natanson C, Danner RL, Elin RJ, et al. Role of endotoxemia in cardiovascular dysfunction and mortality. *J Clin Invest* 1989;83:243–251.
14. Parker JL, Adams HR. Pathophysiology of the heart in shock. In: Balazs T, ed. *Cardiac toxicology*, vol I. Boca Raton, FL: CRC Press; 1981:137–157.
15. Parker JL, Adams HR. Isolated cardiac preparations: models of intrinsic myocardial dysfunction in circulatory shock. *Circ Shock* 1985;15:227–245.
16. Parker JL, Jones CE. The heart in shock. In: Hardaway R, ed. *Shock: the reversible step toward death*. Littleton, MA: PSG Publishing; 1988:348–366.
17. Adams HR, Parker JL, Laughlin MH. Intrinsic myocardial dysfunction during endotoxemia: dependent or independent of myocardial ischemia? *Circ Shock* 1990;30:63–76.
18. Parrillo JE. The cardiovascular pathophysiology of sepsis. *Annu Rev Med* 1989;40:469–485.
19. Cunnion RE, Parrillo JE. Myocardial dysfunction in sepsis. *Crit Care Clinics* 1989;5:99–118.
20. Abel FL. Does the heart fail in endotoxin shock? *Circ Shock* 1990;30:5–13.
21. Abel FL. Myocardial function in sepsis and endotoxin shock. *Am J Physiol* 1989;257:R1265–R1281.
22. Goldfarb RD. Evaluation of ventricular performance in shock. *Circ Shock* 1985;15:281–301.
23. Archer LT. Myocardial dysfunction in endotoxin and *E. coli*-induced shock: pathophysiological mechanisms. *Circ Shock* 1985;15:261–280.
24. Hess ML, Hastillo A, Greenfield LJ. Spectrum of cardiovascular function during gram-negative sepsis. *Prog Cardiovasc Dis* 1981;23:279–298.
25. Udhoji VN, Weil MH. Hemodynamic and metabolic studies on shock associated with bacteremia. *Ann Intern Med* 1965;62:966.
26. Siegel JH, Farrell EJ, Goldwyn RM, et al. Myocardial function in human septic shock states. In: Forscher BK, Lillehei RC, Stubbs SS, eds. *Shock in low- and high-flow states*. Amsterdam: Excerpta Medica; 1972:250–262.
27. Siegel JH, Greenspan M, Del Guercio RRM. Abnormal vascular tone, defective oxygen transport and myocardial failure in human septic shock. *Ann Surg* 1967;165:504–517.
28. Shoemaker WC. Pathophysiology and therapy of shock states. In: Berk JL, Sampliner JE, Artz JS, et al., eds. *Handbook of critical care*. Boston: Little Brown & Co; 1976:205–224.
29. Vincent JL, Weil MH, Puri V, et al. Circulatory shock associated with purulent peritonitis. *Am J Surg* 1981;142:262–270.
30. Weil MH, Nishijima H. Cardiac output in bacterial shock. *Am J Med* 1978;64:920–922.
31. Siegel JH, Goldwyn RM, Del Guercio LRM. Patterns of cardiovascular response in septic shock. In: Hershey SG, Del Guercio LRM, McConn R, eds. *Septic shock in man*. Boston: Little Brown & Co; 1971:173–190.
32. Weisel RD, Vito L, Dennis RC, et al. Myocardial depression during sepsis. *Am J Surg* 1977;133:512–521.
33. Groeneveld ABJ, Bronsveld W, Thijs LG. Hemodynamic determinants of mortality in human septic shock. *Surgery* 1986;99:140.
34. Parker MM, Shelhamer JH, Natanson C, Alling DW, Parrillo JE. Serial cardiovascular variables in survivors and nonsurvivors of human septic shock: heart rate as an early predictor of prognosis. *Crit Care Med* 1987;15:923–929.
35. D'Orio V, Mendes P, Saad G, Marcelle R. Accuracy in early prediction of prognosis of patients with septic shock by analyis of simple indices: prospective study. *Crit Care Med* 1990;18:1339–1345.
36. Jardin F, Brunney D, Auvert B, Beauchet A, Bourdarias FP. Sepsis-related cardiogenic shock. *Crit Care Med* 1990;18:1055–1060.
37. Reinhart K, Hannemann L, Kuss B. Optimal oxygen delivery in critically ill patients. *Intensive Care Med* 1990;16(suppl):S149–S155.

38. Mammana RB, Hiro S, Levitsky S, Thomas PA, Plachetka J. Inaccuracy of pulmonary capillary wedge pressure when compared to left atrial pressure in the early post-surgical period. *J Thorac Cardiovasc Surg* 1982;84:420–425.
39. Lefcoe MS, Sibbald WJ, Holliday RL. Wedged balloon catheter angiography in the critical care unit. *Crit Care Med* 1979;7:449–453.
40. Snyder JV. Cardiac function in septic shock. *Lett Corrections* 1984;879.
41. Hardaway RM. Pulmonary artery pressure versus pulmonary capillary wedge pressure and central venous pressure in shock. *Resuscitation* 1982;10:47–56.
42. Vincent JC, Reuse C, Frank N, Contempré B, Kahn RJ. Right ventricular dysfunction in septic shock: assessment by measurements of right ventricular ejection fraction using the thermo dilution technique. *Acta Anaesthesiol Scand* 1989;33:34–38.
43. Bell H, Thal A. The peculiar hemodynamics of septic shock. *Postgrad Med* 1970; 48:106–118.
44. Clowes GHA Jr. Pulmonary abnormalities in sepsis. *Surg Clin North Am* 1974;54:993–1002.
45. Krausz MM, Perel A, Eimerl D, et al. Cardiopulmonary effects of volume loading in patients in septic shock. *Surg Clin North Am* 1974;54:993–1002.
46. Kimchi A, Ellrodt G, Berman DS, et al. Right ventricular performance in septic shock: a combined radionuclide and hemodynamic study. *J Am Coll Cardiol* 1984;4:945–951.
47. Dhainaut JF, Lanore JJ, de Gournay JM, et al. Right ventricular dysfunction in patients with septic shock. *Intensive Care Med* 1988;14:488–491.
48. Schneider AJ, Teule GJJ, Groeneveld ABJ, Nauta J, Heidendal GAK, Thijs LG. Biventricular performance during volume loading in patients with early septic shock with emphasis on the right ventricle: a combined hemodynamic and radionuclide study. *Am Heart J* 1988;116:103–112.
49. Gunnar RM, Loeb HS, Winslow EJ. Hemodynamic measurements in bacteremia and septic shock in man. *J Infect Dis* 1973;128:S295–S298.
50. Clowes GHA Jr, O'Donnell TF Jr, Ryan NT, et al. Energy metabolism in sepsis: treatment based on different patients in shock and high output stage. *Ann Surg* 1974; 179:684–696.
51. Weil WH, Maclean LD, Visscher MB, et al. Studies on the circulatory changes in the dog produced by endotoxin from gram-negative micro-organisms. *J Clin Invest* 1956; 35:1101–1198.
52. Goodyer AVN. Left ventricular function and tissue hypoxia in irreversible hemorrhagic and endotoxin shock. *Am J Physiol* 1967;212:444–460.
53. Lefer AM. Mechanisms of cardiodepression in endotoxin shock. *Circ Shock* 1979; 1(suppl):1–8.
54. Coleman B, Kallal JE, Feigen LP, et al. Myocardial performance during hemorrhagic shock in the pancreatectomized dog. *Am J Physiol* 1975;228:1462–1468.
55. Abel FL, Kessler DP. Myocardial performance in hemorrhagic shock in the dog and primate. *Circ Res* 1973;32:492–500.
56. Rothe CF, Selkurt EE. Cardiac and peripheral failure in hemorrhagic shock in the dog. *Am J Physiol* 1964;207:203–214.
57. Guntheroth WG, Kawabori I, Stevenson JG, et al. Pulmonary vascular resistance and right ventricular function in canine endotoxin shock. *Proc Soc Exp Biol Med* 1978; 157:610–614.
58. Hinshaw LB. Role of the heart in the pathogenesis of endotoxin shock: a review of clinical findings and observations on animal species. *J Surg Res* 1974;17:134–145.
59. Hinshaw LB, Archer LT, Greenfield LJ, et al. Effects of endotoxin on myocardial hemodynamics, performance and metabolism. *Am J Physiol* 1971;221:504–510.
60. Hinshaw LB, Greenfield LJ, Archer LT, et al. Effects of endotoxin on myocardial hemodynamics, performance, and metabolism during beta adrenergic blockade. *Proc Soc Exp Biol Med* 1971;137:1217–1224.
61. Hinshaw LB, Greenfield LJ, Owen SE, et al. Cardiac response to circulating factors in endotoxin shock. *Am J Physiol* 1972;222:1047–1053.
62. MacLean LD, Weil MH. Hypotension (shock) in dogs produced by *Escherichia coli* endotoxin. *Circ Res* 1956;4:546–556.
63. Brockman SK, Thomas CS Jr, Vasco JS. The effect of *Escherichia coli* endotoxin on the circulation. *Surg Gynecol Obstet* 1967;125:663–774.

64. Wangensteen SL, Geissinger WT, Lovett WL, et al. Relationship between splanchnic blood flow and a myocardial depressant factor in endotoxin shock. *Surgery* 1971; 69:410–418.
65. Priano LL, Wilson RD, Traber DL. Cardiorespiratory alterations in unanesthetized dogs due to gram-negative bacterial endotoxin. *Am J Physiol* 1971;220:705–711.
66. Miller TH, Priano LL, Jorgenson JH, et al. Cardiorespiratory effects of *Pseudomonas* and *E. coli* endotoxins in the awake dog. *Am J Physiol* 1977;232:H682–H689.
67. Solis RT, Downing SE. Effects of *E. coli* endotoxemia on ventricular performance. *Am J Physiol* 1966;211:307–313.
68. Hinshaw LB, Archer LT, Black MR, et al. Myocardial function in shock. *Am J Physiol* 1974;226:357–366.
69. Hinshaw LB, Archer LT, Spitzer JJ, et al. Effects of coronary hypotension and endotoxin on myocardial performance. *Am J Physiol* 1974;227:1051–1057.
70. Hinshaw LB, Greenfield LJ, Owens SE, et al. Precipitation of cardiac failure in endotoxin shock. *Surg Gynecol Obstet* 1972;135:39–48.
71. Archer LT, Black MR, Hinshaw LB. Myocardial failure with altered response to adrenaline in endotoxin shock. *Br J Pharmacol* 1975;54:145–155.
72. David D, Rogel S. Mechanical and humoral factors affecting cardiac function in shock. *Circ Shock* 1976;3:65–75.
73. Elkins RC, McCurdy JR, Brown PP, et al. Effects of coronary perfusion pressure on myocardial performance during endotoxin shock. *Surg Gynecol Obstet* 1973;137:991–996.
74. Goldfarb RD. Cardiac mechanical performance in circulatory shock: a critical review of methods and results. *Circ Shock* 1982;9:633–653.
75. Sagawa K. The ventricular pressure volume loop revisited. *Circ Res* 1978;43:677–687.
76. Guntheroth WG, Jacky JP, Kawabori I, Stevenson JG, Morena AH. Left ventricular performance in endotoxin shock in dogs. *Am J Physiol* 1982;242:H172–H176.
77. Guntheroth WG, Kawabori I, Stevenson JG, Chlorin NR. Pulmonary vascular resistance and right ventricular function in canine endotoxin shock. *Proc Soc Exp Biol Med* 1978;157:610–614.
78. Goldfarb RD, Lee KJ, Dziuban SW. End-systolic elastance as an evaluation of myocardial function in shock. *Circ Shock* 1990;30:15–26.
79. Goldfarb RD, Tambolini W, Wiener SM, Weber PB. Canine left ventricular performance during LD$_{50}$ endotoxemia. *Am J Physiol* 1983;244:H370–H377.
80. Goldfarb RD, Nightingale LM, Kish P, Weber PB, Ooegering DJ. Left ventricular function during lethal and sublethal endotoxemia in swine. *Am J Physiol* 1986;251:H364–H373.
81. Lee KL, van der Zee H, Dziuban SW, Luhmann K, Goldfarb RD. Left ventricular function during chronic endotoxemia in swine. *Am J Physiol* 1988;254:H324–H330.
82. Lee KL, Dziuban SW, van der Zee H, Goldfarb RD. Cardiac function and coronary flow in chronic endotoxemic pigs. *Proc Soc Exp Biol Med* 1988;189:245–252.
83. Kober PM, Thomas J, Raymond RM. Increased myocardial contractility during endotoxin shock in dogs. *Am J Physiol* 1985;249:H715–H722.
84. Raymond RM, King N, Thomas JX, Gordey J. Differential effects of acute endotoxin shock on myocardial contractility and performance. In: *Perspectives in shock research: metabolism, immunology, mediators, and models.* New York: Alan R Liss; 1989:123–129.
85. Law WR, McLane MP, Raymond RM. Substantiation of myocardial resistance to the inotropic action of insulin during endotoxin shock. *Circ Shock* 1988;24:237(abstract).
86. Adams HR, Izenberg SD, Baxter CR. Adrenergic aspects of endotoxin shock. In: Procter RA, Hinshaw LB, eds. *Handbook of endotoxin, vol II: pathophysiology of endotoxin.* Amsterdam: Elseiver Biomedical; 1985:145–172.
87. Papadakis EJ, Abel FL. Left ventricular performance in canine endotoxic shock. *Circ Shock* 1988;24:123–131.
88. Abel FL, Sutherland AE, Haleby K. Comparative measurements of left-ventricular performance produced by rapid changes in blood volume in dogs. *Ann Biomed Eng* 1972;1:9–22.
89. Abel FL, Beck RR. Canine peripheral vascular response to endotoxin shock at constant cardiac output. *Circ Shock* 1988;2225:267–274.

90. Coalson JJ, Hinshaw LB, Guenter CA, et al. Pathophysiologic responses of the subhuman primate in experimental septic shock. *Lab Invest* 1975;32:561–569.
91. Geocaris TV, Quebbeman E, Dewoskin R, et al. Effects of gram-negative endotoxemia on myocardial contractility in the awake primate. *Ann Surg* 1973;178:715–720.
92. Cavanagh D, Rao PS, Sutton DMC, et al. Pathophysiology of endotoxin shock in the primate. *Am J Obstet Gynecol* 1970;108:705–722.
93. Greenfield LJ, Jackson RH, Elkins RC, et al. Cardiopulmonary effects of volume loading of primates in endotoxin shock. *Surgery* 1974;76:560–572.
94. Snow TR, Dickey DT, Tapp T, Hinshaw LB, Taylor FB. Early myocardial dysfunction induced with endotoxin in rhesus monkeys. *Can J Cardiol* 1990;6:130–136.
95. Natanson C, Fink MP, Ballantyne HK, MacVittie TJ, Conklin JJ, Parrillo JE. Gram-negative bacteremia produces both severe systolic and diastolic cardiac dysfunction in a canine model that simulates human septic shock. *J Clin Invest* 1986;78:259–270.
96. Natanson C, Danner RL, Fink MP, MacVittie TJ, Walker RI, Conklin JJ, Parrillo JE. Cardiovascular performance with *E. coli* challenges in a canine model of human sepsis. *Am J Physiol* 1988;254:H558–H569.
97. Momomura S, Iizuka M, Serizawa T, Sugimoto T. Separation of rate of left ventricular relaxation from chamber stiffness in rats. *Am J Physiol* 1988;255:H1468–H1475.
98. Glantz SA, Parmley WW. Factors which affect the diastolic pressure–volume curve. *Circ Res* 1978;42:171–180.
99. Lewis BS, Gotsman MS. Current concepts of left ventricular relaxation and compliance. *Am Heart J* 1980;99:101–112.
100. Ognibene FP, Parker MM, Natanson C, Parrillo JE. Depressed left ventricular performance in response to volume infusion in patients with sepsis and septic shock. *Chest* 1988;93:903–910.
101. Stahl TJ, Alden PB, Ring WS, Madoff RC, Cerra FB. Sepsis-induced diastolic dysfunction in chronic canine peritonitis. *Am J Physiol* 1990;258:H625–H633.
102. Parker JL, Keller RS, Behm LL, Adams HR. Left ventricular dysfunction in early *E. coli* endotoxemia: effects of naloxone. *Am J Physiol* 1990;259:H504–H511.
103. Field BE, Rackow EC, Astiz ME, Weil MH. Early systolic and diastolic dsyfunction during sepsis in rats. *J Crit Care* 1989;4:3–8.
104. Walley KR, Cooper DJ. Diastolic stiffness impairs left ventricular function during hypovolemic shock in pigs. *Am J Physiol* 1991;260:H702–H712.
105. Archer LT, Benjamin BA, Beller-Todd BK, Brackett DJ, Wilson MF, Hinshaw LB. Does LD$_{100}$ *E. coli* shock cause myocardial failure? *Circ Shock* 1982;9:7–16.
106. Adams HR, Baxter CR, Parker JL. Reduction of intrinsic contractile reserves of the left ventricle by *Escherichia coli* endotoxin shock in guinea pigs. *J Mol Cell Cardiol* 1985;17:575–585.
107. Adams HR, Parker JL, Baxter CR, Watts NB. Contractile function and rhythmicity of cardiac preparations isolated from *Escherichia coli* endotoxin shocked guinea pigs. *Circ Shock* 1984;13:241–253.
108. Parker JL, Adams HR. Myocardial dysfunction during endotoxin shock in the guinea pig. *Am J Physiol* 1981;240:H954–H962.
109. Parker JL. Contractile function of heart muscle isolated from endotoxin-shocked guinea pigs and rats. *Adv Shock Res* 1983;9:133–145.
110. Miller H, Parker JL. The guinea pig as a model in shock/trauma research. In: *Perspectives in shock research, immunology, mediators, and models*. New York: Alan R Liss; 1989:277–286.
111. Parker JL, Daily CS, Adams HR. Effects of endotoxin shock on pause-induced inotropy in cardiac muscle. *Circ Shock* 1980;7:191(abstract).
112. Parker JL, Jamison TS. Dissimilarities of arterial and ventricular contractile dysfunction in endotoxin shock. *Circ Shock* 1981;8:224(abstract).
113. Parker JL, Adams HR. Development of myocardial dysfunction in endotoxin shock. *Am J Physiol* 1985;248:H818–H826.
114. Parker JL, Adams HR, Defazio PL. Development of left-ventricular dysfunction in endotoxin shock. *Fed Proc* 1984;43:325(abstract).
115. Parker JL, Adams HR. Myocardial effects of endotoxin shock: characterization of an isolated heart muscle model. *Adv Shock Res* 1979;2:162–175.

116. McDonough KH, Lang CH, Spitzer JJ. Depressed function of isolated hearts from hyperdynamic septic rats. *Circ Shock* 1984;12:241–251.
117. McDonough KH, Lang CH, Spitzer JJ. Effect of cardiotropic agents on the myocardial dysfunction of hyperdynamic sepsis. *Circ Shock* 1985;17:1–19.
118. McDonough KH, Burke EC, Smith LW. *In vitro* cardiac function in early sepsis. *J Med* 1990;21:27–49.
119. McDonough KH, Lang CH, Spitzer JJ. The effect of hyperdynamic sepsis on myocardial performance. *Circ Shock* 1985;15:247–259.
120. Smith LW, Winbery SL, Barker LA, McDonough KH. Cardiac function and chronotropic sensitivity to β-adrenergic stimulation in sepsis. *Am J Physiol* 1986;251(*Heart Circ Physiol* 20):H405–H412.
121. Smith LW, McDonough KH. Inotropic sensitivity to β-adrenergic stimulation in early sepsis. *Am J Physiol* 1988;255(*Heart Circ Physiol* 24):H699–H703.
122. Barker LA, Winbery SL, Smith LW, McDonough KH. Supersensitivity and changes in the active population of beta adrenoceptors in rat right atria in early sepsis. *J Pharmacol Exp Ther* 1989;252:675–682.
123. Fish RE, Burns AH, Lang CH, Spitzer JA. Myocardial dysfunction in a nonlethal, nonshock model of chronic endotoxemia. *Circ Shock* 1985;16:241–252.
124. Shepherd RE, McDonough KH, Burns AH. Mechanism of cardiac dysfunction in hearts from endotoxin-treated rats. *Circ Shock* 1986;19:371–384.
125. Romanosky AJ, Giaimo ME, Shepherd RE, Burns AH. The effect of *in vivo* endotoxin on myocardial function *in vitro*. *Circ Shock* 1986;19:1–12.
126. Shepherd RE, Lang CH, McDonough KH. Myocardial adrenergic responsiveness after lethal and nonlethal doses of endotoxin. *Am J Physiol* 1987;252(*Heart Circ Physiol* 21):H410–H416.
127. Spitzer JA, Rodriquez de Turco EB, Deaciuc IV, Roth BL, Hermiller JB, Mehegan JP. Receptor changes in endotoxemia. In: *Perspectives in shock research: metabolism, immunology, mediators, and models*. New York: Alan R Liss; 1989:95–106.
128. Burns AH, Summer WR, Racey Burns LA, Shepherd RE. Inotropic interactions of dichloroacetate with amrinone and ouabain in isolated hearts from endotoxin-shocked rats. *J Cardvasc Pharmacol* 1988;11:379–386.
129. DeBlieux PMC, McDonough KH, Barbee RW, Shepherd RE. Exercise training attenuates the myocardial disfunction induced by endotoxin. *J Appl Physiol* 1989; 66(6):2805–2810.
130. Hess ML, Krause SM. Myocardial subcellular function in shock. *Tex Rep Biol Med* 1979;39:193–207.
131. Hess ML, Krause SM. Contractile protein dysfunction as a determinant of depressed cardiac contractility during endotoxin shock. *J Mol Cell Cardiol* 1981;13:715–723.
132. Bruni FD, Komwatana P, Soulsbe ME, et al. Endotoxin and myocardial failure: role of the myofibril. *Am J Physiol* 1978;225:H150–H156.
133. Krause SM, Kleinman W, Hess ML. Cardiogenic endotoxin shock: coronary flow and contractile protein dysfunction as determinants of depressed cardiac contractility. *Adv Shock Res* 1980;3:105–116.
134. Hess ML. Concise review: subcellular function in the acutely failing myocardium. *Circ Shock* 1979;6:119–136.
135. Soulsby ME, Bruni FD, Looney TJ, et al. Influence of endotoxin on myocardial calcium transport and the effect of augmented venous return. *Circ Shock* 1978;5:23–34.
136. Hess ML, Krause SM, Komwatana P. Myocardial failure and excitation–contraction uncoupling in canine endotoxin shock: role of histamine and sarcoplasmic reticulum. *Circ Shock* 1980;7:277–287.
137. Warner M, Smith JM, Eaton R, et al. The excitation–contraction coupling system of the myocardium in canine hemorrhagic shock. *Circ Shock* 1981;8:563–572.
138. McCallister LP, Daiello DC, Tyers GFO. Morphometric observation of the effects of normothermic ischemic arrest on dog myocardial ultrastructure. *J Mol Cell Cardiol* 1978;10:67–80.
139. Bhagat B, Beaumont M, Rawson L, et al. Calcium metabolism and contractility of isolated cardiac muscle from endotoxin-treated guinea pig. In: Dhalla NS, ed. *Recent advances in studies on cardiac structure and metabolism, vol 4: myocardial biology.* Baltimore: University Park Press; 1974:305–328.

140. Bhagat B, Rao PS, Cavanagh D. Contractility of endotoxic atria. In: Tajuddin M, Bhatia B, Siddiqui HH, Rona G, eds. *Advances in myocardiology,* vol 2. Baltimore: University Park Press; 1980:199–207.
141. Dhalla NS, Singh JN, Fedelesova M, et al. Biochemical basis of heart function XII. Sodium–potassium stimulated adenosine triphosphatase activity in the perfused rat heart made to fail by substrate lack. *Cardiovasc Res* 1974;8:227–236.
142. Beller GA, Conroy J, Smith TW. Ischemia-induced alterations in myocardial (Na$^+$ + K$^+$)–ATPase and cardiac glycoside binding. *J Clin Invest* 1976;57:341–350.
143. Rabinowitz B, Kligerman M, Parmley WW. Alterations in myocardial and plasma cyclic adenosine monophosphate in experimental myocardial ischemia. In: Roy PE, Harris P, eds. *The cardiac sarcoplasm.* Baltimore: University Park Press; 1975:251–261.
144. Liu MS, Spitzer JJ. *In vitro* effects of *E. coli* endotoxin on fatty acid and lactate oxidation in canine myocardium. *Circ Shock* 1977;4:181–190.
145. Mela L, Hinshaw LB, Coalson JJ. Correlation of cardiac performance, ultra-structural morphology, and mitochondrial function in endotoxemia in the dog. *Circ Shock* 1974;1:265–272.
146. Reeves JP, Hale CC. The stoichiometry of the cardiac sodium–calcium exchange system. *J Biol Chem* 1984;259:7733–7739.
147. Reeves JP. The sarcolemmal sodium–calcium exchange system. In: Shamoo AE, ed. *Current topics in membranes and transport: regulation of calcium transport across muscle membranes.* Orlando, FL: Academic Press; 1985:77–127.
148. Bershon MM, Philipson KS, Fukushima JY. Sodium–calcium exchange and sarcolemmal enzymes in ischemic rabbit hearts. *Am J Physiol* 1982;242:C288–C295.
149. Liu MS, Xuan YT. Mechanisms of endotoxin-induced impairment in Na$^+$–Ca^{2+} exchange in canine myocardium. *Am J Physiol* 1986;251:R1078–R1085.
150. Hale CC, Allert JA, Keller RS, Adams HR, Parker JL. Gram-negative endotoxemia: effects on cardiac Na–Ca exchange and stoichiometry. *Circ Shock* 1989;29:133–142.
151. Kutsky P, Parker JL. Calcium fluxes in cardiac sarcolemma and sarcoplasmic reticulum isolated from endotoxin-shocked guinea pigs. *Circ Shock* 1990;30:349–364.
152. Hale CC, Novela L, Adams HR, Parker JL. Cardiac sarcolemma in endotoxin shock phospholipid profiles. *Circ Shock* 1990;31:15(abstract).
153. McDonough KH. Calcium uptake by sarcoplasmic reticulum isolated from hearts of septic rats. *Circ Shock* 1988;25:291–297.
154. Liu MS, Wu LL. Reduction in the Ca^{2+}-induced Ca^{2+} release from canine cardiac sarcoplasmic reticulum following endotoxin administration. *Biochem Biophys Res Commun* 1991;174:1248–1254.
155. Estes JE, Farley PE, Goldfarb RD. Effect of shock on calcium accumulation by cardiac sarcoplasmic reticulum. *Adv Shock Res* 1980;3:229–237.
156. McDonough KH, Henry JJ, Lang CH, Spitzer JJ. Substrate utilization and high energy phosphate levels of hearts from hyperdynamic septic rats. *Circ Shock* 1986;18:161–170.
157. Laughlin MH, Smyk-Randall EM, Novotny MJ, Brown OR, Adams HR. Coronary blood flow and cardiac adenine nucleotides in *E. coli* endotoxemia in dogs: effects of oxygen radical scavengers. *Circ Shock* 1988;25:173–185.
158. Cunnion RE, Schaer GL, Parker MM, Yatanson C, Parrillo JE. The coronary circulation in human septic shock. *Circulation* 1986;73:637–644.
159. Elkins RC, McCurdy JR, Brown PP, Greenfield LJ. Effects of coronary perfusion pressure on myocardial performance during endotoxin shock. *Surg Gynecol Obstet* 1973;137:991–996.
160. Peyton MD, Hinshaw LB, Greenfield LJ, Elkins RC. The effects of coronary vasodilation on cardiac performance during endotoxin shock. *Surg Gynecol Obstet* 1976;143:533–538.
161. Cho YW. Direct cardiac action of *E. coli* endotoxin. *Proc Soc Exp Biol Med* 1972;141:705–707.
162. Bohs CT, Turbow ME, Kolmen SN, Traber DL. Coronary blood flow alterations in endotoxin shock and the response to dipyridamole. *Circ Shock* 1976;2:281–287.
163. Kleinman WM, Krause SM, Hess ML. Differential subendocardial perfusion and injury during the course of gram-negative endotoxemia. *Adv Shock Res* 1980;4:139–152.

164. Bond RF. Peripheral circulatory responses to endotoxin. *Handbook Endotoxin* 1985;2:36–75.
165. Feigl EO. Coronary physiology. *Physiol Rev* 1983;63:1–205.
166. Bronsveld W, Van Lambalgen AA, Van den Bos GC, Thijs LG, Koopman PAR. Regional blood flow and metabolism in canine endotoxin shock before, during and after infusion of glucose–insulin–potassium (GIK). *Circ Shock* 1986;18:31–42.
167. Bronsveld W, Van Lambalgen AA, Van Veleen D, Van den Bos GC, Koopman PAR, Thijs LG. Myocardial metabolic and morphometric changes during canine endotoxin shock before and after glucose–insulin–potassium. *Cardiovasc Res* 1985;19:455–464.
168. Novotny MJ, Laughlin MH, Adams HR. Evidence for lack of importance of oxygen free radicals in *Escherichia coli* endotoxemia in dogs. *Am J Physiol* 1988;254:H954–H962.
169. Somani P, Saini RK. A comparison of the cardiovascular, renal and coronary effects of dopamine and monensin in endotoxic shock. *Circ Shock* 1981;8:451–464.
170. Nishijima MK, Breslow MJ, Miller CF, Traystman RJ. Effect of naloxone and ibuprofen on organ blood flow during endotoxin shock in pig. *Am J Physiol* 1988;255:H177–H184.
171. Brand ED, Lefer AM. Myocardial depressant factor in plasma from cats in irreversible postoligemic shock. *Proc Soc Exp Biol Med* 1966;122:200–203.
172. Baxter CR, Cook WA, Shires GT. Serum myocardial depressant factor of burn shock. *Surg Forum* 1966;17:1–2.
173. Lefer AM. Properties of cardioinhibitory factors produced in shock. *Fed Proc* 1978; 37:2734–2740.
174. Lefer AM. Role of a myocardial depressant factor in the pathogenesis of circulatory shock. *Fed Proc* 1970;29:1836–1847.
175. Thalinger AR, Lefer AM. Cardiac actions of a myocardial depressant factor isolated from shock plasma. *Proc Soc Exp Biol Med* 1971;136:354–358.
176. Lefer AM, Rovetto MJ. Influence of a myocardial depressant factor on physiologic properties of cardiac muscle. *Proc Soc Biol Med* 1970;134:269–273.
177. Lefer AM. Role of a myocardial depressant factor in shock states. *Mod Concepts Cardiovasc Dis* 1973;42:59–64.
178. Carli A, Auclair MC, Benassayag C, et al. Evidence for an early lipid soluble cardiodepressant factor in rat serum after a sublethal dose of endotoxin. *Circ Shock* 1981;8:301–312.
179. Carli A, Auclair MC, Bleichner G, et al. Inhibited response to isoproterenol and altered action potential of beating rat heart cells by human serum in septic shock. *Circ Shock* 1978;5:85–94.
180. Carli A, Auclair MC, Vernimmen C, et al. Reversal by calcium of rat heart cell dysfunction induced by human sera in septic shock. *Circ Shock* 1979;6:147–157.
181. Goldfarb RD. Cardiac dynamics following shock: role of circulating cardiodepressant substances. *Circ Shock* 1982;9:317–334.
182. Lundgren O, Haglund U, Isaksson O, et al. Effects on myocardial contractility of blood-borne material released from feline small intestine in simulated shock. *Circ Res* 1976;8:307–315.
183. Goldfarb RD, Weber P, Estes JE. Characterization of circulating shock-induced cardiodepressant substances. *Fed Proc* 1978;37:2724–2728.
184. Lefer AM, Spath JA Jr. Pharmacologic basis of the treatment of circulatory shock. In: Antonaccio MJ, ed. *Cardiovascular pharmacology.* New York: Raven Press; 1977:377–428.
185. Lefer AM, Spath JA Jr. Pancreatic hypoperfusion and the production of a myocardial depressant factor in hemorrhagic shock. *Ann Surg* 1974;179:868–876.
186. Litvin Y, Leffler JN, Barenholz Y, et al. Factors influencing the *in vitro* production of a myocardial depressant factor. *Biochem Med* 1973;8:199–212.
187. Green LF, Shapanka R, Glenn RM, et al. Isolation of myocardial depressant factor (MDF) from plasma of dogs in hemorrhagic shock. *Biochim Biophys Acta* 1977; 491:275–285.
188. Wangensteen SL, Geissinger WT, Lovett WL, et al. Relationship between splanchnic blood flow and a myocardial depressant factor in endotoxin shock. *Surgery* 1971; 69:410–418.

189. Haglund U, Lundgren O. Intestinal ischemia and shock factors. *Fed Proc* 1978; 37:2729–2733.
190. Beardsley AC, Lefer AM. Impairment of cardiac function after splanchnic artery occlusion shock. *Circ Shock* 1974;1:123–130.
191. Lefer AM. Interaction between myocardial depressant factor and vasoactive mediators with ischemia and shock. *Am J Physiol* 1987;252:R193–R205.
192. Stahl GL, Lefer AM. Mechanisms of platelet-activating factor-induced cardiac depression in the isolated perfused rat heart. *Circ Shock* 1987;23:165–177.
193. Hinshaw LB. Myocardial function in endotoxin shock. *Circ Shock* 1979 (suppl 1); 6:43–51.
194. Parrillo JE, Burch C, Shelkamer JH, Parker MM, Natanson C, Schuette W. A circulating myocardial depressant substance in humans with septic shock. *J Clin Invest* 1985;76:1539–1553.
195. Holaday JW, Faden AI. Naloxone reversal of endotoxin hypotension suggests role of endorphins in shock. *Nature* 1978;275:450–451.
196. Faden AI, Holaday JW. Opiate antagonists: a role in the treatment of hypovolemic shock. *Science* 1979;205:317–318.
197. Holaday JW. Commentary. Cardiovascular consequences of endogenous opiate antagonism. *Biochem Pharmacol* 1983;32:573–585.
198. Holaday JW, O'Hara M, Faden AI. Hypophysectomy alters cardiorespiratory variables: central effects of pituitary endorphins in shock. *Am J Physiol* 1981;241:H479–H485.
199. Faden AI, Holaday JW. Naloxone treatment of endotoxin shock: stereospecificity of physiologic and pharmacologic effects in rats. *J Pharmacol Exp Ther* 1980;212:441–447.
200. Faden AI, Holaday JW. Experimental endotoxin shock: the pathophysiologic function of endorphins and treatment with opiate antagonists. *J Infect Dis* 1980;142:229–238.
201. Reynolds DG, Guril NJ, Vargish T, et al. Blockade of opiate receptors with naloxone improves survival and cardiac performance in canine endotoxic shock. *Circ Shock* 1980;7:39–48.
202. Vargish T, Reynolds DG, Guril NJ, et al. Naloxone reversal of hypovolemic shock in dogs. *Circ Shock* 1980;7:31–38.
203. Curtis MT, Lefer AM. Protective actions of naloxone in hemorrhagic shock. *Am J Physiol* 1980;239:H416–H421.
204. Wright DJM, Weller MPI. Inhibition by naloxone of endotoxin-induced reactions in mice. *Br J Pharmacol* 1980;70:99–100P.
205. Raymond RM, Harkema JM, Stoffs WV, et al. Effects of naloxone therapy on hemodynamics and metabolism following a superlethal dosage of *Escherichia coli* endotoxin in dogs. *Surg Gynecol Obstet* 1981;152:159–162.
206. Rees M, Payne JG, Bowen JC. Naloxone reverses tissue effects of live *Escherichia coli* sepsis. *Surgery* 1982;91:81–86.
207. Schadt JC, York DH. The reversal of hemorrhagic hypotension by naloxone in conscious rabbits. *Can J Physiol Pharmacol* 1981;59:1208–1213.
208. Thijs LG, Balk E, Tuynman HARE, et al. Effects of naloxone on hemodynamics, oxygen transport and metabolic variables in canine endotoxin shock. *Circ Shock* 1983; 10:147–160.
209. Gadhos FN, Chiu RCJ, McArdle AH, et al. Role of endorphins in septic shock after receptor blockade with naloxone. *Surg Forum* 1980;31:17–19.
210. Traber DL, Thomson PD, Blalock JE, et al. Action of an opiate receptor blocker on ovine cardiopulmonary responses to endotoxin. *Am J Physiol* 1983;245:H189–H193.
211. Janssen HF, Lutherer LO. Ventriculocisternal administration of naloxone protects against severe hypotension during endotoxin shock. *Brain Res* 1980;194:608–612.
212. Koyama S, Santiesteban HL, Ammons WS, et al. The effects of naloxone on the peripheral sympathetics in cat endotoxin shock. *Circ Shock* 1983;10:7–13.
213. Young WS, Wamsley JK, Zarbin MA, et al. Opioid receptors undergo axonal flow. *Science* 1980;210:76–77.
214. Lefer AM, Curtis MT. Peripheral effects of opiate antagonists in shock. *Adv Shock Res* 1983;10:83–86.

215. Wessglas IS. The role of endogenous opiates in shock: experimental and clinical studies *in vitro* and *in vivo. Adv Shock Res* 1983;10:87–94.
216. Caffrey JL, Gaugl JS, Jones CE. Local endogenous opiate activity in dog's myocardium: receptor blockade with naloxone. *Am J Physiol* 1985;48:H382–H388.
217. Riggs TR, Yano Y, Vargish T. Morphine depression of myocardial function. *Circ Shock* 1986;19:31–38.
218. Riggs TR, Yano Y, Vargish T. Opiate agonist depression of myocardial function is dose related and independent of pentobarbital or chloral hydrate anesthesia. *Am Surg* 1986; 52(12):654–658.
219. Vargish T, Beamer KC, Daly T, Head R. Myocardial opiate receptor activity is stereospecific, independent of muscarinic receptor antagonism, and may play a role in depressing cardiac function. *Surgery* 1987;102(2):171–177.
220. Vargish T, Beamer KC, Daly T, Riggs TR. Morphine sulfate depression of cardiac function is attenuated by opiate receptor antagonism with naloxone. *Circ Shock* 1987; 23:189–195.
221. Vargish T, Beamer KC. Delta and mu receptor agonists correlate with greater depression of cardiac function than morphine sulfate in perfused rat hearts. *Circ Shock* 1989;27:245–251.
222. Hathorne LF, Caffrey JL, Kutsky P, Parker JL. *In vitro* effects of opiate peptides in guinea pig myocardium. *Circ Shock* 1985;16:73(abstract).
223. Parker JL, Wehmeier KR, Gaddis RR, Keller RS. Myocardial functional insensitivity to opioid peptides and naloxone *in vitro. Circ Shock* 1986;18:365–366(abstract).
224. Ruth JA, Eiden LE. Lucine–enkephalin modulation of catecholamine positive chronotrophy in rat atria is receptor-specific and calcium-dependent. *Neuropeptides* 1984;4:101–108.
225. Caffrey JL, Hathorne LF, Carter GC, Sinclair RJ. Naloxone potentiates contractile responses to epinephrine in isolated canine arteries. *Circ Shock* 1990;31:317–332.
226. Caffrey JL, Wooldridge CB, Gaugl JF. Naloxone enhances myocardium responses to isoproterenol in the dog isolated heart–lung. *Am J Physiol* 1986;250:H749–H754.
227. Gu H, Gaugl JF, Barron BA, Caffrey JL. Naloxone enhances cardiac contractile responses to epinephrine without altering epinephrine uptake from plasma. *Circ Shock* 1990;32:257–271.
228. Del Maestro RF. An approach to free radicals in medicine and biology. *Acta Physiol Scand [Suppl]* 1980;492:153–168.
229. Sacks T, Moldow CF, Craddock PR, et al. Oxygen radicals mediate endothelial cell damage by complement-stimulated granulocytes. *J Clin Invest* 1978;61:1161–1167.
230. Kontos HA, Wei EP, Povlishock JT, et al. Oxygen radicals mediate the cerebral arteriolar dilation from arachidonate and bradykinin in cats. *Circ Res* 1984;55:295–303.
231. Rosenblum WI. Effects of free radical generation on mouse pial arterioles: probable role of hydroxyl radicals. *Am J Physiol* 1983;245:H139–H142.
232. Parks DA, Bulkley GB, Granger DN, et al. Ischemic injury in the cat small intestine: role of superoxide radicals. *Gastroenterology* 1982;82:9–15.
233. Fong KL, McCay PB, Poyer JL, et al. Evidence that peroxidation of lysosomal membranes is initiated by hydroxyl free radicals produced during flavin enzyme activity. *J Biol Chem* 1973;248:7792–7797.
234. Lynch RC, Fridovich I. Permeation of the erythrocyte stroma by superoxide radical. *J Biol Chem* 1978;253:4697–4699.
235. Mead JR. Free radical mechanisms of lipid damage and consequences for cellular membranes. *Free Rad Biol* 1976;1:51–67.
236. Demopoulos HB, Flamm ES, Pietronigro DD, et al. The free radical pathology and the microcirculation in the major central nervous system disorders. *Acta Physiol Scand [Suppl]* 1980;492:91–119.
237. Hess ML, Okabe E, Kontos HA. Proton and free oxygen radical interaction with the calcium transport system of cardiac sarcoplasmic reticulum. *J Mol Cell Cardiol* 1981; 13:767–772.
238. Manson NH, Hess ML. Interaction of oxygen free radicals and cardiac sarcoplasmic reticulum: proposed role in the pathogenesis of endotoxin shock. *Circ Shock* 1983; 1:205–213.

239. Hess ML, Manson NH. The paradox of steroid therapy: inhibition of oxygen free radicals. *Circ Shock* 1983;10:1–5.
240. Rowe GT, Manson NH, Caplan M, et al. Hydrogen peroxide and hydroxyl radical mediation of activated leucocyte depression of cardiac sarcoplasmic reticulum. *Circ Res* 1983;53:584–591.
241. Kuehl FA Jr, Humes JL, Ham EZ, et al. Inflammation: the role of peroxidase-derived products. In: Samuelsson B, Ramwell PW, Paoletti R, eds. *Advances in prostaglandin and thromboxane research.* New York: Raven Press; 1980:77–86.
242. Loschen G, Azzi A, Richter C, et al. Superoxide radicals as precursor of mitochondrial hydrogen peroxide. *FEBS Lett* 1974;43:68–72.
243. Lefer AM, Araki H, Okamatsu S. Beneficial actions of a free radical scavenger in traumatic shock and myocardial ischemia. *Circ Shock* 1981;8:273–282.
244. Guarnieri C, Flamigni F, Caldarera CM. Role of oxygen in the cellular damage induced by reoxygenation of hypoxic heart. *J Mol Cell Cardiol* 1980;12:797–808.
245. Traber DL, Adams T, Sziebert L, Stein M, Traber L. Potentiation of lung vascular response to endotoxin by superoxide dismutase. *J Appl Physiol* 1985;58:1005–1009.
246. Parker JL, Keller RS, DeFily DV, Laughlin MH, Novotny MJ, Adams HR. Coronary vascular smooth muscle function in *E. coli* endotoxemia in dogs. *Am J Physiol* 1991; 260:H832–H841.
247. Lefer AM. Eicosanoids as mediators of ischemia and shock. *Fed Proc* 1985;44:275–280.
248. Feuerstein G, Hallenbeck JM. Prostaglandins, leukotrienes and platelet activating factor in shock. *Annu Rev Pharmacol Toxicol* 1987;27:301–313.
249. Altura BM, Lefer AM, Schumer W. Role of prostaglandins and thromboxanes in shock states. In: Altura BM, Lefer AM, Schumer W, eds. *Handbook of shock and trauma, vol 1: basic science.* New York: Raven Press; 1983:355–376.
250. Ball HA, Cook JA, Wise WC, Halushka PV. Role of thromboxane, prostaglandins, and leukotrienes in endotoxic and septic shock. *Intensive Care Med* 1986;12:116–126.
251. Sprague RS, Stephenson AH, Dahms TE, Lonigro AJ. Proposed role for leukotrienes in the pathophysiology of multiple systems organ failure. *Crit Care Med* 1989;5:315–329.
252. Stahl GL, Lefer AM. Mechanisms of platelet-activating factor-induced cardiac depression in the isolated perfused rat heart. *Circ Shock* 1987;23:165–177.
253. Roth DM, Hock CE, Lefer DJ, Lefer AM. Cardiac effects of peptidoleukotrienes. In: Bailey JM, ed. *Prostaglandins, leukotrienes, and lipoxins.* New York: Plenum; 1985:371–378.
254. Roth DM, Lefer DJ, Hock CE, Lefer AM. Effects of peptide leukotrienes on cardiac dynamics in rat, cat, and guinea pig hearts. *Am J Physiol* 1985;249:H477–H484.
255. Burke JA, Levi R, Guo ZG, Corey EJ. Leukotrienes C_4, D_4, and E_4: effects on human and guinea pig cardiac preparations *in vitro*. *J Pharmacol Exp Ther* 1982;221: 235–241.
256. Hattori Y, Levi R. Negative inotropic effect of leukotrienes: leukotriene C_4 and D_4 inhibit calcium-dependent contractile responses in potassium-depolarized guinea pig myocardium. *J Pharmacol Exp Ther* 1984;230:646–651.
257. Michelassi F, Castorena G, Hill RD, et al. Effects of leukotrienes B_4 and C_4 on coronary circulation and myocardial contractility. *Surgery* 1983;94:267–275.
258. Karmazyn M, Moffat MP. Positive inotropic effects of low concentrations of leukotrienes C_4 and D_4 in rat hearts. *Am J Physiol* 1990;259:H1239–H1246.
259. Myers PR, Wright RF, Parker JL, Adams HR. Interactions of tumor necrosis factor α (TNF_α), interleukin 1 β (IL1) and endotoxin: effects on endothelium-derived relaxing factor (EDRF) and nitric oxide production in vascular endothelial cells. *Circulation* 1991;84:77(abstract).
260. Adams HR, Parker JL, Zhong Q, Wright TF, Myers PR. Impaired endothelium dependent relaxation of vascular smooth muscle by endotoxin: *ex vivo* and *in vitro* evidence. *Circulation* 1991;84;274.
261. Myers PR, Wright TF, Tanner MA, Adams HR. Endothelial-derived relaxing factor and nitric oxide production in cultured endothelial cells: direct inhibition by *E. coli* endotoxin. *Am J Physiol* 1992; 262:H710–H718.

262. Romano FD, Jones SB. Alteration in β-adrenergic stimulation of myocardial adenylate cyclase in endotoxic rats. *Am J Physiol* 1986;250:R358–R364.
263. Romano FD, Jones SB. Characteristics of myocardial β-adrenergic receptors during endotoxicosis in the rat. *Am J Physiol* 1986;251:R359–R364.
264. Burns AH, Giamo ME, Summer WR. Dichloroacetic acid improves *in vitro* myocardial function following *in vivo* endotoxin administration. *J Crit Care* 1986;1(1):11–17.
265. McDonough KH, Barbee RW, Dobiescu C, Long CH, Spitzer JJ. Enhanced myocardial depression in diabetic rats during *E. coli* sepsis. *Am J Physiol* 1987;252:H410–H416.
266. Liu MS, Takeda H. Endotoxin-induced stimulation on phospholipase A activities in dog hearts. *Biochem Med* 1982;28:62–69.
267. Liu MS, Ghosh S. Myocardial sodium pump activity in endotoxin shock. *Circ Shock* 1986;19:177–184.
268. Groeneveld ABJ, van Lambalgen AA, van den Bos GC, Bronsveld W, Nauta JJP, Thijs LG. Maldistribution of heterogenous coronary blood flow during canine endotoxin shock. *Cardiovasc Res* 1991;25:80–88.

Cardiovascular Toxicology, Second Edition,
edited by Daniel Acosta, Jr.
Raven Press, Ltd., New York © 1992.

10

Cardiotoxicity of Catecholamines and Related Agents

Naranjan S. Dhalla, John C. Yates, Barbara Naimark,
Ken S. Dhalla, Robert E. Beamish, and *Bohuslav Ostadal

*Division of Cardiovascular Sciences, St. Boniface General Hospital Research
Centre, and Department of Physiology, University of Manitoba, Winnipeg,
Manitoba, Canada R2H 2A6; and *Institute of Physiology, Czechoslovak Academy
of Sciences, Prague, Czechoslovakia*

Catecholamines such as adrenaline (epinephrine) and noradrenaline (norepinephrine) are synthesized in the adrenal medulla, and norepinephrine is also synthesized in the sympathetic nervous system. Low concentrations of circulating catecholamines exert positive inotropic action on the myocardium and thus are considered beneficial in regulating heart function. On the other hand, high concentrations of these hormones over a prolonged period produce deleterious effects on the cardiovascular system. In this regard, it has been known for many years that epinephrine (1,2) and norepinephrine (3) can cause cardiac lesions when administered in large doses. Subsequently, Rona et al. (4) discovered that a synthetic catecholamine, isoproterenol, is capable of producing consistent myocardial lesions when injected at dose levels far below the lethal dosage for this agent. Injection of catecholamines in animals also produces a number of dramatic pharmacological effects including changes in hemodynamic factors such as peripheral resistance, arterial blood pressure, cardiac output, venous return, and coronary flow; increases heart rate and cardiac work, thereby causing increased myocardial oxygen demand; releases further amounts of catecholamines from the adrenergic nerve endings; produces alterations in lipid and carbohydrate metabolism; and results in the accumulation of exogenous lipids in the heart. As a consequence of these factors it has been difficult to determine whether catecholamines do in fact exert a direct toxic influence on the myocardium, or whether myocardial cell damage is in some way secondary to other actions of catecholamines as proposed by some investigators (4–10). On the other hand, evidence and arguments have been presented to the effect that cardiovascular, hemodynamic, and other changes following administration of catecholamines cannot completely account for the occurrence of myocardial necrosis in different experimental models (11–18). Detailed studies showing changes in sarcolemmal permeability as the primary event leading to the development of catecholamine-induced cardiac cell injury have also appeared in the literature (19,20). A further complicating factor in this problem is the fact that catecholamines readily undergo oxidation and it has been suggested that the oxidation products of catecholamines rather than catecholamines *per se* are responsible for the cardiotoxicity observed following administration of these agents (21,22). Furthermore, other workers have claimed that the products of catecholamine metabolism, especially those produced during the monoamine oxidase reaction, may be involved in the induction of myocardial necrosis (23). Thus, in spite of a considerable research effort by many investigators devoted to elucidating these mechanisms (24–32), there is as yet no clear-cut explanation of the sequence of events by which cardiac cell necrosis results from an injection of catecholamines. In this chapter, an attempt has been made to synthesize the existing information on diverse problems related to cardiovascular effects of sympathomimetic agents in order to formulate a unifying concept regarding the pathophysiology and clinical significance of catecholamine-induced cardiotoxicity.

CARDIOTOXICITY OF EPINEPHRINE, NOREPINEPHRINE, AND ISOPROTERENOL

The cardiotoxic properties of catecholamines have been known since 1905 when the occurrence of cardiac lesions after epinephrine administration was reported by Ziegler (2); these lesions were subsequently described in detail by Pearce (1) and Josue (33). Fleisher and Loeb (34–37) reported that injection of sparteine sulfate or caffeine sodium benzoate followed by epinephrine provided an easy and certain method of producing myocardial lesions in rabbits. Lesions visible to the naked eye occurred in 60% of the animals; microscopic examination revealed further lesions in a still larger percentage. These investigators suggested that excessive mechanical strain was at least one of the factors responsible for producing the lesions. Christian et al. (38) confirmed these findings and further demonstrated that sparteine sulfate alone did not produce myocardial lesions. In 1913 a full histological account of these epinephrine-induced myocardial changes was provided by Anitschkow (39) and epinephrine was thereafter shown to produce cardiac lesions in humans as well (40,41). While most of these reports dealt with relatively high dose levels of epinephrine, small endocardial lesions were also observed in the left ventricle of dog hearts following continuous infusion for 120–289 hr of epinephrine at a rate considered to be well below the maximum physiological rate of secretion by the adrenal gland (42).

Within a few years after norepinephrine came into widespread use as a primary pressor agent, reports of norepinephrine-induced myocardial lesions began to appear. In the course of a study on the effects of prolonged infusion of norepinephrine on arterial pressure of rabbits, Blacket et al. (43) found that the hypertension resulting from norepinephrine infusion could not be maintained, even with increasing dose levels, and that blood pressure fell drastically when infusion was discontinued. Although the possible release of vasodilator substances was discussed in connection with these findings, these investigators apparently did not consider the possibility of impaired cardiac function. Norepinephrine did not increase the survival rate of dogs in hemorrhagic shock when compared with controls (44), and in fact this agent was found to show a higher incidence of cardiac lesions in this condition (45). The observation of an increased frequency of nonspecific myocarditis and an apparent common denominator of norepinephrine therapy in humans prompted Szakacs and Cannon (3) to study the effects on the heart of continuous intravenous infusions of therapeutic doses of norepinephrine in dogs. Focal myocarditis was found to be uniformly present in the hearts of these animals in association with subendocardial and subepicardial hemorrhages.

Being aware of the epinephrine-induced myocardial lesions previously reported (46), Nahas et al. (47) conducted a series of experiments with both epinephrine and norepinephrine using a heart–lung preparation in which the heart was isolated from all secondary hormonal or nervous influences. All hearts that had been perfused with epinephrine, norepinephrine, or both proved to have extensive lesions of the myocardium. In a quantitative study of the pathological effects of norepinephrine, Szakacs and Mehlman (48) found that dosages considered physiologic and indeed harmless, if administered for short periods of time, might become lethal after prolonged infusion. Thus duration of infusion appears to be an important factor in determining whether a particular dose of norepinephrine is likely to produce myocardial lesions. In addition to myocardial cell damage, norepinephrine was also demonstrated to produce derangements of metabolic processes in the heart. For example, Maling and Highman (49) reported a fatty degeneration of the myocardium under the influence of high doses of norepinephrine. In subsequent studies (50,51), remarkable similarities were found in heart triglyceride content and serum enzyme levels after large doses of epinephrine and norepinephrine as well as following myocardial infarction produced by coronary artery occlusion. However, these studies did not attempt to examine the relationship between changes in lipid metabolism and the occurrence of myocardial necrosis due to catecholamines.

The discovery that severe myocardial necrosis could be consistently produced in rats with doses of isoproterenol that constitute an amazingly small fraction of the median lethal dose (4,52) opened the way for a systematic examination of catecholamine-induced myocardial lesions. Although the

LD_{50} of isoproterenol in rats was reported to be 680 mg/kg, doses as low as 0.02 mg/kg produced microscopic focal necrotic lesions. The severity of myocardial damage was closely related to the dosage of isoproterenol used and varied from focal lesions affecting single cells to massive infarcts involving large portions of the left ventricle. Lesions were generally found to be localized in the apex and left ventricular subendocardium, being observed less frequently in the papillary muscle and right ventricle. A comparison of the cardiotoxic effects of epinephrine, norepinephrine, and isoproterenol in rats (53) showed the lesions produced to be qualitatively similar, but the lesions that were seen after isoproterenol treatment were more severe than those produced by epinephrine or norepinephrine. Whereas the median lethal doses of isoproterenol, epinephrine, and norepinephrine were found in this study to be 581, 6.1, and 8.6 mg/kg, respectively, isoproterenol was found to be 29–72 times more potent in producing myocardial lesions of equal severity than epinephrine or norepinephrine. Isoproterenol was also found to produce apical lesions and disseminated focal necrosis in dogs (54); however, these lesions were frequently fatal to these animals and the median lethal dosage was much lower. Myocardial lesions similar to those produced by catecholamine injections have also been reported in patients with pheochromocytoma (3,55–57), subarachnoid hemorrhage, and various other intracranial lesions (58–61), as well as following electrical stimulation of the stellate ganglion (62,63) or hypothalamus (64) in experimental animals. These studies not only demonstrate that catecholamines are capable of producing myocardial necrosis but also suggest that myocardial cell damage seen in patients may be the result of high levels of circulating catecholamines.

MORPHOLOGICAL AND BIOCHEMICAL CHANGES ASSOCIATED WITH CATECHOLAMINE-INDUCED MYOCARDIAL NECROSIS

Although a number of long-term studies have been conducted on the development and healing of catecholamine-induced infarcts, the present discussion is limited to early events, that is, less than 48 hr after injection, in the production of necrosis.

Ultrastructural Changes

The time course of ultrastructural changes following isoproterenol injections in rats has been studied extensively. The earliest changes, evident within 4–6 min, are disorientation of myofilaments, irregular sarcomere length, occasional regions of contracture or rupture of myofilaments, and some slight dilatation of the sarcoplasmic reticulum (65–67). By 10 min mitochondrial swelling is evident, with the occasional occurrence of electron-dense bodies (67); disorganization and fragmentation of myofibrils are prominent. It has been reported (66,68) that there is no correlation between mitochondrial damage and disruption of myofilaments; normal appearing mitochondria are found among fragmented filaments, and swollen mitochondria with ruptured cristae and electron-dense deposits are found among apparently undamaged sarcomeres. Within 30 min to 1 hr, electron-dense granular deposits are frequently noted within mitochondria, numerous lipid droplets appear, margination of nuclear chromatin is observed, disappearance of glycogen granules is noted, and various degrees of swelling and disruption of transverse and longitudinal tubules as well as mitochondria are seen. At this time there also occurs a spectrum of damage to the contractile filaments, ranging from irregular bands of greater or less than normal density in sarcomeres of irregular length, to fusion of sarcomeres into confluent masses and granular disintegration of the myofilaments (65–67,69). Over the course of the next few hours all these changes become progressively more widespread throughout the myocardium, and more severe (69,70). Interstitial and intracellular edema as well as extensive inflammation also becomes evident (60,69). Herniation of intercalated discs and extensive vacuolization were also seen within several hours of isoproterenol injection (66). Comparison of the effects of norepinephrine and epinephrine with isoproterenol has shown the effects of these three agents to be qualitatively identical at the cellular level (68–73), with the exception that glycogen depletion (69,71) and fat deposition (73) were much more extensive with epinephrine than with isoproterenol or norepinephrine. Maruffo (11) has also reported similar alterations following isoproterenol administration in monkeys.

From the foregoing discussion it appears that alterations of the contractile filaments begin with irregularities in length and disalignment of the sarcomeres, which are usually associated with an increased thickness and density of the Z band. Contracture ensues, with the Z bands becoming indistinct; actin and myosin filaments can no longer be distinguished. Granular disintegration of the sarcomeres follows with the appearance of large empty spaces within the muscle cells, and this fragmentation likely contributes to swelling of the cell. The tubular elements and mitochondria commence swelling very soon after catecholamine injection, and the mitochondrial matrix is subsequently decreased in electron density. Swelling of the transverse tubules and sarcoplasmic reticulum is not as consistent a finding as the mitochondrial swelling and may not be evident with certain fixatives. Following norepinephrine injection the T-system is dilated and much more extensively branched than in normal animals. Rupture of the cristae and deposition of electron-dense material in mitochondria represent the final stage in the disruption of these organelles. Accumulation of lipid droplets and disappearance of glycogen granules are not usually evident until these other changes have occurred to some degree and are probably due to well-known metabolic effects of catecholamines. Herniation of intercalated discs and vacuolization are probably secondary to the swelling and disruption of sub-cellular organelles and the disintegration of myofilaments.

Histological and Histochemical Changes

The earliest change that can be visualized under the light microscope is the appearance of darkly stained contraction bands at 10 min after isopro-terenol injection in thin sections from Araldite-embedded ventricle pieces (11). Focal myocardial degeneration, characterized by loss of striations with sarcoplasmic smudging, lipid accumulation, margination of nuclear chro-matin, and increased cytoplasmic eosinophilia are evident in 2–6 hr following injection of isoproterenol (10,11) or 4–5 hr after beginning infusion of nor-epinephrine (74). Capillary dilatation and interstitial edema are evident by this time in isoproterenol-treated hearts (11) and have been observed much earlier with norepinephrine (68). Interstitial edema is usually associated with subendocardial and subepicardial hemorrhages following administration of catecholamines and is characteristically present in damaged areas of the myocardium even after 72 hr (4,14,54,68,69,74). Rosenblum et al. (14) and Ferrans et al. (69) have made comparative studies that indicate that intersti-tial edema and inflammation are much more prominent following epineph-rine or norepinephrine injections even though isoproterenol is more potent in producing cellular damage. Accordingly, it has been suggested that edema and inflammation result from mechanisms different from those causing ne-crotic tissue damage during the development of catecholamine-induced cardiomyopathy.

Within 12–24 hr, myocardial tissue damage is readily apparent and char-acterized by certain histological staining properties. Fibers with highly eo-sinophilic cytoplasm alternate with normal fibers, giving the myocardium a mottled appearance (4). Swelling, segmentation and fragmentation, and hy-alinization of fibers are evident. Fibers become homogeneous, strongly eo-sinophilic, periodic acid–Schiff (PAS) positive, and stain pink or deep red with Cason's trichrome (4,10,54,69,72). Fat deposition is usually evident as well (72). Histochemical alterations subsequent to administration of lesion-producing doses of catecholamines have also been reported in detail (69–71,74). A marked loss of glycogen, as visualized by PAS reaction, is seen within 30 min and is most marked following epinephrine administration. Ac-cumulation of PAS-positive material is seen at 1 hr and in an increasing num-ber of fibers over the next 24 hr. This is associated with loss of normal stria-tions and appearance of clear vacuoles. A metachromatic substance is usually observed in areas of interstitial edema and inflammation.

All three catecholamines produce a biphasic change in the activity of the oxidative enzymes succinic dehydrogenase, NAD diaphorase, lactic dehy-drogenase, isocitric dehydrogenase, malic dehydrogenase, β-hydroxybu-tyric dehydrogenase, α-glycerophosphate dehydrogenase, glutamic dehydrogenase, and ethanol dehydrogenase. There is a rapid increase in the activity of the enzymes evident within 5 min in various individual fibers followed by a gradual decline in activity 6–12 hr; certain areas of the myocardium having markedly diminished oxidative enzyme activity are interspersed with fibers of normal activity. Decline in oxidative enzyme activity of certain fibers progresses until frank necrosis is evident and there is complete loss of activity. In each case the degree of change of activity is proportional to the normal level of activity of the enzyme involved. Cytochrome oxidase activity is unchanged until evidence of early necrosis is seen after 6–12 hr, at which time activity of this enzyme decreases as well. An increased number of lipid droplets is observed at 30 min. Fatty change is more evident in the endocardial region than elsewhere and has been reported by Ferrans et al. (69) to be least apparent with epinephrine, which is in direct contradiction to the findings of Lehr et al. (73). The reason for this discrepancy in these results is not clear; however, fibers that contain large lipid droplets show decreased activity of oxidative enzymes and cytochrome oxidase. Furthermore, all three agents cause a slight increase in the staining of cytoplasm for lysosomal esterase activity (73).

Biochemical Changes

Following catecholamine administration, coronary blood flow, myocardial oxygen uptake, and cardiac respiratory quotient were increased (75). Blood content of glucose, triglycerides, and nonesterified fatty acids increased markedly without any change in blood cholesterol levels, whereas total serum protein content was decreased (15,76–78). Glycogen and lactate content of the heart decreased rapidly after an injection of isoproterenol. Glycogen levels then rose above control levels over about 5 hr (79). Within 24 hr after the isoproterenol injection, aldosterone levels increased, whereas glucocorticoids and total steroids were decreased (77,78). Serum levels of glutamate–pyruvate transaminase, glutamate–oxaloactetate transaminase (aspartate aminotransferase), lactate dehydrogenase, and creatine phosphokinase were all greatly elevated during the acute phase of necrotization following catecholamine administration (75,77,78,80).

The extraction of nonesterified fatty acids by the heart has been reported to be decreased in comparison with controls following epinephrine infusion, whereas the extraction of triglycerides was increased (75). Likewise, there was no significant increase in the contents of free fatty acids or phospholipids in the left ventricle while there was a significant increase in the triglyceride content of every layer of the left ventricular wall following epinephrine infusion; the greatest increase in triglyceride content occurred in the endocardium (13). The uptake of ^{14}C-labeled triglycerides has also been found to increase during norepinephrine infusion and was associated with a small but significant increase in $^{14}CO_2$ production, whereas synthesis of triglycerides from ^{14}C-acetate or palmitate was unchanged (81). These findings are consistent with the appearance of numerous lipid droplets reported in histological and ultrastructural studies.

The myocardial content of hexosamines became greatly elevated within 24 hr after an injection of isoproterenol and this increase in mucopolysaccharide could not be attributed to fibroblasts or other infiltrating cells (82). Cardiac aspartate aminotransferase (glutamate–oxaloacetate transaminase) activity decreased in a time- and dose-dependent manner following isoproterenol injection (83). This decrease in activity correlates well with the occurrence and severity of macroscopic lesions. Total cardiac lactate dehydrogenase activity fell as well following isoproterenol injection (84). This depression of activity is long term, lasting several days, and appears to be due to a decrease in the ratio of H to M isoenzymes. These findings are consistent with the loss of these enzymes from the heart as evidenced by the increase in plasma concentrations of transaminases and lactate dehydrogenase.

Sobel et al. (22) have reported that a single, large subcutaneous dose of epinephrine, norepinephrine, or isoproterenol produced uncoupling of oxidative phosphorylation in rat heart mitochondria, although these catecholamines *in vitro* did not affect normal rat heart mitochondria. A reduced respiratory control index of heart mitochondria 24 hr after isoproterenol injection has also been reported by Stanton and Schwartz (85) and Vorbeck et al. (86). The results of several studies on cardiac adenine nucleotides following isoproterenol injection in rats are somewhat contradictory. Hattori et al. (87) reported a decrease in the level of all adenine nucleotides, but no change in relative amounts of ATP, ADP, and AMP. Kako (88), on the other hand, found a 26–34% decrease in ATP, an 18–30% decrease in creatine phosphate levels, and a decrease in both the ATP/ADP and the ATP/AMP ratios, but no significant difference in the levels of ADP, AMP, glycogen, lactate, pyruvate, lactate/pyruvate ratio, triglycerides, cholesterol, or phospholipids. Studies of this sort are difficult to evaluate, firstly because the results are expressed in terms of gram wet heart weight, which increases following catecholamine administration due to a large increase in extracellular fluid volume (88,89), and secondly because the scattered portions of the myocardium undergoing necrotic change are "diluted" within a very large mass of cardiac tissue, which has been affected only slightly or not at all. The work of Fleckenstein (90,91), in which he showed a very large decrease in both ATP and creatine phosphate stores of the myocardium, appears to be the best representation of changes in high-energy phosphates presently available. A large increase in the orthophosphate content of the myocardium was also found. These results suggest lowering of the energy state of myocardium due to high doses of catecholamines and this change appears to be at least partly due to an impairment in the process of energy production. On the other hand, relatively little information regarding changes in the process of energy utilization during catecholamine-induced myocardial cell damage is available in the literature. In this regard, Pelouch et al. (92,93) have found that myosin extracted from rat hearts following isoproterenol injections contained a large component consisting of a stable aggregated form of myosin, whereas only the monomeric form of myosin was extracted from control animals. The first phase of aggregation involved a low polymer, probably a dimer, and there is no evidence of proteolytic damage to the myosin; the aggregated form of myosin did not possess any ATPase activity. Fedelesova et al. (94) have reported that injection of a lesion-producing dose of isoproterenol caused an elevation of cardiac myofibrillar ATPase activity and decreased high-energy phosphate stores. However, studies in our laboratory (95) did not reveal any change in myofibrillar Ca^{2+}-stimulated ATPase, whereas the basal ATPase activity was depressed. Thus it appears that further investigations are needed for reaching a meaningful conclusion regarding changes in the process of energy utilization in hearts of animals treated with toxic doses of catecholamines.

Electrolyte Changes

The earliest and most significant changes in tissue ion content following catecholamine administration were found to be a decrease in both magnesium and phosphate, which was evident by 3 hr and persisted beyond 24 hr (72,73,96,97). An increase in myocardial calcium content was observed as well but was not as pronounced in the earlier stages of necrosis, prior to about 6 hr after catecholamine injection. Further studies have shown the uptake of extracellular ^{45}Ca to increase six- to sevenfold with isoproterenol (90,91), although the absolute increase in myocardial content was only of the order of 50–100%. The sodium content of the myocardium did not change until about 24 hr, at which time it was increased, which may be a reflection of an increased interstitial fluid volume (72,73,96,97). Alterations of myocardial potassium content are less certain. Although a transient loss of myocardial potassium has frequently been reported (89,98–100), this is a short-term phenomenon not lasting more than 1–5 min and may be a result of the increased frequency of contraction (101). In this regard, Daggett et al. (102) have reported that norepinephrine caused a dose-dependent uptake of potassium by the isolated heart. In studies concerned with the cardiotoxicity of epinephrine, both an increase (73) and a decrease (13) in the potassium content of the myocardium have been reported. Stanton and Schwartz (85) have also reported a decrease of myocardial potassium content following isoproterenol injection. As mentioned previously, myocardial content determinations are complicated by both the increase of interstitial fluid volume that accompanies necrosis and by the admixture of necrotic and normal fibers that characterizes "multifocal disseminated" necrosis.

Measurements of serum levels of electrolytes 3 hr after isoproterenol injection have revealed an increase of serum magnesium and a decrease of calcium and sodium levels (97). By 7 hr, magnesium returned to control levels and serum potassium was increased, while calcium and sodium levels remained significantly depressed. By 24 hr all serum electrolyte levels returned to normal with the exception of calcium, which remained slightly low. Regan et al. (75) have reported that, after an initial period of uptake of potassium and phosphate, loss of these ions from the left ventricle was evident. Thus serum electrolyte measurements appear to confirm the loss of magnesium and phosphate from the heart and the uptake of calcium as early, important events in the etiology of catecholamine-induced necrosis. Since both net increases and decreases of myocardial and serum potassium have been found at different times, it is possible that potassium may be taken up by more or less undamaged myocardial cells while it is being released from fibers undergoing necrotic changes.

Membrane Changes

By virtue of their ability to regulate Ca^{2+} movements in the myocardial cell, different membrane systems such as sarcolemma, sarcoplasmic reticulum, and mitochondria are considered to determine the status of heart function in health and disease (103–106). Accordingly, alterations in sarcoplasmic reticular, mitochondrial, and sarcolemmal membranes were observed in myocardium from animals treated with high doses of catecholamines (107,108). In order to investigate the role of these membrane changes in the development of contractile dysfunction and myocardial cell damage due to catecholamines, rats were injected intraperitoneally with high doses of isoproterenol (40 mg/kg) and the hearts were removed at 3, 9, and 24 hr later (95,109–115). The cardiac hypertrophy as measured by the heart/body weight ratio and depression in contractile function were seen at 9 and 24 hr, whereas varying degrees of myocardial cell damage occurred within 3–24 hr of isoproterenol injection (Table 1). Alterations in heart membranes were evident from the fact that phospholipid contents in sarcolemma and mitochondria were increased at 3 and 9 hr, whereas the sarcoplasmic reticular phospholipid contents increased at 3, 9, and 24 hr of injecting isoproterenol. It was interesting to observe that phospholipid N-methylation, which has been shown to modulate the Ca^{2+}-transport activities (110), exhibited an increase at 3 hr and a decrease at 24 hr in both sarcolemma and sarcoplasmic reticulum, while no changes were observed in mitochondria (Table 1). These studies (95,109–111) suggest that changes in heart membranes during the development of catecholamine-induced cardiomyopathy are of crucial importance in determining the functional and structural status of the myocardium.

TABLE 1. *Contractile function, structure, and membrane phospholipid changes in myocardium at different times of injecting high doses of isoproterenol (40 mg/kg, ip) in rats*

	Time after isoproterenol injection		
	3 hr	9 hr	24 hr
Heart/body weight ratio	No change	Increase	Increase
Contractile force development	No change	Decrease	Decrease
Myocardial cell damage	Slight	Moderate	Severe
Sarcolemmal phospholipid contents	Increase	Increase	No change
Sarcoplasmic reticular phopholipid contents	Increase	Increase	Increase
Mitochondrial phospholipid contents	Increase	Increase	No change
Sarcolemmal phospholipid methylation	Increase	No change	Decrease
Sarcoplasmic reticular phospholipid methylation	Increase	No change	Decrease
Mitochondrial phospholipid methylation	No change	No change	No change

The information in this table is taken from papers by Dhalla et al. (95,111), Panagia et al. (109), and Okumura et al. (110).

An analysis of results described in various investigations (95,112–114) revealed that the activities of sarcolemmal Ca^{2+} pump (ATP-dependent Ca^{2+} uptake and Ca^{2+}-stimulated ATPase), which is concerned with the removal of Ca^{2+} from the cytoplasm, were increased at 3 hr and decreased at 24 hr of isoproterenol injection (Table 2). On the other hand, Na^+-dependent Ca^{2+} uptake, unlike the Na^+-induced Ca^{2+} release, was decreased at 3, 9, and 24 hr of isoproterenol administration. The sarcolemmal ATP-independent Ca^{2+} binding, which is considered to reflect the status of superficial stores of Ca^{2+} at the cell membrane, and sarcolemmel sialic acid residues, which bind Ca^{2+}, were increased at 9 and 24 hr (Table 2). All these sarcolemmal alterations were not associated with any changes in the nitrendipine binding (an

TABLE 2. *Sarcolemmal changes in myocardium at different times of injecting high doses of isoproterenol (40 mg/kg, ip) in rats*

	Time after isoproterenol injection		
	3 hr	9 hr	24 hr
ATP-dependent Ca^{2+} uptake	Increase	No change	Decrease
Ca^{2+}-stimulated ATPase	Increase	No change	Decrease
Na^+-dependent Ca^{2+} uptake	Decrease	Decrease	Decrease
Na^+-induced Ca^{2+} release	No change	No change	No change
ATP-independent Ca^{2+} binding	No change	Increase	Increase
Sialic acid content	No change	Increase	Increase
Nitrendipine binding	No change	No change	No change
Na^+/K^+–ATPase	No change	No change	No change
Ca^{2+}/Mg^{2+}–ATPase	No change	No change	No change

The information in this table is taken from papers by Makino et al. (112,113), Panagia et al. (114), and Dhalla et al. (95).

index of Ca^{2+} channels), Na^+/K^+-ATPase (an index of Na^+ pump), and Ca^{2+}/Mg^{2+}-ATPase (an index of Ca^{2+}-gating mechanism). An early increase in the sarcolemmal Ca^{2+} pump may help the cell to remove Ca^{2+}, whereas depressed Na^+–Ca^{2+} exchange can be seen to contribute to the occurrence of intracellular Ca^{2+} overload. Likewise, an increase in the entry of Ca^{2+} from the elevated sarcolemmal superficial Ca^{2+} stores as well as a depressed sarcolemmal Ca^{2+} pump may contribute to the occurrence of intracellular Ca^{2+} overload at a late stage of catecholamine-induced cardiomyopathy.

It is now well known that relaxation of the cardiac muscle is mainly determined by the activity of the Ca^{2+} pump located in the sarcoplasmic reticulum, whereas the interaction of Ca^{2+} with myofibrils determines the ability of myocardium to contract. On the other hand, mitochondria, which are primarily concerned with the production of ATP, are also known to accumulate Ca^{2+} in order to lower the intracellular concentration of Ca^{2+} under pathological conditions. Data from different studies (95,109,111), as summarized in Table 3, indicate biphasic changes in the sarcoplasmic reticular Ca^{2+}-pump (ATP-dependent Ca^{2+} uptake and Ca^{2+}-stimulated ATPase) activities during the development of catecholamine-induced cardiomyopathy. Mitochondrial Ca^{2+} uptake, unlike mitochondrial ATPase activity, was increased at 9 and 24 hr of isoproterenol injection. Although no change in myofibrillar Ca^{2+}-stimulated ATPase activity was apparent, the myofibrillar Mg^{2+} ATPase activity was depressed at 9 and 24 hr of isoproterenol injection (Table 3). Time-dependent changes in the adrenergic receptor mechanisms (115), which are also concerned with the regulation of Ca^{2+} movements in myocardium, were also seen during the development of catecholamine-induced cardiomyopathy (Table 4). In particular, the number of beta-adrenergic receptors were decreased at 9 hr, whereas the number of alpha-adrenergic receptors decreased at 24 hr of isoproterenol injection. The basal adenylate cyclase activities were not changed, whereas stimulation of adenylate cyclase by epinephrine was depressed at 3 and 9 hr. Activation of adenylate cyclase by a nonhydrolyzable analog of guanine nucleotide (Gpp(NH)p)

TABLE 3. *Subcellular alterations in myocardium at different times of injecting high doses of isoproterenol (40 mg/kg, ip) in rats*

	Time after isoproterenol injection		
	3 hr	9 hr	24 hr
Sarcoplasmic reticular Ca^{2+} uptake	Increase	No change	Decrease
Sarcoplasmic reticular Ca^{2+}-stimulated ATPase	Increase	No change	Decrease
Mitochondrial Ca^{2+} uptake	No change	Increase	Increase
Mitochondrial ATPase	No change	No change	No change
Myofibrillar Ca^{2+}-stimulated ATPase	No change	No change	No change
Myofibrillar Mg^{2+} ATPase	No change	Decrease	Decrease

The information in this table is taken from papers by Dhalla et al. (95,111) and Panagia et al. (109).

TABLE 4. *Changes in adrenergic receptor mechanisms in myocardium at different times of injecting high doses of isoproterenol (40 mg/kg, ip) in rats*

	Time after isoproterenol injection		
	3 hr	9 hr	24 hr
Beta-adrenergic receptors	No change	Decrease	No change
Alpha-adrenergic receptors	No change	No change	Decrease
Adenylate cyclase activity	No change	No change	No change
Epinephrine-stimulated adenylate cyclase	Decrease	Decrease	No change
Gpp(NH)p-stimulated adenylate cyclase	Decrease	Decrease	Decrease
NaF-stimulated adenylate cyclase	Decrease	Decrease	Decrease

The information in this table is taken from papers by Corder et al. (115).

and NaF was decreased at 3, 9, and 24 hr of isoproterenol injection (Table 4). These results suggest that subcellular mechanisms concerned with the regulation of Ca^{2+} movements are altered in catecholamine-induced cardiomyopathy.

In summary, it appears that some of the changes in heart membranes are adaptive in nature, whereas others contribute to the pathogenesis of myocardial cell damage and contractile dysfunction. The early increase in sarcolemmal and sarcoplasmic reticular Ca^{2+}-pump mechanisms as well as late changes in mitochondrial Ca^{2+} uptake seems to help the myocardial cell in lowering the intracellular concentration of Ca^{2+}. On the other hand, the early depression in sarcolemmel Na^+–Ca^{2+} exchange and late decrease in the sarcolemmal and sarcoplasmic reticular Ca^{2+} pump may lead to the development of intracellular Ca^{2+} overload. This change may result in the redistribution and activation of lysosomal enzymes (116) and other mechanisms for the disruption of the myocardial cell due to high levels of circulating catecholamines.

Coronary Spasm and Ventricular Arrhythmias

Under a wide variety of stressful conditions, where circulating levels of catecholamines are markedly elevated, occurrence of coronary spasm and arrhythmias have been well recognized (117). In fact, coronary spasm is considered to result in arrhythmias, myocardial ischemia, and myocardial cell damage due to catecholamines. In order to understand the mechanisms of coronary spasm, changes in coronary resistance were monitored upon infusion of norepinephrine in the isolated perfused rat heart preparations (118). A biphasic change in coronary resistance was evident; however, when norepinephrine infusion was carried out in the presence of a beta-adrenergic blocking agent, propranolol, only a marked increase in coronary resistance (coronary spasm) was evident. This coronary spasm was dependent on the extracellular concentration of Ca^{2+} and was prevented by alpha-adrenergic blocking agents as well as Ca^{2+} antagonists (118). On the other hand, indomethacin and acetylsalicylic acid, which interfere with prostaglandin metabolism, did not modify the norepinephrine-induced coronary spasm (118). In another set of experiments, intravenous injection of epinephrine in rats was found to elicit varying degrees of arrhythmias depending on the time and dose of the hormone (119,120). Pretreatment of animals with vitamin E, reducing agent (cysteine), or oxygen free-radical scavenger (superoxide dismutase) was found to markedly reduce the incidence of arrhythmias due to epinephrine. These results indicate the importance of free radicals in the generation of cardiotoxic effects of high concentrations of catecholamines.

MODIFICATION OF CATECHOLAMINE CARDIOTOXICITY

Pharmacological Interventions

Monoamine oxidase inhibitors (MAOIs) of the hydrazine type have been found to decrease the incidence and severity of myocardial lesions following catecholamine administration (79,85,121–125) and to antagonize increases in myocardial water, sodium, and chloride as well as loss of potassium (85). The hydrazine-type inhibitors investigated include isocarboxazide, iproniazide, pivaloylbanzhydrazine, and phenylzine. On the other hand, the non-hydrazine-type MAO inhibitors such as tranylcypromine, pargyline, and R05-7071 have been reported by some workers to be ineffective (79,124,125), although Leszkovsky and Gal (126) reported a reduction of the severity of isoproterenol-induced lesions with pargyline and another nonhydrazine MAOI identified as E-250. Muller (23) also found that hydrazine-type MAOIs protected the heart, whereas nonhydrazine-type MAOIs did not, but pointed out that hydrazine-type inhibitions are long lasting in their effects whereas tranylcypromine is a competitive blocker with an intensive but transient effect and thus the inhibition produced by this drug may be of insufficient duration to afford protection.

The beta-receptor blocking compounds, propranolol, pronethalol, and dichloroisoproterenol were found to reduce the incidence and severity of myocardial lesions induced by isoproterenol (96,97,121,127–129), although Wenzel and Lyon (84) found pronethalol to be ineffective. In another study, Wenzel and Chau (83) have reported that pronethalol afforded some protection against the loss of myocardial aspartate aminotransferase (AAT) activity caused by epinephrine, norepinephrine, and high doses of isoproterenol but potentiated the loss of AAT activity with moderate lesion-producing doses of isoproterenol. Propranolol has also been found to ameliorate or completely prevent electrolyte shifts (increased myocardial Ca^{2+}; decreased Mg^{2+} and P^-) associated with isoproterenol-induced necrosis (97,127), thus producing an apparent dichotomy between the occurrence of lesions and elctrolyte shifts since myocardial lesions were still seen, although less severe (127). In view of the proportion of the ventricle not undergoing necrotic damage in these experiments, it is difficult to know whether the alterations of electrolytes are truly and completely prevented. Kako (130) has reported that propranolol reduced the amount by which myocardial ATP declined following isoproterenol-induced damage. Propranolol appears to have a more selective action on endocardial versus midmyocardial or epicardial changes in metabolism due to catecholamines (131). One can thus conclude that the beta-adrenergic blocking agents are capable of modifying certain cardiotoxic effects of catecholamines.

The alpha-adrenergic blocking compounds, such as azapetine, phentolamine, dibenamine, dihydroergocryptin, phenoxybenzamine, and tolazoline were ineffective against isoproterenol (79,84,128,129,132), but reduced somewhat the incidence and severity of lesions caused by alpha-receptor agonists, such as phenylephrine (96,132), epinephrine (84,96,132,133), and norepinephrine (84,132). The alpha-blockers also ameliorated the loss of myocardial AAT and lactic dehydrogenase activity and shifts of electrolytes caused by epinephrine and norepinephrine (73,84,134). These agents were usually more effective against epinephrine lesions when used in combination with a beta-blocker (73,96,132). It should be pointed out that isoproterenol has been shown to reduce the endogenous norepinephrine stores from the nerve endings (135) and it is possible that the endogenously released norepinephrine may also be participating in producing the cardiotoxic effects upon injecting the animals with isoproterenol.

The postganglionic blocker guanethidine has been reported to be ineffective (79,129) or to increase the severity (126) of necrosis caused by isoproterenol. Another postganglionic blocker, isocaramidine, has also been found to have no effect on isoproterenol-induced necrosis (79). Reserpine, which is known to decrease catecholamine stores, has been reported to be without effect (79,125) or to increase the severity (23,126) of isoproterenol-induced lesions. Pyrogallol, a catechol-O-methyl transferase inhibitor, increased the severity of lesions (23). Serotonin and nialimide administered together reduced the severity and incidence of myocardial lesions (136). Other drugs found not to influence the production of lesions by isoproterenol are the vasodilators sodium nitrite, aminophylline, dipyridamole, and hexobendine, and the psychosedative chlorpromazine, chlordiazepoxide, meprobamate, amitriptyline as well as creatinol O-phosphate and zinc (79,137–139). In this regard, it is worth mentioning that most of these drugs are not specific with respect to their site of action and conclusions drawn from such studies should be interpreted with some caution.

Inhibition of lipolysis by nicotinic acid or β-pyridyl carbinol decreased the amount by which isoproterenol infusion increased the myocardial oxygen consumption (140). Chronic administration of nicotine in high doses tended to increase the severity and incidence of lesions produced by isoproterenol

(141). The calcium blockers, verapamil, D600, prenylamine, and vascoril, reduced the severity of lesions and prevented the decrease in high-energy phosphate stores and accumulation of calcium by the myocardium caused by isoproterenol injections (90,91,142). Another Ca^{2+} antagonist, diltiazem, also prevented isoproterenol-induced changes in myocardial high-energy phosphate stores in rats (143).

Hormonal, Electrolyte, and Metabolic Interventions

The mineralocorticoids such as deoxycorticosterone and 9-α-fluorocortisol increased the severity of myocardial lesions (52,91,121,122,144), the level of ^{45}Ca accumulation by the heart (90,91), and the severity of high-energy phosphate depletion (91) caused by isoproterenol. Among the other steroids, estrone and testosterone also increased the severity of necrotic lesions (121,122), whereas estrogen, progesterone, glucocorticoids, cortisone, and 9-α-fluoro-16 hydrocortisol were without effect, as were ACTH or adrenalectomy (121,122,145). High sodium or low potassium diets were similar to mineralocorticoid therapy in increasing the severity of lesions, whereas low sodium or high potassium diets reduced the incidence and severity of lesions (121,122,144). Administration of KCl, $MgCl_2$, or NH_4Cl_2 reduced the severity of lesions (74,91,146) and protected against the electrolyte shifts and reduction of high-energy phosphate stores (81,91,146). On the other hand, if plasma Mg^{2+}, K^+, or H^+ concentrations were low, isoproterenol-induced lesions were potentiated (147). Administration of K^+,Mg^{2+}–aspartate together with isoproterenol has also been found to prevent or reduce the changes in myofibrillar ATPase activity, Ca^{2+} accumulation by mitochondria and microsomes, and high-energy phosphates stores (94), and to decrease the severity of ultrastructural damage to the myocardium (148).

Thyroxine and hyperthyroidism increased the severity of lesions (53, 121,122), whereas thyroidectomy, thiouracil, or propylthiouracil decreased the extent of necrosis with isoproterenol (53,121,122,125). Calciferol and another antirachitic agent, dihydrotachysterol, increased the severity of necrotic lesions, as did $NaHPO_4$ (90,91,121). The increased severity of the lesions was associated with a further increase in the uptake of ^{45}Ca and a greater fall of high-energy phosphate stores of the heart. Likewise, thyrocalcitonin and reduction of plasma calcium with EDTA decreased the extent of both lesions and electrolyte shifts (91).

Administration of glucose, lactate, or pyruvate had no effect on the extent and severity of catecholamine-induced lesions (79). Sex and breed in rats did not influence the severity of the myocardial damage, although the severity was increased with increased body weight and excess body fat (121,122, 149,150). The severity of lesions did increase with age, but this is probably an indirect effect related to the increase of body weight with age (151). Starvation or restricted food intake likewise tended to reduce the severity of lesions (121,122,152).

Previous myocardial damage markedly reduced the severity of lesions produced by high doses of isoproterenol (153–155). This protective effect disappeared with time, was independent of the part of the heart previously damaged, and did not result from necrosis of extracardiac tissues. Similarly, previous isoproterenol injections (49,156,157) and coronary arteriosclerosis (78,158) increased the resistance of the heart to isoproterenol-induced damage. Cardiac hypertrophy (153) or a simultaneous hypoxia (124) increased the extent and severity of lesions. A higher ambient temperature also potentiated the necrotic effect of isoproterenol, possible due to the increased workload of the heart during thermoregulatory vasodilation (159) as well as changes in the calcium transport mechanisms (107). On the other hand, high altitude acclimation or hyperbaric oxygen tended to protect the heart against necrotic damage (160–162). Isolation stress or cold exposure both increased the severity of isoproterenol-induced lesion and electrolyte shifts (121,122, 149,163,164), although this may be an indirect result of increased mineralocorticoid production, which occurs under these conditions (163–165).

Thus it would appear that factors tending to increase the workload of the heart, increase the metabolic rate of the heart, interfere with oxygen supply to myocardial cells, favor the electrolyte change, or favor mobilization of lipids aggravate the necrotic influence of catecholamine administration. On the other hand, factors that block the stimulatory effects of catecholamines, thereby reducing cardiac work, or otherwise reduce myocardial metabolic rate, aid in the supply of oxygen to the myocardium, limit the mobilization of lipids, or counteract the ionic shifts can at least reduce the severity of necrotic changes. In particular, interventions that promote the occurrence of intracellular Ca^{2+} overload have been shown to aggravate and those that reduce the intracellular Ca^{2+} overload have been reported to prevent the catecholamine-induced cardiotoxicity. Although the protective effect of MAOI compounds is still enigmatic, it is clear from the above discussion that an imbalance between oxygen availability and work, the metabolism of lipids, and the alteration of electrolyte balance are all crucial factors contributing to the etiology of catecholamine lesions. The evidence available in the existing literature does not permit the identification of a single molecular lesion that can be considered responsible for the pathogenesis of myocardial necrosis due to catecholamines.

MECHANISMS BY WHICH CATECHOLAMINES ELICIT CARDIAC LESIONS

It has been for the most part assumed that the cardiac cell necrosis that occurs following administration of catecholamines in large amounts is due to a defect in the supply of energy for the maintenance of essential cellular processes. Various theories have been proposed with regard to the cause of the energy deficiency and the nature of the irreversible step following decreased energy availability. The major hypotheses include: a relative cardiac hypoxemia due to increased cardiac work and myocardial oxygen demands, aggravated by hypotension in the case of isoproterenol (10,54); coronary arterial vasoconstriction (spasm) causing endocardiac ischemia (7,8); inadequate perfusion of the endocardium due to impaired venous drainage of the heart (166); hypoxia due to direct oxygen wasting effects of catecholamines or their oxidation products (21); interference with mitochondrial oxidative phosphorylation by free fatty acids (140,167); massive calcium influx (91); or formation of adrenochromes (22). Potassium depletion (168), altered permeability of the myocardial cell membrane through elevation of plasma nonesterified free fatty acids (169), and depletion of intracellular magnesium required for many ATP-dependent enzymatic processes (96,146) have also been suggested to explain myocardial necrosis due to catecholamines.

Relative Hypoxia and Hemodynamic Changes

The concept of a relative cardiac hypoxemia due to increased cardiac work and myocardial oxygen demands was advanced by Rona et al. (10,54) following their discovery of the cardiotoxicity of isoproterenol. It was found that both high and low doses of isoproterenol produced similar increases in heart rate in dogs, but a much more profound fall in blood pressure was seen with higher lesion-producing doses of isoproterenol, and it was suggested that the fall in aortic blood pressure was of such a degree that a reduced coronary flow could be inferred. It was further postulated that the necrotic lesions are an ischemic infarct due to a decreased coronary flow during a time when both amplitude and frequency of cardiac contractions are increased. Thus the greater cardiotoxicity of isoproterenol as compared to epinephrine or norepinephrine was attributed to the dramatic hypotension produced by this agent, and various factors, such as previous myocardial damage or previous isoproterenol injections, activate metabolic processes that provide cardiac muscle cells with an enhanced adaptation to withstand the increased demand and relative hypoxia produced by isoproterenol (170).

On the other hand, Rosenblum et al. (14) found that mephenteramine, dl-ephedrine, and d-amphetamine produced lesions in less than 50% of animals, although these agents increase blood pressure while ephedrine and amphetamine have a positive inotropic effect. Accordingly, drugs with both positive inotropic and chronotropic actions may not produce cardiac lesions. Also, methoxamine, which has no positive inotropic effect, was found to produce cardiac lesions. In another study (15), the hemodynamic effects of "pharmacologic" and "lesion-producing" doses of sympathomimetics were compared in cats. It was found that lesion-producing doses of isoproterenol caused a decrease in aortic flow and heart rate as compared to pharmaco-logic doses, but these were still above control values. Stroke work was greater with lesion-producing doses as compared to pharmacologic doses, but mean aortic pressure, which determines the coronary perfusion pressure, was not reduced by lesion-producing doses of isoproterenol. Thus there is evidence of impaired function of the myocardium but the hemodynamic change does not appear adequate to produce insufficient myocardial perfusion. As a result of these findings it was suggested that the effects of isoproterenol were due to some direct action on the myocardial cell and not solely to the hemodynamic effects. Maruffo (11) also considered it unlikely that, in experiments on monkeys, the coronary flow could have been greatly reduced by isoproterenol, since blood pressure remained above that found in shock and was associated with increased cardiac output. Strubelt and Siegers (171) concluded that hypotension is nonessential for production of cardiac necrosis by isoproterenol after finding that verapamil was effective in protecting the heart from isoproterenol-induced necrosis even though blood pressure fell almost twice as much when verapamil was administered together with isoproterenol as it did following administration of isoproterenol alone.

Coronary Spasm and Hemodynamic Alterations

Another hypothesis closely related to that of coronary insufficiency of hemodynamic origin is that of a relative ischemia resulting from coronary vascular changes. Handforth (7) injected India ink at a pressure of 50 mm Hg into the aorta of heart excised from hamsters 5–30 min after isoproterenol injection. The dye failed to penetrate large areas of the endocardium in 6 out of 14 hearts from isoproterenol-injected hamsters, although uniform filling of capillaries was seen in control hearts. It was suggested that dilatation of arteriovenous shunts might be responsible for the endocardiac ischemia, since coronary flow is usually found to be increased with isoproterenol. In a subsequent study (8), however, it was noted that the superficial veins draining these areas were also not filled with ink. A similar experiment was performed with bismuth oxychloride in which these larger particles did not reach the veins. This evidence was interpreted to indicate a true endocardiac ischemia, postulated to be due to arterial constriction rather than arteriovenous shunts. More consistent evidence of endocardiac ischemia was seen at 1 hr than had been observed at 5–30 min; therefore coronary artery constriction was considered to be more important than peripheral vasodilation since the drop in peripheral resistance occurred within minutes of injection. A coronary arteritis was also found 1–3 days after isoproterenol injection (8), which was considered to support the concept of a vascular component in the etiology of necrosis. Ostadal and Poupa (172) repeated these experiments and reported a marked occlusion of coronary vessels in

69% of animals at 30 min, 33% at 60 min, and practically no occlusion at 24 hr after isoproterenol injection. These workers assumed this to be due to spasm of the coronary vessels, but the importance of peripheral resistance change is emphasized by their observation that whereas occlusion was evident with injection of India ink at 50 mm Hg, uniform filling of capillaries was seen even in isoproterenol-treated animals if an injection pressure of 100 mm Hg was used. Jasmin (166) found that it was possible to reproduce essentially similar pathological changes by surgical occlusion of efferent vessels, and on this basis suggested that impairment of venous drainage via venospasm largely accounts for the adverse effects of sympathomimetic amines.

The occurrence of coronary arterial or venous spasm is of course only conjectural, and a somewhat simpler explanation of the impaired perfusion of the endocardium can be inferred from certain other studies of the circulation in the heart. Blood flow to left ventricular subendocardial muscle has been suggested to be compromised during systole and to occur mainly during diastole because intramyocardial compressive forces are greatest in this region (173,174). Furthermore, it has been shown (175) that when aortic diastolic pressure was lowered or diastole shortened (by pacing) and myocardial oxygen demands simultaneously raised, myocardial performance was found to be impaired. In a subsequent study (176), coronary flow distribution was determined by scintillation counting of the distribution of [141]Ce,[85]Sr, and [46]Sc labeled microspheres (12–15 μm diameter) injected into the left atrium during isoproterenol infusion. When isoproterenol was infused at a rate that failed to maintain an increase in contractile force, it was found that subendocardial flow fell by 35% while subepicardial flow increased by 19%. Thus, although spasm of coronary arteries and/or veins may well occur, it is possible that increased cardiac activity, reduced aortic pressure, and greatly decreased diastole could also be responsible for an underperfusion of the endocardium.

A serious challenge to the concept of impaired ventricular perfusion as the primary cause of necrosis was presented by the findings of Regan et al. (13) who used [85]Kr clearance methods to study perfusion of the ventricle during epinephrine infusion in dogs. Evidence of cardiac necrosis was obtained by 75 min after the start of epinephrine infusion, but [85]Kr clearance studies showed no difference in the rate of clearance from inner, middle, and outer layers of the left ventricle in either the control or epinephrine-treated hearts. Thus there was no evidence for ischemia of subendocardial tissue as a causal factor in the epinephrine-induced necrosis. On the other hand, in a study by Boutet et al. (5) in which isoproterenol was infused in rats at a low concentration, a decreased passage of the trace substance horseradish peroxidase from the capillaries to the myocardial interstitium was observed. Thus this controversy still remained to be resolved. The hypothesis that the previously described vascular factors are the primary cause of necrotic lesions has also been tested by Ostadal et al. (12) using the turtle heart as a unique model in which perfusion of the endocardium is avascular. In the turtle heart, the internal spongy vasculature is supplied by diffusion from the ventricular lumen via intertrabecular spaces, while the outer compact layer is supplied by the coronary artery branching off the aorta. Isoproterenol injections were found to produce necrotic lesions in the spongy layer of the turtle heart, which does not support the opinion that isoproterenol-induced cardiac necrosis is due to a vascular mechanism.

Metabolic Effects

As Bajusz (177) has pointed out in his careful survey of data on various types of cardiac necrosis, catecholamine-induced necrosis must be considered to be a mixed pathogenesis involving both direct metabolic actions on the fibers as well as factors secondary to vascular and hemodynamic effects. Although cardiac lesions induced by epinephrine, methoxamine, and isoproterenol are indistinguishable as regards both distribution and histologic characteristics, it would appear that the methoxamine-induced lesion is a typical secondary cardiomyopathy, while that due to epinephrine and isoproterenol is of a mixed type in which both hypoxia secondary to vascular and hemodynamic effects as well as direct metabolic effects on the heart muscle have a role. It is not then unreasonable to regard vascular and hemodynamic effects as complicating factors, which greatly aggravate some more direct toxic influence of catecholamines on myocardial cells, in view of which it is readily understood how a reduction in the extent and severity of catecholamine-induced lesions is brought about by interventions that specifically block the peripheral vascular change, that prevent the positive inotropic and chronotropic effects of these drugs on the heart, or that improve the delivery of oxygen to the myocardium.

Many years ago Raab (21) attributed the cardiotoxic actions of catecholamines to their oxygen wasting effect. According to him:

> The most conspicuous reaction of myocardial metabolism to the administration of adrenaline is an intense enhancement of local oxygen consumption which, in certain dosages, by far exceeds the demand of simultaneously increased myocardial muscular work, and which is only partially compensated by a simultaneous increase of coronary blood flow. In this respect adrenaline is able, so to speak, to mimic the anoxiating effects of coronary insufficiency in the absence of any real coronary anomaly. It should be emphasized, however, that the tissue anoxia resulting from the administration of adrenaline is probably not caused by adrenaline itself but by an oxidation product of adrenaline (Bruno Kisch's omega) which acts as an oxidation catalyst even in very high dilutions.

In a later study (178) it was found that identical electrocardiographic changes occurred during cardiac sympathetic nerve stimulation, electrically induced muscular exercise, or intravenous injection of norepinephrine or epinephrine, when coronary artery dilatability is impaired and during exogenous anoxia or partial occlusion of the coronary arteries. This was taken as evidence that the increased O_2 consumption caused by catecholamines produced a relative hypoxia if coronary flow could not be sufficiently increased. A crucial point in this concept concerns the origin of the increased O_2 consumption with catecholamines—whether it is due to a decreased efficiency of oxygen utilization or to increased demand. Lee and Yu (179) found the oxgen consumption of resting papillary muscle not to be increased by catecholamines even in concentrations 10 times higher than those effective in stimulating oxygen consumption of contracting papillary muscles, and they concluded that the increased oxygen consumption of the intact heart following administration of epinephrine or norepinephrine is secondary to the increased contractility. On the other hand, Weisfeldt and Gilmore (180) reported that low doses of norepinephrine exerted a maximal inotropic effect with little or no increase of O_2 consumption, while larger doses had no further inotropic effect but did increase O_2 consumption, indicating that it is excessive catecholamine concentrations that cause "oxygen wasting." Klocke et al. (181) studied the increase in oxygen consumption produced by catecholamine in the isolated dog heart. It was found that the increase of oxygen consumption of the potassium-arrested heart caused by catecholamines was 5–20% of that found in the beating heart, and thus they concluded that most, but not all, of the increased oxygen consumption was secondary to hemodynamic alterations and increased cardiac work. In a similar comparison of the effects of epinephrine on oxygen consumption in beating and arrested hearts, Challoner and Steinberg (182) found that about one-third of the increment in oxygen consumption in beating hearts was accounted for by a metabolic effect dissociable from increased work. Hauge and Oye (183) confirmed an increased oxygen consumption in arrested heart with epinephrine and reported that this effect could be blocked by dichloroisoproterenol but not by phentolamine. From these studies it is evident that catecholamines can cause an increase in oxygen consumption that is not related to increased cardiac work or activity and the concept of decreased efficiency or "oxygen-wasting" is therefore justified. Furthermore, Raab (21) has suggested that this oxygen-wasting effect was actually due to an oxidation product of epinephrine, and one such oxidation product, adrenochrome, has been shown to uncouple mitochondria (184). The uncoupling of mitochondria by adrenochrome was antagonized by glutathione in high concentration, probably due to a direct reduction of adrenochrome since the characteristic red color of adrenochrome was lost when glutathione was added in the presence or absence of mitochondria, whereas oxidized glutathione did not affect uncoupling by adrenochrome.

Sobel et al. (22) found the P/O ratio of heart mitochondria from animals given norepinephrine, epinephrine, or isoproterenol to be significantly lower than controls. RCI and QO_2 were similar to control, but unfortunately the control RCI values in these experiments were very low. A good relationship between elevation of myocardial catecholamine content and depression of P/O ratio in mitochondria was observed. Whereas propranolol pretreatment enhanced the increase in myocardial catecholamines and caused a more marked depression of mitochondrial P/O ratios, dibenzyline inhibited both the increase in catecholamine content and the decrease in the mitochondrial P/O ratio. Reserpine pretreatment caused a depletion of myocardial catecholamines and prevented the depression of the mitochondrial P/O ratio. Since the three catecholamines used did not affect the P/O ratio of normal rat heart mitochondria *in vitro* at a concentration of 10^{-3} M, it was concluded that this was not a direct action of the catecholamines on the mitochondria, and it was suggested that adrenochrome or one of its metabolites might be responsible for the observed effects (22). Stanton and Schwartz (85) also studied the oxidative phosphorylation of heart mitochondria from isoproterenol-treated rats but found the RCI was reduced without affecting the P/O ratio. It is not possible to draw any definite conclusions from these studies as regard the effects of catecholamines on mitochondrial respiration, although uncoupling of oxidative phosphorylation is certainly indicated and would explain both the "oxygen-wasting" effect and the depletion of myocardial high-energy phosphate stores caused by large doses of catecholamines. Likewise, the possibility that the agent producing this uncoupling might be adrenochrome or some one of its metabolites is intriguing.

Having found that heart mitochondria from catecholamine-treated rats were uncoupled, Sobel et al. (22) determined the free fatty acid levels of the mitochondria since free fatty acids are known to uncouple mitochondria. No differences in mitochondrial free fatty acid content or composition was found and it was thus concluded that the observed uncoupling was not due to accumulation of fatty acids. Furthermore, ephedrine, which produced no significant changes in plasma nonesterified free fatty acids, can cause cardiac lesions (169). Nevertheless, Mjos (140) found that inhibition of lipolysis by nicotinic acid, β-pyridyl carbinol, or high plasma glucose concentrations during infusion of isoproterenol could substantially reduce the increase in myocardial oxygen consumption, possibly by preventing an uncoupling action of high intracellular concentrations of free fatty acid in the heart following catecholamine administration. Hoak et al. (167) have also postulated a causal relationship between the increase in plasma free fatty acids following norepinephrine administration and the occurrence of cardiac lesions. Although the evidence fails to implicate elevated levels of free fatty acids as primary agents in mitochondrial uncoupling following administration of catecholamines, the findings of Mjos (140) as well as the previous correlation of severity of lesions with the amount of body fat (121) suggest that metabolism of free fatty acids in some way aggravates the cardiotoxic effects of catecholamines.

Electrolyte Shifts and Intracellular Ca^{2+} Overload

In view of the close relationship between electrolyte shifts and the occurrence of necrotic lesions, Lehr (96) has suggested that changes in myocardial electrolyte content initiated by altered ionic transfer ability of myocardial cells at the plasma membrane and subcellular membrane sites contribute to irreversible failure of cell function. It was the loss of cellular magnesium, in particular, that he suggested (146) is most critical in the pathogenesis of irreversible damage. In this regard, it was pointed out that Mg^{2+} is an important prosthetic or activator ion participating in the function of many enzymes involved in phosphate transfer reactions, including utilization of ATP. Unfortunately, this mechanism is not adequate to explain the reduction of high-energy phosphate content in the myocardium (91) since interference with utilization would have the opposite effect. On the other hand, magnesium is reported to cause a decrease in the respiration-supported uptake of calcium by isolated heart mitochondria (185) and could thus be important in regulating mitochondrial function in terms of oxidative phosphorylation versus calcium uptake. Raab (168) has similarly argued that it is the derangement of myocardial electrolyte balance, most specifically the loss of K^+ and Mg^{2+} ions from the myocardium, that is the central mechanism in a variety of cardiomyopathies. But this derangement of electrolyte balance was considered to be secondary to an inadequate supply of energy for transmembrane ion pumps required for maintenance of electrolyte equilibrium, which occurs with oxygen deficiency or impaired energy production. Bajusz (177) has also suggested that electrolyte shifts are an important component in the development of irreversible damage produced by both direct and indirect pathogenic mechanisms, and that myocardial resistance is related to the ability of the heart to maintain a normal electrolyte balance in the face of potentially cardiotoxic episodes.

Fleckenstein et al. (91) found that the isoproterenol-induced necrosis and decline in high-energy phosphates were associated with a six- to sevenfold increase in the rate of radioactive calcium uptake and a doubling of net myocardial calcium content, and they suggested that isoproterenol causes a greatly increased influx of calcium that overloads the fiber. It was postulated that the intracellular calcium overload initiates a high-energy phosphate deficiency by excessive activation of Ca-dependent intracellular ATPase and by impairing mitochondrial oxidative phosphorylation. When high-energy phosphate exhaustion reaches a critical level, fiber necrosis results. This hypothesis attempts to explain why myocardium can be sensitized to isoproterenol-induced necrosis by factors, such as 9-α-fluorocortisol acetate, dihydrotachysterol, NaH_2PO_4, high extracellular calcium, or increased blood pH, which favor calcium overload. Consistent with this hypothesis, K and Mg salts, low extracellular calcium, thyrocalcitonin, low blood pH, or specific blockers of transmembrane calcium fluxes protect the heart against isoproterenol, presumably by preventing calcium overload. In support of this concept of a central role for Ca^{2+} in the pathogenesis of necrosis is the finding that spontaneous necrotization of cardiac tissues of myopathic hamster, which exhibit high levels of circulating catecholamines, is prevented by treatment with the calcium blocker verapamil (186,187). Also, necrosis of skeletal muscle fibers can be induced through mechanical injury of the cell membrane, permitting Ca^{2+} influx, and can be prevented by elimination of Ca^{2+} from the Ringer solution or by an outward electric current, which blocks Ca^{2+} influx (188).

Unfortunately, there is no direct evidence that it is in fact calcium that produces the decline of high-energy phosphate in the hearts of animals given isoproterenol, and therefore a causal relationship has not yet been established. Furthermore, Bloom and Davis (127) have found that myocardial calcium content increased in a manner well correlated to isoproterenol dose in the range from 0.1 to 10 μg/kg but did not further increase with higher dose levels required to produce myocardial lesions. Thus it was suggested that the inotropic response is related to calcium entry, but that necrosis is due to some other factor, possibly including the intracellular metabolism of calcium. It was also shown by these workers that propranolol could completely block the increase of calcium content of the myocardium but would only reduce the incidence of lesions rather than preventing them. Bloom and Davis (127) have interpreted their results to indicate a mechanism other than calcium influx in isoproterenol-induced necrosis, but the dramatic modification of necrosis by factors influencing transmembrane calcium fluxes clearly suggests the involvement of calcium at some level in the etiology of necrosis caused by catecholamines.

Muller (23) has suggested that, on the basis of coincidence of localization of isoproterenol-induced myocardial lesions and the highest myocardial MAO activity, the accumulation of amines metabolically formed during deamination of catecholamines may be the cause of necrosis in the heart. It is further pointed out that in young rats, heart MAO activity is less than in older rats, and that isoproterenol sensitivity is also less. None of the hypotheses discussed so far account for these findings as well as the protective effect of MAOIs. Likewise, no specific explanation has been offered for the changes in contractile proteins, which are seen to occur in catecholamine-induced necrotic lesions, except for the suggestion by Pelouch et al. (93) that a direct interaction of catecholamine or some metabolite with the heavy meromyosin region of the myosin molecule is involved. It is possible that MAOIs may inhibit the oxidation of catecholamines and thus decrease the formation of toxic substances such as free radicals and adrenochrome and subsequent myocardial necrosis. It may very well be that lysosomes (116) are activated due to calcium and decreased energy state of the myocardium after catecholamine injection and this may produce cellular damage. Furthermore, catecholamines are known to markedly increase the concentration

TABLE 5. *Possible mechanisms for cardiotoxic effects of high levels of circulating catecholamines*

1. Functional hypoxia
   a. Increased cardiac work
   b. Excessive demand for O_2
2. Coronary insufficiency
   a. Coronary spasm
   b. Hemodynamic effects
3. Increased membrane permeability
   a. Electrolyte shift
   b. Loss of intracellular contents
4. Decreased levels of high-energy phosphate stores
   a. Excessive hydrolysis of ATP
   b. Uncoupling of mitochondrial oxidative phosphorylation
5. Alterations in lipid metabolism
   a. Increased lipolysis
   b. Increased accumulation of fatty acids
6. Intracellular Ca^{2+} overload
   a. Excessive Ca^{2+} entry and intracellular release
   b. Depressed Ca^{2+} efflux and intracellular uptake
7. Oxidative stress
   a. Formation of free radicals
   b. Formation of adrenochrome

of cyclic AMP in the heart, and it is likely that this agent in high concentrations may represent an important factor for causing catecholamine-induced myocardial necrosis.

In summary, the majority of the factors found to influence the severity of catecholamine-induced lesions can be understood in terms of their effects on hemodynamic factors, delivery of oxygen to the myocardium, electrolyte balance, or the metabolism of calcium and lipids. It would thus appear that hemodynamic and coronary vascular factors contribute significantly to the severity of myocardial damage following catecholamine administration, but that some primary pathogenic mechanism acting directly on the myocardial cell is probably involved as well. Furthermore, it is clear that exhaustion of high-energy phosphate stores and disruption of electrolyte balance are crucial events in the etiology of irreversible cell damage. Although the metabolism of lipids and calcium is involved, the nature of the direct pathogenic influence following injection of catecholamines is still unknown. Some of the possible mechanisms that have been proposed to explain the cardiotoxic effects of catecholamines are given in Table 5.

SIGNIFICANCE OF ADRENOCHROME AND RELATED OXIDATION PRODUCTS IN CATECHOLAMINE-INDUCED CARDIOTOXICITY

The oxidation products of epinephrine, adrenochrome, and adrenolutin have been identified in the heart, skeletal muscle, liver, brain, and kidney of rabbits (189–191) by paper chromatography and by their fluorescent properties. In addition to the spontaneous oxidation of epinephrine to adrenochrome by an autocatalytic process (192), adrenochrome is enzymatically formed in mammalian tissues. These enzymes include tyrosinases (193–198) and polyphenol oxidases from various sources (198–202), particularly in guinea pig and rat muscles (202). Other enzyme systems shown to actively convert epinephrine to adrenochrome are xanthine oxidase (203), leukocyte myeloperoxidase (204,205), heart muscle cytochrome *c* oxidase (206–208), a cyanide-insensitive system present in heart and skeletal muscle (209), the cytochrome–indophenol oxidase system present in all tissues (209,210), and an unidentified enzyme in cat salivary gland (211). The oxidation of epinephrine has also been reported to be catalyzed by cytochrome *c* and by methamyoglobin (212), to stabilize with the formation of adrenochrome in the presence of bicarbonate buffer regardless of the oxidizing system used (213), and to occur in blood (214,215). Recently, a method for the measurement of adrenolutin, as an oxidation product of catecholamines, in plasma has been developed by using the reverse-phase high performance liquid chromatography (216).

Much of the work in the literature dealing with the physiological and pharmacological effects of epinephrine oxidation products was carried out before the structure of adrenochrome was known, and still more before a relatively pure preparation could be obtained, as has been discussed by Osmond and Hoffer in their review of this subject (217). Furthermore, due to the inherent instability of adrenochrome in solution, one cannot be certain whether reports attributing either specific effects or the absence of certain effects can truly be considered as an accurate assessment of the adrenochrome activity. Nevertheless, it is well worth reviewing the broad spectrum of physiological activities that have been found to result from adrenochrome or at least from some closely related epinephrine oxidation product to which adrenochrome is converted.

Oxidized epinephrine solutions have been found to inhibit cardiac inotropism and chronotropism (194,195,199,218–220) and to increase rather than decrease the tone of rabbit intestinal strips (221). Adrenochrome has been reported to increase blood pressure (222,223), to be effective as a vasoconstrictor (224), to be a powerful hemostatic agent, and to greatly diminish capillary permeability (225,226). Adrenochrome has frequently been reported to reduce blood sugar levels and potentiate the effects of insulin and has been described as an anti-insulinase (217,227), although this claim has been disputed (228). Administration of adrenochrome either by injection or by feeding can result in an increased oxygen consumption in humans and guinea pigs (229,230) and has been reported to increase tissue oxygen consumption *in vitro* (231,232). On the other hand, other workers have found that adrenochrome may stimulate, inhibit, or have no effect on tissue oxygen consumption, depending on the metabolic substrate used (233) or the adrenochrome concentration (234). These studies may explain that adreno-chrome did not affect the oxygen uptake of rat muscle (235) and inhibited oxygen uptake and lactic acid production in dog heart slices (236).

Adrenochrome has also been reported to uncouple mitochondrial oxidative phosphorylation, depressing P/O ratios (184,237,238), and it has been suggested that adrenochrome may act as a hydrogen carrier between substrate and molecular oxygen with the formation of water and regeneration of adrenochrome after each cycle (237). It was also reported to be much more effective in inhibiting pyruvate oxidation than succinate oxidation (238). Adrenoxyl, a closely related epinephrine oxidation product, has been found to lower mitochondrial potassium content, decrease ATPase activity, and alter mitochondrial P/O ratio (239). Adrenochrome also inhibited hexokinase and phosphofructokinase, thus inhibiting glucose phosphorylation and glycolysis, while stimulating glycogen synthesis (209,240–243) and the hexose monophosphate shunt (244,245). Adrenochrome and adrenoxyl have both been found to be inhibitors of myosin ATPase activity in heart and smooth muscle (246–249). Adrenochrome and oxidized epinephrine solutions inhibited not only monoamine oxidase in a variety of tissues (250–252) but the enzyme alkaline phosphatase also (253). It was thought that inhibition of all of the above enzymes is at least partly due to the reversible oxidation of sulfhydryl groups in the enzymes (248,250). Other effects attributed to adrenochrome and adrenoxyl include antimitotic activity (254), reduction of coenzyme A levels in heart, kidney, and brain (255), antihistaminic properties (217), and an increase in mitochondrial material of cultured cells (256). Thus it can be appreciated that adrenochrome is a highly reactive molecule chemically, and it not only is capable of oxidizing protein sulfhydryl groups but is also a dynamic catalyst for the deamination of a variety of amines and amino acids (257–261). Furthermore, it may likely be capable of functioning as an oxidative hydrogen carrier acting on either metabolic substrates (237) or $NADP^+$ (245) and thus altering or disrupting essential metabolic pathways.

The metabolism of adrenochrome and related epinephrine oxidation products has been studied in rabbits, cats, and dogs (262–264). Adrenochrome injected into rabbits rapidly disappeared from the blood and was transformed in the liver to adrenolutin, which was removed from the system via the kidney (262). Most of it was excreted in the urine as adrenolutin (both free and conjugated) or in the form of a fluorescent brown pigment, while a small amount was excreted unchanged. In cats and dogs, approximately 70% was excreted in the form of a variety of adrenochrome reduction products and other indoles (263). An unstable yellow pigment has been observed in the urine of rats after injection of ^{14}C labeled adrenochrome (265).

To summarize, there is evidence both for the presence of and the formation of adrenochrome in mammalian tissues, and adrenochrome has been shown to be capable of producing a wide variety of metabolic changes by interfering with numerous enzyme systems. Thus adrenochrome and/or other catecholamine oxidation products may be regarded as possible candidates that are involved in toxic manifestation occurring in conjunction with catecholamine excess or altered catecholamine metabolism. The injection of catecholamine into animals can be conceived to result in the formation of oxidation products such as adrenochrome in the circulating blood as well as in the myocardial cell. The accumulation of these oxidation products in myocardium could then directly or indirectly, acting by themselves or in conjunction with other effects of catecholamines, initiate processes leading to myocardial necrosis. Accordingly, experiments were undertaken to understand the problem of whether or not catecholamines, their oxidation products or metabolites are indeed capable of a direct toxic influence on the heart. For this purpose, the isolated perfused rat heart preparation was employed as this appears to be an ideal model for several reasons. These include elimination of hemodynamic factors, neural mechanisms, availability of exogenous lipids, and other physiological parameters that tend to complicate the production of heart lesions in intact animals. Furthermore, changes in contractile events can be monitored concomitantly and the heart can readily be fixed at a desired time for ultrastructural examination. Fresh isoproterenol, oxidized isoproterenol, fresh epinephrine, adrenochrome, and various metabolites of epinephrine were used for investigating changes in the ultrastructure and contractile functions of the isolated perfused rat hearts. In addition to studying the time course and dose–responses to the cardiotoxic agents, attempts were made to elucidate the mechanisms subserving the functional and morphological alterations. The hearts were perfused in the absence or presence of the cardiotoxic substance with media of different cationic compositions or containing various pharmacologic agents that are known to influence the catecholamine-induced myocardial necrosis *in vivo*.

When the isolated rat hearts were perfused with high concentrations of isoproterenol for 1 hr, no depression in contractile activity or myocardial cell damage was evident (266). These observations were confirmed by other investigators (267). On the other hand, perfusion of the isolated hearts with oxidized isoproterenol produced dramatic cardiac contractile, morphological, and subcellular alterations (266,268). Toxic effects of isoproterenol on cultured cardiac muscle cells were also shown to be due to its oxidation (269). In fact, the contractile dysfunction and myocardial cell damage in the isolated perfused rat hearts due to adrenochrome were shown to depend on its concentration as well as time of perfusion (270). Various pharmacological agents and cations, which prevent the occurrence of intracellular Ca^{2+} overload, were observed to reduce the cardiac contractile failure and cell damage due to adrenochrome (271,272). Adrenochrome was suggested to affect Ca^{2+} movements in the myocardial cell due to its action on the sarcolemmal, sarcoplasmic reticular, and mitochondrial membranes (273–276). In fact, adrenochrome was found to be accumulated in the myocardium and localized at different organelles (276,277). Adrenochrome was also shown to be a potent coronary artery constrictor in the isolated rat heart preparations (278). Although administration of adrenochrome to rats was found to induce arrhythmias, myocardial cell damage, and heart dysfunction under *in vivo* conditions (279–281), oxidation products other than adrenochrome have also been suggested to be involved in the genesis of catecholamine-induced cardiotoxicity (282).

Since the oxidation of catecholamines results in the formation of aminochromes (such as adrenochrome) and free radicals, it is possible that free radicals may also be involved in the development of catecholamine-induced cardiotoxicity. Pretreatment of rats with vitamin E, a well-known free-radical scavenger, was found to prevent the isoproterenol-induced arrhythmias, lipid peroxidation, myocardial cell damage, and loss of high-energy phosphates, whereas vitamin E deficiency was shown to increase the sensitivity of animals to the cardiotoxic actions of isoproterenol (120,283,284). Other antioxidants such as ascorbic acid and sodium bisulfite were also shown to prevent the cytotoxic effects of isoproterenol in cultured rat myocardial cells (285–287). Exercise training, which is considered to increase the antioxidant reserve, has also been reported to decrease the myocardial cell damage due

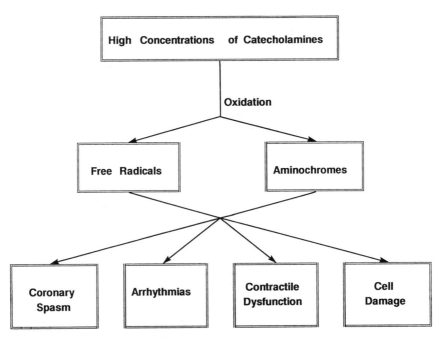

FIG. 1. Schematic representation of the mechanism for the genesis of cardiotoxic effects of high concentrations of catecholamines.

to catecholamines (288,289). In this regard, it should be pointed out that oxygen free radicals have been shown to exert cardiotoxic effects such as myocardial cell damage, contractile failure, subcellular alterations, and intracellular Ca^{2+} overload (290–295). Thus it appears that the generation of free radicals, in addition to the formation of aminochromes, may play an important role in the pathogenesis of cardiotoxicity under conditions associated with high levels of circulating catecholamines. A scheme indicating the involvement of both free radicals and adrenochrome in the development of catecholamine-induced arrhythmias, coronary spasm, contractile failure, and myocardial cell damage is depicted in Fig. 1.

SUMMARY AND CONCLUSIONS

It is well known that massive amounts of catecholamines are released from the sympathetic nerve endings and adrenal medulla under stressful situations. Initially, these hormones produce beneficial effects on the cardiovascular system to meet the energy demands of various organs in the body and their actions on the heart are primarily mediated through the stimulation of the beta-adrenergic receptors–cyclic AMP system in the myocardium. However, prolonged exposure of the heart to high levels of catecholamines results in coronary spasm, arrhythmias, contractile dysfunction, cell damage, and myocardial necrosis. Different pharmacological, hormonal, and metabolic interventions, which are known to reduce the occurrence of intracellular Ca^{2+} overload, have been shown to prevent the cardiotoxic actions of catecholamines, whereas interventions that promote the development of intracellular Ca^{2+} overload promote the catecholamine-induced cardiotoxicity. Several mechanisms such as relative hypoxia, hemodynamic alterations, coronary insufficiency, changes in lipid and energy metabolism, electrolyte imbalance, and membrane alterations have been suggested to explain the cardiotoxic effects of high concentrations of catecholamines. Recent studies have shown that oxidation of catecholamines results in the formation of highly toxic substances such as aminochromes (e.g., adrenochrome) and free radicals, and these then, by virtue of their actions on different types of heart membranes, cause intracellular Ca^{2+} overload and myocardial cell damage. Hemodynamic and metabolic actions of catecholamines may aggravate toxic effects of the oxidation products of catecholamines. Thus it appears that antioxidant therapy in combination with some Ca^{2+} antagonist and/or metabolic intervention may be most effective in preventing the catecholamine-induced cardiotoxicity.

ACKNOWLEDGMENTS

The authors wish to thank Dr. George Rona of Montreal, Canada for his continued advice and inspiration and are most pleased to dedicate this chapter in his honor. The research work from our laboratory presented in this chapter was supported by a grant from the Heart and Stroke Foundation of Manitoba.

REFERENCES

1. Pearce RM. Experimental myocarditis: a study of the histological changes following intravenous injections of adrenaline. *J Exp Med* 1906;8:400–409.
2. Ziegler K. Uber die Wirkung intravenoser Adrenalin injektion auf das Gefasssystem und ihre Beziehungen zur Arterisclerose. *Beitr Path Anat Allg Path* 1905;38:229–254.
3. Szakacs JE, Cannon A. l-Norepinephrine myocarditis. *Am J Clin Pathol* 1958;30:425–430.
4. Rona G, Chappel CI, Balazs T, Gaudry R. An infarct-like myocardial lesion and other toxic manifestations produced by isoproterenol in the rat. *Arch Pathol* 1959;67:443–455.
5. Boutet M, Huttner I, Rona G. Aspect microcirculatoire des lesions myocardiques provoquees par l'infusion de catecholamines. Etude ultrastructural a l'aide de traceurs de diffusion. I. Isoproterenol. *Pathol Biol (Paris)* 1973;21:811–825.
6. Boutet M, Huttner I, Rona G. Aspect microcirculatoire des lesions myocardiques provoquees par l'infusion de catecholamines. Etude ultrastructural a l'aide de traceurs de diffusion. II. Norepinephrine. *Pathol Biol (Paris)* 1974;22:377–387.
7. Handforth CP. Isoproterenol-induced myocardial infarction in animals. *Arch Pathol* 1962;73:161–165.
8. Handforth CP. Myocardial infarction and necrotizing arteritis in hamsters, produced by isoproterenol (Isuprel). *Med Serv J Can* 1962;18:506–512.
9. Rona G, Boutet M, Hutter I, Peters H. Pathogenesis of isoproterenol induced myocardial alterations: functional and morphological correlates. In: Dhalla NS, ed. *Recent advances in studies on cardiac structure and metabolism,* vol. 3. Baltimore: University Park Press; 1973:507–525.
10. Rona G, Kahn DS, Chappel CI. Studies on infarct-like myocardial necrosis produced by isoproterenol: a review. *Rev Can Biol* 1963;22:241–255.
11. Maruffo CA. Fine structural study of myocardial changes induced by isoproterenol in rhesus monkeys *(Macaca mulatta). Am J Pathol* 1967;50:27–37.
12. Ostadal B, Rychterova V, Poupa O. Isoproterenol-induced acute experimental cardiac necrosis in the turtle. *Am Heart J* 1968;76:645–649.
13. Regan TJ, Markov A, Kahn MI, Jesrani MJ, Oldewurtel HA, Ettinger PO. Myocardial ion and lipid exchanges during ischemia and catecholanine induced necrosis: relation to regional blood flow. In: Bajusz E, Rona G, eds. *Recent advances in studies on cardiac structure and metabolism,* vol 1. Baltimore: University Park Press; 1972:656–664.
14. Rosenblum I, Wohl A, Stein AA. Studies in cardiac necrosis. I. Production of cardiac lesions with sympathomimetic amines. *Toxicol Appl Pharmacol* 1965;7:1–8.
15. Rosenblum I, Wohl A, Stein AA. Studies in cardiac necrosis. II. Cardiovascular effects of sympathomimetic amines producing cardiac lesions. *Toxicol Appl Pharmacol* 1965;7:9–17.
16. Bhagat B, Sullivan JM, Fisher VW, Nadel EM, Dhalla NS. cAMP activity and isoproterenol-induced myocardial injury in rats. In: Kobayashi T, Ito Y, Rona G, eds. *Recent advances in studies on cardiac structure and metabolism,* vol 12. Baltimore: University Park Press; 1978:465–470.
17. Todd GL, Baroldi G, Pieper GM, Clayton FC, Eliot RS. Experimental catecholamine-induced myocardial necrosis. I. Morphology, quantification and regional distribution of acute contraction band lesions. *J Mol Cell Cardiol* 1985;17:317–338.
18. Todd GL, Baroldi G, Pieper GM, Clayton FC, Elliot RS. Experimental catecholamine-induced myocardial necrosis. II. Temperal development of isoproterenol-induced contraction band lesions correlated with ECG, hemodynamic and biochemical changes. *J Mol Cell Cardiol* 1985;17:647–656.

19. Boutet M, Huttner I, Rona G. Permeability alterations of sarcolemmal membrane in catecholamine-induced cardiac muscle cell injury. *Lab Invest* 1976;34:482–488.
20. Todd GL, Cullan GE, Cullan GM. Isoproterenol-induced myocardial necrosis and membrane permeability alterations in the isolated perfused rabbit heart. *Exp Mol Pathol* 1980;33:43–54.
21. Raab W. Pathogenic significance of adrenalin and related substances in heart muscle. *Exp Med Surg* 1943;1:188–225.
22. Sobel B, Jequier E, Sjoerdsma A, Lovenberg W. Effect of catecholamines and adrenergic blocking agents on oxidative phosphorylation in rat heart mitochondria. *Circ Res* 1966;19:1050–1061.
23. Muller E. Histochemical studies on the experimental heart infarction in the rat. *Naunyn Schmiedebergs Arch Pharmacol Exp Pathol* 1966;254:439–447.
24. Blaiklock RG, Hirsh EM, Lehr D. Effect of cardiotoxic doses of adrenergic amines on myocardial cyclic AMP. *J Mol Cell Cardiol* 1978;10:499–509.
25. Balazs T, ed. *Cardiac toxicology,* vol 1. Boca Raton, FL: CRC Press; 1981.
26. Horak AR, Opie LH. Energy metabolism of the heart in catecholamine-induced myocardial injury. In: Chazov E, Saks V, Rona G, eds. *Advances in myocardiology,* vol 4. New York: Plenum Press; 1983:23–43.
27. Joseph X, Bloom S, Pledger G, Balazs T. Determinants of resistance to the cardiotoxicity of isoproterenol in rats. *Toxicol Appl Pharmacol* 1983;69:199–205.
28. Waldenstrom AP, Hjalmarson AC, Thornell L. A possible role of noradrenaline in the development of myocardial infarction: an experimental study in the isolated rat heart. *Am Heart J* 1978;95:43–51.
29. Rona G, Huttner I, Boutet M. Microcirculatory changes in myocardium with particular reference to catecholamine-induced cardiac muscle cell injury. In: Meeson H, ed. *Handbuck der allgemeinen pathologie III/7, microcirculation.* Berlin: Springer; 1977:791–888.
30. Rona G. Catecholamine cardiotoxicity. *J Mol Cell Cardiol* 1985;17:291–306.
31. Ostadal B, Beamish RE, Barwinsky J, Dhalla NS. Ontogenetic development of cardiac sensitivity to catecholamines. *J Appl Cardiol* 1989;4:467–486.
32. Ganguly PK, ed. *Catecholamines and heart disease.* Boca Raton, FL: CRC Press; 1991.
33. Josue O. Hypertrophie cardiaque causee par l'adrenaline et la toxine typhique. *C R Soc Biol (Paris)* 1907;63:285.
34. Fleisher MS, Loeb L. Experimental myocarditis. *Arch Intern Med* 1909;3:78–91.
35. Fleisher MS, Loeb L. The later stages of experimental myocarditis. *JAMA* 1909;53:1561–1571.
36. Fleisher MS, Loeb L. Uber experimentelle Myocarditis. *Centr Allg Path Path Anat* 1909;20:104–106.
37. Fleisher MS, Loeb L. Further investigations in experimental myocarditis. *Arch Intern Med* 1910;6:427–438.
38. Christian HA, Smith RM, Walker IC. Experimental cardiorenal disease. *Arch Intern Med* 1911;8:468–551.
39. Anitschkow N. Uber die Histogenese der Myokardveranderungen bei einigen Intoxikationen. *Virchows Arch Pathol Anat Physiol Klin Med* 1913;211:193–232.
40. Franz G. Eine seltene Form von toxischer Myokardschadeging. *Virchows Arch Path Anat* 1937;298:742–743.
41. Gormsen H. Case of fatal epinephrine intoxication. *Ugeskr Laeger* 1939;101:242–245.
42. Samson PC. Tissue changes following continuous intravenous injection of epinephrine hydrochloride into dogs. *Arch Pathol* 1932;13:745–755.
43. Blacket RB, Pickering GW, Wilson GM. The effects of prolonged infusion of noradrenaline and adrenaline on arterial pressure of rabbit. *Clin Sci* 1950;9:247–257.
44. Catchpole BN, Hacket DB, Simeone FA. Coronary and peripheral blood flow in experimental hemorrhagic hypotension treated with l-norepinephrine. *Ann Surg* 1955;142:372–380.
45. Hackel DB, Catchpole BN. Pathologic and electrocardiographic effects of hemorrhagic shock in dogs treated with l-norepinephrine. *Lab Invest* 1958;7:358–368.
46. Vishnevskaya OP. Reflex mechanisms in the pathogenesis of adrenaline myocarditis. *Bull Exp Biol Med* 1956;41:27–31.

47. Nahas GG, Brunson JG, King WM, Cavert HM. Functional and morphological changes in heart lung preparations following administration of adrenal hormones. *Am J Pathol* 1958;34:617–729.
48. Szakacs JE, Mehlman B. Pathologic change induced by l-norepinephrine. Quantitative aspects. *Am J Cardiol* 1960;5:619–627.
49. Maling HM, Highman B. Exaggerated ventricular arrhythmias and myocardial fatty changes after large doses of norepinephrine and epinephrine in unanesthetized dogs. *Am J Physiol* 1958;194:590–596.
50. Highman B, Maling HM, Thompson EC. Serum transaminase and alkaline phosphatase levels after large doses of norepinephrine and epinephrine in dogs. *Am J Physiol* 1959;196:436–440.
51. Maling HM, Highman B, Thompson EC. Some similar effects after large doses of catecholamine and myocardial infarction in dogs. *Am J Cardiol* 1960;5:628–633.
52. Chappel CI, Rona G, Balazs T, Gaudry R. Severe myocardial necrosis produced by isoproterenol in the rat. *Arch Int Pharmacodyn* 1959;122:123–128.
53. Chappel CI, Rona G, Balazs T, Gaudry R. Comparison of cardiotoxic actions of certain sympathomimetic amines. *Can J Biochem Physiol* 1959;37:35–42.
54. Rona G, Zsoter T, Chappel C, Gaudry R. Myocardial lesions, circulatory and electrocardiographic changes produced by isoproterenol in the dog. *Rev Can Biol* 1959;18:83–94.
55. Kline IK. Myocardial alterations associated with phenochromocytoma. *Am J Pathol* 1961;38:539–551.
56. Szakacs JE, Dimmette RM, Cowart EC Jr. Pathologic implication of the catecholamines, epinephrine and norepinephrine. *US Armed Forces Med J* 1959;10:908–925.
57. van Vliet PD, Burchell HB, Titus JL. Focal myocarditis associated with pheochromocytoma. *New Engl J Med* 1966;274:1102–1108.
58. Connor RCR. Focal myocytolysis and fuchsinophilic degeneration of the myocardium of patients dying with various brain lesions. *Ann NY Acad Sci* 1969;156:261–270.
59. Greenhoot JH, Reichenbach DD. Cardiac injury and subarachnoid hemorrhage. A clinical, pathological and physiological correlation. *J Neurosurg* 1969;30:521.
60. Reichenbach DD, Benditt EP. Catecholamines and cardiomyopathy: the pathogenesis and potential importance of myofibrillar degeneration. *Hum Pathol* 1970;1:125–150.
61. Smith RP, Tomlinson BE. Subendocardial hemorrhages associated with intracranial lesions. *J Path Bacteriol* 1954;68:327–334.
62. Kaye MP, McDonald RH, Randall WC. Systolic hypertension and subendocardial hemorrhages produced by electrical stimulation of the stellate ganglion. *Circ Res* 1961;9:1164–1170.
63. Klouda MA, Brynjolfson G. Cardiotoxic effects of electrical stimulation of the stellate ganglia. *Ann NY Acad Sci* 1969;156:271–279.
64. Melville KI, Garvey HL, Sluster HE, Knaack J. Central nervous system stimulation and cardiac ischemic change in monkeys. *Ann NY Acad Sci* 1969;156:241–260.
65. Bloom S, Cancilla PA. Myocytolysis and mitochondrial calcification in rat myocardium after low doses of isoproterenol. *Am J Pathol* 1969;54:373–391.
66. Csapa Z, Dusek J, Rona G. Early alterations of cardiac muscle cells in isoproterenol induced necrosis. *Arch Pathol* 1972;93:356–365.
67. Kutsuna F. Electron microscopic studies on isoproterenol-induced myocardial lesions in rats. *Jpn Heart J* 1972;13:168–175.
68. Ferrans VJ, Hibbs RG, Cipriano PR, Buja LM. Histochemical and electron microscopic studies of norepinephrine-induced myocardial necrosis in rats. In: Bajusz E, Rona G, eds. *Recent advances in studies on cardiac structure and metabolism*, vol 1. Baltimore: University Park Press; 1972:495–525.
69. Ferrans VJ, Hibbs RG, Walsh JJ, Burch GE. Histochemical and electron microscopic studies on the cardiac necrosis produced by sympathomimetic agents. *Ann NY Acad Sci* 1969;156:309–332.
70. Ferrans VJ, Hibbs RG, Black WC, Weilbaecher DG. Isoproterenol-induced myocardial necrosis. A histochemical and electron microscopic study. *Am Heart J* 1964;68:71–90.
71. Ferrans VJ, Hibbs RG, Weiley HS, Weilbaecher DG, Walsh JJ, Burch GE. A histochemical and electron microscopic study of epinephrine-induced myocardial necrosis. *J Mol Cell Cardiol* 1970;1:11–22.

72. Lehr D. Healing of myocardial necrosis caused by sympathomimetic amines. In: Bajusz E, Rona G, eds. *Recent advances in studies on cardiac structure and metabolism*, vol 1. Baltimore: University Park Press; 1972:526–550.
73. Lehr D, Krukowshi M, Chau R. Acute myocardial injury produced by sympathomimetic amines. *Israel J Med Sci* 1969;5:519–524.
74. Schenk EA, Moss AJ. Cardiovascular effects of sustained norepinephrine infusions. II. Morphology. *Circ Res* 1966;18:605–615.
75. Regan TJ, Moschos CB, Lehan PH, Oldewurtel HA, Hellems HK. Lipid and carbohydrate metabolism of myocardium during the biphasic inotropic response to epinephrine. *Circ Res* 1966;19:307–316.
76. Wexler BC, Judd JT, Kittinger GW. Myocardial necrosis induced by isoproterenol in rats: changes in serum protein, lipoprotein, lipids and glucose during active necrosis and repair in arteriosclerotic and nonarteriosclerotic animals. *Angiology* 1968;19:665–682.
77. Wexler BC, Judd JT, Lutmer RF, Saroff J. Pathophysiologic change in arteriosclerotic and nonarteriosclerotic rats following isoproterenol-induced myocardial infarction. In: Bajusz E, Rona G, eds. *Recent advances in studies on cardiac structure and metabolism,* vol 1. Baltimore: University Park Press; 1972:463–472.
78. Wexler BC, Kittinger GW. Myocardial necrosis in rats: serum enzymes, adrenal steroid and histopathological alterations. *Circ Res* 1963;13:159–171.
79. Zbinden G, Moe RA. Pharmacological studies on heart muscle lesions induced by isoproterenol. *Ann NY Acad Sci* 1969;156:294–308.
80. Wexler BC. Serum creatine phosphokinase activity following isoproterenol-induced myocardial infarction in male and female rats with and without arteriosclerosis. *Am Heart J* 1970;79:69–79.
81. Regan TJ, Passannante AJ, Oldewurtel HA, Burke WM, Ettinger PO. Metabolism of ^{14}C labelled triglycerides by the myocardium during injury induced by norepinephrine. *Circulation* 1968;38(suppl VI):162.
82. Judd JT, Wexler BC. Myocardial connective tissue metabolism in response to injury: histological and chemical studies of mucopolysaccharides and collagen in rat hearts after isoproterenol-induced infarction. *Circ Res* 1969;25:201–214.
83. Wenzel DG, Chau RYP. Dose–time effect of isoproterenol on aspartate aminotransferase and necrosis of the rat heart. *Toxicol Appl Pharmacol* 1966;8:460–463.
84. Wenzel DG, Lyon JP. Sympathomimetic amines and heart lactic dehydrogenase isoenzymes. *Toxicol Appl Pharmacol* 1967;11:215–228.
85. Stanton HC, Schwartz A. Effects of hydrazine monoamine oxidase inhibitor (phenelzine) on isoproterenol-induced myocardiopathies in the rat. *J Pharmacol Exp Ther* 1967;157:649–658.
86. Vorbeck ML, Malewski EF, Erhart LS, Martin AP. Membrane phospholipid metabolism in the isoproterenol-induced cardiomyopathy of the rat. In: Fleckenstein A, Rona G, eds. *Recent advances in studies on cardiac structure and metabolism,* vol 6. Baltimore: University Park Press; 1975:175–181.
87. Hattori E, Yatsaki K, Miyozaki T, Nakamura M. Adenine nucleotides of myocardium from rats treated with isoproterenol and/or Mg- or K-deficiency. *Jpn Heart J* 1969; 10:218–224.
88. Kako K. Biochemical changes in the rat myocardium induced by isoproterenol. *Can J Physiol Pharmacol* 1965;43:541–549.
89. Robertson WVB, Peyser P. Changes in water and electrolytes of cardiac muscle following epinephrine. *Am J Physiol* 1951;166:277–283.
90. Fleckenstein A. Specific inhibitors and promoters of calcium action in the excitation–contraction coupling of heart muscle and their role in the prevention or production of myocardial lesions. In: Harris P, Opie LH, eds. *Calcium and the heart*. London: Academic Press; 1971:135–188.
91. Fleckenstein A, Janke J, Doering HJ. Myocardial fiber necrosis due to intracellular Ca-overload. A new principle in cardiac pathophysiology. In: Dhalla NS, ed. *Recent advances in studies on cardiac structure and metabolism,* vol 4. Baltimore: University Park Press; 1974:563–580.
92. Pelouch V, Deyl Z, Poupa O. Experimental cardiac necrosis in terms of myosin aggregation. *Physiol Bohemoslov* 1968;17:480–488.

93. Pelouch V, Deyl Z, Poupa O. Myosin aggregation in cardiac necrosis induced by iso-proterenol in rats. *Physiol Bohemoslov* 1970;19:9–13.
94. Fedelesova M, Ziegelhoffer A, Luknarova O, Kostolansky S. Prevention by K⁺, Mg⁺⁺-aspartate of isoproterenol-induced metabolic changes in myocardium. In: Fleckenstein A, Rona G, eds. *Recent advances in studies on cardiac structure and metabolism,* vol 6. Baltimore: University Park Press; 1975:59–73.
95. Dhalla NS, Dzurba A, Pierce GN, Tregaskis MG, Panagia V, Beamish RE. Membrane changes in myocardium during catecholamine-induced pathological hypertrophy. In: Alpert NR, ed. *Perspectives in cardiovascular research,* vol 7. New York: Raven Press; 1983:527–534.
96. Lehr D. Tissue electrolyte alteration in disseminated myocardial necrosis. *Ann NY Acad Sci* 1969;156:344–378.
97. Lehr D, Krukowski M, Colon R. Correlation of myocardial and renal necrosis with tissue electrolyte changes. *JAMA* 1966;197:105–112.
98. Melville KI, Korol B. Cardiac drug responses and potassium shifts. Studies on the interrelated effects of drugs on coronary flow, heart action and cardiac potassium movement. *Am J Cardiol* 1958;2:81–94.
99. Melville KI, Korol B. Cardiac drug responses and potassium shifts. Studies on the interrelated effect of drugs on coronary flow, heart action and cardiac potassium movement. *Am J Cardiol* 1958;2:189–199.
100. Nasmyth PA. The effect of corticosteroids on the isolated mammalian heart and its response to adrenaline. *J Physiol* 1957;139:323–336.
101. Langer GA. Ion fluxes in cardiac excitation and contraction and their relation to myocardial contractility. *Physiol Rev* 1968;48:708–757.
102. Daggett WM, Mansfield PB, Sarnoff SJ. Myocardial K⁺ changes resulting from inotropic agents. *Fed Proc* 1964;23:357.
103. Dhalla NS, Ziegelhoffer A, Harrow JAC. Regulatory role of membrane systems in heart function. *Can J Physiol Pharmacol* 1977;55:1211–1234.
104. Dhalla NS, Das PK, Sharma GP. Subcellular basis of cardiac contractile failure. *J Mol Cell Cardiol* 1978;10:363–385.
105. Dhalla NS, Pierce GN, Panagia V, Singal PK, Beamish RE. Calcium movements in relation to heart function. *Basic Res Cardiol* 1982;77:117–139.
106. Dhalla NS, Dixon IMC, Beamish RE. Biochemical basis of heart function and contractile failure. *J Appl Cardiol* 1991;6:7–30.
107. Varley KG, Dhalla NS. Excitation–contraction coupling in heart. XII. Subcellular calcium transport in isoproterenol-induced myocardial necrosis. *Exp Mol Pathol* 1973; 19:94–105.
108. Fedelesova M, Dzurba A, Ziegelhoffer A. Effect of isoproterenol on the activity of Na⁺,K⁺–adenosine triphosphatase from dog heart. *Biochem Pharmacol* 1974;23:2887–2893.
109. Panagia V, Pierce GN, Dhalla KS, Ganguly PK, Beamish RE, Dhalla NS. Adaptive changes in subcellular calcium transport during catecholamine-induced cardiomyopathy. *J Mol Cell Cardiol* 1985;17:411–420.
110. Okumura K, Panagia V, Beamish RE, Dhalla NS. Biphasic changes in the sarcolemmel phosphatidylethanolamine N-methylation in catecholamine-induced cardiomyopathy. *J Mol Cell Cardiol* 1987;19:357–366.
111. Dhalla NS, Ganguly PK, Panagia V, Beamish RE. Catecholamine-induced cardiomyopathy: alterations in Ca²⁺ transport systems. In: Kawai C, Abelman WH, eds. *Pathogenesis of myocarditis and cardiomyopathy.* Tokyo: University of Tokyo Press; 1987:135–147.
112. Makino N, Dhruvarajan R, Elimban V, Beamish RE, Dhalla NS. Alterations of sarcolemmal Na⁺–Ca²⁺ exchange in catecholamine-induced cardiomyopathy. *Can J Cardiol* 1985;1:225–232.
113. Makino N, Jasmin G, Beamish RE, Dhalla NS. Sarcolemmal Na⁺–Ca²⁺ exchange during the development of genetically determined cardiomyopathy. *Biochem Biophys Res Commun* 1985;133:491–497.
114. Panagia V, Elimban V, Heyliger CE, Tregaskis M, Beamish RE, Dhalla NS. Sarcolemmal alterations during catecholamine induced cardiomyopathy. In: Beamish RE, Pan-

agia V, Dhalla NS, eds. *Pathogenesis of stress-induced heart disease.* Boston: Martinus Nijhoff; 1985:121–131.

115. Corder DW, Heyliger CE, Beamish RE, Dhalla NS. Defect in the adrenergic receptor–adenylate cyclase system during development of catecholamine-induced cardiomyopathy. *Am Heart J* 1984;107:537–542.

116. Roman S, Kutryk MJB, Beamish RE, Dhalla NS. Lysosomal changes during the development of catecholamine-induced cardiomyopathy. In: Beamish RE, Panagia V, Dhalla NS, eds. *Pathogenesis of stress-induced heart disease.* Boston: Martinus Nijhoff; 1985:270–280.

117. Selye H. *The pluicausal cardiopathies.* Springfield, IL: Charles C Thomas; 1961.

118. Beamish RE, Dhalla NS. Involvement of catecholamines in coronary spasm under stressful conditions. In: Beamish RE, Singal PK, Dhalla NS, eds. *Stress and heart disease.* Boston: Martinus Nijhoff; 1985:129–141.

119. Lown B. Clinical management of ventricular arrhythmias. *Hosp Pract* 1982;17:73–86.

120. Singal PK, Kapur N, Beamish RE, Das PK, Dhalla NS. Antioxidant protection against epinephrine-induced arrhythmias. In: Beamish RE, Singal PK, Dhalla NS, eds. *Stress and heart disease.* Boston: Martinus Nijhoff; 1985:190–201.

121. Kahn DS, Rona G, Chappel CI. Isoproterenol-induced cardiac necrosis. *Ann NY Acad Sci* 1969;156:285–293.

122. Rona G, Chappel CI, Kahn DS. The significance of factors modifying the development of isoproterenol-induced myocardial necrosis. *Am Heart J* 1963;66:389–395.

123. Zbinden G. Inhibition of experimental myocardial necrosis by the monoamine oxidase inhibitor isocarboxazid (Marplan). *Am Heart J* 1960;60:450–453.

124. Zbinden G. Effects of anoxia and amino oxidase inhibitors on myocardial necrosis induced by isoproterenol. *Fed Proc* 1961;20:128.

125. Zbinden G, Bagdon RE. Isoproterenol-induced heart necrosis, an experimental model for the study of angina pectoris and myocardial infarct. *Rev Can Biol* 1963;22: 257–263.

126. Leszkovsky GP, Gal G. Observations on isoprenaline-induced myocardial necroses. *J Pharm Pharmacol* 1967;19:226–230.

127. Bloom S, Davis D. Isoproterenol myocytolysis and myocardial calcium. In: Dhalla NS, ed. *Myocardial biology: recent advances in studies on cardiac structure and metabolism,* vol 4. Baltimore: University Park Press; 1974:581–590.

128. Dorigotti L, Gaetani M, Glasser AH, Turollia E. Competitive antagonism of isoproterenol-induced cardiac necrosis by β-adrenoreceptor blocking agents. *J Pharm Pharmacol* 1969;21:188–191.

129. Mehes G, Rajkovits K, Papp G. Effect of various types of sympathicolytics on isoproterenol-induced myocardial lesions. *Acta Physiol Acad Sci Hung* 1966;29:75–85.

130. Kako K. The effect of beta-adrenergic blocking agents on chemical changes in isoproterenol-induced myocardial necrosis. *Can J Physiol Pharmacol* 1966;44:678–682.

131. Pieper GM, Clayton FC, Todd GL, Eliot RS. Temporal changes in endocardial energy metabolism following propranolol and the metabolic basis for protection against isoprenaline cardiotoxicity. *Cardiovasc Res* 1979;13:207–214.

132. Mehes G, Papp G, Rajkovits K. Effect of adrenergic- and β-receptor blocking drugs on the myocardial lesions induced by sympathomimetic amines. *Acta Physiol Acad Sci Hung* 1967;32:175–184.

133. Waters LL, deSuto-Nagy GI. Lesions of the coronary arteries and great vessels of the dog following injection of adrenaline. Their prevention by Dibenamine. *Science* 1950;111:634–635.

134. Wenzel DG, Chau RY. Effect of adrenergic blocking agents on reduction of myocardial aspartate–aminotransferase activity by sympathomimetics. *Toxicol Appl Pharmacol* 1966;9:514–520.

135. Dhalla NS, Balasubramanian V, Goldman J. Biochemical basis of heart function. III. Influence of isoproterenol on the norepinephrine stores in the rat heart. *Can J Physiol Pharmacol* 1971;49:302–311.

136. Bajusz E, Jasmin G. Protective action of serotonin against certain chemically and surgically induced cardiac necroses. *Rev Can Biol* 1962;21:51–62.

137. Okumura K, Ogawa K, Satake T. Pretreatment with chlorpromazine prevents phos-

pholipid degradation and creatine kinase depletion in isoproterenol-induced myocardial damage in rats. *J Cardiovasc Pharmacol* 1983;5:983–988.
138. Godfraind T, Strubois X. The prevention by creatinol *O*-phosphate of myocardial lesions evoked by isoprenaline. *Arch Int Pharmacodyn Ther* 1979;237:288–297.
139. Singal PK, Dhillon KS, Beamish RE, Dhalla NS. Protective effects of zinc against catecholamine-induced myocardial changes. Electrocardiographic and ultrastructural studies. *Lab Invest* 1981;44:426–433.
140. Mjos DD. Effect of inhibition of lipolysis on myocardial oxygen consumption in the presence of isoproterenol. *J Clin Invest* 1971;50:1869–1873.
141. Wenzel DG, Stark LG. Effect of nicotine on cardiac necrosis induced by isoproterenol. *Am Heart J* 1966;71:368–370.
142. Sigel H, Janke J, Fleckenstein A. Restriction of isoproterenol-induced myocardial Ca uptake and necrotization by a new Ca-antagonistic compound (ethyl-4(3,4,5-trimethoxycinnamoyl) piperazinyl acetate (Vascoril). In: Fleckenstein A, Rona G, eds. *Recent advances in studies on cardiac structure and metabolism*, vol 6. Baltimore: University Park Press; 1975:121–126.
143. Takeo S, Takenaka F. Effects of diltiazem on high-energy phosphate content reduced by isoproterenol in rat myocardium. *Arch Int Pharmacodyn Ther* 1977;228:205–212.
144. Rona G, Chappel CI, Gaudry R. Effect of dietary sodium and potassium content on myocardial necrosis elicited by isoproterenol. *Lab Invest* 1961;10:892–897.
145. Chappel CI, Rona G, Gaudry R. The influence of adrenal cortical steroids on cardiac necrosis produced by isoproterenol. *Acta Endocrinol* 1959;32:419–424.
146. Lehr D, Chau R, Kaplan J. Prevention of experimental myocardial necrosis by electrolyte solutions. In: Bajusz B, Rona G, eds. *Recent advances in studies on cardiac structure and metabolism*, vol 1. Baltimore: University Park Press; 1972:684–698.
147. Janke J, Fleckenstein A, Hein B, Leder O, Sigel H. Prevention of myocardial Ca overload and necrotization by Mg and K salts or acidosis. In: Fleckenstein A, Rona G, eds. *Recent advances in studies on cardiac structure and metabolism*, vol 6. Baltimore: University Park Press; 1975:33–42.
148. Slezak J, Tribulova N. Morphological changes after combined administration of isoproterenol and K^+, Mg^{++}–aspartate as a physiological Ca^{2+} antagonist. In: Fleckenstein A, Rona G, eds. *Recent advances in studies on cardiac structure and metabolism*, vol 6. Baltimore: University Park Press; 1975:75–84.
149. Balazs T. Cardiotoxicity of isoproterenol in experimental animals. Influence of stress, obesity, and repeated dosing. In: Bajusz B, Rona G, eds. *Recent advances in studies on cardiac structure and metabolism*, vol 1. Baltimore: University Park Press; 1972:770–778.
150. Balazs T, Sahasrabudhe MR, Grice HC. The influence of excess body fat on cardiotoxicity of isoproterenol rats. *Toxicol Appl Pharmacol* 1962;4:613–620.
151. Rona G, Chappel CI, Balazs T, Gaudry R. The effect of breed, age and sex on myocardial necrosis produced by isoproterenol in the rat. *J Gerontol* 1959;14:169–173.
152. Balazs T, Arena E, Barron CN. Protection against the cardiotoxic effect of isoproterenol HCl by restricted food intake in rats. *Toxicol Appl Pharmacol* 1972;21:237–243.
153. Dusek J, Rona G, Kahn DS. Myocardial resistance. A study of its development against toxic doses of isoproterenol. *Arch Pathol* 1970;89:79–83.
154. Dusek J, Rona G, Kahn DS. Myocardial resistance to isoprenaline in rats: variations with time. *J Pathol* 1971;105:279–282.
155. Selye H, Veilleux R, Grasso S. Protection by coronary ligation against isoproterenol-induced myocardial necrosis. *Proc Soc Exp Biol Med* 1960;104:343–345.
156. Balazs T, Ohtake S, Noble JF. The development of resistance to the ischemic cardiopathic effect of isoproterenol. *Toxicol Appl Pharmacol* 1972;21:200–213.
157. Turek Z, Kalus M, Poupa O. The effect of isoprenaline pretreatment on the size of acute myocardial necrosis induced by the same drug. *Physiol Bohemoslov* 1966;15:353–356.
158. Wexler BC, Kittinger GW, Judd JT. Responses to drug-induced myocardial necrosis in rats with various degrees of arteriosclerosis. *Circ Res* 1967;20:78–87.
159. Faltova E, Poupa P. Temperature and experimental acute cardiac necrosis. *Can J Physiol Pharmacol* 1969;47:295–299.
160. Kennedy JH, Alousi M, Homi J. The protective effect of hyperbaric oxygenation upon

isoproterenol-induced myocardial necrosis in Syrian hamsters. *Med Thorac* 1966; 23:169–175.

161. Poupa O, Krofta K, Prochazka J, Turek Z. Acclimation to simulated high altitude and acute necrosis. *Fed Proc* 1966;25:1243–1246.
162. Poupa O, Turek Z, Kaluz M, Krofta K. Acute infarct-like necrosis in high altitude adapted rats. *Physiol Bohemoslov* 1965;14:542–545.
163. Balazs T, Murphy JG, Grice HC. The influence of environmental changes on the cardiotoxicity of isoprenaline in rats. *J Pharm Pharmacol* 1962;14:750–755.
164. Raab W, Bajusz E, Kimura H, Henlich HC. Isolation, stress, myocardial electrolytes and epinephrine cardiotoxicity in rats. *Proc Soc Exp Biol Med* 1968;127:142–147.
165. Hatch AM, Wiberg GS, Zawidzka Z, Cann M, Airth JM, Grice GC. Isolation syndrome in the rat. *Toxicol Appl Pharmacol* 1965;7:737–745.
166. Jasmin G. Morphologic effects of vasoactive drugs. *Can J Physiol Pharmacol* 1966; 44:367–372.
167. Hoak JC, Warner ED, Connor WE. New concept of levarterenol-induced acute myocardial ischemic injury. *Arch Pathol* 1969;87:332–338.
168. Raab W. Myocardial electrolyte derangement: crucial feature of plusicausal, so-called coronary, heart disease. *Ann NY Acad Sci* 1969;147:627–686.
169. Rosenblum I, Wohl A, Stein A. Studies in cardiac necrosis. III. Metabolic effects of sympathomimetic amines producing cardiac lesions. *Toxicol Appl Pharmacol* 1965; 7:344–351.
170. Rona G, Dusek J. Studies on the mechanism of increased myocardial resistance. In: Bajusz E, Rona G, eds. *Recent advances in studies on cardiac structure and metabolism,* vol 1. Baltimore: University Park Press; 1972:422–429.
171. Strubelt O, Siegers CP. Role of cardiovascular and ionic changes in pathogenesis and prevention of isoprenaline-induced cardiac necrosis. Pathophysiology and morphology of myocardial cell alteration. In: Fleckenstein A, Rona G, eds. *Recent advances in studies on cardiac structure and metabolism,* vol 6. Baltimore: University Park Press; 1975:135–142.
172. Ostadal B, Poupa O. Occlusion of coronary vessels after administration of isoprenaline, adrenalin and noradrenalin. *Physiol Bohemoslov* 1967;16:116–119.
173. Brandi G, McGregor M. Intramural pressure in the left ventricle of the dog. *Cardiovasc Res* 1969;3:472–475.
174. Cutarelli R, Levy MN. Intraventricular pressure and the distribution of coronary blood flow. *Circ Res* 1963;12:322–327.
175. Buckberg GD, Fixler DE, Archie JP, Hoffmann JIE. Experimental subendocardial ischemia in dogs with normal coronary arteries. *Circ Res* 1972;30:67–81.
176. Buckberg GD, Ross G. Effects of isoprenaline on coronary blood flow: its distribution and myocardial performance. *Cardiovasc Res* 1973;7:429–437.
177. Bajusz E. The terminal electrolyte-shift mechanism in heart necrosis: its significance in the pathogenesis and prevention of necrotizing cardiomyopathies. In: Bajusz E, ed. *Electrolytes and cardiovascular diseases.* Basel: S. Karger; 1975.
178. Raab W, van Lith P, Lepeschkin E, Herrlich HC. Catecholamine-induced myocardial hypoxia in the presence of impaired coronary dilatability independent of external cardiac work. *Am J Cardiol* 1962;9:455–470.
179. Lee KS, Yu DH. Effects of epinephrine on metabolism and contraction of cat papillary muscle. *Am J Physiol* 1964;206:525–530.
180. Weisfeldt ML, Gilmore JP. Apparent dissociation of the inotropic and O_2 consumption effects of norepinephrine. *Fed Proc* 1964;23:357.
181. Klocke FJ, Kaiser GA, Ross J Jr, Braunwald E. Mechanism of increase of myocardial oxygen uptake produced by catecholamines. *Am J Physiol* 1965;209:913–918.
182. Challoner DR, Steinberg D. Metabolic effect of epinephrine on the QO_2 of the arrested isolated perfused rat heart. *Nature* 1965;205:602–603.
183. Hauge A, Oye I. The action of adrenaline in cardiac muscle. II. Effect on oxygen consumption in the asystolic perfused rat heart. *Acta Physiol Scand* 1966;68:295–303.
184. Park JH, Meriwether BP, Park CR, Mudd SH, Lipmann F. Glutathione and ethylene-diamine-tetraacetate antagonism of uncoupling of oxidative phosphorylation. *Biochim Biophys Acta* 1956;22:403–404.
185. Sordahl LA, Sliver BB. Pathological accumulation of calcium by mitochondria: mod-

ulation by magnesium. In: Fleckenstein A, Rona G, eds. *Recent advances in studies on cardiac structure and metabolism,* vol 6. Baltimore: University Park Press; 1975: 85–93.

186. Lossnitzer K, Janke J, Hein B, Stauch M, Fleckenstein A. Disturbed myocardial calcium metabolism: a possible pathogenetic factor in the hereditary cardiomyopathy of the Syrian hamster. In: Fleckenstein A, Rona G, eds. *Recent advances in studies on cardiac structure and metabolism,* vol 6. Baltimore: University Park Press; 1975:207–217.

187. Jasmin G, Bajusz E. Prevention of myocardial degeneration in hamsters with hereditary cardiomyopathy. In: Fleckenstein A, Rona G, eds. *Recent advances in studies on cardiac structure and metabolism,* vol 6. Baltimore: University Park Press; 1975: 219–229.

188. Fleckenstein A, Janke J, Doering HJ, Leder O. Key role of Ca in the production of noncoronarogenic myocardial necroses. In: Fleckenstein A, Rona G, eds. *Recent advances in studies on cardiac structure and metabolism,* vol 6. Baltimore: University Park Press; 1975:21–32.

189. Osinskaya VO. Catecholamines and compounds with the properties of their oxidation products in the animal organisms. In: *Adrenalin: noradrenalin.* Regulyatsii: Akad Nauk SSSR, Lab Neiro-Gumoralin; 1964:118–123 *(Chem Abstr* 1965;63:869).

190. Osinskaya VO. Adrenalin and noradrenalin metabolism in animal tissues. *Biokhimiya* 1957;22:537–545 *(Chem Abstr* 1958;52:2211).

191. Utevskii AM, Osinskaya VO. The nature, properties and significance of fluorescing substances formed in the processes of adrenaline and noradrenaline oxidation. *Ukr Biokhim Zh* 1955;27:401–406 *(Chem Abstr* 1956;50:1948).

192. Kisch B. Die autokatalyse der adrenalinoxydation. *Biochem Z* 1930;220:84–91.

193. Okagawa M, Ichitsubo H. Oxidation and reduction of adrenaline in the body. *Proc Jpn Pharmacol Soc* 1935;9:155.

194. Heirman P. L'adrenoxine, adrenaline oxydee inhibitrice. *CR Soc Biol (Paris)* 1937; 126:1264–1266.

195. Heirman P. Action de la Tyrosinase sur l'oxidation et les effets cardiaques de l'adrenaline et de la tyramine. *CR Soc Biol (Paris)* 1937;124:1250–1251.

196. Hogeboom GH, Adams MH. Mammalian tyrosinase and dopa oxidase. *J Biol Chem* 1942;145:272–279.

197. Mason HS. The chemistry of melanin. II. The oxidation of dihydroxyphenylalanine by mammalian dopa oxidase. *J Biol Chem* 1947;168:433–438.

198. von Euler US. *Noradrenaline—chemistry, physiology, pharmacology and clinical aspects.* Springfield, IL: Charles C Thomas; 1956.

199. Heirman P. Modifications of the cardiac action of adrenaline in the course of its oxidation by phenolases. *Arch Intern Physiol* 1938;46:404–415.

200. Blaschko H, Schlossman H. The inactivation of adrenaline by phenolases. *J Physiol* 1940;98:130–140.

201. Derouaux G. The *in vitro* oxidation of adrenaline and other diphenol amines by phenol oxidase. *Arch Intern Pharmacodyn Ther* 1943;69:205–234.

202. Wajzer J. Oxydation de l'adrenaline. *Bull Soc Chim Biol* 1946;28:341–345.

203. Valerno DM, McCormack JJ. Xanthine oxidase-mediated oxidation of epinephrine. *Biochem Pharmacol* 1971;20:47–55.

204. Vercauteren R. Sur la cytochimie des granulocytes eosinophiles. *Bull Soc Chim Biol* 1951;33:522–525.

205. Odajima T. Myeloperoxidase of the leukocyte of normal blood. II. Oxidation–reduction reaction mechanism of the myeloperoxidase. *Biochim Biophys Acta* 1971;235:52–60.

206. Philpot FJ. Inhibition of adrenaline oxidation by local anaesthetics. *J Physiol* 1940; 97:301–307.

207. Slater EC. The measurement of the cytochrome oxidase activity of enzyme preparations. *Biochem J* 1949;44:305–318.

208. Iisalo E, Rekkarinen A. Enzyme action on adrenaline and noradrenaline. Studies on heart muscle *in vitro. Acta Pharmacol Toxicol* 1958;15:157–174.

209. Green DE, Richter D. Adrenaline and adrenochrome. *Biochem J* 1937;31:596–616.

210. Bacq ZM. Metabolism of adrenaline. *Pharmacol Rev* 1949;1:1–26.

211. Axelrod J. Enzymic oxidation of epinephrine to adrenochrome by the salivary gland. *Biochim Biophys Acta* 1964;85:247–254.
212. Falk JE. The formation of hydrogen carriers by haemitin-catalyzed peroxidations. *Biochem J* 1949;44:369–373.
213. Chaix P, Pallaget C. Comparative characteristics of the oxidation of adrenaline and noradrenaline. *Congr Int Biochim Resumes Commun 2nd Congr* 1952;54 (*Chem Abstr* 1954;48:12851).
214. Chikano M, Kominami M. Uber die spaltung des adreanlins im serum. *Biochem Z* 1929;205:176–179.
215. Hoffer A. Adrenochrome and adrenolutin and their relationship to mental disease. In: Garattini S, Ghetti V, eds. *Psychotropic drugs*. Amsterdam: Elsevier; 1957:10–25.
216. Dhalla KS, Ganguly PK, Rupp H, Beamish RE, Dhalla NS. Measurement of adrenolutin as an oxidation product of catecholamines in plasma. *Mol Cell Biochem* 1989; 87:85–92.
217. Osmond H, Hoffer A. Schizophrenia: a new approach continued. *J Ment Sci* 1959; 105:653–673.
218. Schweitzer A. Comparative investigations of the action of *p*-benzoquinone and omega on the function of the frog heart. *Arch Ges Physiol* 1931;228:568–585.
219. Sanders E. The inhibiting effect of oxidized adrenalin. *Arch Exp Pathol Pharmacol* 1939;193:572–575.
220. Webb WR, Dodds RP, Unal MO, Karow AM, Cook WA, Daniel CR. Suspended animation of the heart with metabolic inhibitors. Effect of magnesium sulfate or fluoride and adrenochrome in rats. *Ann Surg* 1966;164:343–350.
221. Yen T. The reversal of the effect of adrenaline upon the rabbit intestine and the toad limb vessels. *Tohoku J Exp Med* 1930;14:415–465.
222. Raab W, Lepeschkin E. Pressor and cardiac effects of adrenochrome (omega) in the atropinized cat. *Exp Med Surg* 1950;8:319–329.
223. Titaev AA. Relation of some metabolites to the sympathetic nervous system in newborn animals. *Chem Abstr* 1964;60:8438.
224. Green S, Mazur A, Shorr E. Mechanism of catalytic oxidation of adrenalin by ferritin. *J Biol Chem* 1956;220:237–255.
225. Parrot JL. Decrease in capillary permeability under the influence of adrenochrome. *CR Soc Biol (Paris)* 1949;143:819–822 (*Chem Abstr* 1950;44:5008).
226. Lecomte J, Fischer P. The effect of trihydroxy-1-methylindole on bleeding time and capillary permeability. *Arch Int Pharmacodyn Ther* 1951;87:225–231.
227. Marquordt P. The pharmacology and chemistry of the adrenochromes. *Z Ges Exp Med* 1944;114:112–126 (*Chem Abstr* 1950;44:2657).
228. Snyder FH, Leva E, Oberst FW. An evaluation of adrenochrome and iodoadrenochrome based on blood-sugar levels in rabbits. *J Am Pharm Assoc* 1947;36:253–255.
229. Kaulla KNV. Uber die beeinflussung des O_2—Verbrauches durch adrenochrom beim meerschweinchen. *Biochem Z* 1949;319:453–456.
230. Parrot JL, Cara M. Action of adrenochrome on oxygen consumption of man and guinea pig. *CR Soc Biol (Paris)* 1951;145:1829–2862 (*Chem Abstr* 1952;46:10415).
231. Kisch B. Katalytische wirkungen oxydierten adrenalins. *Klin Wochenschr* 1930;9: 1062–1064.
232. Gaisinska MY, Utevskii AM. Effect of catecholamines on oxidative processes under normal conditions and in experimental hypertension. *Ukr Biokhim Zh* 1962;34:237–242 (*Chem Abstr* 1962;57:3986).
233. Radsma W, Golterman HL. Influence of adrenaline and adrenochrome on oxygen consumption of liver homogenates. *Biochim Biophys Acta* 1954;13:80–86.
234. Kisch B, Leibowitz J. Die beeinflussung der gewebsatmung der omega und durch chinon. *Biochem Z* 1930;220:97–116.
235. Issekutz B Jr, Lichtneckert I, Hetenyi G Jr, Bedo M. Metabolic effects of noradrenaline and adrenochrome. *Arch Int Pharmacodyn Ther* 1950;84:376–384.
236. Itasaka K. Tissue respiration and substrate utilization of heart muscle slices. *Fukuoka Igaku Zasshi* 1958;49:3347–3367 (*Chem Abstr* 1959;53:7436).
237. Wieland O, Suyter M. Der stoffwechselwirkung des adrenochroms. *Klin Wochenschr* 1956;34:647–648.

238. Krall AR, Siegel GJ, Goznaski DM, Wagner FL. Adrenochrome inhibition of oxidative phosphorylation by rat brain mitochondria. *Biochem Pharmacol* 1964;12:1519–1525.

239. Sudovtsov VE. Effect of adrenoxyl on the oxidative phosphorylation and potassium and sodium permeability of mitochondria. In: Severin SE, ed. *Mitokhondrii, bioklium,* vol 4. Moscow: Funkts, Sist Kletochnykh Organell, Mater, Simp; 1969:83–88. (*Chem Abstr* 1971;74:2436).

240. Wajzer J. Effet pasteur du muscle de grenouille et adrenochrome. *Bull Soc Chim Biol* 1946;28:345–349.

241. Wajzer J. Synthese dur glycogene en presence d'adrenochrome. *Bull Soc Chim Biol* 1947;29:237–239.

242. Meyerhof O, Randall LO. Inhibitory effects of adrenochrome on cell metabolism. *Arch Biochem* 1948;17:171–182.

243. Walaas E, Walaas O, Jervell K. Action of adrenochrome on glucose phosphorylation in the rat diaphragm. *Congr Int Biochim Resumes Commun 2nd Congr Paris* 1952;67 (*Chem Abstr* 1955;49:5632).

244. Pastan I, Herring B, Johnson P, Field JB. Mechanisms by which adrenaline stimulates glucose oxidation in the thyroid. *J Biol Chem* 1962;237:287–290.

245. Dumont JE, Hupka S. Action of neuromimetic amines on the metabolism of thyroid incubated *in vitro*. *CR Soc Biol (Paris)* 1962;156:1942–1946 (*Chem Abstr* 1963;59:5434).

246. Dickens F, Glock GE. Mechanism of oxidative inhibition of myosin. *Biochim Biophys Acta* 1951;7:578–584.

247. Inchiosa MA Jr, Van Demark NL. Influence of oxidation products of adrenaline on adenosinetriphosphatase activity of a uterine muscle preparation. *Proc Soc Exp Biol Med* 1958;97:595–597.

248. Denisov VM. Effect of the oxidation products of catecholamines on the ATPase activity of myosin. *Ukr Biokhim Zh* 1964;36:711–717 (*Chem Abstr* 1965;62:2930).

249. Denisov VM, Rukavishnikova SM. Influence of adrenoxyl on the activity of heart adenosine-triphosphatase and phosphorylase. *Ukr Biokhim Zh* 1968;40:384–387 (*Chem Abstr* 1968;69:105000).

250. Friedenwald JS, Heniz H. Inactivation of amine oxidase by enzymatic oxidative products of catechol and adrenaline. *J Biol Chem* 1942;146:411–419.

251. Usdin VR, Su X, Usdin E. Effects of psychotropic compounds on enzyme systems. II. *In vitro* inhibition of monoamine oxidase (MAO). *Proc Soc Exp Biol Med* 1961;108:461–463.

252. Petryanik VD. Effect of adrenochrome and vikasol on monoamine oxidase of some rabbit organs. *Ukr Biokhim Zh* 1971;43:225–228 (*Chem Abstr* 1971;75:47117).

253. Anderson AB. Inhibition of alkaline phosphatase by adrenaline and related dihydroxyphenols and quinones. *Biochim Biophys Acta* 1961;54:110–114.

254. Heacock RA. The chemistry of adrenochrome and related compounds. *Chem Rev* 1959;59:181–237.

255. Shebeko GS. Effect of adrenaline and adrenoxyl on the level of coenzyme A in some organs of albino rats. *Ukr Biokhim Zh* 1970;42:596–599 (*Chem Abstr* 1971;74:72333).

256. Frederick J. Cytologic studies on the normal mitochondrion and those submitted to experimental procedures in living cells cultured in vitro. *Arch Biol* 1958;69:167–349.

257. Blix G. Adrenaline as an oxidation catalyzer. Oxidative deamination of amino acids by some means of adrenaline or some simple hydroxygenzenes. *Scand Arch Physiol* 1929;56:131–172.

258. Kisch B, Leibowitz J. Die omegakatalyze der oxydativen glykokollspaltung. *Biochem Z* 1930;220:370–377.

259. Kisch B. Die omegakatalyze der oxydativen glykokollspaltung. Neue untersuchungen. *Biochem Z* 1931;236:380–386.

260. Kisch B. *O*-Chinone als fermentmodell. II. Mitteilung: Versuch mit verschiedened substraten. *Biochem Z* 1932:244:440–450.

261. Aberhalden E, Baertich E. Deamination of glycine by "omega" (adrenaline oxidation product). *Fermentforschung* 1937;15:342–347 (*Chem Abstr* 1938;32:3431).

262. Fischer P, Landtsheer L. The metabolism of adrenochrome and trihydroxymethylindole in the rabbit. *Experientia* 1950;6:305–306.

263. Fischer P, Lecomte J. Metabolisme de l'adrenochrome, de ses produits de reuction et

du trihydroxy-*N*-methylindol chez le lapin, le chat et le chien. *Bull Soc Chim Biol* 1951;33:569–600.

264. Noval JJ, Sohler A, Stackhouse SP, Bryan AC. Metabolism of adrenochrome in experimental animals. *Biochem Pharmacol* 1962;11:467–473.

265. Schayer RW, Smiley RL. The metabolism of epinephrine containing isotropic carbon. III. *J Biol Chem* 1953;202:425–430.

266. Yates JC, Dhalla NS. Induction of necrosis and failure in the isolated perfused rat heart with oxidized isoproterenol. *J Mol Cell Cardiol* 1975;7:807–816.

267. Steen EM, Noronha-Dutra AA, Woolf N. The response of isolated rat heart cells to cardiotoxic concentrations of isoprenaline. *J Pathol* 1982;137:167–176.

268. Dhalla NS, Yates JC, Lee SL, Singh A. Functional and subcellular changes in the isolated rat heart perfused with oxidized isoproterenol. *J Mol Cell Cardiol* 1978;10: 31–41.

269. Severin S, Sartore S, Schiaffino S. Direct toxic effects of isoproterenol on cultured muscle cells. *Experientia* 1977;33:1489–1490.

270. Yates JC, Beamish RE, Dhalla NS. Ventricular dysfunction and necrosis produced by adrenochrome metabolite of epinephrine: relation to pathogenesis of catecholamine cardiomyopathy. *Am Heart J* 1981;102:210–221.

271. Yates JC, Taam GML, Singal PK, Beamish RE, Dhalla NS. Protection against adrenochrome-induced myocardial damage by various pharmacological interventions. *Br J Exp Pathol* 1980;61:242–255.

272. Yates JC, Taam GML, Singal PK, Beamish RE, Dhalla NS. Modification of adrenochrome-induced cardiac contractile failure and cell damage by changes in cation concentrations. *Lab Invest* 1980;43:316–326.

273. Takeo S, Fliegel L, Beamish RE, Dhalla NS. Effects of adrenochrome on rat heart sarcolemmal ATPase activities. *Biochem Pharmacol* 1980;29:559–564.

274. Takeo S, Taam GML, Beamish RE, Dhalla NS. Effects of adrenochrome on calcium accumulating and adenosine triphosphate activities of the rat heart microsomes. *J Pharmacol Exp Ther* 1980;214:688–693.

275. Takeo S, Taam GML, Beamish RE, Dhalla NS. Effect of adrenochrome on calcium accumulation by heart mitochondria. *Biochem Pharmacol* 1981;30:157–163.

276. Taam GML, Takeo S, Ziegelhoffer A, Singal PK, Beamish RE, Dhalla NS. Effect of adrenochrome of adenine nucleotides and mitochondrial oxidative phosphorylation in rat heart. *Can J Cardiol* 1986;2:88–93.

277. Fliegel L, Takeo S, Beamish RE, Dhalla NS. Adrenochrome uptake and subcellular distribution in the isolated perfused rat heart. *Can J Cardiol* 1985;1:122–127.

278. Karmazyn M, Beamish RE, Fliegel L, Dhalla NS. Adrenochrome-induced coronary artery constriction in the rat heart. *J Pharmacol Exp Ther* 1981;219:225–230.

279. Singal PK, Dhillon KS, Beamish RE, Dhalla NS. Myocardial cell damage and cardiovascular changes due to I.V. infusion of adrenochrome in rats. *Br J Exp Pathol* 1982;63:167–176.

280. Beamish RE, Dhillon KS, Singal PK, Dhalla NS. Protective effect of sulfinpyrazone against catecholamine metabolite adrenochrome-induced arrhythmias. *Am Heart J* 1981;102:149–152.

281. Beamish RE, Singal PK, Dhillon KS, Karmazyn M, Kapur N, Dhalla NS. Effects of sulfinpyrazone on adrenochrome-induced changes in the rat heart. In: Hirsch J, Steele PP, Verrier RL, eds. *Effects of platelet-active drugs on the cardiovascular system*. Denver: University of Colorado; 1981:131–146.

282. Singal PK, Yates JC, Beamish RE, Dhalla NS. Influence of reducing agents on adrenochrome-induced changes in the heart. *Arch Pathol Lab Med* 1981;105:664–669.

283. Singal PK, Kapur N, Dhillon KS, Beamish RE, Dhalla NS. Role of free radicals in catecholamine-induced cardiomyopathy. *Can J Physiol Pharmacol* 1982;60:1390–1397.

284. Singal PK, Beamish RE, Dhalla NS. Potential oxidative pathways of catecholamines in the formation of lipid peroxides and genesis of heart disease. In: Spitzer JJ, ed. *Myocardial injury*. New York: Plenum Press; 1983:391–401.

285. Ramos K, Acosta D. Prevention by l(-)ascorbic acid of isoproterenol induced cardiotoxicity in primary culture of rat myocytes. *Toxicology* 1983;26:81–90.

286. Ramos K, Combs AB, Acosta D. Cytotoxicity of isoproterenol to cultured heart cells:

effects of antioxidants on modifying membrane damage. *Toxicol Appl Pharmacol* 1983;70:317–323.

287. Acosta D, Combs AB, Ramos K. Attenuation by antioxidants of Na^+/K^+ ATPase inhibition by toxic concentrations of isoproterenol in cultured rat myocardial cells. *J Mol Cell Cardiol* 1984;16:281–284.

288. Rupp H, Bukhari AR, Jacob R. Modulation of catecholamine synthesizing and degrading enzymes by swimming and emotional excitation in the rat. In: Jacob R, ed. *Cardiac adaptation to hemodynamic overload, training and stress.* Berlin: Steinkopff Verlag; 1983:267–273.

289. Mitova M, Bednarik B, Cerny E, Foukal T, Dratky J, Popousek F. Influence of physical exertion on early isoproterenol-indued heart injury. *Basic Res Cardiol* 1983; 78:131–139.

290. Burton KP, McCord JM, Ghai G. Myocardial alterations due to free radical generation. *Am J Physiol* 1984;246:H1776–H1783.

291. Blaustein AS, Schine L, Brooks WW, Fanburg BL, Bing OHL. Influence of exogenously generated oxidant species on myocardial function. *Am J Physiol* 1986; 250:H595–H599.

292. Gupta M, Singal PK. Time course of structure, function and metabolic changes due to an exogenous source of oxygen metabolites in rat heart. *Can J Physiol Pharmacol* 1989;67:1549–1559.

293. Kaneko M, Beamish RE, Dhalla NS. Depression of heart sarcolemmal Ca^{2+}-pump activity by oxygen free radicals. *Am J Physiol* 1989;256:H368–H374.

294. Rowe GT, Manson NH, Caplan M, Hess ML. Hydrogen peroxide and hydroxyl radical mediation of activated leukocyte depression of cardiac sarcoplasmic reticulum: participation of cyclooxygenase pathway. *Circ Res* 1983;53:584–591.

295. Hata T, Kaneko M, Beamish RE, Dhalla NS. Influence of oxygen free radicals on heart sarcolemmal $Na^+–Ca^{2+}$ exchange. *Coronary Artery Disease* 1991;2:397–407.

Cardiovascular Toxicology, Second Edition,
edited by Daniel Acosta, Jr.
Raven Press, Ltd., New York © 1992.

11

Chemical Agent Actions on Ion Channels and Electrophysiology of the Heart

Nicholas Sperelakis

*Department of Physiology and Biophysics, University of Cincinnati,
College of Medicine, Cincinnati, Ohio 45267*

The unique electrical properties of cardiac muscle determine most of the special mechanical properties of the heart. The heart is an effective pump for circulating the blood. The entire ventricle is rapidly activated, within several hundredths of a second, by the rapidly conducting (2–3 m/sec) specialized pathways (e.g., the Purkinje fiber system of mammals) and by propagation through the myocardium proper (0.3–0.5 m/sec). The ventricle usually contracts in an all-or-none fashion, not tetanically (i.e., it is not held in a sustained contracted state), because of a long functional refractory period that is dependent on the duration of the action potential (AP) and on the recovery kinetics of the ionic channels. The long-duration plateau component of the cardiac AP keeps the heart actively contracted for a relatively long period.

The heart can be made to pump more forcefully when the conditions require this, by various mechanisms, including action of the neurotransmitter norepinephrine on the myocardial cell membrane. One action of norepinephrine is to increase the number of slow Ca^{2+} channels available for voltage activation through which Ca^{2+} ions can pass into the cell during the AP. A larger Ca^{2+} influx during the AP plateau causes a greater force of contraction. The mechanism of the norepinephrine action on the slow Ca^{2+} channels is mediated by elevation of cAMP (1–5). The neurotransmitter acetylcholine counteracts the membrane effects of the catecholamines (6–15).

Thus the autonomic innervation and the myocardial cell membrane exert tight control over the contractile machinery by regulating the amount of Ca^{2+} influx per cardiac impulse. The Ca^{2+} entering across the cell membrane is directly involved in elevating the myoplasmic Ca^{2+} concentration ($[Ca]_i$) to the level necessary to activate the myofilaments and, in addition, brings about the further release of Ca^{2+} from the internal Ca^{2+} stores within the sarcoplasmic reticulum (SR). The steps in this overall control process comprise excitation–contraction coupling (or electromechanical coupling). Relaxation of the heart is produced by lowering $[Ca]_i$ due to resequestration of Ca^{2+} by the SR and to extrusion of Ca^{2+} across the cell membrane (by Ca–Na exchange and by a Ca–ATPase pump).

Some cardiotoxic agents affect the heart by acting on the ion channels and electrical properties of the cell membrane (Table 1) or on other steps of the excitation–contraction coupling sequence. Some drugs block the slow Ca^{2+} channels selectively and thereby depress the force of contraction or even completely uncouple contraction from excitation. Toxins, such as the Japanese puffer fish poison tetrodotoxin (TTX), selectively block the fast Na^+ channels in the heart (also in nerve and skeletal muscle) and thereby cause cardiac standstill (and respiratory paralysis). Substances such as the tetraethylammonium (TEA^+) ion depress the kinetics of activation of the K^+ channels, thereby prolonging the cardiac AP and having important repercussions on the physiology of the heart. Some agents, like veratridine, prolong the AP by a different mechanism, namely, by depressing the kinetics of spontaneous inactivation of the voltage-activated fast Na^+ channels (i.e., the closing of the inactivation gate is slowed). Other agents can directly or indirectly, via a metabolic action, affect the release or uptake of Ca^{2+} from the SR. Therefore for an understanding of the mode of action of cardiotoxic agents, it is important for the reader to review the electrical properties and behavior of the myocardial cell membrane (e.g., see refs. 16 and 17) (Tables 1–3).

TABLE 1. *Some agents that affect contractility of the myocardium*

Positive inotropic agents	Negative inotropic agents	Contracture-inducing agents
ATX	Tricyclic antidepressants	Volvatoxin A
Veratridine	Phenothiazines	Metabolic poisons
Catecholamines (high concentration)	Chlorpromazine	Cardiac glycosides
Methylxanthines	Barbiturates	GTX
Adriamycin (low dose)	Adriamycin (high dose)	BTX
Cardiac glycosides (low dose)	Chlorinated solvents	ATX
Vanadate	Quinidine	
Histamine	Local anesthetics	
Angiotensin II	Metabolic poisons; hypoxia	
Increased $[Ca]_o$	Acidosis	
GTX-1	Cardiac glycosides (high dose)	
	Verapamil; D600	
	Nifedipine	
	Papaverine	
	Mn^{2+}, Co^{2+}, La^{3+}	
	Aminoglycoside antibiotics	
	Endotoxin	
	ACh	

TABLE 2. *Effects of some agents on contraction, automaticity, and rhythm*

Conduction slowed	A-V conduction depressed or blocked	SA nodal and ectopic automaticity		Arrhythmias	
		Depressed	Enhanced	Suppressed	Developed
Quinidine	ACh	Quinidine	Ba²⁺	Quinidine	Cardiac glycosides
Local anesthetics (high doses)	Tricyclic antidepressants	Local anesthetics	TEA⁺	Local anesthetics	Tricyclic antidepressants
TTX, STX	Cd²⁺	Verapamil	Catecholamines	Verapamil	Chlorpromazine
Tricyclic antidepressants	Verapamil	Mn²⁺	Adriamycin	Bepridil	Adriamycin
Phenothiazines		Increased [K]ₒ	Marijuana		Emetine
					Chloroquine
					Aconitine
					Phenothiazines
					Ischemia

Excitability		Heart Rate	
Enhanced	Depressed	Slowed	Accelerated
Low [Ca]ₒ	Quinidine	Cardiac glycosides	Beta-adrenergic agonists
Ba²⁺ (low dose)	Local anesthetics	Tricyclic antidepressants (high doses)	Tricyclic antidepressants (low doses)
TEA⁺	TTX, STX	Cd²⁺	Emetine; chloroquine
4-AP	Ba²⁺ (high dose)	ACh	Ba²⁺ (low dose)
9-AA	Cardiac glycosides (high dose)	TTX, STX	Methylxanthines
Veratridine	High [Ca]ₒ	All slow-channel blockers	Marijuana
BTX (low dose)	Veratridine (high dose, long time)		
GTX (low dose)			
Cardiac glycosides (low dose)			

Note: Lidocaine and phenytoin increase max dV/dt at low doses, as does elevated [Ca]ₒ. ACh also has the same effect, secondary to the hyperpolarization. Lidocaine and phenytoin increase conduction velocity at low doses.

TABLE 3. Effects of some agents on the resting potential and action potential

Depolarization	max dV/dt and responsiveness depressed	Action potential duration		Functional refractory period	
		Prolonged	Shortened	Prolonged	Shortened
Veratridine	Quinidine	Ba^{2+}	TTX	Quinidine	TTX
Aconitine	Local anesthetics (high doses)	TEA^+	ACh	Local anesthetics	ACh
GTX	TTX, STX	4-AP	Verapamil		Verapamil
BTX	Trichloroethylene	9-AA	Mn^{2+}		Mn^{2+}
ATX	Tricyclic antidepressants	Veratridine	Valinomycin		Valinomycin
Trichloroethylene		GTX	Hypoxia (long times)		Hypoxia (long times)
Adriamycin	Chlorpromazine	BTX	High $[Ca]_o$		High $[Ca]_o$
Ba^{2+}	Depolarizing agents	ATX	Local anesthetics		
Cardiac glycosides (high doses, long times)	Salicylates	CTX	Gentamycin		
		Salicylates	Alcohol		
Local anesthetics (high doses, long times)		Adriamycin	Increased $[K]_o$		
Metabolic depression		Cyclophosphamide	Metabolic depression		
Agents that decrease g_K		Nicotine			
Increased $[K]_o$		Depolarizing agents			
Endotoxin					

Heart damage is associated with the administration of many therapeutic drugs and with exposure to a variety of chemicals. Potentially cardiotoxic drugs include antineoplastic agents, antibiotics, psychological antidepressant agents, antimalarials and emetine, analgesics, antiarrhythmics, local anesthetics, general anesthetics, barbiturates, sympathomimetic amines, antihypertensives, and cardiac glycosides. Cardiotoxic chemicals that people are exposed to include alcohol, marijuana, nicotine, endotoxins, insecticides, fungicides, heavy metals, chlorinated solvents, fluorocarbons, and the natural toxins produced by a variety of poisonous animals and plants. This chapter presents only some representative cardiotoxic substances from many of these chemical groups.

Focus is on the changes in myocardial membrane electrical properties that these drugs and chemicals produce and the mechanism(s) of action is given when known. Considerable findings are presented from the giant axons of invertebrates, because these are the excitable membrane preparations in which the most information is known. However, as a general rule (with a few notable exceptions), the actions of drugs are similar in all excitable membranes whether they be from nerve, skeletal muscle, or heart, and whether in vertebrates or invertebrates. When there are differences, they most often deal with the relative sensitivity of the various membranes to the agent.

EFFECTS OF SOME CARDIOTOXIC AGENTS

Metabolic Poisons, Hypoxia, Ischemia, and Acidosis

Inhibitors of metabolism and hypoxia can produce a great number of nonspecific toxic effects on the heart. For example, lowering of the ATP level will depress the rate of Na–K pumping, and so the cells may depolarize because of (a) inhibition of V_{pump} and (b) gradual rundown of the ionic gradients (e.g., decrease in $[K]_i$). However, the degree of depolarization produced is reduced because the contribution of V_{pump} to the resting E_m may be increased, thus tending to hold the resting E_m constant; this protects against the repercussions of a substantial depolarization. For example, very little depolarization is produced after 1 hr of severe hypoxia. On the other hand, with more prolonged and severe metabolic interference, the myocardial cells do depolarize. During ischemia, in addition to the resultant hypoxia, other factors are involved, including K^+ accumulation in the interstitial space, which itself produces depolarization.

Metabolic inhibition and lowering of the ATP level (in hypoxia, the ATP level declines to about 25% of the control value within 20 min) (18–21) also may lower the cAMP level, since ATP is the substrate for adenylate cyclase. This in turn could affect the activity of cAMP–protein kinase and the number of available slow channels in the myocardial membrane. This reduces or abolishes the inward slow Ca^{2+} current and so depresses contraction and blocks the Ca^{2+}-dependent slow APs. The quick effect produced is to slightly depress the overshoot and plateau duration of the AP. However, the slower effect of metabolic interference is to markedly shorten the plateau, due to unmasking of an ATP-regulated K^+ channel.

With ischemia, a large and rapid acidosis is produced, intracellularly and extracellularly (22–24). The same might be expected by hypoxia or metabolic poisons, such as cyanide, that block oxidative metabolism and thereby promote anaerobic glycolysis and lactic acid production. Acidosis is known to depress contractility, with only little effect on the normal cardiac AP; one mechanism for this effect is the selective blockade of the slow Ca^{2+} channels at acid pH (25–27). Blockade of the slow Ca^{2+} channels (Fig. 1), and hence the slow Ca^{2+} current, inhibits Ca^{2+} influx and contractions, causing excitation–contraction uncoupling. Acidosis also depresses metabolism (28).

Acidosis protects against the deleterious effects of hypoxia, with respect to the degree of recovery of contractility that occurs after a period of hypoxia (29,30). The mechanism of this protective effect of acidosis was suggested to be the blockade of the slow Ca^{2+} channels (Fig. 1) by acidosis,

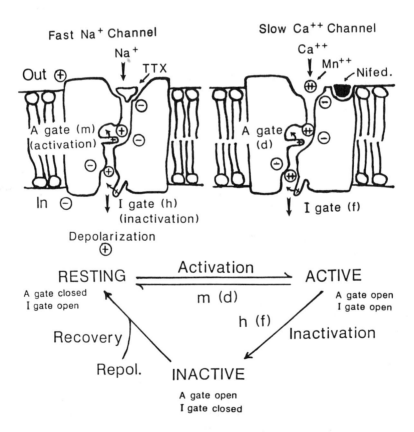

thus inhibiting Ca^{2+} influx and depressing the contractions, and so sparing ATP (4,24,31). That is, acidosis further weakens contraction during hypoxia but allows greater recovery afterward. When the Ca^{2+}-dependent slow APs are blocked during hypoxia, suddenly changing the pH of the perfusing solution to pH 8.0 ("pH clamp") rapidly reverses (partially) the effect of hypoxia; the slow APs reappear, but the rate of rise and force of contraction are lower compared to the control (prehypoxic) period (31). The reversal by alkalosis is temporary in that, with continued hypoxia, the force of contraction and maximum dV/dt of the slow AP progressively diminish. These results suggest that an important factor in blocking of the slow Ca^{2+} channels during hypoxia is the accompanying acidosis, because the ATP level was not so far depressed that slow APs accompanied by contractions could not be produced.

The effects of some metabolic poisons, such as valinomycin (an uncoupler of oxidative phosphorylation, like dinitrophenol), or of hypoxia can be re-

---

FIG. 1. Top: Cartoon models for a fast Na^+ channel (*left diagram*) and for a slow Ca^{2+} channel (*right diagram*) in myocardial cell membrane. As depicted, there are two gates associated with each type of channel: an activation (A) gate and an inactivation (I) gate. The gates are presumably charged positively so that they can sense the membrane potential. The I gate moves more slowly than the A gate. The fast Na^+ channel is depicted in the resting state (A gate closed, I gate open) and just beginning the process of activation. Depolarization causes the A gate to open quickly, so that the channel becomes conducting (the active state). However, the I gate slowly (within 1–2 msec) closes during depolarization and inactivates the channel (the inactive state). During recovery upon repolarization, the A gate recloses and the I gate reopens (returns to the resting state). Tetrodotoxin (TTX) blocks the fast Na^+ channel from the outside, presumably by binding in the channel mouth. In addition, the gates of the slow channels operate over a less negative (more depolarized) voltage range. The gates of the slow channels, on a population basis, appear to be kinetically much slower than those of the fast Na^+ channels. Not depicted is the hypothesis that a protein constituent of the slow Ca^{2+} channel must be phosphorylated in order for the channel to be in a functional state available for voltage activation. Diltiazem and nifedipine block the slow channels, perhaps by binding to the outer surface of the channel protein. Mn^{2+} may block by displacing Ca^{2+} from a binding site in the outer mouth of the channel. **Bottom:** Diagram of the three states of the fast Na^+ channels and slow channels in the myocardial cell membrane. Conversion from the resting state to the active state by depolarization is known as activation and corresponds to the m factor of Hodgkin and Huxley (or d factor for myocardial slow channels): $g_{Na} = g_{Na} m^3 h$. The active state spontaneously converts to the inactive state, even though the membrane potential remains depolarized. This process is known as inactivation and corresponds to the h factor of Hodgkin and Huxley (or f factor for slow channels). The inactivated channel can be converted back to the resting state, from which it can be reactivated again only by repolarization of the membrane toward the resting potential. This process is known as recovery. The conversions from one state to another occur rapidly for the fast Na^+ channels (e.g., over a few milliseconds) but appear to be slow (on a population basis) for the slow channels (e.g., over tens of milliseconds). The inactivation time constant for the slow channel conductance is long, being up to 200 msec. The process of activation is reversible. Once in the inactivated state, the channel can only go into the active state again by first passing through the resting state. In the resting state, the activation (A) gate is closed and the inactivation (I) gate is open. In the active state, both A gate and I gate are open (I gate beginning to close, but with a longer time constant compared to the movement of the A gate). In the inactive state, the A gate is open but the I gate is closed. The gates are presumably charged positively, and their movements reflect changes in the transmembrane potential.

versed or prevented by elevation of glucose several-fold above normal (e.g., from 10 to 50 mM). This was demonstrated both for the plateau shortening that occurs in the normal fast APs (32–34) and for the blockade of the slow APs (33,34). The high glucose reversal presumably results from stimulation of glycolysis and elevation of the cellular ATP level.

Catecholamines and Caffeine

High doses of catecholamines are known to produce cardiomyopathies. One proposed mechanism for this catecholamine-induced myocardial necrosis is a direct effect on the heart resulting from an increased Ca^{2+} influx through the slow channels. For example, it was shown that agents that increase Ca^{2+} influx, such as catecholamines, increase the size of experimental myocardial infarcts, whereas agents that depress Ca^{2+} influx, such as verapamil, tend to decrease the degree of catecholamine-induced necrosis (35, 36).

It has even been proposed that the ischemic release of myocardial norepinephrine (37,38), brought about by the transient constriction of a coronary artery, may play an important role in the myocardial infarction process (39). It was proposed that a vicious cycle is started between the catecholamine-induced increase in O_2 demand and the catecholamine-induced vasoconstriction and ischemic damage. It was suggested (39,40) that coronary artery thrombosis could be secondary to the deleterious effects of catecholamines, which are known to cause thrombocyte aggregation. Perfusion of isolated rat hearts with NE (10^{-7} to 10^{-4} M) caused (a) leakage of several myocardial enzymes, (b) depression of ATP level, and (c) ultrastructural changes (39). Pretreatment with a beta-adrenergic blocker, a Ca^{2+} antagonist (verapamil), or a membrane stabilizer (lidocaine) prevented these effects. Tyramine (to rapidly release myocardial catecholamines) caused the same damage as NE.

The deleterious effects of catecholamines may result from activation of the beta-adrenergic receptor, stimulation of the adenylate cyclase, and elevation of cAMP. The latter activates cAMP-dependent protein kinase and increases the state of phosphorylation of the slow Ca^{2+} channels (Fig. 1). This would make a greater fraction of the Ca^{2+} channels become available for voltage activation. Thus the Ca^{2+} influx per beat would increase, and possibly lead to Ca^{2+} overload of the myocardial cells (the "stone heart" syndrome) (41). Ca^{2+} overload occurs because the Ca^{2+} influx is greater than the efflux (i.e., greater than what the cells can handle). The bailout of Ca^{2+} from the cell is primarily via the sarcolemmal Ca^{2+}–ATPase pump and the Ca_i–Na_o exchange reaction. The high internal $[Ca^{2+}]$ caused by the catecholamines can produce a variety of functional and morphological changes, including contracture, swollen SR, Ca^{2+} precipitates in the mitochondria, altered enzyme activities, and altered membrane electrical properties. The high $[Ca]_i$ also can overtax the cells metabolically, thus causing the ATP level to be lowered, further hampering the efflux of Ca^{2+} and leading to cellular necrosis.

The methylxanthines, such as caffeine, theophylline (aminophylline), and methyl isobutyl xanthine (MIX) are also positive inotropic agents and thus exert effects similar to the catecholamines, namely, increase of I_{si} and hence Ca^{2+} influx. The methylxanthines act to elevate cAMP by inhibiting the phosphodiesterase that destroys cAMP. The methylxanthines also exert some effects directly on the SR to cause Ca^{2+} release.

Cholera Toxin and Pertussis Toxins

Cholera toxin is an oligometric protein secreted by *Vibrio cholerae* bacteria with an M_r of 84,000 (42). It is composed of two types of subunits (A and B). The B subunits have been shown to bind to ganglioside GM_1 in the cell membrane, followed by insertion of the A subunits into the cell. The A subunit of cholera toxin ADP-ribosylates the G_s (the GTP-binding protein, which is coupled to adenylate cyclase) and results in a maintained activation of adenylate cyclase, and the consequent accumulation of cAMP (43). The elevated levels of cAMP activate cAMP–protein kinase, which may then phosphorylate and thereby activate the Ca^{2+} channels. Cholera toxin injected into ventricular myocytes has been shown to induce Ca^{2+}-dependent slow APs (44).

Pertussis toxin is a bacterial exotoxin produced by *Bordetella pertussis*. Like cholera toxin, pertussis toxin contains an A and a B chain; the B chain binds to glycoprotein surface receptors, which facilitates the insertion of the A chain into the cell. Pertussis toxin ADP-ribosylates the α-subunit of the G-proteins G_i and G_o, and this action results in an inhibition of the activity of the associated adenylate cyclase. Pertussis toxin has also been shown to directly block K^+ ion channels in heart that are opened by acetylcholine (43).

Okadaic Acid

Okadaic acid (OA) is a protein phosphatase inhibitor isolated from marine sponges of the genus *Halichondria*. This toxin is a positive inotrope in isolated cardiac papillary muscle, and it has also been shown to increase the duration of the cardiac AP (45). Recently, it was found that OA (5–100 μM) produced a twofold increase in I_{Ca} recorded from voltage-clamped guinea pig cardiac myocytes (46). Small increases in the delayed rectifier current (I_K) were also observed with OA. The results suggest OA may act to prevent the dephosphorylation of the Ca^{2+} channel protein, thereby enhancing the probability of channel opening, and hence current flow through these channels.

Ca^{2+} Antagonists

Ca^{2+} antagonists depress Ca^{2+} influx through excitable membranes by blocking the slow Ca^{2+} channels (47–50) (Fig. 1). Some of these agents also block slow channels that allow Na^+ to pass through. For example, verapamil and its more active cogener D600 block the slow Na^+ channels found in some hearts (51). The Ca^{2+} antagonists also block the slow Ca^{2+} channels of vascular smooth muscle cells, and so act as vasodilators and antianginal agents. Their action on the myocardial cells bestows negative inotropic action on them. Some of these drugs, particularly those that have strong use dependency, possess some antiarrhythmic properties.

The effect of verapamil and D600 is use dependent; that is, the effect is more pronounced and more rapid in onset with higher frequencies of stimulation. For example, a dose of bepridil that produced complete blockade of the Ca^{2+}-dependent slow APs at a stimulation rate of 1 Hz had virtually no effect at 0.1 Hz or if a rest period of 0.5 min was given (52). Thus it appears that one factor in the blockade is a slowed recovery of the slow Ca^{2+} channels from inactivation.

The effect of verapamil and D600 are slow to reverse upon washing. However, elevating $[Ca]_o$ can antagonize the effect of the drug (47). In cultured heart cells, verapamil also depolarizes (53).

The effect of the dihydropyridine, nifedipine, is less use dependent than is verapamil, and its effect can be more easily washed out. Nifedipine does not affect any of the kinetics of the slow channels (54). Nifedipine is about 10 times more potent than verapamil in blocking slow Ca^{2+} channels in cardiac muscle.

Diltiazem, the third major class of organic Ca^{2+} antagonist drugs, blocks myocardial slow Ca^{2+} channels and current ($I_{Ca(s)}$ or I_{si}) with an IC_{50} value close to verapamil (about 10^{-7} M). Like verapamil and bepridil, diltiazem is strongly use dependent. This compound has the lowest lipid solubility of the Ca^{2+} antagonist drugs and so presumably confines its action to the outer surface of the cell membrane (55). Its effects can be rapidly washed out.

The Ca^{2+} antagonist drugs block only the slow Ca^{2+} channels and current ($I_{Ca(s)}$ or I_{si}) and not the fast Ca^{2+} channel or current ($I_{Ca(f)}$). The slow Ca^{2+} channel is responsible for the long-lasting (L-type), slowly inactivating, high-threshold current, whereas the Ca^{2+} fast channel is responsible for the transient (T-type), rapidly inactivating, low-threshold current.

Papaverine, a vasodilating drug that has some structural similarities to verapamil, also blocks myocardial slow channels (56). However, papaverine also has at least one other effect; namely, it acts as a phosphodiesterase (PDE) inhibitor and thereby elevates cAMP. The slow channel blocking effect predominates in determining the overall response of cardiac muscle to this drug. The vasodilating effect can result from both properties of papaverine, namely, PDE inhibition and Ca^{2+} slow channel blockade.

Because the Ca^{2+} antagonists depress or block Ca^{2+} influx into the myocardial cells, they produce excitation–contraction uncoupling. That is, the APs are only slightly affected (due to loss of the Ca^{2+} slow current), whereas the contractions may be completely suppressed. The fast inward Na^+ current and the K^+ currents are much less affected by Ca^{2+} antagonists (57,58). However, at higher doses, verapamil and bepridil do affect the fast Na^+ current and K^+ currents (52,59–61).

Bepridil, a fourth class of Ca^{2+} antagonist drug and antianginal agent, blocks myocardial slow Ca^{2+} channels (52). However, bepridil was less potent than verapamil in blockade of the slow channels. Bepridil also exerted a second internal effect, which was thought to be depression of Ca^{2+} release from the SR. Thus bepridil was unusual in that it was capable of producing excitation–contraction uncoupling during slow APs.

Various heavy metal cations, such as Mn^{2+}, Co^{2+}, and La^{3+}, also act as Ca^{2+} antagonists that are not use dependent. These cations presumably compete with Ca^{2+} ions for binding sites on the outer surface of the slow channels, thereby displacing Ca^{2+} ions from these sites and preventing their passage through the channels.

Heavy Metals

A number of heavy metals exert potent toxic effects on cardiovascular tissues. The mitochondria are affected by heavy metals, such as Pb^{2+} and Hg^{2+}, including inhibition of Ca^{2+} accumulation and inhibition of oxidative phosphorylation. Many enzymes are sensitive to heavy metals. However, this discussion is limited to some heavy metal ions that directly affect ion channels in excitable membranes.

Manganese (Mn^{2+}) and cobalt (Co^{2+}) ions, at 1 mM, block the Ca^{2+} slow channels (1,62–64). These divalent cations do not block the slow Na^+ channels. In higher concentrations (e.g., >5 mM), these cations are less specific and block other channels, including the fast Na^+ channels (65). Mn^{2+} and Co^{2+} may block the slow Ca^{2+} channels by competition with Ca^{2+} for binding to the outer mouth of the channel, since the first step in penetration of the Ca^{2+} ion through a channel is binding to such a site. In high concentrations (e.g., 10 mM) (and zero Ca^{2+}), Mn^{2+} actually can carry inward current through the slow channels (66,67).

Cardiomyopathy was caused by some beer, which contained added Co^{2+} as a foam stabilizer. In rats, a single ip injection of $CoCl_2$ (30 mg/kg) produced lesions of the myocardial cells, including contracture, myocytolysis, and disintegration of the myofibrils (68). Ischemic lesions (sequelae of thrombosis) also occurred.

Lanthanum (La^{3+}) ions, at 1 mM, also selectively block Ca^{2+} slow channels (1,60,64,69). La^{3+} displaces Ca^{2+} from binding sites on the outer surface of the cell membrane (70,71). La^{3+} does not normally enter into the cells but has been reported to penetrate into hypoxic heart cells (72,73) and into neuraminidase-treated cells (74).

Barium ions (Ba^{2+}), between 0.05 and 2 mM, decrease g_K in a dose-dependent manner and thereby depolarize (75–77). The Ba^{2+} depolarization occurs rapidly in cells in which g_{Cl} is relatively low, like heart cells. The kinetics of activation of g_K are also depressed, so that the AP is greatly prolonged. Sometimes repetitive firing of APs occurs on the prolonged plateau of the first AP (78). Ba^{2+} also can carry inward current through the slow Ca^{2+} channels even better than Ca^{2+} ion (75).

The effect of strontium ion (Sr^{2+}) is more similar to that of Ca^{2+} ion. Sr^{2+} has little or no effect on g_K but can carry current through the slow Ca^{2+} channels better than Ca^{2+} (75,79).

Calcium ion (Ca^{2+}) has potent effects on membrane excitability. In low $[Ca]_o$, the membrane becomes hyperexcitable and spontaneously active; g_{Na} is increased. Therefore any chemical (such as EGTA) or drug that chelates or binds Ca^{2+} will have profound effects on membrane excitability. Ca^{2+} binds to fixed negative charges on the outer surface of the cell membrane and so alters the surface charge or zeta potential. Changes in surface charge (at the outer or inner surface of the membrane) alters the true transmembrane potential, and so alters a variety of electrical properties, such as threshold potential and mechanical threshold. Ca^{2+} also binds to fixed charges in the cell coat (mucopolysaccharides) coating the cell membrane. Ca^{2+} is also required for the release of neurotransmitter from the autonomic nerves supplying the heart and vascular smooth muscle.

Cadmium (Cd^{2+}), an environmental pollutant, exerts powerful cardiotoxic effects. Cd^{2+} depresses contractility of the heart (80). In isolated frog heart, $CdCl_2$ markedly shortened the AP and increased the P-R interval; larger doses caused the heart to stop in diastole (81). In isolated rabbit atria, 0.1 mM Cd^{2+} markedly depressed the AP amplitude and duration, and 0.5 mM abolished the AP, with only a slight reduction in RP. Since the inhibitory effect of Cd^{2+} was partly reversed by cysteine (1 mM) (or elevated $[Ca]_o$), it appears that Cd^{2+} acts on membrane SH groups (82). In rat atrium, 10^{-4} M Cd^{2+} (and Cu^{2+}) shortened the AP and decreased contractile force; the negative inotropic effect was reversed by high $[Ca]_o$; these effects on contraction were produced with little or no effect on the RP or on the AP overshoot (80). However, a positive inotropic effect was produced by Hg^{2+} (about 10^{-5} M) (in normal $[Ca]_o$). Contractility was depressed by Mg^{2+} (8.2 mM), Mn^{2+} (0.5 mM), Zn^{2+} (0.6 mM), Co^{2+} (7×10^{-5} M), and Ni^{2+} (0.5 mM).

Cd^{2+} (0.5 mM) was more potent than Zn^{2+}, $Mn,^{2+}$, or La^{3+} in depressing contractile force in perfused neonatal rat papillary muscle (83), and it was concluded that the cation sequence for depression of contraction was in the same order as their ability to displace Ca^{2+} from extracellular rapidly exchangeable Ca^{2+} binding sites: La > Cd > Zn > Mn > Mg.

In isolated perfused rat hearts, Cd^{2+} (3×10^{-5} M) caused a progressive increase in the P-R interval of the ECG, and then partial or complete A-V block; heart rate was decreased (84). Rats given Cd^{2+} in their drinking water also developed prolonged P-R intervals and other signs of marked changes in cardiac conduction (85). There was hypertrophy and vacuolization of the cells of the His–Purkinje system.

Vanadate ion (VO_4^{3-}), a known inhibitor of the Na/K–ATPase (see Table 6), exerts a positive inotropic effect in ventricular (papillary) muscle (ED_{50} of about 100 μM) but a negative inotropic effect in atrial muscle of several mammalian species (IC_{50} of about 3–30 μM) (86). The atrial APs were markedly shortened, whereas those of the ventricular muscle were slightly lengthened. Since the inhibition of the Na/K–ATPase was about the same in atria and ventricles, it was concluded that vanadate exerts its inotropic effects by some mechanism other than by inhibition of the Na–K pump, namely, by altering the AP duration. Vanadate did not produce arrhythmias. In cultured chick heart (ventricular) cells, vanadate (0.5 mM) produced repetitive firing of spikes on a lengthened plateau (P. Jourdon and N. Sperelakis, *unpublished observations*).

K⁺ Channel Blockers

Agents that depress the K^+ channels in all excitable membranes, including heart cells, include tetraethylammonium ion (TEA^+, 5–15 mM), aminopyridines (2-AP, 3-AP, and 4-AP, 1 mM), Ba^{2+} ion (0.05–2.0 mM), Cs^+ ion (1–10 mM), Rb^+ ion (1–10 mM), and local anesthetics (10^{-5} to 10^{-3} M) (see Table 5). Most of these agents depress both the resting g_K and the excitable K^+ channels (depress the voltage-dependent activation of g_K). The kinetics of turn-on of the K^+ channels is also slowed. The steady-state voltage–current curve is linearized by the K^+ channel blockers, indicative of suppression of the inward-rectifying K^+ channel (I_{K1}). Because resting g_K is lowered (R_m increased), the ratio of g_{Na}/g_K is increased and depolarization results.

Ba^{2+} ion is one of the most potent K^+ channel blockers. Ba^{2+} raises R_m by decreasing resting g_K and depolarizes cardiac muscle in a dose-dependent manner (75,77). In skeletal muscle bathed in Cl^--free solution to lower g_{Cl}, Ba^{2+} depolarizes and induces automaticity (spontaneous production of Ca^{2+}-dependent slow APs) (76).

TEA^+ blocks the voltage-dependent K^+ channels from the inner surface of the membrane by lodging inside the activation gate of the channel (87). Thus the suppression of K^+ activation by TEA^+ is use dependent (or frequency dependent), because TEA^+ can only enter the K^+ channel to bind when the gate is open. If a large driving force is applied for K^+ ion to enter the K^+ channel from the outside, the blocking TEA^+ molecule can be dislodged, thus relieving the block. A number of longer acyl chain TEA analogs can also enter the K^+ channel and block (88).

The aminopyridines were effective in squid giant axon when applied to either internal or external membrane surfaces (89). Repetitive depolarizing voltage-clamp pulses relieve the steady-state block of the K^+ channels in a manner dependent on the magnitude of the clamp pulse and the duration of the interval between pulses. It was concluded that the aminopyridine molecules bind to closed K^+ channels but are released from open channels in a voltage-dependent manner. Similar effects of 4-aminopyridine were observed in frog skeletal muscle (90).

9-Aminoacridine (0.1–1 mM) has an effect similar to that of Ba^{2+}, namely, an inhibition of P_K. For example, 9-aminoacridine inhibits K^+ efflux (increasing $[K]_i$) and augments and prolongs the depolarizing afterpotential in skeletal muscle (91).

The K^+ channel blockers, such as TEA^+ and Ba^{2+}, also greatly prolong the APs, even prior to any significant depolarization. This is due to their slowing of K^+ activation (g_K turn-on) that terminates the AP. Thus the plateau is lengthened and/or prominent depolarizing afterpotentials are developed. In cultured heart cells, for example, Ba^{2+} (1 mM) greatly prolonged the AP plateau and often small regenerative spikes were superimposed on the plateau component (78).

The depression of g_K and K^+ activation by agents such as Ba^{2+} and TEA^+ also causes them to increase excitability. For example, arterial vascular smooth muscle, that is usually electrically inexcitable *in vitro,* can be made to respond to electrical stimulation or even to fire APs spontaneously by Ba^{2+} or TEA^+ (79,92,93). The mechanism for this action presumably is the decrease in outward I_K, which allows the net inward current to be greater, and thereby to support regenerative activity.

Charybdotoxin (ChTX), a peptide inhibitor from scorpion venom, has been shown to be a highly potent inhibitor of the high-conductance Ca^{2+}-activated K^+ channel ($g_{K(Ca)}$) of mammalian skeletal muscle (94). Apamin, a polypeptide toxin in bee venom, has a similar effect (95).

K^+ Channel Openers

There is a new class of compounds that open K^+ channels. These compounds include pinacidil, nicorandil, chromakalim, and lemakalim (optical isomer of chromakalin). These drugs activate several types of K^+ channels, including those that are Ca^{2+} dependent ($g_{K(Ca)}$), both large-conductance and small-conductance types, ATP regulated ($g_{K(ATP)}$), and delayed rectifier type ($g_{K(del)}$) (96). Opening K^+ channels in VSM cells increases g_K and therefore the g_{Na}/g_K ratio is decreased, resulting in hyperpolarization (5–25 mV) of the cells (97). Such hyperpolarization decreases the excitability of the cell membrane and brings E_m more negative than the mechanical threshold voltage. This results in muscle relaxation and hence vasodilation. Such drugs thereby have potent antihypertensive effects. The action of the K^+ channel openers/ vasodilators is blocked by glibenclamide, 4-aminopyridine, and TEA^+, but not by apamin or charybdotoxin (98). In VSM cells of rat portal vein, the glibenclamide-sensitive K^+ channel had a small single-channel conductance of 10 pS and was sensitive to both Ca^{2+} and ATP. In cat cerebral artery VSM cells, the glibenclamide-sensitive K^+ channel was 98 pS and was sensitive to Ca^{2+} (99). Glibenclamide also prevented the hypoxic increase in mean open time and open probability of the 98-pS K^+ channel (and hence vaso-dilation). In canine renal artery VSM cells, lemakalin activated a large-con-ductance (217 pS) K^+ channel by increasing $N \cdot P_o$ (number of channels ac-tive in a patch times the open probability).

Bretylium and Bethanidine

Bretylium, an antifibrillatory and antiarrhythmic drug, was reported to produce K^+ channel blockade in heart cells (100). When applied intracellu-larly in squid giant axon, bretylium blocked the fast inward Na^+ current (I_{Na}) as well as I_K. Using the patch pipette technique in single isolated ven-tricular cells from old embryonic chick hearts, extracellular (bath) applica-tion of bretylium decreased I_K but had no effect on the fast I_{Na} (101,102). Introducing bretylium intracellularly inhibited I_{Na} as well as I_K.

Bethanidine, another antifibrillatory drug, was also found to inhibit I_K in single embryonic chick heart cells; however, it also potentiated the slow Ca^{2+} current ($I_{Ca(s)}$) and fast Na^+ current (I_{Na}) (101). This drug also exerted, as predicted, a positive inotropic effect. Intracellular application of bethan-idine inhibited I_{Na}, as in the case of bretylium.

In single vascular smooth muscle cells from rabbit aorta, bethanidine (10^{-4} M) decreased the early outward K^+ current ($I_{K(to)}$), but increased the delayed rectifier K^+ current ($I_{K(del)}$) (103). The resting potential was hyper-polarized and contraction was inhibited. It was suggested that the vasodila-tory effect of bethanidine is associated with activation of K^+ channels, caus-ing hyperpolarization.

Cardiac Glycosides

The digitalis compounds exert potent effects on the heart, including their well-known positive inotropic action. The cardiac glycosides increase the maximal force generated and the rate at which the force is developed. There is a fine line between the therapeutic effects (e.g., for congestive heart fail-ure) of the cardiac glycosides and the toxic effects. It is widely believed that the therapeutic and toxic effects act by the same mechanism, the toxic man-ifestations being to a greater degree. The major specific action of the cardiac glycosides is the inhibition of the Na/K–ATPase and Na–K pump in the cell membrane (see Table 6). Although there is some degree of variability from tissue to tissue with respect to the dose–response curves, in general, 50% inhibition of the enzyme occurs at 10^{-7} to 10^{-6} M ouabain.

The therapeutic effect of digitalis on cardiac contractility is presumably due to partial inhibition of the Na–K pump, thus causing an elevation in $[Na]_i$, and this in turn produces a steady-state elevation of $[Ca]_i$ because of the Ca–Na exchange system. The elevation in $[Ca]_i$ may allow the SR to load more with Ca^{2+}, for a greater release in subsequent beats. That is, there may be a shift in Ca^{2+} balance so that more Ca^{2+} is retained by the myocardial cells. In this view, the therapeutic action of digitalis is to make more Ca^{2+} available to the myofilaments (104).

The toxic effect of the cardiac glycosides is presumably due to a greater degree of inhibition of the Na–K pump that causes the ionic gradients to run down too far and cause a Ca^{2+} overload. The Ca^{2+} overload produces a number of deleterious functional and morphological changes, and the rundown of the Na^+ and K^+ gradients leads to partial depolarization and all of its repercussions. In addition, overloading the SR with Ca^{2+} causes uncontrolled Ca^{2+} release and resulting delayed afterdepolarizations (DADs) and triggered arrhythmias.

Release of catecholamines from nerve terminals, another effect of the cardiac glycosides (which may be mediated by inhibition of the Na–K pump and elevation of $[Ca]_i$), could contribute to their overall cardiotoxicity. The catecholamines may act primarily to increase Ca^{2+} influx and augment the Ca^{2+} overload. The therapeutic positive inotropic effect of digitalis is not dependent on catecholamine release.

The cardiac glycosides do not increase the inward slow current in myocardial cells but instead, at high doses, they act to depress the slow current (3,105). This means that their positive inotropic action in heart cannot be explained by such a mechanism. However, in the case of vascular smooth muscle (dog coronary arteries), the inward slow current (Ca^{2+} influx) is greatly increased by cardiac glycosides (106). This action may explain the known coronary vasoconstrictor effect of the cardiac glycosides, which also could contribute to their cardiotoxicity.

The cardiac glycosides also could have an internal site of action that may contribute to their therapeutic or toxic actions on the heart. For example, the SR was shown histochemically to have some ouabain-sensitive ATPase activity (107), and the glycosides are known to be able to penetrate intracellularly.

The cardiac glycosides also can induce cardiac arrhythmias, which can lead to dire consequences. One mechanism proposed for genesis of the arrhythmias concerns the fact that the glycosides increase the incidence and magnitude of the depolarizing afterpotentials (DADs) that follow the hyperpolarizing afterpotential and spike (108,109). The DAD, if it reaches the threshold potential, triggers a spike. This mechanism has been proposed as one basis for generation of ectopic foci in the myocardium. The DAD are due to a transient release of Ca^{2+} ion from the SR, which activates a mixed conductance channel ($g_{Na,K(Ca)}$). The DADs are suppressed by Ca antagonist drugs because they reduce Ca^{2+} overload of the SR.

Digitalis increases the automaticity of ectopic pacemakers due to the increase in slope of the pacemaker potential (accompanying the depolarization) (110). For example, there is an acceleration of the latent pacemaker activity of the Purkinje fibers. Ectopic impulse generation can be exposed in early digitalis intoxication by vagal stimulation that allows time for the ectopic impulse to escape (111). Although the early digitalis toxicity is due to such an enhanced ectopic pacemaker mechanism, as the toxicity advances and further depolarization occurs, conduction velocity is depressed. The two effects combine to set the stage for reentrant activity, culminating in ventricular fibrillation (110). Part of the toxic effect of digitalis on automaticity is mediated by the autonomic nervous system, and beta-adrenergic blocking agents provide some protection against the digitalis-induced arrhythmias.

The electrical excitability of the atrium and ventricle is slightly increased by low doses of digitalis, but depressed by higher doses (110). The enhanced excitability is due to a lower RP, hence smaller critical depolarization required to reach the threshold potential. Depressed excitability is produced presumably by greater depolarization and inactivation of fast Na^+ channels. Digitalis-induced depression of excitability decreases progressively from atrium to Purkinje to ventricular fibers (i.e., the ventricular muscle is most resistant). Since conduction velocity is a function of rate of rise and amplitude of the AP, conduction is impaired or fails because of the decreased RP. Conduction through the A-V node is also depressed (reflected by increases in the P-R and A-H intervals). High doses also cause slowing of conduction in the Purkinje fibers (reflected by increases in the H-V and P-R intervals), and even complete A-V block.

Digitalis also slows the heart rate (in patients with congestive heart failure who have reflex tachycardia) and dramatically slows the ventricular rate in atrial fibrillation (110). The slowing of the heart rate is mediated in part by the vagus nerve and in part by a direct action on the heart. Pacemaker suppression by ACh is enhanced by digitalis, and pacemaker stimulation by NE is reduced (an anti-adrenergic action). In the direct action, digitalis prolongs the refractory period of the A-V node, resulting in a decrease in the proportion of "concealed" impulses that can pass through the node during atrial fibrillation (or flutter). (In concealed A-V conduction, most of the high-frequency impulses in the atria are extinguished by decremental conduction within the node and thus fail to emerge, but leave the upper margin refractory to the passage of subsequent impulses.) Thus the ventricular frequency is slowed under these conditions because the atrial margin of the A-V node is left refractory by the concealed impulses. In addition, an increase in vagal activity caused by digitalis can reduce the ventricular rate during atrial fibrillation by reducing the duration of the atrial refractory period (shortened APs), and so increasing the fibrillation frequency and causing the atrial margin of the node to be refractory more often. Thus there are some beneficial antiarrhythmic actions of digitalis.

Local Anesthetics, Phenytoin

Local anesthetics block excitable membranes without appreciably affecting the resting E_m. Both the peak transient inward current (I_{Na}) and the steady-state outward current (I_K) are suppressed by local anesthetics (112). The time to peak current (i.e., kinetics of Na^+ activation) is only slightly affected by the local anesthetics. The local anesthetics may block the AP from inside the membrane. The tertiary amine local anesthetics (e.g., lidocaine and procaine) penetrate through the membrane in the un-ionized form and block from inside in the ionized form; thus they are about equally effective when applied to either side of the membrane. The quarternary amine local anesthetics, which penetrate less readily because of their net charge, block much more effectively when applied inside.

The fast Na^+ channels (Fig. 1) and slow Na^+ channels of cultured chick heart cells are both blocked by local anesthetics (Table 3). The normal (fast) AP (dependent on fast I_{Na}) and slow AP (dependent on I_{Ca}) had similar dose–response curves (50% depression of max dV/dt at about 10^{-4} M) (113). However, the depressed fast AP (in 10 mM $[K]_o$ to lower max dV/dt) is more sensitive to blockade by the local anesthetics (114). In summary, the local anesthetics depress both the resting and voltage-activated membrane conductances, including the fast inward Na^+ current, slow Ca^{2+} current, and K^+ outward current; that is, they act as nonspecific membrane stabilizers. The local anesthetics also depolarize heart cells, and this effect may result from a decrease in resting g_K and depression of the Na/K-ATPase (115–117).

Several local anesthetics (e.g., lidocaine and procainamide) are also used as cardiac antiarrhythmic agents. The mechanism of the antiarrhythmic action is not fully understood. Procainamide depresses the excitability of the atrium and ventricle (118). Conduction is slowed, and pacemaker potentials (phase 4 depolarization) are suppressed. Procainamide usually prolongs the functional refractory period more than the AP; that is, recovery of the ionic channels is slowed. The ECG changes, reflecting these effects of the drug, include widening of the QRS complex and prolongation of the P-R and Q-T intervals. Ventricular extrasystoles are suppressed. These properties of the drugs contribute to their antifibrillatory and antiarrhythmic qualities. Contractility of the heart is also depressed. The effects of quinidine are much like those of procainamide. At low concentrations (10^{-5} M), lidocaine and diphenylhydantoin (but not procaine or cocaine) actually increase max dV/dt (113,119,120), and this action had been used to partly explain their antiarrhythmic properties (121,122).

Lidocaine is used in the treatment of ventricular arrhythmias (118). Its antiarrhythmic action develops very rapidly and declines quickly when discontinued. Like procainamide, lidocaine shortens the APs of both Purkinje fibers and myocardial cells and reduces the functional refractory period of Purkinje fibers; but the AP duration is decreased more than the refractory period is decreased. The membrane responsiveness curve is depressed at high concentrations of lidocaine ($>>3$ μg/ml). Lidocaine depresses automaticity (the pacemaker current) that occurs at high levels of E_m (e.g., in Purkinje cells) (123,124) but has little effect on the automaticity that occurs at low levels of E_m (e.g., in nodal cells) (114).

Diphenylhydantoin (phenytoin) abolishes ventricular tachycardias due to ectopic foci and antagonizes digitalis arrhythmias (118). In low concentrations, phenytoin depresses pacemaker activity in Purkinje fibers and has a similar effect on the SA nodal cells at higher concentrations (e.g., 10^{-4} M). Phenytoin can cause fatal cardiac arrest due to oversuppression of automaticity. Excitability is not depressed and the functional refractory period is not prolonged. The AP duration of Purkinje fibers is shortened, but the functional refractory period is not shortened in proportion. Phenytoin produces a striking increase in max dV/dt of Purkinje fibers, particularly when this parameter is depressed (e.g., by digitalis). This reduces the chance of impaired conduction and block, and hence of reentrant rhythms.

Yohimbine

Yohimbine, a naturally occurring indole–alkylamine alkaloid with alpha-adrenergic blocking properties, depresses both the fast Na^+ current and the delayed rectifier K^+ current in a use-dependent manner (125,126). Yohimbine also is a competitive inhibitor of the BTX-induced increase in P_{Na} (127). In perfused old embryonic chick hearts, yohimbine depressed max dV/dt and overshoot and prolonged the AP; complete blockade of the AP and fast Na^+ channels occurred at 5×10^{-4} M (128). At 10^{-5} to 10^{-4} M, yohimbine induced and enhanced Ca^{2+}-dependent slow APs; at 10^{-3} M, it depressed and blocked the slow APs. Consistent with this dual action, yohimbine exerted a small positive inotropic action at low concentration and a larger negative inotropic action at high concentration. Thus yohimbine exerts a local anesthetic-like effect on myocardial cells, blocking both fast Na^+ channels and slow Ca^{2+} channels (fast Na^+ channels being more sensitive) and blocking K^+ channels.

Quinidine and Amiodarone

Quinidine is the d-isomer of quinine found in the bark of the cinchona tree; both alkaloids are antimalarial. They depress the contractions of cardiac muscle. Quinidine is used in treatment of atrial fibrillation and certain other cardiac arrhythmias (118). It depresses excitability of the heart, prolongs the functional refractory period, and decreases max dV/dt of the AP with resultant decrease in conduction velocity. Quinidine produces a significant shift of the max dV/dt versus E_m curve (membrane responsiveness curve), such that greater inactivation occurs at more negative E_m values. This has the effect of requiring the membrane to become more completely repolarized following one AP before another propagated AP can occur. Thus a premature AP initiated during the relative refractory period (during phase 3) may fail to propagate. Hence quinidine tends to abolish premature APs caused by a reentrant circuit.

The APs of the SA node are prolonged by quinidine, but those of myocardial cells and Purkinje fibers are not. That is, the prolongation of the functional refractory period is not accompanied by a comparable increase in AP duration, the tissue remaining refractory for an appreciable period after full restoration of the resting E_m. This suggests that the drug depresses the recovery process of the ionic channels (Fig. 1).

In addition, quinidine decreases the slope of the pacemaker potential of the SA node; that is, it depresses automaticity. Ectopic pacemaker activity is also suppressed, perhaps due to both depression of automaticity and to elevation of threshold, and it is this action that is probably most responsible for its antiarrhythmic effect. Quinidine also exerts an anticholinergic action, preventing the cardiac slowing produced by vagal stimulation.

In summary, quinidine acts to abolish premature APs initiated by a reentrant circuit or by ectopic pacemaker activity, thus giving the drug antiarrhythmic properties. The cardiac actions of quinidine are similar to those produced by procainamide.

With respect to cardiotoxicity, quinidine may cause cardiac asystole or paroxysms of ventricular tachycardia and fibrillation. Quinidine is not recommended in cases of incomplete or complete A-V block and in the treatment of digitalis intoxication. Quinidine (10^{-5} to 10^{-3} M) may also depress the contraction of cardiac muscle by inhibiting the Ca–ATPase of the SR (129) (see Table 6).

Amiodarone, an antiarrhythmic and antianginal agent, increases coronary flow, reduces O_2 consumption by the heart, and antagonizes the actions of catecholamines. This agent also protects against ouabain-induced ventricular fibrillation (130). It markedly prolongs the cardiac AP (130).

Barbiturates

Pentobarbital, a general anesthetic agent, causes marked depression of myocardial contractility within 15 min after administration (30 mg/kg iv) (131). Pentobarbital, when applied from either side of the membrane, depresses (reversibly) both the Na^+ and K^+ conductance activations that occur during excitation in squid axon (132). The kinetics of g_{Na} turn-on were unaffected, but the peak g_{Na} versus E_m curve was shifted in the depolarizing direction. Similar findings were obtained in lobster giant axon. Pentobarbital decreased both the peak transient inward current (I_{Na}) and late steady-state outward current (I_K), and the maximum conductances for Na^+ and K^+; the g_{Na} versus E_m curve was shifted in the depolarizing direction (133). However, the barbiturate also slowed the rate at which g_{Na} turns on. From the relative effectiveness at different pH values, it was concluded that the anionic form of the drug was the active form and it became inserted into the lipid bilayer of the membrane.

General Anesthetics

Halothane has a negative inotropic effect (134). For example, 2% halothane markedly depressed myocardial contractility (131). Halothane inhibits Ca^{2+} uptake by the SR in mechanically skinned myocardial fibers and in microsomal fractions, consistent with the myocardial depression (135,136) (see Table 6). Halothane had little or no effect on the Ca^{2+}-induced release of Ca^{2+} from the SR or on the pCa versus tension relationship. In isolated cardiac SR, the depression of Ca^{2+} uptake was paralleled by depression of the Ca–ATPase activity (137). However, the concentration of halothane required to inhibit Ca^{2+} uptake was much greater than that required to depress contraction. Halothane also inhibits actomyosin ATPase (136,138) and alters the conformation of proteins.

The effects of halothane on the membrane electrical properties seem to vary from one species to another, and from one tissue of the heart to another. For example, rabbit atrial fibers were not very sensitive to halothane (1–2%), whereas sheep Purkinje fibers were hyperpolarized (by 5 mV), and the AP was shortened and its overshoot diminished (139). The rate of rise was significantly reduced by 2% halothane and conduction velocity was decreased. In sheep ventricular muscle, 2% halothane did not alter the RP, but shortened the AP and reduced overshoot. In rabbit SA node, the slope of the pacemaker potential was markedly decreased by 2% halothane, thus depressing the frequency of firing; the maximum diastolic potential and the AP overshoot were also decreased (140). The depression of nodal automaticity by halothane is not prevented by atropine, thus indicating that the effect is not mediated by the cholinergic receptor (141).

Methyoxyflurane had a negative chronotropic action similar to that of halothane, with the exception that there was an initial brief positive chronotropic effect. In Purkinje fibers (latent pacemaker cells), phase 4 depolarization was enhanced by methyoxyflurane (as with cyclopropane) and depressed by halothane. The effects of these agents were reversible.

In papillary muscles, halothane (0.5–4% gas mixtures) caused an early positive inotropic action and a late negative inotropic action (142). Halothane did not affect max dV/dt of the normal AP or the RP. High concentrations of halothane (4–5%) caused complete electromechanical uncoupling. Elevation of Ca^{2+} did not reverse the effects, but washout of halothane gave nearly full recovery. With Ca^{2+}-dependent slow APs (in 26 mM K^+ solution and 10^{-7} M isoproterenol), halothane (4%) abolished the contractions and depressed the slow APs. Thus halothane affects the functioning of the slow Ca^{2+} channels. The small early positive inotropic action of halothane could be due to an augmented release of Ca^{2+} from the SR, and the later sustained negative inotropic action could be due to inhibition of the slow Ca^{2+} channels and to depletion of the SR store.

In summary, halothane shortens the cardiac AP, depresses automaticity, and inhibits the slow Ca^{2+} channels. It may also increase g_K and/or enhance the kinetics of K^+ activation, thereby explaining the small hyperpolarization produced. Halothane also has internal effects (e.g., on the SR) that may contribute to its negative inotropic action.

Enflurane (1–6%) did not affect max dV/dt and amplitude of the normal fast AP, but AP duration was shortened in >3% enflurane (143). In contrast, the contractions and Ca^{2+}-dependent slow APs were greatly depressed, and it was concluded that enflurane inhibits the slow Ca^{2+} channels, which may contribute to the negative inotropic effect of enflurane.

Trichloroethylene (20–50% saturated solution) depolarizes due to a decrease in resting P_K (144). At 30%, the anesthetic greatly depressed the AP rate of rise and overshoot. The peak transient conductance (g_{Na}) during voltage clamp was suppressed, and the reversal potential for the peak I_{Na} was shifted to a less positive value due to accumulation of Na^+ inside and to decrease in channel selectivity. The steady-state fast Na^+ channel inactivation curve was also shifted in the hyperpolarizing direction.

Enflurane (1.5–5%) and methoxyflurane (0.5–1%) substantially reduced (reversibly) postdrive hyperpolarization in Purkinje fibers (145,146). These effects of the anesthetics resembled that of cardiac glycosides, and it was suggested that enflurane and methyoxyflurane inhibited the electrogenic Na/K–ATPase and pump potential.

Chlorinated Solvents, Fluorocarbons, and Polychlorinated Biphenyls

The chlorinated solvents include carbon tetrachloride and chloroform. The most toxic chlorinated solvent is trichloroethylene, and the least toxic is methylene chloride (147). The primary action of the chlorinated solvents is depression of myocardial contractility, which reduces cardiac output, coronary flow, and blood pressure. The latter, by activation of the baroreceptors, increases the sympathetic discharge to the heart. Persons that inhale the chlorinated solvents can develop circulatory shock and cardiac arrest. The chlorinated solvents also sensitize the heart to arrhythmias (147). The cardiotonic agent and coronary vasodilator, inosine, counteracts the myocardial depressant effect of methylene chloride without sensitizing the heart to arrhythmias (147).

Fluorocarbons can produce cardiac arrhythmias and depress contractility (147). The fluorocarbon, trichloromonofluoromethane, induces cardiac arrhythmias at concentrations of 0.25% and above, and the sensitivity of the heart is increased during ischemia. The mechanisms proposed (147) for fluorocarbon induction of arrhythmias include (a) reflex increase in sympathetic and parasympathetic impulses to the heart caused by irritation of the respiratory tract mucosa, (b) sensitization of the heart to the arrhythmogenic effects of catecholamines, and (c) reduction in cardiac output and coronary blood flow.

Polychlorinated biphenyls (PCBs) are a major environmental contaminant, for example, in inland waters. Significant amounts of PCBs are found in fish and humans, the highest concentrations being in adipose tissue. Addition of PCBs to heart mitochondria inhibits some mitochondrial enzymes and oxidative phosphorylation (148). Such mitochondrial alterations could lead to cardiomyopathy.

Tricyclic Antidepressants

The tricyclic antidepressants, such as amitriptyline-HCl, nortriptyline-HCl, or doxepin-HCl, have potent cardiotoxic effects and anticholinergic action (149). Imipramine enhanced myocardial contractility and heart rate at low doses (0.3 mg/kg, iv), in anesthetized dogs; at higher doses (1–8 mg/kg), it depressed contractility, lowered heart rate, markedly lowered blood pressure, decreased coronary blood flow, and diminished cardiac output (150,151). Many of these effects are thought to be directly on the heart.

The cardiac electrophysiological symptoms in patients having plasma levels of tricyclic antidepressants of over 1.0 μg/ml include QRS durations greater than 100 msec, heart rate of over 120 beats/min (sinus tachycardia), cardiac arrhythmias, bundle-branch block, and A-V block (152). Cardiac arrest and hypotension also can occur. Similar observations were made in another study (153) in which the average ingestion of tricyclic antidepressants was 100 mg: QRS durations greater than 110 msec (indicative of slowed conduction in the ventricle), QT prolongation (indicative of a longer duration AP plateau), prolonged P-Q time (indicative of slowed conduction through the A-V node and/or Purkinje system), heart rate greater than 90 beats/min, and arrhythmias. These drugs impaired distal conduction in the His–Purkinje system (prolonged the His–ventricular interval by over 100 msec and widened the QRS complexes), similar to the effects of quinidine and procainamide (154). The authors suggested that the prolongation of conduction, and its usually associated unidirectional block, may induce reentrant ventricular arrhythmias, and that this could explain the increased incidence of sudden death in patients being treated with tricyclic antidepressant drugs.

Phenothiazines

Phenothiazines, such as chlorpromazine, have a direct effect on the heart to depress myocardial contractility and cardiac output (155,156). Hypotension commonly occurs. These effects are qualitatively similar to the tricyclic antidepressant, imipramine, and have some similarity to quinidine. Chlorpromazine also decreases peripheral vascular resistance and impairs cardiovascular reflex mechanisms. Focal interstitial myocardial necrosis occurs with mucopolysaccharide deposition, particularly near the conduction system (151). Cardiac catecholamine depletion may occur, and there is a tendency to cardiac arrhythmias. The ECG changes include S-T segment changes, prolongation of P-R and Q-T intervals, decrease in T-wave amplitude, appearance of prominent U-waves, and conduction disturbances. The T-wave changes were returned to normal by K^+ administration. It was suggested that slowed conduction and nonhomogeneous repolarization set the stage for reentrant arrhythmias (151).

The beta-adrenergic blocker, propranolol, by reducing heart rate, reversed the QRS prolongation produced by chlorpromazine (157). Chlorpromazine ($0.5–10$ μg/ml) reduced the AP rate of rise in ventricular muscle and Purkinje fibers when the pacing frequency was increased (158). There was no change in RP, and the max dV/dt versus E_m curve was shifted. The drug also decreased the AP overshoot and the plateau duration and amplitude. All effects were more pronounced in Purkinje fibers than in ventricular muscle. The QRS prolongation (indicative of decreased ventricular conduction velocity) produced by chlorpromazine (1–20 mg/kg, iv, in anesthetized dogs) was due to slowed recovery of the fast Na^+ channels (159). That is, the slowed recovery kinetics caused a smaller maximum Na^+ conductance (max g_{Na}) available for the subsequent AP. The more rapid the rate of pacing, the greater the degree of QRS prolongation. It was suggested that this action of chlorpromazine was responsible for its induction of ventricular arrhythmias and susceptibility to reentry.

Doxyrubicin (Adriamycin)

The anthracycline antibiotic doxyrubicin (adriamycin) (isolated from cultures of *Streptomyces peucetius* var. *caesius*) is a widely used antineoplastic agent. Daunorubicin has actions similar to doxyrubicin. However, these agents are very toxic to the heart. Doxyrubicin causes serious cardiac dysrhythmias and a certain incidence of sudden death. ECG changes have been observed in 9–26% of patients undergoing adriamycin therapy (160). The acute cardiotoxic effects of doxyrubicin, including hypotension, tachycardia, and arrhythmias, develop within minutes after intravenous administration (161,162). The chronic cardiotoxic effects include congestive heart failure. Adriamycin also produces cardiomyopathy in most regions of the heart

(163–165). The cardiomyopathy becomes severe and often fatal when cumulative dose levels are reached greater than 500 mg/m^2 of body surface area.

With administration of doxyrubicin at a high dose for a short term (80 mg/ m^2/day × 3 days in dogs), 50% of the animals developed ventricular arrhythmias, including tachycardias (166). When administered a low dose for a long term (25 mg/m^2/week × 20 weeks), all animals developed ventricular dysrhythmias and ectopic foci. Atrial fibrillation, second-degree A-V block, and sinus tachycardia occurred often. The time courses of the progression of the dysrhythmias and cardiomyopathy were similar. Doxyrubicin was reported to enhance automaticity of latent pacemaker cells in the His–Purkinje system (167). Doxyrubicin also increased the duration of the Purkinje AP, produced some depolarization, and depressed conduction. Thus the drug could cause arrhythmias based on accelerated automaticity and reentry.

The mechanisms whereby adriamycin exerts its pathological effects are not known, but several facts may be relevant. (a) Hearts exhibit impaired synthesis of nucleic acids and proteins (168). (b) Coenzyme Q-dependent electron transfer reactions are inhibited (presumably because of the quinone structure), thereby uncoupling oxidative phosphorylation in mitochondria (169). (c) Anthracycline compounds cause superoxide free radicals to be formed that convert unsaturated fatty acids in the membrane to lipid peroxides (170). The free-radical scavenger, tocopherol, increases the adriamycin concentration required to produce cardiomyopathy, without decreasing its antineoplastic activity (171). (d) Adriamycin (1.7 μM for 3 hr) inhibited growth of cultured heart cells, decreased the ATP and phosphocreatine levels, and spontaneous beating ceased by 24–48 hr (172). (e) Verapamil and propranolol provided some protection against adriamycin-induced cardiomyopathy (173). (f) Adriamycin (20 μg/ml) elevated cAMP and potentiated the slow Ca^{2+} current (presumably by making more functional slow channels available) in perfused chick embryonic hearts (174). It was suggested that augmented Ca^{2+} influx could be a factor in the Ca^{2+} overload associated with the cardiomyopathy. However, higher doses (100–500 μg/ ml) depressed and blocked the slow Ca^{2+} channels within 10–30 min and produced a pronounced negative inotropic action (175).

The effect of adriamycin was studied on organ cultured 3-day-old chick embryonic hearts that were spontaneously active and had a max dV/dt of about 30 V/sec (S. M. Vogel and N. Sperelakis, *unpublished observations*). In acute experiments in the presence of TTX (10^{-6} M) (for blockade of any fast Na$^+$ channels present), adriamycin (3.8 × 10^{-5} to 3.8 × 10^{-4} M) caused depression and sometimes blockade of the slow APs within 15–30 min; these effects were fully reversed by prolonged washout (e.g., 2 hr). Incubation with adriamycin (3.8 × 10^{-6} to 1.9 × 10^{-5} M) for 72 hr caused severe depolarization (the RPs were less than −20 mV), and there were no APs. At 3.8 × 10^{-7} M, there was little or no effect on the RPs and APs over the 72-hr period.

Adriamycin (10^{-6} to 10^{-4} M) had a positive inotropic action in papillary muscles, but neither induced nor augmented the slow APs (S. M. Vogel and N. Sperelakis, *unpublished observations*). Thus adriamycin, like cardiac glycosides, augments the contractions without increasing the slow Ca^{2+} current, but depresses the slow current at high concentrations.

Adriamycin (10 mg/liter) depolarized isolated Purkinje fibers to a mean value of -69 mV (from a control value of -87 mV) within 5 hr (166). Automaticity was enhanced and small oscillations appeared. The APs were increased in duration. Conduction was slowed, and local block occurred with reentrant type of activity. The free-radical scavenger, tocopherol, partially protected.

Another agent used in cancer treatment, cyclophosphamide, also causes heart damage, including myocardial necrosis and ECG changes. Cyclophosphamide (500 mg/kg in a single dose to dogs) produced ECG evidence of myocardial damage, including falling QRS voltage, prolonged Q-T interval (longer ventricular APs), and some T-wave changes, and they died within 4–6 hr with acute pulmonary edema (176). Cyclophosphamide is metabolized by the liver to produce highly toxic active (alkylating) metabolites. Capillary damage and thrombosis was also observed in the heart of a patient who died of acute heart failure following treatment with cyclophosphamide (163).

Antibiotics

In general, all antibiotics produce myocardial depression (177). The aminoglycoside antibiotics, gentamicin and neomycin, depressed ^{45}Ca uptake and contractility in vascular smooth muscle and cardiac muscle (178). In perfused guinea pig hearts, gentamicin, in concentrations greater than 0.4 mM, produced dose-dependent decreases in left ventricular developed pressure and dP/dt within 5 min. Contractions were abolished at 6.4 mM. Elevation of $[Ca]_o$ rapidly reversed the effects, as did washout of the drug. In isolated left atria of guinea pigs, gentamicin (2–4 mM) greatly depressed contractile force within 15 min, and elevation of $[Ca]_o$ (to 8–14 mM) counteracted the depressant effect (177).

In guinea pig hearts paced at a constant rate, gentamicin rapidly depressed the contractions and shortened the normal AP, but max dV/dt was unaffected, thus indicating that gentamicin does not affect the fast Na^+ channels (S. M. Vogel and N. Sperelakis, *unpublished observations*). Since gentamicin (0.5–6 mM) rapidly depressed and abolished the isoproterenol-induced slow APs along nearly the same time course as its negative inotropic action, blockade of the slow Ca^{2+} channels can explain the electromechanical uncoupling caused by gentamicin. The effect of gentamicin could be counteracted by elevation of $[Ca]_o$ and reversed by washout.

Other types of antibiotics increase ionic permeability (179). For example, valinomycin increases P_K rather selectively, whereas gramicidin D increases both P_K and P_{Na}. The fungicide amphotericin B (Fungizone, Greseofulvin) produces a general increase in permeability to both cations and anions.

Insecticides

Some insecticides exert pronounced effects on excitable membranes. For example, DDT, an agent that produces hyperactivity and convulsions, prolongs the depolarizing afterpotential that follows the nerve spike, and repetitive afterdischarges follow a single stimulus. These effects are due to inhibition of both Na^+ inactivation (veratridine-like effect) (Fig. 1) and K^+ activation (TEA$^+$-like effect) (see Table 5) during excitation (180).

Allethrin (a pyrethroid) also increases the depolarizing afterpotentials and induces repetitive afterdischarges like DDT, but, in addition, allethrin depolarizes slightly and eventually blocks the AP (181). The conduction block is due primarily to an inhibition and slowing of Na^+ activation kinetics and to a shift of the steady-state fast Na^+ channel inactivation curve in the hyperpolarizing direction (see Table 5). The pyrethroids stimulate Na^+ entry through the Na^+ channels by slowing of the inactivation kinetics but act on a different site than do BTX and GTX (182). The mean open time of single Na^+ channels is greatly prolonged by the pyrethroids. It has been reported that these toxins transform fast Na^+ channels into slower channels (180). Only partial recovery occurs with washing.

Aldrin trans-diol, a metabolite of dieldrin (a cyclodiene) and possibly its active form, depresses and blocks the nerve AP by primarily suppressing the inward fast Na^+ current (inhibits Na^+ activation) (180). The K^+ activation mechanism is only slightly depressed. These effects were not reversible.

Emetine and Chloroquine

Cardiac toxicity is common in patients treated with emetine for amebiasis (antimalarial) and schistosomiasis because of the small margin of safety between the therapeutic and toxic doses (151). Similar, but milder, toxicity occurs with chloroquine. The myocardial mitochondria become damaged and there is necrosis of some heart cells. Among the heart electrophysiological changes are sinus tachycardia, arrhythmias, Q-T interval prolongation, S-T segment displacement, precordial T-wave inversion, and conduction disturbances. Ventricular fibrillation may occur.

Salicylates

These analgesic, antipyretic, and anti-inflammatory agents have effects on excitable membranes. For example, 5-bromosalicyclic acid (0.1–0.5 mM) prolonged the repolarizing phase of the nerve AP and, above 1.5 mM, blocked conduction (183). Both the peak transient Na^+ conductance and steady-state K^+ conductance increases were reduced, and the curves relating these conductances to E_m were shifted in the depolarizing direction. The time constant for fast Na^+ channel inactivation (τ_h) was greatly increased, thus accounting for the AP prolongation. The steady-state fast Na^+ channel inactivation curve (h_∞) was shifted in the hyperpolarizing direction, indicating a greater fractional Na^+ inactivation at the normal resting potential and hence depressed max dV/dt. The Na^+ inactivation gate rate constants (α_h and β_h) were decreased, and the rate of activation of the K^+ channels (α_n) was reduced. These effects were largely reversed by washing. The site of action of the salicylates may be on the inner surface of the membrane. In Purkinje fibers, salicylate (10 mM) depresses the pacemaker current and automaticity and shifts the activation curve to more negative potentials (184,185).

Alcohol

Ethyl alcohol is a myocardial depressant when administered acutely. In some alcoholic patients, there is a full-blown cardiomyopathy and dilated heart failure (163,186). Intoxicating amounts of ethanol cause leakage of myocardial cell components, and there is significant depression of oxidative phosphorylation of the heart mitochondria (187). Cardiac arrhythmias and thromboembolism also may occur in alcoholics.

Alcohol depressed the AP amplitude and duration in squid giant axon. Ethanol (3% by volume) reduced the maximum conductances for both Na^+ (max g_{Na}) and K^+ (max g_K) during activation (to about 80%), and 6% ethanol reduced max g_{Na} and max g_K to about 65% (188). The activation and inactivation kinetic parameters were not affected. It was concluded that ethanol mainly reduces max g_{Na} and max g_K, that is, the number of available channels or the conductance per channel.

Similar results were obtained on squid axon in another study (87), except the depression of max g_{Na} was greater than that of the max g_K. The alcohol concentration required to affect the membrane properties decreased greatly as the number of carbon atoms (lipid solubility) increased (e.g., 0.50 M for ethanol, 0.13 M for n-propyl, 0.06 M for isobutyl, and 0.037 mM for octyl). The short-chain alcohols (C_2 through C_5) depolarized by a few millivolts, due to a decrease in resting g_K, and the depolarization preceded any changes in the AP.

Nicotine

In addition to its well-known effects on autonomic ganglia (to stimulate and then paralyze) and neuromuscular junctions, nicotine also has a potent local anesthetic type of action on membrane. For example, nicotine (1 mM) applied internally in squid giant axon suppresses the K^+ conductance activation without having much effect on the Na^+ conductance increase; at 10 mM, both conductances are completely suppressed (189). Nicotine is less effective when added to the outside, suggesting that its site of action is near the inner surface of the membrane. Since nicotine exerts a greater effect on the K^+ conductance mechanism than on the Na^+ conductance mechanism, nicotine should, at lower concentrations, prolong the AP and give rise to repetitive afterdischarges.

Marijuana

Levo delta-9-tetrahydrocannabinol (Δ-9-THC), the pharmacologically active substance in marijuana, has different effects on the heart in humans compared to smaller mammals. In anesthetized dogs, cats, and rats, Δ-9-THC decreases heart rate, whereas in human patients the iv administration of Δ-9-THC, in a dose approximating that delivered by one marijuana cigarette, increased heart rate and cardiac pump performance (190). The effect of the drug was mediated through the sympathetic and parasympathetic nervous systems. In humans, the drug also causes premature ventricular contractions due to enhanced ventricular automaticity and ventricular ectopy. There was also facilitation of SA conduction and AV nodal conduction, as indicated by decrease in the A-H interval and in A-V nodal refractoriness (190). In contrast, in experimental animals, Δ-9-THC in high doses (>100 μg/kg) causes P-R prolongation and second degree A-V block.

Endotoxin

Gram-negative bacterial endotoxin (mol wt of about 10^6) released from ischemic splanchnic bed during circulatory shock (hypotension) may have a direct effect on the heart, causing depression of contractility, especially during the later stages of shock (191). In addition, there are depressed inotropic and chronotropic responses of the heart to norepinephrine, tyramine, and histamine (192). Pathological morphological changes of the heart also occur during shock (193) and myocardial enzymes are released (194).

The Ca–ATPase activity of Ca^{2+} uptake into isolated dog SR vesicles were found to be depressed in animals in endotoxin shock, secondary to poor coronary perfusion (195). It was proposed that the depressed myocardial contractility in endotoxin shock could result partially from the lower Ca^{2+} sequestration by the SR, causing less Ca^{2+} release from the SR by subsequent APs. Therefore inadequate coronary perfusion due to hypotension is thought to play a significant role in heart dysfunction after endotoxin (196). However, a direct toxic effect of endotoxin on the heart has been described. In rat myocardial cell cultures, sera taken from patients in septic shock (after

4–5 hr) caused (after 24 hr) some depolarization (about 10 mV) and prolonged the AP (197). In addition, the shock sera blocked the positive chronotropic response of the cells to isoproterenol (i.e., a beta-blocker-like effect).
In isolated cat papillary muscle, a myocardial depressant factor isolated
from plasma hemorrhagic-shocked cats was reported to decrease contractility but not to affect the resting potential or AP amplitude over an 11-min
period, but did prolong the AP plateau (198). It was found that, in skeletal
muscle of dogs placed into endotoxin shock, a depolarization averaging 32
mV was produced, with the expected resultant effect on max dV/dt and AP
duration (199). The fibers also gained Na^+ and Cl^- and lost K^+.

Guinea pigs treated with *E. coli* endotoxin (4–8 mg/kg) went into severe
circulatory shock within 18 hr (200): atrial muscle isolated from these animals showed greatly depressed force development. Elevation of $[Ca]_o$ was
able to counteract the contractile depression produced by the endotoxin (administered *in vivo*).

Toxins Acting on Fast Na^+ Channels

The ion channel toxins have been used by a number of investigators as
tools to isolate and purify fast Na^+ channels (Fig. 1) and postsynaptic channels (e.g., the nicotinic receptor–ion channel complex) (201–203). Similar
uses may be forthcoming for other types of ion channels. The toxins have
also been used to identify subtypes of Na^+ channels. For example, some
Na^+ channels are TTX sensitive and are blocked in the nanomolar range,
whereas others are TTX resistant (blocked in the micromolar range) or TTX
insensitive. Finally, toxins are useful to study the appearance of ion channels
during development. For example, TTX sensitivity of the APs and TTX
binding have been used to follow the appearance of fast Na^+ channels during embryonic development of heart (16,204–206). A complete discussion of
such uses and the results therefrom have been given (207,208).

There appears to be at least four or five separate binding sites for toxins
on the fast Na^+ channels: (a) one site for TTX and STX; (b) one site for the
lipid-soluble toxins BTX, GTX, veratridine, and aconitine; (c) one site for
the polypeptide toxins, scorpion toxin (ScTXs) and sea anemone toxin-II
(ATXs-II); (d) one site for the small polypeptide *Goniopora* toxin (GPTX);
and (e) one site for the polyether ciguatoxin (CgTX).

TTX and STX block the channels by binding in the outer mouth and plugging the channel (Table 4). All the other toxins open and/or cause persistent
activation of the channel primarily by slowing inactivation (i.e., inactivation
gate held open) (Table 4). The main evidence for separate binding sites for
toxin categories (a)–(e) consists of lack of competition for binding and synergistic effects. The reader is referred to a review chapter by Renaud and
Lazdunski (207) for a more detailed discussion.

TABLE 4. *Some major classes of agents that act on the fast Na$^+$ channel*

Class	Effect
1. TTX, STX	Channel blocker
2. Veratridine, aconitine; BTX, GTXs	Channel openers; persistent activation
3. ScTXs, ATXs	Inhibit (slow) inactivation of channel
4. ScTXs	Block early Na$^+$ current
5. Pyrethroids	Modify channel closing

The physiological consequences of the action of these toxins are as follows: (a) TTX/STX depress max dV/dt of the AP and propagation velocity, resulting in a negative inotropic effect and depressed excitability; (b) toxins in categories (a)–(e) (e.g., BTX, GTX, veratridine, aconitine, ScTX, ATX-II, GPTX, and CgTX) prolong the AP and produce a positive inotropic effect (because of the increase in [Na]$_i$ producing an increased [Ca]$_i$ via the Ca–Na exchange). However, at higher concentrations and longer times, these toxins depolarize, and thereby depress excitability and contraction, and induce arrhythmias.

Tetrodotoxin and Saxitoxin

Many of the neurotoxins also have potent effects on the heart. For example, tetrodotoxin (TTX), the toxin isolated from the Japanese puffer fish (mainly from the ovaries and liver) and from the California newt (*Taricha torosa*) (eggs), blocks the fast Na$^+$ channels in most excitable membranes rather selectively (209) (see Fig. 1, Table 5). In nerve, TTX blocks in a dose-dependent manner between 10^{-9} and 10^{-7} M, the ED$_{50}$ being about 10^{-8} M. In skeletal muscle and cardiac muscle, higher concentrations are usually required to block the fast Na$^+$ channels (e.g., 10^{-8} to 10^{-6} M), with an ED$_{50}$ of about 10^{-7} M. In some species, and in some cardiac tissues such as Purkinje fibers, even still higher doses are required (e.g., 10^{-5} to 10^{-4} M) for complete blockade. On the other hand, in some species (e.g., chick and frog), the myocardial cells are about equally sensitive to TTX as nerve is (210).

Not all fast Na$^+$ channels are sensitive to blockade by TTX. For example, the nerve fast Na$^+$ channels of the California and the Japanese puffer fish are relatively insensitive to TTX. However, these nerves are highly sensitive to saxitoxin (STX). The nerves from some clams and shellfish are not blocked by TTX or STX (179). In addition, when mammalian skeletal muscle is denervated, a new population of fast Na$^+$ channels begins to appear that are insensitive to TTX but still sensitive to STX (211). Some tissues have no (or very few) functional fast Na$^+$ channels and so these tissues are insensitive to (or only slightly affected by) TTX. Such tissues include visceral

TABLE 5. *Some agents that affect the state of the ionic channels in myocardial cells*

Type of action	Voltage-dependent channels		
	Fast Na$^+$ channels	Slow Ca^{2+} channels	K$^+$ channels

Blockers	TTX
	STX
	Local anesthetics
	Barbiturates
	Alcohol
	Scorpion toxins
	Trichloroethylene
	Allethrin
	Aldrin trans-diol
	Chlorpromazine[a]
		Verapamil, D600
		Papaverine
		Nifedipine
		Bepridil
		Mn^{2+}, Co^{2+}
		La^{3+}
		Acidosis
		Metabolic poisons:
		  valinomycin,
		  hypoxia, ischemia
		Local anesthetics
		Phenytoin (high dose)
		Gentamycin
		Adriamycin
		Cardiac glycosides
		  (high doses)
			Ba^{2+}
			Cs$^+$, Rb$^+$
			TEA$^+$
			4-Aminopyridine
			9-Aminoacridine
			Local
			  anesthetics
			Barbiturates
			Alcohol
			Salicylates
			Scorpion toxins
			DDT
			Nicotine

Openers	BTX GTX Veratridine Aconitine	ATX-II	ACh$^+$ Low ATP [Ca]$_i$
Inactivation inhibitors	ATX CTX DDT Scorpion toxin I BTX[b] Veratridine[b] Aconitine[b] GTX[b] DDT Salicylates Buthus tamalus toxin	—	—
Stimulators	—	Catecholamines Methylxanthines Histamine Angiotensin II Cyclic AMP F$^-$	Cyclic AMP

[a]Also depresses rate of recovery of the ion channels.
[b]Also shifts voltage-dependence of inactivation in hyperpolarizing direction.

smooth muscle (212), vascular smooth muscle (92,93), cardiac A-V and S-A nodal cells (213–215), young embryonic hearts (204), and cultured heart cell monolayers (75,216).

TTX also has been found to decrease the resting g_{Na} in a variety of nerve membranes, producing a hyperpolarization of 2–7 mV (179). In Na$^+$-free solution, TTX no longer hyperpolarizes, as expected if TTX suppresses the resting P_{Na}.

TTX acts on the outer surface of the membrane and not on the inner surface (209). The TTX molecule contains a guanidinium group that is required for activity, and it is generally believed that the positively charged guanidinium group sticks into the mouth of the fast Na$^+$ channel (binding to a negative charge near the selectivity filter of the channel) and acts to physically block the passage of Na$^+$ ions through the channel, like a plug. The channel gates are not blocked by TTX because the gating current is unaffected by TTX (223). However, recent studies with TTX analog molecules and chemical modifications of the fast Na$^+$ channels suggest that TTX may not block by sitting in the mouth of the channel, but rather by binding to an adjacent site ("receptor") and producing a conformational change in the channel protein (C.Y. Kao, *personal communication;* 224, 225).

Saxitoxin (STX) is isolated from the Alaska butter clam (*Saxidomas giganteus*), but the toxin is derived from a dinoflagellate parasite (*Gonyaulax catanella*) (179). STX is chemically different from TTX and contains two guanidinium groups. However, STX has an action nearly identical to that of TTX. One major difference from TTX is that washout of STX occurs faster than for TTX.

It was reported that the TTX sensitivity of the fast Na$^+$ channels in rat papillary muscle was increased when the membrane was partly depolarized; that is, there was a voltage dependence of TTX block (226). However, others have reported that there was no voltage dependence for steady-state TTX block of the fast Na$^+$ current (227,228).

Binding studies on cultured heart cells from neonatal rats showed presence of both high-affinity (K_d = 1.6 nM) and low-affinity (K_d = 130 nM) binding sites, the number of low-affinity binding sites being 45 times greater than the high-affinity sites (229). It was concluded that, although both high-affinity and low-affinity binding sites coexist in mammalian heart cells, the Na$^+$ channels with low affinity for TTX predominate electrically (207). TTX binding is inhibited at acid pH, half-inhibition occurring at pH 6.2 (230). The relevant ionizable group on the Na$^+$ channel was postulated to be carboxylate. Monovalent cations displayed TTX binding in the sequence: guanidinium$^+$ > Tl$^+$ > NH$_4$ > Li$^+$ > Na$^+$ > K$^+$ > Rb$^+$ > Cs$^+$. Mg^{2+} (K_d = 1.3 mM) and Ca^{2+} (K_d = 3.2 mM) had a similar action (207). Photoactivatable TTX derivatives have been prepared that can irreversibly bind to and block the fast Na$^+$ channel upon irradiation (231).

Sea Anemone Toxins

A series of neurotoxins was isolated from the sea anemone (*Anemonia sulcata*). One of these sea anemone toxins (ATX-II) has been purified and sequenced. ATX-II is a small polypeptide containing 47 amino acids (mol wt of about 50,000) and cross-linked by three disulfide bridges; the molecule is positively charged (at pH 7.4). It has potent effects on many excitable mem-

branes including nerve and cardiac muscle. ATX-II also releases neurotransmitters from the nerve terminals (similar to the effect of veratridine, batrachotoxin, and scorpion toxin), presumably due to its depolarizing action.

On crayfish giant axons and frog myelinated fibers, ATX-II (10^{-7} to 10^{-6}
M) was shown by Romey et al. (220) to selectively affect the closing (inactivation) of the Na^+ channels by slowing down this process considerably.
The nerve AP was greatly prolonged, with the appearance of a marked plateau component within 1–2 min; pronounced depolarization occurred at
longer times (10–30 min). ATX-II was found to act only on the outer surface
of the membrane. It was difficult to reverse these effects by washing the
toxin out. However, both effects of ATX-II were rapidly antagonized by
TTX (10^{-7} M).

In cultured embryonic chick hearts (monolayers), ATX-II (10^{-7} to 3×10^{-6} M) greatly increased ^{45}Ca uptake (maximum stimulation of 12-fold) and
^{85}Sr uptake (249). The toxin only slightly increased (by 1.5-fold) the rate of
^{22}Na uptake; there was no effect on the rates of efflux for ^{45}Ca, ^{22}Na, or ^{86}Rb.
Mn^{2+}, Co^{2+}, Ni^{2+}, and La^{3+} blocked the ^{45}Ca influx stimulated by ATX-II;
verapamil, D600, and local anesthetics also blocked, and TTX antagonized
the ATX-II effect. The ATX-II-stimulated ^{45}Ca influx was dependent on
$[Na]_o$; Li^+ could not replace Na^+. The authors proposed that ATX-II opens
or holds open a Ca^{2+} entry system or channel blockable by cations, verapamil, and local anesthetics.

In a subsequent study on cultured embryonic chick heart cells (reaggregates and monolayers), ATX-II was shown by Romey et al. (250) to exert
effects on cells derived from both 16-day-old hearts and 3-day-old hearts.
The toxin (0.1–1.0 µM) greatly prolonged the AP plateau, slowed down the
rate of spontaneous firing (negative chronotropic effect), and increased the
amplitude and duration of the contractions (positive inotropic effect) recorded by a photoelectric method. These effects were reversed by washing
or by TTX (0.1 µM), and the ATX-II actions were dependent on $[Na]_o$. Verapamil, D600, or Mn^{2+} (2 mM), however, did not prevent the ATX-II effects, and the ATX-II effects occurred even in low $[Ca]_o$ (10% of normal).
The uptake of ^{22}Na and ^{45}Ca was stimulated by ATX-II. The effects of ATX-
II were synergistic with those of veratridine, subthreshold doses of both
agents causing pronounced effects. It was suggested that the positive inotropic effect of ATX-II was due to the holding open of the Na^+ channels causing an increased $[Na]_i$ and therefore $[Ca]_i$ via the Ca–Na exchange system.

In nonexcitable cells also, namely, a cultured cell line (C-9) derived from
rat tumor cells, ATX-II stimulated ^{22}Na uptake, depolarized, and induced
spontaneous slow-wave oscillations, all of which were blocked by TTX
(251).

Another anemone toxin, obtained from the tentacles of the Bermuda
anemone *Condylactis gigantea,* is a polypeptide with a molecular weight of
about 13,000 (179). *Condylactis* toxin (CTX) greatly prolongs the repolariz-

ing phase of the AP of lobster and crayfish giant axons. In voltage-clamp experiments, CTX prolonged the falling phase of the transient fast inward current (I_{Na}) and caused only a small suppression of the steady-state outward current (I_K). CTX caused the total ionic conductance (in the steady state) to exceed the control conductance either during the transient inward Na$^+$ current or during the steady-state K$^+$ outward current. CTX was ineffective on the squid giant axon.

Veratridine and Aconitine

The veratrum alkaloids are steroids found in certain plants, such as those belonging to the genus *Veratrum*. Aconitine is a steroidal alkaloid found in the plant *Aconitum napellus*. The veratrine alkaloids and their most active principle, veratridine, also have an effect similar to that of grayanotoxin, namely, a specific increase in Na$^+$ permeability resulting in depolarization with the expected consequences on the AP rate of rise and duration (221,232–234). At low concentrations and short times, veratridine can be shown to prolong greatly the AP of nerve, skeletal muscle, and cardiac muscle before depolarizing (235). This effect is reversed by TTX. The APs develop very prominent depolarizing ("negative") afterpotentials. The mechanism of this effect is presumably by the drug holding open the fast Na$^+$ channels longer; that is, the inactivation process (closing of the inactivation or I gates) is greatly slowed (Table 5). Since these agents seem to bind to the open (active) form of the fast Na$^+$ channel, this suggests that there is a use dependency of their action. In addition, veratridine (as well as batrachotoxin, grayanotoxin, and aconitine) is believed to modify the voltage dependence of the activation curve (m_∞) for fast Na$^+$ channels in a hyperpolarizing direction, such that there is a persistent activation of a fraction of these channels (235). This causes depolarization to occur (ratio of g_{Na}/g_K increases).

Hence the steady-state depolarization produced by veratridine can result from a permanent holding open of the I gates of the fast Na$^+$ channels and/or the shift of the voltage-dependency of the activation (A) gate, such that many channels are conducting (open) in the resting condition. In addition, there may be an opening of the resting (voltage-independent) Na$^+$ channels (and K$^+$ channels).

Veratridine also was suggested to increase K$^+$ permeability, as well as the Na$^+$ permeability, in cultured heart cells (221). This was suggested on the basis (a) that the E_m never went positive in high concentrations of the drug as would be expected from a selective and large increase in g_{Na}, (b) that membrane resistance decreased more than what would be expected from only an increase in g_{Na}, and (c) that in the presence of TTX, veratridine actually hyperpolarized. That is, veratridine had an effect similar to that of acetylcholine at the postsynaptic membrane of the neuromuscular junction.

The depolarizing effect of veratridine (and GTX, BTX, and ATX) is reversed or prevented by TTX (221,235–239). In the prior presence of TTX, veratridine may actually hyperpolarize slightly (221). If TTX acts on the outer surface of the membrane, and if veratridine acts at the I gate located at the inner surface of the membrane, then it is difficult to explain the antagonism between TTX and veratridine unless both of these drugs are capable of acting at more than one site. However, in any tissue that agents like veratridine, grayanotoxins, batrachotoxin, sea anemone toxin, and scorpion toxin depolarize by opening and/or slowing the inactivation of Na^+ channels, TTX prevents or reverses the effects of these agents. For example, this was shown for cultured heart cell monolayers that do not possess functional fast Na^+ channels (221). Therefore veratridine may open and slow the inactivation of the voltage-dependent fast and slow Na^+ channels, and that TTX blocks both of these actions (221). Veratridine has been used to unmask "silent" (nonfunctional) fast Na^+ channels that may be present in such tissues (222).

Aconitine, another highly toxic alkaloid, has an effect similar to that of veratridine; that is, it increases Na^+ permeability (channel opener). It has been used to induce cardiac arrhythmias in experimental animals. The induction of and enhancement of automaticity by aconitine and veratridine presumably are a consequence of the depolarization due to the increase in g_{Na} (213). The increase in $[Na]_i$ that follows from the increased g_{Na}, coupled with the Ca–Na exchange reaction, may be the mechanism of the positive inotropic effect of veratridine (235,239,240).

Grayanotoxins; Batrachotoxin

Grayanotoxins

Grayanotoxins (GTX) are the toxic principles extracted from the leaves of various species, including *Rhododendran Ericacea,* which chemically are tetracyclic diterpenoids (perihydroazulene skeleton). These toxins act specifically to increase Na^+ permeability, perhaps by opening the voltage-dependent Na^+ channels (presumably both the fast and the slow Na^+ channels) in excitable membranes (see Table 5). The action of GTX is prevented or reversed by tetrodotoxin (TTX). The effect of GTX is also reversed by washout of the toxin.

In cardiac muscle, GTX-I was shown to exert a positive inotropic action in guinea pig atrium (241,242). A similar positive inotropic effect (tension increased two- to threefold) produced by GTX-I (30 μM) was also observed in rabbit atrial muscle (243). This effect was explained on the basis of a greater Na^+ influx leading to a higher $[Na]_i$, and this in turn, because of the

Ca–Na exchange reaction (see Cardiac Electrophysiology), leads to a higher [Ca]$_i$ and hence greater force of contraction (243). At 100 μM, GTX caused contracture to occur.

In rabbit atrial muscle, GTX-I (100 μM) depolarized by a mean of 26 mV, whereas in rabbit SA nodal cells, the same dose of GTX-I depolarized by only 3.6 mV (243). TTX (10 μM) reversed the depolarization, as did withdrawal of Na$^+$ ions from the bathing medium. The depolarization produced by GTX has repercussions with respect to the AP rate of rise and duration as discussed in the section on Cardiac Electrophysiology. GTX-I (50 μM) also had the effect of shifting the h$_\infty$ versus E$_m$ curve (for the fast Na$^+$ channels) in a hyperpolarizing direction by 7 mV.

In squid axon also, the grayanotoxins increase Na$^+$ permeability (244) and affect the kinetics of the Na$^+$ conductance change (245). GTX-I caused a shift of the m and h parameters for the Na$^+$ gating mechanism toward the hyperpolarizing direction, thus increasing the steady-state Na$^+$ current at rest and generating a "slow" (i.e., sustained) inward Na$^+$ current during the plateau (245).

Batrachotoxin

Batrachotoxin (BTX) is a steroidal alkaloid (pyrrole carboxylic ester) obtained from the skin secretion of the Columbian frog *(Pyllobates aurotaenia)*. BTX is very toxic; for example, the LD$_{50}$ for rabbits is about 1 μg (fatal within 1 hr). The cause of death is the development of ventricular arrhythmias and fibrillation (246). Batrachotoxin has an effect similar to that of grayanotoxin, namely, a specific increase in resting Na$^+$ permeability (see Tables 4 and 5). The depolarizing action of BTX was almost entirely prevented by pretreatment of the membrane with various sulfhydryl reagents such as *N*-ethylmaleimide, dithiothreitol, and *p*-chloromercuribenzene sulfonic acid, suggesting that the toxin acts on a protein constituent of the Na$^+$ channel (247).

BTX was shown to decrease the resting potential of Purkinje fibers and cat ventricular myocardial cells (217,248). The depolarization produced by BTX (1–5×10^{-9} g/ml) in dog Purkinje fibers is very large, the E$_m$ going to nearly zero potential (range of -30 to $+20$ mV) within 1–2 hr (248); about half of the total depolarization produced occurred within the first 20 min. Low Na$^+$ (1 mM) solution or TTX reversed the depolarization. Even prior to onset of the depolarization, BTX caused an increased in duration of the plateau, and the AP was followed by a prominent depolarizing afterpotential.

In cat papillary muscle, Shotzberger et al. (217) reported that BTX depolarized to about -50 mV at 2×10^{-9} M and to -12 mV at 2×10^{-7} M. At 2×10^{-9} M, spontaneous APs and contractions were produced. TTX (2×10^{-7} M) antagonized all the effects of BTX. BTX also exerted a positive inotropic effect (contractile force increased about 50%). The authors suggested that the increased force of contraction was produced by the increase in [Na]$_i$ and hence in [Ca]$_i$ via the Ca–Na exchange system.

In contrast to the depolarization described above, Honerjager and Reiter (218) found that isolated guinea pig papillary muscles were not depolarized by BTX in concentrations up to 1.2 μM for 30 min. Instead, they only observed the prolongation of the AP caused by BTX (about 1–60 nM); this was accompanied by an increase in contractility (including increase in rate of force development). Sometimes there occurred a secondary regenerative AP arising from the repolarizing phase of the first AP and producing an extrasystole. This effect appeared (progressively) only after a series of APs were elicited; that is, the effect was actively dependent. Washout of the effect of BTX required several hours. TTX antagonized the effect of BTX. It was suggested that the positive inotropic effect of BTX was caused by the prolongation of g$_{Na}$ during the AP leading to an increase in [Na]$_i$, and therefore [Ca]$_i$ via the Ca–Na exchange reaction.

In skeletal muscle of the rat (given a subarachnoid injection of 20 ng of BTX), there was differential sensitivity of fast muscles (extensor digitorum longus, EDL) and slow muscles (soleus) to BTX, the EDL muscle becoming depolarized by about 9 mV after 24 hr (no significant depolarization at 6 hr), whereas the soleus muscle was only slightly depolarized (219).

Ciguatoxin

Ciguatoxin, an oxygenated polyether synthesized by a dinoflagellate, increases Na$^+$ permeability and depolarization, that is prevented by TTX (noncompetitively), due to activation of the fast Na$^+$ channels (252). However, ciguatoxin does not act on the same sites as GTX, BTX, and veratridine. Ciguatoxin may belong to a new class of fast Na$^+$ channel toxins (207).

Coral Toxins and *Goniopora* Toxin

Two polypeptide toxins have been isolated from corals *(Goniopora)*, one with an M$_r$ of 9000 and the second having an M$_r$ of 19,000. The first toxin acts similar to sea anemone toxin (ATX), namely, to slow inactivation of the fast Na$^+$ channels (253). The second toxin stimulates Ca^{2+} influx in myocardial cells, and this effect is prevented by Ca antagonist drugs (254). Since this toxin also competes for binding on the dihydropyridine binding site, it was suggested that this toxin is a Ca^{2+} channel activator (agonist) (207).

Goniopora toxin (GPTX), isolated from a coral *(Goniopora* sp.), is a small polypeptide having a molecular weight of 1200. It produces positive inotropic effects that are inhibited by TTX, presumably by stimulating Na$^+$ influx

(253). The mechanism of the effect is thought to be by slowing inactivation of the fast Na^+ channels. GPTX potentiates the persisting activation/opening of fast Na^+ channels by veratridine, suggesting that GPTX binds to a different site (255).

ω-Conotoxin

ω-Conotoxin is extracted from the venom of the cone snail *Conus geographus*. It has been demonstrated that this toxin blocks voltage-dependent Ca^{2+} channels at the frog neuromuscular junction (256) and the high threshold Ca^{2+} currents in chick dorsal root ganglion cells. It does not, however, appear to block Ca^{2+} currents in guinea pig or frog heart cells, or in chick myotubes (257). It is thought that this toxin blocks the N-type Ca^{2+} channel.

Apamin and Melittin

Several toxins have been isolated from bee venom. One of these is the polypeptide apamin. This toxin was found to block the Ca^{2+}-activated K^+ conductance channel ($g_{K(Ca)}$) in several types of cells (258). Apamin binding was inhibited by quinidine. It was also reported that apamin blocks the Ca^{2+} slow channels in cardiac muscle, and that this effect was reversed by quinidine (259).

A second bee venom toxin is melittin, a polypeptide. This toxin was reported to inhibit adenylate cyclase and, therefore, cAMP production (260) and to inhibit two types of protein kinases (PK-C and calmodulin-PK) (261). It was also reported that melittin, in very low concentrations, inhibited a fast Ca^{2+} channel current (transient, T-type, low-threshold) in young embryonic chick hearts (262). This current was insensitive to Ca antagonist drugs. In much higher concentrations, melittin inhibited the slow Ca^{2+} channels (sustained, L-type, high-threshold, Ca antagonist-sensitive) as well.

Scorpion Neurotoxins

Several neurotoxins have been isolated from the venom of the highly poisonous scorpion, *Androctonus australis hector*. These toxins are single-chain proteins composed of 63–64 amino acids and eight cysteine residues. The scorpion toxins are also highly cardiotoxic. One of these toxins, scorpion toxin 1, has been shown by Romey et al. (263) to slow the closing of the Na^+ channel and the opening of the K^+ channel in giant axons of crayfish and lobster. In squid giant axon, the same toxin blocks both the Na^+ and K^+ conductances (263). TTX prevents the action of scorpion toxin only if it is added prior. The toxin from *Androctonus* was reported to increase the rate of beating of cultured heart cells and induce fibrillation and contraction at high concentration (1 μM) (264). The toxin from *Androctonus* also causes neurotransmitter release, and this action of the toxin is quasi-irreversible (265).

Another scorpion *(Leirus quinquestriatus)* venom was found to decrease Na^+ conductance (by 60%), to slow Na^+ inactivation, and to reduce K^+ activation in myelinated nerve fibers of *Xenopus* (266). Similarly, the venom from the scorpion *Buthus tamalus* was found by Narahashi et al. (267) to greatly prolong Na^+ inactivation and to suppress the steady-state K^+ current in squid giant axon.

Two polypeptide toxins from Central American/South American scorpions have been examined: (a) Tityus-γ toxin (from *Tityus serrulatus*) and (b) CssTX (from *Centruroides suffisus*). Tityus-γ toxin contains 61 amino acids in a coiled arrangement with four disulfide bridges. This toxin shifts the voltage dependence of activation and inactivation or the fast Na^+ channel in the negative direction, and the K_d value is about 2 pM. It was reported that *Centruroides* toxin selectively blocks the sarcolemmal fast Na^+ channels compared to the T-tubular Na^+ channels in skeletal muscle (268). TTX has no effect on *Tityus* toxin binding (207).

Ervatamine

Ervatamine, an alkaloid isolated from an Australian tree *(Ervatamina orientalis)*, produces a frequency-dependent block of fast Na^+ channels and slow Na^+ channels (207,269). Like TTX, ervatamine inhibits the effects of veratridine, BTX, GTX, ScTXs, and ATXs on the fast Na^+ channels but does not bind to the TTX receptor or the ScTX receptor. However, ervatamine is a competitive inhibitor of BTX, indicating a common receptor site. Like TTX, ervatamine blocks the cardiac AP (K_d = 20 μM), and slows the rate of reactivation of the Na^+ channel (269).

Maitotoxin

Maitotoxin (MTX), a large molecular weight nonprotein toxin isolated from a dinoflagellate *(Gambierdiscus toxicus)*, is presumably the most potent marine toxin known. It is thought to be an activator of the V-dependent Ca^{2+} channels, acting at a site different from the dihydropyridines (270). MTX increases Ca^{2+} influx, produces a positive inotropic effect, and contracts smooth muscle. MTX was also reported to stimulate IP_3 production in rat aortic smooth muscle cells (271). Kobayashi et al. (272) showed that, in addition to a positive inotropic effect, MTX produced a positive chronotropic effect in isolated right atria, which was almost abolished by Co^{2+} or verapamil, and increased tissue Ca^{2+} content. In isolated cardiomyocytes, MTX exerted an arrhythmogenic effect and caused irreversible rounding of the cells. Maitotoxin is a large molecular weight substance purified from the dinoflagellate *Gambieridiscus toxicus* (273). The highly potent toxin has a positive inotropic effect on cardiac muscle and it has been shown to increase the plateau duration of the rat ventricular AP (274). These findings are consistent with the possibility that maitotoxin acts to increase the Ca^{2+} current. The specific mechanism(s) for the positive inotropic effect of maitotoxin may also involve an inhibitor of the Na/K–ATPase (275), which would lead to an enhanced $[Ca]_i$ via the Na–Ca exchange mechanism. In the whole animal maitotoxin produces arrhythmias and tachycardias leading to cardiac failure (274).

Spider Toxins

Spiders produce numerous toxins, some of high molecular weight (proteinaceous) and many of low molecular weight (< 1 kDa). Some of the low molecular weight toxins act as potent noncompetitive antagonists of glutamate receptors (GluRs), particularly the L-quisqualate-sensitive GluRs, in both invertebrates and vertebrates (276). For example, a toxin isolated from the venom of the Joro spider (JSTX) suppressed the excitatory postsynaptic potentials (EPSPs) (and postjunctional glutamate depolarization) at excitatory neuromuscular junctions of lobster skeletal muscle (277). The threshold concentration is about 10^{-10} M, and at high concentrations, the antagonism of GluR was irreversible. The quisqualate-sensitive postjunctional GluRs (D-receptors) gate nonselective cation channels. The venom from North American spiders (*Argiope trifasciata* and *A. lobata*) contain a 636-Da toxin, argiotoxin, which has similar effects on GluRs. The argiotoxins have a marked use dependency (278). It was suggested that argiotoxin produces open-channel block of the GluR channel.

Several araneid spider venoms also block transmission at the frog motor endplate (nicotinic AChR), and they inhibit glutamate binding in rat brain (276). One of the toxins in the venom of the North American spider *Agelenopsis aperta* acts presynaptically to produce spontaneous EPSPs and repetitive firing. Other toxins (AG1 and AG2) from *Agelenopsis* produce block of neuronal and cardiac Ca^{2+} channels (279,280). AG1 (6 kDa) produces a persistent block of Ca^{2+} channels in vertebrate CNS. AG2 blocks slow Ca^{2+} channels in cardiac muscle and competes with dihydropyridines for binding sites. A 16-kDa toxin from *Hololena curta* venom produces irreversible presynaptic blockade of neuromuscular transmission in *Drosophila* due to block the presynaptic Ca^{2+} channels. Thus some spider toxins block slow Ca^{2+} channels and some block fast Ca^{2+} channels.

Volvatoxin A, Cobra Venom Cardiotoxin, and Palytoxin

Volvatoxin A

Volvatoxin A, a cardiotoxic protein from a species of mushroom *(Volvariella volvacea)*, causes cardiac arrest in systole. The toxin is composed of two subunits (in a ratio of 1:3) having molecular weights of 50,000 and 24,000, and their amino acid compositions have been determined (281). The effect of the toxin is dose dependent and time dependent. From experiments on isolated guinea pig heart muscle, Fassold et al. (282) determined that the mechanism of action of this toxin (10–50 μg/ml) was to make the SR membrane leaky to Ca^{2+} ion so that the SR cannot adequately sequester the myoplasmic Ca^{2+} (Table 6). The Ca–ATPase of the SR was not inhibited, nor was the Na/K–ATPase activity. The toxin also altered the ultrastructure of the mitochondria and inhibited their ability to accumulate Ca^{2+}. These findings can explain why the toxin increases the diastole resting tension of cardiac muscle because of the predicted rise in $[Ca]_i$, causing Ca overload. The possible metabolic impairment of the mitochondria would contribute to the Ca^{2+} overload.

Cobra Venom Cardiotoxin

Two toxins isolated from the venom of the Indian cobra *(Naja nigricollis)* are polypeptides; one is a neurotoxin and the other is a cardiotoxin (283,284). The cardiotoxin has a molecular weight of about 6500 (60–62 amino acids) and causes systolic arrest. The toxin lacks phospholipase activity. In experiments on SR fractions isolated from guinea pig hearts, Nayler et al. (285) found that the cobra cardiotoxin (10–50 μg/ml) depressed Ca^{2+} accumulation by the SR (Table 6). This effect was due to inhibition of the Ca–ATPase and to release of previously sequestered Ca^{2+}; that is, the SR

TABLE 6. *Some agents that affect the sarcoplasmic reticulum (SR) or the Na–K pump of the sarcolemma*

Depress Ca^{2+} uptake by SR		Inhibit Na/K–ATPase
Inhibit Ca–ATPase	Increase g_{Ca} of SR membrane	
Cobra venom toxin	Volvatoxin A	Cardiac glycosides
Halothane	Cobra venom toxin	Vanadate
Endotoxin		Local anesthetics
Quinidine		Sulfhydryl reagents
		Phlorizin
		Oligomycin
		Chlorpromazine free radical
		Ethanol (acutely)

membranes become more leaky. The toxin also depressed Ca^{2+} accumulation by isolated mitochondria. When isolated papillary muscles or perfused hearts were exposed to the cardiotoxin, extensive ultrastructural damage was observed including disruption of the cell membrane, vacuolated mitochondria, and disrupted myofibrils and contracture bands. Thus the mode of action of the cobra cardiotoxin is quite different from volvatoxin A, although both toxins have an effect on the SR. It was postulated by Nayler et al. (285) that the cobra cardiotoxin first disrupts the myocardial cell membranes, and then both the toxin and Ca^{2+} enter the cells, where the toxin suppresses the uptake of Ca^{2+} by the SR and mitochondria, thereby causing an elevated $[Ca]_i$ with all the consequences of such Ca^{2+} overload.

Palytoxin

Palytoxin, isolated from zoanthids (genus *Palythoa*), is a potent marine toxin. It depolarizes cells, and the depolarization is Na^+ dependent and TTX resistant (286,287). Palytoxin produces contracture, associated with Ca^{2+} uptake, of isolated cardiac muscle in below nanomolar concentrations (288). In patch clamp studies on isolated single ventricular cells from guinea pig, it was found that palytoxin (2×10^{-11} M) induces (within a few minutes) a type of Na^+-selective ionic channel having unique gating behavior (289). The single-channel inward current was resistant to TTX and Co^{2+} and was present in Ca^{2+}-free solution but not in Na^+-free solution. Thus the palytoxin-induced channel has a high selectivity for Na^+, and thereby depolarizes. Inactivation is not produced when the membrane is depolarized. The authors suggested that palytoxin forms a unique type of channel.

SUMMARY AND CONCLUSIONS

In surveying the cardiotoxic agents to be discussed, it was not possible to cover all or even most of such agents, but representative agents of a wide variety of chemical structures that exerted a variety of mechanisms of action were examined. A summary of the effects of the various agents is given in Tables 1–6.

Some agents blocked various ionic channels, whereas other agents opened and held open certain ionic channels. The kinetics of opening and closing of the channel gates were sometimes affected (slowed). Some agents (e.g., verapamil) also depressed the recovery kinetics of the slow channels. We saw that some agents, such as the cardiac glycosides, exerted their therapeutic and toxic effects by inhibiting the Na–K pump. In other cases, the primary site of action of the cardiotoxin did not appear to be on the electrical properties of the cell membrane, but instead affected the uptake or release of Ca^{2+} by the SR. We discussed why agents that affect metabolism of the heart will indirectly have effects on the membrane electrical properties, as, for example, a rapid depression of the inward slow (Ca–Na) current, and later an acceleration of the g_K turn-on kinetics (delayed rectification) perhaps due to an increase in $[Ca]_i$.

Changes in the electrical properties of the cell membrane produced by the cardiotoxic agents have important repercussions on the mechanical activity of the heart and its usefulness as a blood pump. The electrical activity exerts tight control over the mechanical activity. Block of the slow channels selectively by some agents depresses the force of contraction directly by reducing the Ca^{2+} influx, whereas the electrical activity remains nearly normal (excitation–contraction uncoupling). Depression of velocity of propagation greatly weakens the heart because the entire heart must be activated quickly (e.g., within 10–20 msec) in order for the heart to be effective as a pump (e.g., series elastic problem). Depressed conduction velocity can also give rise to arrhythmias (reentrant type) that can lead to ventricular fibrillation, thus making the heart completely ineffectual as a pump. Similar problems can arise by agents that cause automaticity in heart cells not normally exhibiting automaticity or enhance automaticity in latent pacemaker cells (e.g., Purkinje fibers) (ectopic foci). Nonuniform changes in duration of the AP, and hence in the refractory periods, by cardiotoxic agents also predisposes to the development of dysrhythmias and fibrillation. Depression of conduction velocity will occur by agents that depolarize or depress the kinetics of turn-on of fast g_{Na}. Prolongation of the AP will occur by agents that inhibit inactivation of the fast g_{Na} (hold open the I gates of the fast Na^+ channels) or that inhibit activation of the g_K (delayed rectification).

The changes in the electrical properties of the cell membrane produced by many cardiotoxic substances can lead indirectly to changes in the ultrastructure of the cells. For example, an agent, such as excessive catecholamines, which increased $[Ca]_i$ directly (e.g., by increasing g_{Ca}) could cause supercontraction of the myofilaments, SR swelling, deposits in the mitochondria, and other evidence of Ca^{2+} overload. The internal [Ca] also exerts control on a number of enzymes, including phospholipases. Other agents, such as BTX or metabolic poisons, that increase $[Ca]_i$ indirectly (e.g., by increasing $[Na]_i$ coupled with the Ca–Na exchange reaction or by lowering the ATP level required for Ca^{2+} or Na^+ pumping and exchange) could produce similar morphological changes.

Vice versa, agents that have their primary site of action on an internal organelle could exert secondary effects on the electrical behavior of the cell membrane. For example, an agent, such as volvatoxin, that caused SR (or mitochondria) not to properly sequester Ca^{2+}, could cause $[Ca]_i$ to rise and this would increase g_K (steady-state and kinetics of turn-on) and hyperpolarize and would reduce I_{Ca} because of a reduced electrochemical driving force and perhaps an effect on g_{Ca}. For another example, an agent, such as hypoxia or cyanide, that depressed metabolism of the mitochondria would lead to depression of Ca^{2+} influx (because of the metabolic dependence of the slow channels) and contraction, and to an increase in steady-state g_K and in g_K turn-on (because of the elevated $[Ca]_i$).

It is obvious that no cardiotoxic agent improves the functioning of the heart. The channel gating mechanisms and kinetics are more or less normally optimal and the toxic agents interfere with the operation of the various component parts. Of the agents that are used therapeutically to treat heart diseases (e.g., cardiac glycosides, local anesthetics, and Ca^{2+} antagonists), they may be therapeutic at one dose, but highly toxic at a higher dose.

ACKNOWLEDGMENTS

The work from the author's laboratory summarized in this chapter was supported by a grant from the U.S. Public Health Service (HL-18711). The author would like to thank Rhonda Hentz for help in preparing the manuscript, Anthony Sperelakis for help with figures, and Dr. Ira Josephson for help with several brief sections.

REFERENCES

1. Shigenobu K, Sperelakis N. Ca^{2+} current channels induced by catecholamines in chick embryonic hearts whose fast Na^+ channels are blocked by TTX or elevated K^+. *Circ Res* 1972;31:932–952.
2. Tsien RW, Giles W, Greengard P. Cyclic AMP mediates the effects of adrenaline on cardiac Purkinje fibers. *Nature (London) New Biol* 1972;240:181.
3. Schneider JA, Sperelakis N. Slow Ca^{2+} and Na^+ responses induced by isoproterenol and methylxanthines in isolated perfused guinea pig hearts exposed to elevated K^+. *J Mol Cell Cardiol* 1975;7:249–273.
4. Sperelakis N, Schneider JA. A metabolic control mechanism for calcium ion influx that may protect the ventricular myocardial cell. *Am J Cardiol* 1976;37:1079–1085.
5. Reuter H, Scholz H. The regulation of the calcium conductance of heart muscle by adrenaline. *J Physiol* 1977;264:49–62.
6. George WJ, Wilkerson RD, Kadowitz PJ. Influence of acetylcholine on contractile force and cyclic levels in the isolated perfused rat heart. *J Pharmacol Exp Ther* 1973; 184:228.
7. Watanabe AM, Besch HR Jr. Interaction between cyclic adenosine monophosphate and cyclic guanosine monophosphate in guinea pig ventricular myocardium. *Circ Res* 1975;37:309.
8. TenEick R, Nawrath H, McDonald TF, Trautwein W. On the mechanism of the negative inotropic action of acetylcholine. *Pflugers Arch Eur J Pharmacol* 1976;361:207.
9. Giles W, Noble SJ. Changes in membrane currents in bullfrog atrium produced by acetylcholine. *J Physiol (Lond.)* 1976;261:103.
10. Inui J, Imamura H. Effects of acetylcholine on calcium-dependent electrical and mechanical responses in the guinea-pig papillary muscle depolarized by potassium. *Naunyn Schmiedebergs Arch Pharmacol* 1977;209:1.
11. Nawrath H. Does cyclic GMP mediate the negative inotropic effect of acetylcholine in the heart? *Nature* 1977;267:72.
12. Ikemoto Y, Goto M. Effects of acetylcholine on slow inward current and tension components of the bullfrog atrium. *J Mol Cell Cardiol* 1977;9:313.
13. Josephson I, Sperelakis N. Acetylcholine blockade of the Ca^{2+}-mediated action potential in cultured heart cells. *Fed Proc Fed Am Soc Exp Biol* 1979;38(3):1387 (abstract).

14. Biegon R, Pappano A. Dual mechanism for acetycholine inhibition of calcium-dependent action potentials (AP) in avian ventricle. *Fed Proc Fed Am Soc Exp Biol* 1979;38(3):986 (abstract).

15. Wahler GM, Sperelakis N. Cholinergic attenuation of the electrophysiological effects of forskolin. *J Cyclic Nucleotide and Prot Phosphorylation Res* 1986;11:1–10.

16. Sperelakis N. Effects of cardiotoxic agents on the electrical properties of myocardial cells. In: Balazs T, ed. *Cardiac toxicology.* Boca Raton, FL: CRC Press; 1981:39–108.

17. Sperelakis N. Physiological principles of cardiac toxicology. In: Baskin SI, ed. *Principles of Cardiac Toxicology.* CRC Press, 1991;71–166.

18. McDonald TF, Hunter EG, MacLeod DP. Adenosinetriphosphate partition in cardiac muscle with respect to transmembrane electrical activity. *Pflugers Arch* 1971;322:95–108.

19. Neely JR, Rovetto MJ, Whitmer JT, Morgan HE. Effects of ischemia on function and metabolism of the isolated working rat heart. *Am J Physiol* 1973;225:651.

20. Neely JR, Whitmer JT, Rovetto MJ. Effect of coronary blood flow on glycolytic flux and intracellular pH in isolated hearts. *Circ Res* 1975;37:733.

21. Bricknell OL, Opie LH. Glycolytic ATP and its production during ischemia in isolated Langendorff-perfused rat hearts. In: Kobayshi T, Sano T, Dhalla NS, eds. *Recent advances in studies on cardiac structure and metabolism.* Baltimore: University Park Press; 1978:509–519.

22. Williamson JR, Schaffer SW, Ford C, Safer B. Contribution of tissue acidosis to ischemic injury in the perfused rat heart. In: Braunwald E, ed. *Protection of the ischemic myocardium.* Washington, DC: CIRC, 1976;53:1–3, 1–14.

23. Poole-Wilson, PA. Measurement of myocardial intracellular pH in pathological states. *J Mol Cell Cardiol* 1978;10:511.

24. Sperelakis N, Belardinelli L, Vogel SM. Electrophysiological aspects during myocardial ischemia. In: Hayase S, Murao S, eds. *Proceedings, VIII World Congress on cardiology.* Amsterdam: Excerpta Medica; 1979:229–236.

25. Kohlhardt M, Haap K, Figulla HR. Influence of low extracellular pH upon the Ca inward current and isometric contractile force in mammalian ventricular myocardium. *Pflugers Arch* 1976;366:31–38.

26. Vogel S, Sperelakis N. Blockade of myocardial slow inward current at low pH. *Am J Physiol* 1977;233:C99–C103.

27. Chesnais JM, Coraboeuf E, Sauviat MP, Vassas JM. Sensitivity to H, Li and Mg ions of the slow inward sodium current in frog atrial fibers. *J Mol Cell Cardiol* 1975;7:627–642.

28. Steenbergen C, DeLeemin G, Rich T, Williamson JR. Effects of acidosis and ischemia on contractility and intracellular pH of rat heart. *Circ Res* 1977;41:849–858.

29. Bing OHL, Brooks WW, Messer JV. Heart muscle viability following hypoxia: protective effect of acidosis. *Science* 1973;180:1297–1298.

30. Bing OHL, Apstein CS, Brook WW. Factors influencing tolerance of cardiac muscle to hypoxia. In: Roy, PE, Rona, G, eds. *Recent Advances in Studies on Cardiac Structure and Metabolism* Baltimore: University Park Press 1975;343–354.

31. Belardinelli L, Vogel SM, Sperelakis N, Rubio R, Berne RM. Restoration of slow responses in hypoxic heart muscle by alkaline pH. *J Mol Cell Cardiol* 1979;11:877–892.

32. McDonald TF, MacLeod DP. Metabolism and the electrical activity of anoxic ventricular muscle. *J Physiol* 1973;229:559–582.

33. Vleugels A, Carmeliet E, Bosteels S, Zaman M. Differential effects of hypoxia with age on the chick embryonic heart. *Pflugers Arch* 1976;365:159.

34. Vogel S, Sperelakis N. Valinomycin blockade of myocardial slow channels is reversed by high glucose. *Am J Physiol* 1978;235:H46–H51.

35. Fleckenstein A. Specific inhibitors and promoters of calcium action in the excitation-contraction coupling of heart muscle and their role in the prevention or production of myocardial lesions. In: Harris P, Opie LH, eds. *Calcium and the Heart,* London: Academic Press, 1971;135.

36. Puri PS. Modification of experimental myocardial infarct size by cardiac drugs. *Am J Cardiol* 1974;33:521–528.

37. Wollenberger A, Krause EG, Shahab L. Endogenous catecholamine mobilization and the shift to anaerobic energy production in the acutely ischemic myocardium. In: Mar-

chetti G, Taccardi B, eds. *Coronary Circulation and Energetics of the Myocardium,* Basel: Karger, 1967;200.

38. Wollenberger A, Shahab L. Anoxia-induced release of noradrenaline from the isolated perfused heart. *Nature (London)* 1965;207:88.

39. Waldenstrom AP, Kjalmarson AC, Thornell L. A possible role of noradrenaline in the development of myocardial infarction. *Am Heart J* 1978;95:43–.

40. Roberts WC, Buja LM. The frequency and significance of coronary arterial thrombi and other observations in fatal acute myocardial infarction. A study of 107 neuropsy patients. *Am J Med* 1972;52:425–443.

41. Fleckenstein A, Janke J, Doring HJ, Pachinger O. Ca overload as the determinant factor in the production of catecholamine-induced myocardial lesions. In: Bajusz E, Rona G, eds. *Recent Advances in Studies on Cardiac Structure and Metabolism* Munich: Urban Schwarzenbertg, 1973;455.

42. Johnson G. Cholera toxin action and the regulation of hormone-sensitive adenylate cyclase. In: Cohen P, VanHeyningen S, eds. *Molecular Action of Toxin and Viruses* New York: Elsevier, 1982;33–49.

43. Allende J. GTP-mediated macromolecular interactions: the common features of different system. *FASEB J.* 1988;2:2356–2367.

44. Li T, Sperelakis N. Stimulation of slow action potentials in guinea pig papillary muscle by intracellular injection of cyclic AMP, GPP(NH)P and cholera toxin. *Circ Res* 1983;52:111–117.

45. Kodama I, Kondo N, Shibata S. Electromechanical effects of okadaic acid isolated from block sponge in guinea-pig ventricular muscle. *J Physiol* 1986;378:359–373.

46. Hechler J, Mieskes G, Ruegg JC, Takai A, Trautwein W. Effects of a protein phosphate inhibitor, okadaic acid, on membrane currents on isolated guinea-pig cardiac myocytes. *Pflugers Arch* 1988;412:248.

47. Sperelakis N. *Calcium antagonists: mechanism of action on cardiac muscle and vascular smooth muscle.* Boston: Martinus Nijhoff Publishers, 1984;1–352.

48. McLean MJ, Shigenobu K. Sperelakis N. Two pharmacological types of slow Na$^+$ channels as distinguished by verapamil blockade. *Eur J Pharmacol* 1974;26:379–382.

49. Nawrath H, TenEick RE, McDonald TF, Trautwein W. On the mechanism underlying the action of D-600 on slow inward current and tension in mammalian myocardium. *Circ Res* 1977;40:408.

50. Kohlhardt M, Mnich Z. Studies on the inhibitory effect of verapamil on the slow inward current in mammalian ventricular myocardium. *J Mol Cell Cardiol* 1978;10:1037–1052.

51. Kojima M, Sperelakis N, Calcium antagonistic drugs differ in ability to block the slow Na$^+$ channels of young embryonic chick hearts. *Eur J Pharmacol* 1983;94:9–18.

52. Vogel S, Crampton R, Sperelakis N. Blockade of myocardial slow channels by bepridil (CERM-1978). *J Pharmacol Exp Ther* 1979;210:378–385.

53. McLean MJ, Shigenobu K, Sperelakis N. Two pharmacological types of cardiac slow Na$^+$ channels as distinguished by verapamil. *Eur J Pharmacol* 1974;26:379–382.

54. Kohldart M, Fleckenstein A. Inhibition of the slow inward current by nifedipine in mammalian ventricular myocardium. *Naunyn Schmiedebergs Arch Pharmacol* 1977; 298:267–272.

55. Pang DC, Sperelakis N. Nifedipine, diltiazem, bepridil, and verapamil uptakes into cardiac and smooth muscles. *Eur J Pharmacol* 1983;87:199–207.

56. Schneider JA, Brooker G, Sperelakis N. Papaverine blockade of an inward slow Ca^{2+} current in guinea pig heart. *J Mol Cell Cardiol* 1975;7:867–876.

57. Kohlhardt M, Bauer B, Krause H, Fleckenstein A. Differentiation of the transmembrane Na and Ca channels in mammalian cardiac fibers by the use of specific inhibitors. *Pflugers Arch* 1972;335:309–322.

58. Shigenobu K, Schneider JA, Sperelakis N. Verapamil blockade of slow Na$^+$ and Ca^{2+} responses in myocardial cells. *J Pharmacol Exp Ther* 1974;190:280–288.

59. Bayer R, Kalusche D, Kauffman R, Mannhold R. Inotropic and electrophysiological actions of verapamil and D600 in mammalian myocardium. III. Effects of optical isomers on transmembrane action potentials. *Naunyn Schmiedebergs Arch Pharmacol* 1975;290:81–97.

60. Kass RS, Tsein RW. Multiple effects of calcium antagonists on plateau currents in cardiac Purkinje fibers. *J Gen Physiol* 1975;66:169–192.

61. Reuter H. Properties of two inward membrane currents in the heart. *Annu Rev Physiol* 1979;41:413–424.
62. Coraboeuf E, Vassort G. Effects of some inhibitors of ionic permeabilities on ventricular action potential and contraction of rat and guinea-pig hearts. *J Electrocardiol* 1968;1:19–29.
63. Kohlhardt M, Bauer B, Krause H, Fleckenstein A. Selective inhibition of the transmembrane calcium conductivity of mammalian myocardial fibers by Ni, Co and Mn ions. *Pflugers Arch Eur J Physiol* 1973;338:115–123.
64. Renaud JF, Sperelakis N. Electrophysiological properties of chick embryonic hearts grafted and organ cultured in vitro. *J Mol Cell Cardiol* 1976;8:889–900.
65. Sperelakis N, Valle R, Orozco C, Martinez-Palomo A, Rubio R. Electromechanical uncoupling of frog skeletal muscle by possible change in sarcoplasmic reticular content. *Am J Physiol* 1973;225:793–800.
66. Delahayes JF. Depolarization-induced movement of Mn^{++} across the cell membrane in the guinea pig myocardium. *Circ Res* 1975;36:713–718.
67. Ochi R. Manganese-dependent propagated action potentials and their depression by electrical stimulation in guinea-pig myocardium perfused by Na^+-free media. *J Physiol* 1976;263:139.
68. Semenova LA, Martyniuk RA, Martsinovich VP. Acute lesion of rat myocardium by a single injection of cobalt dichloride. *Cor Vasa* 1975;17:145–150.
69. Kymoto Y, Saito M, Goto M. Effects of caffeine on the membrane potentials, membrane currents, and contractility of the bullfrog atrium. *Jpn J Physiol* 1974;240:531–542.
70. Langer GA, Frank JA. Lanthanum in heart cells culture. Effect on calcium exchange correlated with its localization. *J Cell Biol* 1972;54:441–455.
71. Langer GA, Frank JS, Nudd LM, Seraydarian K. Sialic acid; effect of removal on calcium exchangeability of cultured heart cells. *Science* 1976;193:1013–1015.
72. Nayler WG, Poole-Wilson PH, Williams A. Hypoxia and calcium. *J Mol Cell Cardiol* 1979;11:683.
73. Burton KP, Hagler HK, Templeton GH, Willerson JT, Buja LM. Membrane permeability alterations induced by hypoxia precede the development of irreversible injury in isolated cardiac muscle. *Circulation* 1976;54(suppl):11.
74. Frank JS, Langer GA, Nudd LM, Seraydarian K. The myocardial cell surface, its histochemistry, and the effect of sialic acid and calcium removal on its structure and cellular ionic exchange. *Circ Res* 1977;41:702.
75. Sperelakis N, Lehmkuhl D. Ionic interconversion of pacemaker and nonpacemaker cultured chick heart cells. *J Gen Physiol* 1966;49:867–895.
76. Sperelakis N, Schneider M, Harris EJ. Decreased K^+ conductance produced by Ba^{2+} in frog sartorius fibers. *J Gen Physiol* 1967;50:1565–1583.
77. Hermsmeyer K, Sperelakis N. Decrease in K^+ conductance and depolarization of frog cardiac muscle produced by Ba^{++}. *Am J Physiol* 1970;219:1108–1114.
78. Kumamoto M, Nakajima A, Horn L. Effect of TEA on membrane excitability of vascular smooth muscle. *Jpn J Smooth Muscle Res* 1973;9:205–207.
79. Vereecke J, Carmeliet E. Strontium action potentials in cardiac Purkinje fibers. II. Dependence of the SR conductance on the external SR concentration and SR–Ca antagonism. *Pflugers Arch Eur J Physiol* 1971;322:73.
80. Kleinfield M, Stein E. Action of divalent cations on membrane potentials and contractility in rat atrium. *Am J Physiol* 1968;215:593–599.
81. Kleinfield M, Greene H, Stein E, Magin J. Effect of cadmium ion on the electrical and mechanical activity of the frog heart. *Am J Physiol* 1955;181:35–38.
82. Toda N. Influence of cadmium ions on the transmembrane potential and contractility of isolated rabbit left atria. *J Pharmacol Exp Ther* 1973;186:60.
83. Langer GA, Serena SD, Nudd LM. Cation exchange in heart cell culture: correlation with effects on contractile force. *J Mol Cell Cardiol* 1974;6:149–161.
84. Kopp SJ, Hawley PL. Factors influencing cadmium toxicity in A-V conduction system of isolated perfused rat heart. *Toxicol Appl Pharmacol* 1976;37:631–644.
85. Kopp SJ, Hawley PL. Cadmium feeding: apparent depression of atrioventricular–His–Purkinje conduction system. *Acta Pharmacol Toxicol* 1978;42:110–116.
86. Borchard U, Fox AAL, Greeff K, Schlieper P. Negative and positive inotropic action of vanadate on atrial and ventricular myocardium. *Nature* 1979;279:339–341.

87. Armstrong C, Binstock L. Anomalous rectification in the squid giant axon injected with tetraethylammonium chloride. *J Gen Physiol* 1965;48:859–872.
88. Armstrong CM. Inactivation of the potassium conductance and related phenomena caused by quarternary ammonium ion injection in squid axon. *J Gen Physiol* 1969;54:553–575.
89. Yeh JZ, Oxford GS, Wu CH, Narahashi T. Dynamics of aminopyridine block of potassium channels in squid axon membrane. *J Gen Physiol* 1976;68:519.
90. Gillespie JI. Voltage-dependent blockade of the delayed potassium current in skeletal muscle by 4-aminopyridine. *J Physiol (Lond.)* 1977;273:64.
91. Volle RL. Actions of acridine compounds and barium ions on action potentials of frog muscle fibers. *Life Sci* 1970;9:753.
92. Harder DR, Sperelakis N. Action potentials induced in guinea pig arterial smooth muscle by tetraethylammonium. *Am J Physiol* 1979;237:C75–C80.
93. Harder DR, Sperelakis N. Action potential generation in reaggregates of rat aortic smooth muscle cells in primary culture. *Blood Vessels* 1979;16:186–201.
94. Miller C, Moczydlowski E, Latorre R, Phillips M. *Nature* 1985;313:316–318.
95. Lazdunski M. Apamin, a neurotoxin specific for one class of Ca^{2+}-dependent K^+ channels. *Cell Calcium* 1983;4:421.
96. Post JM, Stevens RJ, Sanders KM, Hume JR. Effect of cromakalim and lemakalim on slow waves and membrane currents in colonic smooth muscle. *Am J Physiol* 1991;260:C375–C382.
97. Erne P, Hermsmeyer K. Modulation of intracellular calcium by potassium channel openers in vascular muscle. *Naunyn Schmiedebergs Arch Pharmacol* 1991;344:706–715.
98. Xiong ZL, Kajioka S, Sakai T, Kitamura K, Kuriyama H. Pinacidil inhibits the ryanodine-sensitive outward current and glibenclamide antagonizes its action in cells from the rabbit portal vein. *Br J Pharmacol* 1991;102:788–790.
99. Bonnet P, Rusch NJ, Harder DR. Characterization of an outward K^+ current in freshly dispersed cerebral arterial muscle cells. *Pflugers Arch* 1991;418:292–296.
100. Bacaner MB, Clay JR, Shrier A, Brochu RM. Potassium channel blockade: a mechanism of suppressing ventricular fibrillation. *Proc Natl Acad Sci USA* 1986;83:2223–2227.
101. Bkaily G, Payet MD, Benabderrazik M, Renaud JF, Sauve R, Bacaner MB, Sperelakis N. Bethanidine increased Na^+ and Ca^{2+} currents and caused a positive inotropic effect in heart cells. *Can J Physiol Pharmacol* 1988;66(3):190–196.
102. Bkaily G, Payet MD, Benabderrazik M, Sauve R, Renaud JF, Bacaner MB, Sperelakis N. Intracellular bretylium blocks Na^+ and K^+ currents in heart cells. *Eur J Pharmacol* 1988;151:389–397.
103. Bkaily G, Caille JP, Payet MD, Peyrow M, Sauve R, Renaud JF, Sperelakis N. Bethanidine increases one type of potassium current and relaxes aortic muscle. *Can J Physiol Pharmacol* 1988;66:731–736.
104. Schwartz A, Lindenmayer GE, Allen JC. The sodium–potassium adenosine triphosphatase: pharmacological, physiological and biochemical aspects. *Pharmacol Rev* 1975;27:3–134.
105. Josephson I, Sperelakis N. Ouabain blockade of inward slow current in cardiac muscle. *J Mol Cell Cardiol* 1977;9:409.
106. Belardinelli L, Harder D, Sperelakis N, Rubio R, Berne RM. Cardiac glycoside stimulation of inward Ca^{++} current in vascular smooth muscle of canine coronary artery. *J Pharmacol Exp Ther* 1979;209:62–66.
107. Forbes MS, Sperelakis N. (Na^+,K^+)-ATPase activity in tubular systems of mouse cardiac and skeletal muscles. *Z Zellforsch Mikrosk Anat* 1972;134:1–11.
108. Ferrier GR, Moe GK. Effect of calcium on acetylstrophanthidin-induced transient depolarizations in canine Purkinje tissue. *Circ Res* 1973;33:508.
109. Kass RS, Lederer WJ, Tsien RW, Weingard R. Role of calcium ions in transient inward currents and aftercontractions induced by strophanthidin in cardiac Purkinje fiber. *J Physiol (Lond)* 1978;281:187.
110. Moe GK, Farah AD. Digitalis and allied cardiac glycosides. In: Goodman LS, Gilman A, eds. *The pharmacological basis of therapeutics*. New York: Macmillan; 1975:653.
111. Vassalle M, Greenspan K, Hoffman BF. Analysis of arrhythmias induced by ouabain in intact dogs. *Circ Res* 1963;13:132.

112. Narahashi T, Frazier DT, Moore JW. Comparison of tertiary and quarternary amine local anesthetics in their ability to depress membrane ionic conductances. *J Neurobiol* 1972;3:267.

113. Josephson I, Sperelakis N. Local anesthetic blockade of Ca^{2+}-mediated action potentials in cardiac muscle. *Eur J Pharmacol* 1976;40:201.

114. Brennan FJ, Cranefield PF, Wit AL. Effect of lidocaine on slow response and depressed fast response action potentials of canine cardiac Purkinje fibers. *J Pharmacol Exp Ther* 1978;204:312–324.

115. Skou JC, Zerahn K. Investigations on the effect of some local anesthetics and other amines on the active transport of sodium through the isolated shortcircuited frog skin. *Biochim Biophys Acta* 1959;35:324.

116. Henn FA, Sperelakis N. Stimulative and protective action of Sr^{2+} and Ba^{2+} on $(Na^{+}-K^{+})$-ATPase from cultured heart cells. *Biochim Biophys Acta* 1968;163:415–417.

117. Riccioppo-Neto F, Sperelakis N. Effects of lidocaine, procainamide and quinidine on electrophysiologic properties of cultured embryonic chick hearts. *Br J Pharmacol* 1985;86:817–826.

118. Moe GK, Abilskov JA. Antiarrhythmic drugs. In: Goodman LS, Gilman A, eds. *The pharmacological basis of therapeutics*. New York: Macmillan; 1975:683.

119. Bigger JT Jr, Bassett AL, Hoffman BF. Electrophysiological effects of diphenylhydantoin in canine Purkinje fibers. *Circ Res* 1968;22:221–236.

120. Bigger JT Jr, Mandel WJ. Effect of lidocaine on the electrophysiological properties of ventricular muscle and Purkinje fibers. *J Clin Invest* 1970;49:63–77.

121. Cranefield PF. *The conduction of the cardiac impulse*. Mt Kisco, NY: Futura; 1975.

122. Brennan FJ, Cranefield PF, Wit AL. Effects of lidocaine and on slow response and depressed fast response action potentials of canine cardiac Purkinje fibers. *J Pharmacol Exp Ther* 1978;204:312–324.

123. Weld FM, Bigger JT Jr. Effect of lidocaine on diastolic transmembrane currents determining pacemaker depolarization in cardiac Purkinje fibers. *Circ Res* 1976;38:203.

124. Davis CD, Temte JV. Electrophysiological actions of lidocaine on canine ventricular muscle and Purkinje fibers. *Circ Res* 1969;24:639–655.

125. Lipicky RJ, Ehrenstein G, Gilbert DL. Mechanism of blockage of sodium channels by yohimbine in squid giant axon. *Biophys J* 1977;17:205a.

126. Lipicky RJ, Gilbert DL, Ehrenstein G. Blockage of ionic currents by yohimbine in squid giant axon. *Biophys J* 1976;16:186a.

127. Huang LM, Ehrenstein G, Catterall WA. Interaction between batrachotoxin and yohimbine in cultured neuroblastoma cells. *Biophys J* 1977;17:208a (Abstr).

128. Azuma J, Vogel S, Josephson I, Sperelakis N. Yohimbine blockade of ionic channels in myocardial cells. *Eur J Pharmacol* 1978;51:109–119.

129. Fuchs S, Gertz EW, Briggs FN. The effect of quinidine on calcium accumulation by isolated sarcoplasmic reticulum of skeletal and cardiac muscle. *J Gen Physiol* 1968; 52:955.

130. Vaughan Williams EM, Polster P. The effect on cardiac muscle of two drugs related to amiodarone, L8040 and L8462. *Eur J Pharmacol* 1974;25:241.

131. Vatner SF. Effects of anaesthesia on cardiovascular control mechanisms. *Environ Health* 1978;26:193.

132. Narahashi T, Moore JW, Poston RN. Anesthetic blocking of nerve membrane conductances by internal and external applications. *J Neurobiol* 1969;1:3.

133. Blaustein MP. Barbiturates block sodium and potassium conductance increases in voltage-clamped lobster axons. *J Gen Physiol* 1968;51:293–307.

134. Ko KC, Paradise RR. The effects of substrates on contractility of rat atria depressed with halothane. *Anesthesiology* 1969;31:532–539.

135. Su JY, Kerrick GL. Effects of halothane on caffeine-induced tension transients in functionally skinned myocardial fibers. *Pflugers Arch* 1979;380:29–34.

136. Lee SL, Alto LE, Dhalla NS. Subcellular effects on some anesthetic agents on rat myocardium. *Can J Physiol Pharmacol* 1979;57:65–70.

137. Lain RF, Hess ML, Gertz EW, Briggs NF. Calcium uptake activity of canine myocardial sarcoplasmic reticulum in the presence of anesthetic agents. *Circ Res* 1968;23:597–604.

138. Merin RG, Kumazawa R, Honig CR. Reversible interaction between halothane and Ca^{++} on cardiac actomyosin adenosine triphosphate conductance in Alpysia nerve cells. *Comp Biochem Physiol* 1974;190:1–14.

139. Hauswirth O. Effects of halothane on single atrial, ventricular, and Purkinje fibers. *Circ Res* 1969;24:745.
140. Hauswirth O, Schaen H. Effects of halothane on the sino-atrial node. *J Pharmacol Exp Ther* 1967;198:36.
141. Reynolds AK, Chiz JF, Pasquet AF. Halothane and methoxyfluorane: a comparison of their effects on cardiac pacemaker fibers. *Anesthesiology* 1970;33:602–610.
142. Lynch C, Vogel S, Sperelakis N. Halothane depression of myocardial slow action potentials. *Anesthesiology* 1981;55:360–368.
143. Lynch C, Vogel S, Pratila MG, Sperelakis N. Enflurane depression of myocardial slow action potentials. *J Pharmacol Exp Ther* 1982;222:405–409.
144. Shrivastav BB, Narahashi T, Kitz RJ, Roberts JD. Mode of action of trichlorethylene on squid axon membranes. *J Pharmacol Exp Ther* 1976;199:179.
145. Pratila M, Vogel S, Sperelakis N. Inhibition by enflurane and methoxyflurane of post-drive hyperpolarization in canine Purkinje fibers. *J Pharmacol Exp Ther* 1984;229:603–607.
146. Pratila MC, Pratilas V. Effects of the volatile anesthetic agents on the heart. In: Sperelakis N, ed. *Physiology and pathophysiology of the heart.* Boston: Kluwer Academic Publishers; 1988:671–690.
147. Aviado DM. Effects of fluorocarbons, chlorinated solvents, and inosine on the cardiopulmonary system. *Environ Health Perspect* 1978;26:207–215.
148. Pardini RS. Polychlorinated biphenyls (PCB): effect on mitochondrial enzyme systems. *Bull Environ Contam Toxicol* 1971;6:539–545.
149. Goodman LS, Gilman A. *The pharmacological basis of therapeutics.* New York: Macmillan, 1970.
150. Sigg EB, Osborne M, Korol B. Cardiovascular effects of imipramine. *J Pharmacol Exp Ther* 1963;141:237.
151. Hurst JW. *The heart.* New York: McGraw-Hill, 1978.
152. Biggs JT, Spiker DG, Petit JM, Ziegler VE. Tricyclic antidepressant overdose: incidence of symptoms. *JAMA* 1977;238:135–138.
153. Thorstrand C. Clinical features in poisonings by tricyclic antidepressants with special reference to the ECG. *Acta Med Scand* 1976;199:337.
154. Vohra J, Burrows G, Hunt D, Sloman G. The effect of toxic and therapeutic doses of tricyclic antidepressant drugs on intracardiac conduction. *Eur J Cardiol* 1975;3:219.
155. Moyer JH, Kent B, Knight R, Morris G, Huggins R, Handley CA. Laboratory and clinical observation on chlorpromazine (SKF-2601): hemodynamic and toxicological studies. *Am J Med Sci* 1954;227:282.
156. Cerletti A, Fanchamps A. Neuroplegie und kontrollierte Hypothermie; Bemerkungen zur Frage der "kunstlichen Hibernation." *Schweiz Wochenschr* 1955;85:141–148.
157. Arita M, Mashiba H. Effects of phenothiazine and propranolol on ECG. The effects of propranolol on the electrocardiographic abnormalities induced by phenothiazine derivatives. *Jpn Circ J* 1970;34:391–400.
158. Arita M, Surawicz B. Electrophysiologic effect of phenothiazines on canine cardiac fibers. *J Pharmacol Exp Ther* 1973;184:619–630.
159. Arita M, Nagamoto Y, Saikawa T. Intraventricular conduction disturbance due to delayed recovery from ventricular inactivation in chlorpromazine-treated dogs. In: Kobayashi T, Sano T, Dhalla NS, eds. *Recent advances in studies on cardiac structure and metabolism.* Baltimore: University Park Press; 1978:85–90.
160. O'Bryan R, Luce J, Talley R, Gottlieb J, Baker L, Bonadonna G. Phase II evaluation of adriamycin in human neoplasia. *Cancer* 1973;32:1.
161. Herman EH, Schen P, Farmar RM. Influence of pharmacologic or physiologic pretreatment on acute daunomycin cardiac toxicity in the hamster. *Toxicol Appl Pharmacol* 1970;16:335.
162. Herman EH, Hatre RM, Lee I, Vick J, Waravdekar V. A comparison of the cardiovascular actions of daunomycin, adriamycin and *N*-acetyl-daunomycin in hamsters and monkeys. *Pharmacology* 1971;6:230.
163. Buja LM, Ferrans VJ, Roberts WC. Drug-induced cardiomyopathies. Comparative pathology of the heart. *Adv Cardiol* 1974;13:330–348.
164. Balazs T, Herman EH. Toxic cardiomyopathies. *Ann Clin Lab Sci* 1976;6:467–476.
165. Balazs T, Ferrans VJ. Cardiac lesions induced by chemicals. *Environ Health Perspect* 1978;26:181–191.
166. Kehoe R, Singer DH, Trapani A, Billingham M, Levandowski R, Elson J. Adriamycin-

induced cardiac dysrhythmias in an experimental dog model. *Cancer Treat Rep* 1977;62:963–978.

167. Kehoe R, Sicotte M. Arrythmogenic properties of adriamycin. *Fed Proc Fed Am Soc Exp Biol* 1977;36:1013.

168. Arena E, Biondo F, D'Allesandro N, Dusonchet L, Beggia N, Gerbasi F. DNA, RNA and protein synthesis in heart, liver and brain of mice treated with daunomycin or adriamycin. *Int Res Commun Syst* 1974;2:1053.

169. Iwamoto Y, Hansen I, Porter T, Rausa L, Sanguedolce R. Inhibition of coenzyme Q10-enzymes, succinoxidase and NADH-oxidase by adriamycin and other quinones having antitumor activity. *Biochem Biophys Res Commun* 1974;58:633.

170. Handa K, Sato S. Generation of free radicals of quinone group-containing anticancer chemicals in NADPH–microsome system as evidenced by initiation of sulfite oxidation. *Gann* 1975;66:43.

171. Myers C, McGuire W, Liss R, Ifrim I, Grotziner K, Young R. Adriamycin: the role of lipid peroxidation in cardiac toxicity and tumor response. *Science* 1977;197:165.

172. Seraydarian MW, Goodman MF. Cardiotoxic effects of adriamycin in mammalian cardiac cells in culture. In: Kobayashi T, Ito Y, Rona G, eds. *Recent advances in studies on cardiac structure and metabolism*. Baltimore: University Park Press; 1978:713–719.

173. Bristow MR, Mason JW, Billingham ME, Daniels JR. Doxorubicin cardiomyopathy: evaluation by phonocardiography, endomyocardial biopsy, and cardiac catheterization. *Ann Intern Med* 1978;88:168–175.

174. Azuma J, Sperelakis N, Hasegawa H, et al. Adriamycin cardiotoxicity: possible pathogenic mechanisms. *J Mol Cell Cardiol* 1981;13:381–397.

175. Azuma J, Ishiyama T, Marita Y, et al. Changes of energy metabolism and electrophysiology in adriamycin-perfused chick hearts. *Proceedings, VIII World Congress on cardiology*. Amsterdam: Excerpta Medica; 1979:297 (Abstr. 0829).

176. O'Connell TX, Berenbaum MC. Cardiac and pulmonary effects of high doses of cyclophosphamide and isophosphamide. *Cancer Res* 1974;34:1586.

177. Adams HR, Parker JL, Durrett LR. Cardiac toxicities of antibiotics. *Environ Health Perspect* 1978;26:217–223.

178. Adams HR, Goodman FR, Weiss GB. Alteration of contractile function and calcium ion movements in vascular smooth muscle by gentamycin and other aminoglycoside antibiotics. *Antimicrob Agents Chemother* 1974;5:640.

179. Narahashi T. Chemicals as tools in the study of excitable membranes. *Physiol Rev* 1974;54:813.

180. Narahashi T. Effects of insecticides on nervous conduction and synaptic transmission. In: Wilkinson CF, ed. *Insecticide biochemistry and physiology*. New York: Plenum Press; 1976:327.

181. Narahashi T, Anderson NC. Mechanism of excitation block by the insecticide allethrin applied externally and internally to squid giant axons. *Toxicol Appl Pharamcol* 1967;10:529.

182. Jacques Y, Romey G, Cavey MT, Kartalovski B, Lazdunski M. Interaction of pyrethroids with the Na^+ channel in mammalian neuronal cells in culture. *Biochim Biophys Acta* 1980;600:882.

183. Neto FR, Narahashi T. Ionic mechanism of the salicylate block of nerve conduction. *J Pharmacol Exp Ther* 1976;199:454.

184. Carmeliet E, Vereece J. Electrogenesis of the action potential and automaticity. In: Berne RM, Sperelakis N, eds. *Handbook of physiology, section 2, the cardiovascular system, vol 1, the heart*. Baltimore: Williams & Wilkins; 1979:269.

185. Eisner DA, Ohba M, Ojeda C. The effect of salicylate on Purkinje fiber pacemaker activity. *J Pharmacol (Lond)* 1977;269:84P–85P.

186. Regan TJ. Ethyl alcohol and the heart. *Circulation* 1971;44:957–963.

187. Gvozdjak A, Bada V, Krutz F, Niederland TR, Gvorzdjak J. Effect of ethanol on the metabolism of the myocardium and its relationship to development of alcoholic myocardiopathy. *Cardiology* 1973;58:290.

188. Moore JW, Ulbricht W, Takata M. Effect of ethanol on the sodium and potassium conductances of the squid axon membranes. *J Gen Physiol* 1964;48:279.

189. Narahashi T, Fraizer DT, Takeno K. Effects of calcium on the local anesthetic suppression of ionic conductances in squid axon membranes. *J Pharmacol Exp Ther* 1976; 197:426.

190. Miller RH, Dhingra RC, Kanakis C Jr, Amat-y-Leon F, Rosen KM. The electrophys-

iological effects of delta-9-tetrahydrocannabinol (cannabis) on cardiac conduction in man. *Am Heart J* 1977;94:740–747.

191. Siegel JH, Greenspan M, Del Guercio LRM. Abnormal vascular tone, defective oxygen transport and myocardial failure in human septic shock. *Ann Surg* 1967;165:504.

192. Bhagat B, Beaumont M, Rawson L, Sulakhe PV, Dhalla NS. Calcium metabolism and contractility of isolated cardiac muscle from endotoxin-treated guinea pig. In: Dhalla, NS, Sano T, eds. *Recent advances in studies on cardiac structure and metabolism.* Baltimore: University Park Press; 1972:305.

193. Hackel DB, Ratliff NB, Mikat E. The heart in shock. *Circ Res* 1974;35:805.

194. Regan TJ, LeForce FM, Teres D, Block J, Hellems HK. Contribution of left ventricle and small bowel in irreversible hemorrhagic shock. *Am J Physiol* 1965;208:938.

195. Soulsby ME, Bruni FD, Looney TJ, Hess ML. Influence of endotoxin on myocardial calcium transport and the effect of augmented venous return. *Circ Shock* 1978;5:23.

196. Hinshaw LB, Archer LT, Spitzer JJ, Black MR, Peyton MD, Greenfield LJ. Effects of coronary hypotension and endotoxin in myocardial performance. *Am J Physiol* 1974;227:1051.

197. Carli A, Auclair MC, Bleichner G, Weber S, Lechat P, Monsallier JF. Inhibited response to isoproterenol and altered action potential of beating rat heart cells by human serum in septic shock. *Circ Shock* 1978;5:85–94.

198. Lefer AM, Rovetto MJ. Influence of a myocardial depressant factor on physiologic properties of cardiac muscle. *Proc Soc Biol Med* 1969;134:269–273.

199. Gibson WH, Cook JJ, Gatipon G, Moses ME. Effect of endotoxin shock on skeletal muscle membrane potential. *Surgery* 1977;81:571.

200. Parker JL, Mathew BP, Adams HR. Shock-induced alterations in cardiovascular responsiveness. *Cir Shock* 1978;5:200.

201. Moore HPH, Fritx LC, Raftery MA, Brockes JP. Isolation and characterization of a monoclonal antibody against the saxitoxin-binding component from the electric organ of eel *Electrophorus electricus. Proc Natl Acad Sci USA* 1982;79:1673–1677.

202. Hartshorne RP, Catterall WA. Purification of the saxitoxin receptor of the sodium channel from rat brain. *Proc Natl Acad Sci USA* 1981;78:4620.

203. Barchi RL, Murphy LE. Size characteristics of the solubilized sodium channel saxitoxin binding site from mammalian sarcolemma. *Biochim biophys Acta* 1980;597:391–398.

204. Sperelakis N, Shigenobu K. Changes in membrane properties of chick embryonic hearts during development. *J Gen Physiol* 1972;60:430–453.

205. Renaud J-F, Romey G, Lombet A, Lazdunski M. Differentiation of the fast sodium channel in embryonic heart cells followed by its interaction with neurotoxins. *Proc Natl Acad Sci USA* 1981;78:5348–5352.

206. Renaud J-F, Scanu AM, Kazazoglou T, Lombet A, Romey G, Lazdunski M. Normal serum and lipoprotein-deficient serum give different expressions of excitability corresponding to different stages of differentiation in chicken cardiac cells in culture. *Proc Natl Acad Sci USA* 1982;79:7768–7772.

207. Renaud J-F, Lazdunski M. Action of natural toxins on cardiac ionic channels. In: Sperelakis N, ed. *Physiology and pathophysiology of the heart.* Boston: Kluwer Academic Press; 1988:551–572.

208. Lazdunski M, Frelin C, Barhanin J, et al. Polypeptide toxins as tools to study voltage-sensitive Na^+ channels. *Ann NY Acad Sci* 1986;479:204–220.

209. Narahashi T, Moore JW, Scott WR. Tetrodotoxin blockage of sodium conductance increase in lobster giant axon. *J Gen Physiol* 1964;47:965.

210. Iijima T, Pappano AJ. Ontogenic increase of the maximum rate of rise of the chick embryonic heart action potential. Relationship of voltage, time, and tetrodotoxin. *Circ Res* 1979;44:358.

211. Redfern P, Thesleff S. Action potential generation in denervated rat skeletal muscle. II. The action of tetrodotoxin. *Acta Physiol Cand* 1971;82:70–78.

212. Bulbring E, Tomita T. Evidence supporting the assumption that the "inhibitory potential" in the taenia coli of the guinea pig is a post-synaptic potential due to nerve stimulation. *J Physiol* 1966;185:24.

213. Irisawa H. Comparative physiology of the cardiac pacemaker mechanism. *Physiol Rev* 1978;58:461.

214. Yamagishi S, Sano T. Effect of tetrodotoxin on the pacemaker action potential on the sinus node. *Proc Jpn Acad* 1966;42:1194.

215. Irisawa, 1972.

216. McLean MJ, Sperelakis N. Rapid loss of sensitivity of tetrodotoxin by chick ventricular myocardia cells after separation from the heart. *Exp Cell Res* 1974;86:315.
217. Shotzberger GS, Albuquerque EX, Daly JW. The effects of batrachotoxin on cat papillary muscle. *J Pharmacol Exp Ther* 1976; 196:433.
218. Honerjager P, Reiter M. The cardiotoxic effect of batrachotoxin. *Naunyn Schmiedebergs Arch Pharmacol* 1977;299:239.
219. Garcia JH, Deshpande SS, Pence RS, Albuquerque EX. Spinal myelopathy induced by subarachnoid batrachotoxin: ultrastructure and electrophysiology. *Brain Res* 1978; 140:75–87.
220. Romey G, Abita JP, Schweitz H, Wunderer G, Lazdunski M. Sea anemone toxin: a tool to study molecular mechanisms of nerve conduction and excitation–secretion coupling. *Proc Natl Acad Sci USA* 1976;73:4055–4063.
221. Sperelakis N, Pappano AJ. Increase in P_{Na} and P_K of cultured heart cells produced by veratridine. *J Gen Physiol* 1969;53:97–114.
222. Lazdunski M, Balerna M, Chiceportiche R, et al. Interaction of neurotoxins with the selectivity filter and the gating system of the sodium channel. In: Ceccarelli B, Clementi F, eds. *Advances in cytopharmacology*. New York: Raven Press; 1979:353–361.
223. Armstrong CM, Bezanilla F. Charge movement associated with the opening and closing of the activation gates of the Na^+ channels. *J Gen Physiol* 1974;63:533–552.
224. Baker PF, Rubinson KA. Chemical modification of crab nerves can make them insensitive to the local anaesthetics tetrodotoxin and saxitoxin. *Nature* 1975;257:412–414.
225. Spalding BC. Properties of toxin-resistant sodium channels produced by chemical modification in frog skeletal muscle. *J Physiol (Lond)* 1980;305:485.
226. Baer M, Best PM, Reuter H. Voltage-dependent action of tetrodotoxin in mammalian cardiac muscle. *Nature* 1976;263:344.
227. Cohen CJ, Bean BO, Colatsky TJ, Tsein RW. Tetrodotoxin block of sodium channels in rabbit purkinje fibers. *J Gen Physiol* 1981;78:383–411.
228. Colatsky TJ, Gadsby DC. Is tetrodotoxin block of background sodium channels in canine cardiac Purkinje fibers voltage-dependent? *J Physiol (Lond)* 1980;306:20.
229. Renaud J-F, Kazazoglou T, Lombet A, Chiceportiche R, Jaimovich E, Romey G, Lazdunski M. The Na^+ channel in mammalian cardiac cells. Two kinds of tetrodotoxin receptors in rat heart membranes. *J Biol Chem* 1983;258:8799–8805.
230. Lombet A, Renaud JF, Chiceportiche M. A cardiac tetrodotoxin binding component: biochemical identification, characterization, and properties. *Biochemistry* 1981; 20:1279.
231. Chiceportiche R, Balerna M, Lombet A, Romey G, Lazdunski M. Synthesis and mode of action on axonal membranes of photoactivable derivatives of tetrodotoxin. *J Biol Chem* 1979;254:1552–1557.
232. Straub R. Die wirkug von veratridin und Ionen auf das ruhepotential markhaltiger nervenfasern des frosches. *Helv Physiol Pharmacol Acta* 1956;14:1.
233. Swain HH, McCarthy DA. Veratrine, protoveratrine, and andromedotoxin arrhythmias in the isolated dog heart. *J Pharmacol Exp Ther* 1957;121:379.
234. Wallon G, Coraboeuf E, Gargouil YM. Action de la veratrine sur les phenomenes mechaniques et electriques d'un coeur isole et perfuse. *CR Soc Biol (Paris)* 1959; 153:2077.
235. Honerjager P, Reiter M. The relation between the effects of veratridine on action potential and contraction in mammalian ventricular myocardium. *Naunyn Schmiedebergs Arch Pharmacol* 1975;289:1.
236. Catterall WA, Niremberg M. Sodium uptake associated with activation of action potential ionophores of cultured neuroblastoma and muscle cells. *Proc Natl Acad Sci USA* 1973;70:3759.
237. Catterall WA. Activation of the action potential Na^+ ionophore of veratridine and batrachotoxin. *J Biol Chem* 1975;250:4053.
238. Catterall WA. Purification of a toxic protein from scorpion venom which activates the action potential Na^+ ionophore. *J Biol Chem* 1976;251:5528.
239. Fossett M, DeBarry J, Lenoir M, Lazdunski M. Analysis of molecular aspects of Na^+ and Ca^{2+} uptakes by embryonic cardiac cells in culture. *J Biol Chem* 1977;252:6112.
240. Horackova M, Vassort G. Excitation–contraction coupling in frog heart. Effects of veratrine. *Pflugers Arch* 1974;352:291.
241. Akera T, Ku DD, Frank M, Brody TM, Twasa J. Effects of grayanotoxin I on cardiac

Na$^+$, K$^+$–adenosine triphosphatase activity, transmembrane potential and myocardial contractile force. *J Pharmacol Exp Ther* 1976;199:247.

242. Ku DD, Akera T, Frank M, Brody TM, Iwasa J. The effects of gray-anotoxin I and α-dihydrograyanotoxin II on guinea-pig myocardium. *J Pharmacol Exp Ther* 1977; 200:363–372.

243. Seyama I. Effect of grayanotoxin I on SA node and right atrial myocardia of the rabbit. *Am J Physiol* 1978;235(3):C136–C142.

244. Seyama I, Narahashi T. Increase in sodium permeability of squid axon membranes by α-dihydrograyanotoxin II. *J Pharmacol Exp Ther* 1973;184:299–307.

245. Seyama I, Narahashi T. Sodium conductance kinetics of squid axon membrane poisoned by grayanotoxin I. *Biophys J* 1976;16:187a.

246. Daly J, Witkop B. Batrachotoxin, an extremely active cardio- and neuro-toxin from the Colombian arrow poison frog. *Clin Toxicol* 1971;4:331–342.

247. Albuquerque EX. The mode of action of batrachotoxin. *Fed Proc Fed Am Soc Exp Biol* 1972;31:1133–1138.

248. Hogan PM, Albuquerque EX. The pharmacology of batrachotoxin. III. Effect on the heart Purkinje fibers. *J Pharmacol Exp Ther* 1971;176:529.

249. DeBarry J, Fosset M, Lazdunzki M. Molecular mechanism of the cardiotoxic action of a polypeptide neurotoxin from sea anemone on cultured embryonic cardiac cells. *Biochemistry* 1977;16:3850–3855.

250. Romey G, Renaud JF, Fosset M, Lazdunski M. Pharmacological properties of the interaction of cardiac cells in culture with a sea anemone polypeptide toxin producing a positive inotropic effect. *J Pharmacol Exp Ther* 1980;213:607–615.

251. Romey G, Jacques Y, Schweitz H, Fosset M, Lazdunski M. The sodium channel in non-impulsive cells: interaction with specific neurotoxins. *Biochim Biophys Acta* 1979;556:344–353.

252. Bidard JN, Vijerberg HPM, Felin C, Chungue E, Legrand AM, Bagnis R, Lazdunski M. Ciguatoxin is a novel type of Na$^+$ channel toxin. *J Biol Chem* 1984;259:8353.

253. Fujiwara M, Muramatsu I, Hidaka H, Ikushima S, Ashida K. Effects of goniopora toxin, a polypeptide isolated from coral, on electromechanical properties of rabbit myocardium. *J Pharmacol Exp Ther* 1979;210:153.

254. Qar J, Schweitz H, Schmid A, Lazdunski M. A polypeptide toxin from the coral *Goniopora*. Purification and action on Ca^{2+} channels. *FEBS Lett* 1986;202:331.

255. Gonoi T, Ashida K, Feller D, Schmidt J, Fujiwara M, Catterall WA. Mechanism of action of a polypeptide neurotoxin from the coral Goniopora on sodium channels in mouse neuroblastoma cells. *Mol Pharmacol* 1986;29:347.

256. Kerr L, Yoshikami D. A venom peptide with a novel presynaptic blocking action. *Nature* 1984;308:282–284.

257. McCleskey EW, Fox AP, Feldman D, Olivera BM, Tsein RW, Yoshikami D. The peptide toxin CgTx blocks particular types of neuronal Ca channels. *Biophys J* 1986; 40:431a.

258. Lazdunski M. Apamin, a neurotoxin specific for one class of Ca^{2+}-dependent K$^+$ channels. *Cell Calcium* 1983;4:421–428.

259. Bkaily G, Sperelakis N, Renaud JF, Payet MD. Apamin, a highly specific Ca^{2+} blocking agent in heart muscle. *Am J Physiol* 1985; 248 (*Heart Circ Physiol* 17):H961–H965.

260. Cook GH, Wolff J. Melittin interactions with adenylate cyclase. *Biochim Biophys Acta* 1977;498:255.

261. Katoh N, Raynor RL, Wise BC, et al. Inhibition by melittin of phospholipid-sensitive and calmodulin-sensitive Ca^{2+}-dependent protein kinases. *Biochem J* 1982;202:217–224.

262. Bkaily G, Jacques D, Yamamoto T, Sculptoreanu A, Payet MD, Sperelakis N. Three types of slow inward currents as distinguished by melittin in 3-day-old embryonic heart. *Can J Physiol Pharmacol* 1988;66:1017–1022.

263. Romey G, Chicheportiche R, Lazdunski M. Scorpion neurotoxin: a presynaptic toxin which affects both Na$^+$ and K$^+$ channels in axons. *Biochem Biophys Res Commun* 1975;64:115–121.

264. Fayet G, Couraud F, Miranda F, Lissitzky S. Electro-optical system for monitoring activity of heart cells in culture: application to the study of several drugs and scorpion toxins. *Eur J Pharmacol* 1974;27:165.

265. Romey G, Abita JP, Chicheportiche R, Rochat H, Lazdunski M. Scorpion neurotoxin:

mode of action on neuromuscular junctions and synaptosomes. *Biochim Biophys Acta* 1976;448:607–619.

266. Koppenhoffer E, Schmidt H. Die Wirkung von Scorpiongift auf die Ionenstrome des Ranvierschen schnurrings. I. Die Permeabilitaten PNa and PA. *Pflugers Arch* 1968;303:133.

267. Narahashi T, Shapiro BI, Deguchi T, Scuka M, Wang CM. Effects of scorpion venom on squid axon membranes. *Am J Physiol* 1972;222:850.

268. Jaimovich E, Ildefonse M, Barhanin J, Rougier O, Lazdunski M. Centruroides toxin, a selective blocker of surface Na$^+$ channels in skeletal muscle: voltage-clamp analysis and biochemical characterization of the receptor. *Proc Natl Acad Sci USA* 1982; 79:3896.

269. Sauviat MP. Effects of ervatamine chlorhydrate on cardiac membrane currents in frog atrial fibers. *J Physiol (Lond)* 1978;280:29.

270. Freedman SB, Miller RJ, Miller DM, Tindall DR. Interactions of maitotoxin with voltage-sensitive calcium channels in cultured neuronal cells. *Proc Natl Acad Sci USA* 1984;81:4582.

271. Berta P, Sladexcek F, Derancourt J, Durand M, Travo P, Haiech J. Maitotoxin stimulates the formation of inositol phosphates in rat aortic myocytes. *FASEB Lett* 1986;197:349.

272. Kobayashi M, Ohizumi Y, Yasumoto T. The mechanism of action of maitotoxin in relation to Ca^{2+} movements in guinea-pig and rat cardiac muscles. *Br J Pharmacol* 1985;86:385.

273. Bagnis R, Charteau S, Chungue Z, Hurtel JM, Yasumoto T, Inoue H. Origins of ciguatera fish poison. *Toxin* 1980;18:199.

274. Legrand AM, Galonnier M, Bagnis R. Studies on the mode of action of ciguateric toxins. *Toxicon* 1982;20:311–315.

275. Bengmann JS, Nechay BR. Maitotoxin inhibits Na$^+$ K$^+$ ATPase in vitro. *Fed Proc Fed Am Soc Exp Biol* 1982;41:1562.

276. Jackson H, Usherwood PNR. Spider toxins as tools for dissecting elements of excitatory amino acid transmission. *Trends Neurosci* 1988;11(6):278.

277. Kawai N, Niwa A, Abe T. *Brain Res* 1982;247:169–171.

278. Usherwood PNR, Duce IR, Bode P. *J Physiol (Paris)* 1984;79:241.

279. Kerr LM, Walmsley SK, Filloux F, Parks TN, Jackson H. *Soc Neurosci Abstr* 1987;13:102.

280. Jackson H, Parks TN. *Soc Neurosci Abstr* 1987;13:1078.

281. Lin JY, Jeng TW, Chen CC, Shi GY, Tung TC. Isolation of a new cardiotoxic protein from the edible mushroom. *Nature* 1973;246:524–525.

282. Fassold E, Slade AM, Lin J-Y, Nayler WG. An effect of the cardiotoxic protein volvatoxin A on the function and structure of heart muscle cells. *J Mol Cell Cardiol* 1976;8:501.

283. Tazieff-Depierre F, Czajka M, Lowagie C. Action pharmacologique des fractions pures de venin de Naja nigricollis et liberation de calcium dans les muscles stries. *CR Acad Sci Ser D* 1969;268:2511.

284. Lee CY. Chemistry and pharmacology of polypeptide toxins in snake venom. *Am Rev Pharmacol* 1972;12:265–286.

285. Nayler WG, Sullivan AT, Dunnett J, Slade AM, Trethewie ER. The effect of a cardiotoxic component of the venom of the Indian cobra *(Naja nigricollis)* on the subcellular structure and function of heart muscle. *J Mol Cell Cardiol* 1976;8:341.

286. DuBois JM, Cohen JB. Effect of palytoxin on membrane potential and current of frog myelinated fibers. *J Pharmacol Exp Ther* 1977;201:148.

287. Muramatsu I, Uemura D, Fujiwara M, Narahasi T. Characteristics of palytoxin-induced depolarization in squid axons. *J Pharmacol Exp Ther* 1984;231:488–494.

288. Rayner MD, Sanders BJ, Harris SM, Lin YC, Morton BE. Palytoxin: effects on contractility and ^{45}Ca^{2+} uptake in isolated ventricle strips. *Res Commun Chem Pathol Pharmacol* 1975;11:55–64.

289. Muramatsu I, Nishio M, Kigoshi S, Uemura D. Single ionic channels induced by palytoxin in guinea-pig ventricular myocytes. *Br J Pharmacol* 1988;93:811.

Cardiovascular Toxicology, Second Edition,
edited by Daniel Acosta, Jr.
Published by Raven Press, Ltd., New York, 1992.

12

The Effect of Centrally Acting Drugs on the Cardiovascular System

Steven I. Baskin

*United States Army Medical Research Institute of Chemical Defense,
Aberdeen Proving Ground, Maryland 21010-5425*

There are many instances of drugs or chemicals whose role was originally thought to interact with the central nervous system and were found to exert considerable action on the cardiovascular system. Initially there is surprise and then rationalization of the finding and occasionally with the passage of time a dimming of the phenomenon until the next time it is rediscovered with another drug, chemical, or toxin with a similar sequelae of events.

Many consider the observations by Harris and Kokernot (1) symbolize a formal recognition that agents which affect CNS function can also affect cardiovascular actions as well. In this study, Harris and Kokernot reasoned that drugs such as phenytoin, which suppress central dysrhythmias (convulsions), will also suppress cardiac arrhythmias. The results that were found supported their contention. Many anticonvulsant drugs such as phenobarbital, phenytoin, and carbamazepine also exert cardiac antiarrhythmic action. This as well as other studies illustrate that CNS-acting drugs and chemicals can affect a number of cardiac functions as well. For example, we found that drugs such as amphetamine, psilocybin, and LSD could also modify effects in the isolated heart. It is the purpose of this chapter to briefly review some of the mechanisms by which this may occur and illustrate some of the classes of compounds providing examples.

RECEPTORS

Control of basic signal communication is maintained by a series of ionic or chemically derived messages. Ionic messages may be regulated by so-

---

The opinions or assertions contained herein are the private views of the author and are not to be construed as official or as reflecting the views of the Army or the Department of Defense.

dium, potassium, calcium, or anion (e.g., chloride) ions. Many but not all of these same or similar systems, gating mechanisms, channels, or ionic receptors occur in the CNS as well as in cardiac tissues. Drugs or chemicals that act by affecting these ionic systems should act on both the CNS and cardiac systems.

The cardiac tissue handles calcium differently than CNS tissue. The reasons are not completely understood but a number of contributory causes participate in these differences. One reason given is that heart mitochondria appear to function quantitatively distinct from brain organelles. However, a number of studies indicate that there are specific calcium pools that exist in the heart that may not be as prominent in other tissues (2). Development of drugs that are calcium agonists or antagonists, for example, may achieve a desired CNS effect in an isolated brain slice preparation but also may produce unwanted cardiac effects, particularly at higher doses. On the other hand, a variety of calcium antagonists may act on the heart or A-V node while others may have vascular effects particularly at low doses (3). Calcium agonists (e.g., A23187) may not only display effects on heart and skeletal muscle but may produce CNS convulsions as well.

Cardiac receptors serve similar functions as receptors in the CNS. They act to modulate responses to hormones. So it is not unreasonable to assume that drugs or chemicals that will affect CNS receptors may also modify cardiac receptors. Several cardiac receptors may respond quantitatively to drugs differently from CNS receptors. Differences for this may include (a) saturability and reversibility of binding, (b) stereospecificity of binding (e.g., high affinity binding), (c) tissue responsiveness or density of receptor binding, (d) altered dose–response relationships, (e) metabolic activation or metabolism to a different species, and (f) blood flow.

Although this chapter may attempt to compare receptors or responses between the CNS and the cardiovascular systems, it is important to remember that all tissues do not respond equally or contain the same cardiac receptors. For example, the responses to acetylcholine in the atria and ventricle are much different. These differences even extend to cell types within a given cardiac tissue as well as in the CNS (i.e., neurons, glia, oligodendrocytes). On the other hand, if a drug is administered to a patient as a CNS antidepressant, one should not be surprised if cardiac effects occur. If the antidepressant acts through adrenergic mechanisms, cardiac adrenergic effects may be observed and if cholinergic CNS effects are expected then cardiac cholinergic effects may also be seen. Many different messengers have been reported to occur in the cardiovascular system (Table 1). Additional hormones are known to interact in some way with components of the cardiovascular system. CNS acting compounds that are thought to interact with receptors of these messengers could also interact with cardiovascular receptors for these same messengers. A hormonal signal that may modulate depression within the CNS may modulate contractile force or the rate of

TABLE 1. *Messengers reported to interact with cardiac receptors*

Epinephrine
Norepinephrine
Histamine
Dopamine
Vasopressin
Glucagon
Thyrotropic hormone
Corticotropic hormone
Luteinizing factor
Opiates
Insulin
Acetylcholine
Follicle stimulating hormone
Corticotropic hormone releasing factor
Endothelial derived releasing factor
Endothelin
Angiotensin II
Atrial natriuretic factor

atrial depolarization in the heart, so the final event will manifest itself differently.

Those who are trying to extrapolate data from one animal to another or to humans using a perceived CNS drug to gain information on proposed cardiac actions may be in for a degree of unprepared difficulty. Cardiac actions of drugs and chemicals are quantally species specific. The same relationships do not follow in the CNS. For example, the rat is used to develop a number of CNS-acting compounds but does not show the same sensitivity to cardiac compounds (4). Rat heart Na/K-activated ATPase is relatively insensitive to the effects of cardiac glycosides (i.e., ouabain), while rat brain enzyme is very sensitive to small concentrations of ouabain. The dog Na/K-activated ATPase from the heart and brain are both relatively sensitive to ouabain.

Other discriminatory factors such as age, sex, diurnal cycle, diet, and pregnancy may further alter the relationship of a central nervous system response to a cardiac one.

Adrenergic Drugs

Cardiovascular tissues contain alpha- and beta-adrenergic receptors. There are subtypes of both of these receptors that appear to exhibit unequal distribution according to tissue type. Separation of the actions has vastly improved with more selective drugs. However, absolute complete selectivity has not been achieved. Agents such as clonidine, which is thought to exert its antihypertensive effects on the central system neurons, may also produce some toxicity at high doses at a peripheral site.

Drugs that act on beta-adrenergic receptors also can produce cardiac toxicity (5). Life-threatening cardiac arrhythmias and cardiac necrosis and death can ensue from overdosage of this type of drug. An example of this class of drug would be isoproterenol. Intranasal administration of this class of chemical for legitimate or illicit use could result in cardiac damage.

Drugs that act on both alpha- and beta-adrenergic receptors centrally should also affect the cardiac receptors. Norepinephrine and epinephrine act on alpha- and beta-adrenergic receptors. Thus compounds that indirectly release endogenous catecholamines and exert CNS changes could produce changes in the EKG either centrally or peripherally and directly produce cardiac toxicity. Examples of this class could include amphetamine and cocaine. Cocaine has been shown to have a variety of cardiac adverse effects, including ischemia (6), myocarditis (7), necrosis (8), and cardiomyopathy (9).

Cholinergic Drugs

Longer acting cholinomimetics, carbamates, and substances that would produce a prolonged cholinergic crisis are known to produce cardiac slowing, cardiac arrhythmias, and death (10). Although the classical pharmacologist claimed at one time there was "no vagal action below the atria," this may not be entirely accurate. Other mechanisms may be the cause of ventricular or conducting fiber "cholinergic" actions (10).

Serotonergic Drugs

Several antidepressants (i.e., spiperone, ketanserin) appear to act by inhibiting one of the transport systems (5-HT2) for 5-HT. The receptors may aid in the regulation of the heart rate (11).

Histaminergic Drugs

The cardiovascular system has been reported to contain both H1 and H2 receptors. The H2 receptors appear to be more important in regulating contractile force and heart rate.

Antipsychotic Drugs

Drugs such as chlorpromazine and thioridazine (and other compounds of this structural class) are known to exert serious cardiac action. Phenothiazines are capable of causing a decrease in systemic blood pressure possibly due to alpha-adrenergic blocking activity and central pressor reflexes

(12,13). Other mechanisms such as an action on cholinergic vagal tone have been proposed. It is also thought that catechol derivatives may play a role due to the toxicity and persistent, potent adrenergic effects (14). Myocardial degeneration and atrophy of myocytes after chronic administration of chlorpromazine has been noted (15). In rare instances, ventricular arrhythmias as torsade de points and ventricular fibrillation have been noted.

Antidepressant Drugs

Drugs such as MAO (monoamine oxidase) inhibitors have been found to produce cardiotoxicity. An acute overdose of drugs such as imipramine or amitriptyline can cause widening of the QRS complex, prolongation of the PR and QT intervals, bundle branch block, supraventricular as well as ventricular arrhythmias, and myocardial depression (16).

Analgesic/Anti-inflammatory Drugs

Heroin, acetaminophen, methylsalicylate, and colchicine have been associated with toxic myocarditis in animals or in humans (17). The mechanism of how these compounds produce these effects is not completely established.

Solvents

Solvents such as alcohol, chloroform, trichloroethane, and other halogenated hydrocarbons are known CNS-acting products. The toxicology of these substances are discussed elsewhere in this book (see chapter by Zakhari). Halothane, methoxyflurane and enflurane and also substituted halogenated hydrocarbons which are used as general anesthetic agents are known to inhibit calcium movement in cardiac cells (18). This action has also been shown with barbiturates in isolated perfused heart preparations.

CONCLUSIONS

Many commonly used central nervous system drugs as well as many chemicals in use which are recognized to exert effects on the central nervous system also appear to have effects on the cardiovascular system. They affect cardiac systems, in part, by interacting with ionic and receptor mechanisms that are similar in other excitable membranes and that transmit electrical and chemically mediated messages.

REFERENCES

1. Harris AS, Kokernot RH. The effects of diphenylhydantoin sodium (dilantin sodium) and phenobarbital sodium upon ectopic ventricular tachycardia in acute myocardial infarction. *Am J Physiol* 1950;163:505–516.
2. Nayler WG. Calcium exchange in cardiac muscle: a basic mechanism of drug action. *Am Heart J* 1967;73:379–394.
3. Reuter H. Membranes. A variety of calcium channels. *Nature* 1985;316:391.
4. Akera T, Baskin SI, Tobin T, Brody TM. Ouabain: temporal relationship between the inotropic effect in the Langendorff preparation and the *in vitro* binding to and dissociation from (Na/K)-activated ATPase. *Naunyn Schmiedebergs Arch Pharmacol Exp Pathol* 1973;277:151–162.
5. Kaldor G, DiBattista WJ, Venus M, Baskin SI. Isoproterenol effects on hearts of aging rats. In: Kaldor G, DiBattista WJ, eds. *Aging in muscle*. New York: Raven Press; 1978:101–140.
6. Mathias D. Cocaine-associated myocardial ischemia: review of clinical and angiographic findings. *Am J Med* 1986;81:675.
7. Virmani R, Rabinowitz M, Smialek JE, Smyth DF. Cardiovascular effects of cocaine: an autopsy study of 40 patients. *Am Heart J* 1988;115:1068.
8. Peng S-K, French WJ, Pelikan PCD. Direct cocaine cardiotoxicity demonstrated by endomyocardial biopsy. *Arch Pathol Lab Med* 1989;113:842.
9. Weiner R, Lockart J, Schwartz R. Dilated cardiomyopathy and cocaine abuse. *Am J Med* 1986;81:568.
10. Baskin SI, Whitmer MP. The cardiac toxicology of organophosphorus agents. In: Baskin SI, ed. *Principles of cardiac toxicology*. Boca Raton, FL: CRC Press; 1991:275–294.
11. Gother M. Serotonin receptors in the circulatory system. *Prog Pharmacol* 1986; 6(2):155–172.
12. Fowler NO, McCall D, Chou TC. Electrocardiographic changes and cardiac arrhythmias in patients receiving psychotropic drugs. *Am J Cardiol* 1976;37:223.
13. Weiss LW. The cardiotoxicity of neuroleptic and tricyclic antidepressant drugs. In: Balazs T, ed. *Cardiac toxicity*, vol 2. Boca Raton, FL: CRC Press; 1981.
14. Akera T, Baskin SI, Tobin T, Brody TM, Manian AA. 7,8-Dihydroxychlorpromazine: (Na/K)-ATPase inhibition and positive inotropic effect in the phenothiazines and structurally-related drugs. In: Forrest IS, Carr CJ, Usdin E, eds. *Phenothiazines and structurally related compounds*. New York: Raven Press; 1974:633–640.
15. Matsumoto O. Toxic damages of various organs induced by chronic administration of chlorpromazine. *Yokohama Med J* 1975;12:1.
16. Braden NJ, Jackson JE, Walson PD. Tricyclic antidepressant overdose. *Pediatr Clin North Am* 1986;33:287.
17. Herman EH, Ferrans VJ. The cardiac toxicology of organophosphorus agents. In: Baskin SI, ed. *Principles of cardiac toxicology*. Boca Raton, FL: CRC Press; 1991:607–681.
18. Porsius AJ, van Zwieten PA. On the mechanism of the negative inotropic action of halothane and propanidide. In: Fleckenstein A, Dhalla NS, eds. *Recent advances in studies on cardiac structure and metabolism*. Baltimore: University Park Press; 1975:413.

Cardiovascular Toxicology, Second Edition,
edited by Daniel Acosta, Jr.
Raven Press, Ltd., New York © 1992.

13

Cardiotoxicity of Acute and Chronic Ingestion of Various Alcohols

*†S. Sultan Ahmed and *‡Timothy J. Regan

Department of *Medicine, †Stress Testing and Cardiovascular Catheterization
Laboratories, and ‡Division of Cardiovascular Diseases, UMDNJ–New Jersey
Medical School, Newark, New Jersey 07103

HISTORY OF THE USE OF ALCOHOL

The origin of alcoholic beverages is lost in the mists of prehistory. Early humans presumably liked the effects, if not the taste, and proceeded to purposeful production. Surviving records of Greek and Roman histories reveal the common and copious use of wine by the gods, as well as by people of all classes. These records also indicate warnings of the evil effects of excess in drinking.

The earliest references in the Bible show that abundant wine was regarded as a blessing. Quite a different kind of religious control was adopted later in Islam: the Quran simply condemned alcohol and the result was an effective prohibition wherever the devout followers of this religion prevailed.

Modern complex societies are troubled by a lack of consensus around many issues of right and wrong, or proper and improper behavior, and drinking. This conflict reflects the complex interactions of individuals and small groups and larger society.

Estimates of the prevalence of alcoholism vary greatly. It is estimated that between 70 and 90% of adults in the United States drink more than occasionally. Approximately 10 million Americans (7.3% of men, 1.3% of women, and 4.2% of adults over age 20) could be classified as alcoholics (1).

The social and economic costs of alcoholism and heavy drinking are essentially incalculable. Crude projections of the annual costs of alcoholism to the national economy of the United States range from 7 to 10 billion dollars annually. An estimated 2 billion dollars are provided to alcoholics in the area of health and welfare services.

The socioeconomic and health consequences of heavy alcohol drinking place alcoholism in the front rank of public health problems (1). Its gravity is underlined by the higher rates of mortality (2.5 times normal) among alcoholics. Suicide rates are 2.5 times higher; accidental death rates are seven times higher; and there is an enormously higher rate of general morbidity among alcoholics.

High number of accidents with fatalities, personal injuries, and property damage are also well documented results of alcohol-impaired driving of motor vehicles.

BRIEF HISTORICAL REVIEW OF CARDIOTOXICITY OF ALCOHOL

Although the toxic effects of ethanol on cerebral and hepatic function have long been known, their contribution to the development of heart disease has only gradually been recognized. Alcohol in modest amounts had traditionally been prescribed as a medicinal agent, and heart disease in alcoholics usually has been attributed to underlying rheumatic, hypertensive, or coronary artery disease, often without good supporting evidence.

In the 1950s, several reports drew attention to the fact that many cardiac patients with a history of long-standing alcoholism had no evidence of significant nutritional deficiency. Eliaser and Giansiracus (2) related the cardiac abnormalities seen in alcoholics to the severity and duration of alcoholism and concluded that a significant number of alcoholics with heart failure had no vitamin deficiency or hepatic disease. Brigden and Robinson (3) reported observations in 40 cardiac patients and noted the difficulty in obtaining a history of alcoholism. But other causes of heart disease—hypertension, coronary artery disease, cor pulmonale, congenital and valvular disease—were excluded. A few patients presented with the high output failure of beriberi and responded to thiamine administration. The others presented with low output heart failure, often complicated by atrial and ventricular arrhythmias. Evans (4) emphasized the occupational diversity of patients with alcoholic cardiomyopathy. Most of the patients in his study held executive positions. A male predominance has been repeatedly observed in these and subsequent series and is believed to be due to the greater prevalence of alcoholism in men. The duration of alcoholism is usually reported to be at least 10 years before cardiac symptoms appear. Therefore if a population study samples predominantly short-term alcohol abusers, relatively few would have clinically detectable disease.

To understand the cardiac effects of ethanol, these effects must be evaluated in a state of adequate nutrition, usually in the experimental model. In the clinical situation, the alcoholic may have associated vitamin and protein deficiencies, cigarette use, or viral infections, which may affect evaluation of the role of ethyl alcohol in cardiomyopathy. The broader question of why the heart, liver, or brain predominates in the pathologic responses of a given patient has not been answered satisfactorily.

Depression of left ventricular function during the acute phase of beriberi heart disease has been described (5). In addition, the persistence of a chronic cardiac abnormality after treatment with thiamine suggests that alcoholism, usually present in subjects with beriberi on the North American continent, may be responsible. The reversible nature of the cardiac abnormalities in subjects who were apparently not alcoholic has been indicated in American prisoners of war in World War II (6). Long-term follow-up failed to reveal a significantly higher incidence of heart disease than in controls.

Moreover, although thiamine is required as a cofactor in the Krebs cycle, oxidative phosphorylation in heart was not found impaired in two patients studied with cardiac beriberi (7). These authors concluded that energy supply to the myocardium in beriberi is largely through metabolism of fats rather than carbohydrates. Thus although depressed myocardial function secondary to impaired energy production is an attractive hypothesis, it has not yet been clearly demonstrated.

RESPONSE TO ACUTE INGESTION IN NORMAL SUBJECTS AND NONALCOHOLIC CARDIACS

Although early investigations of the toxicity of ethanol were largely focused on the liver, in recent years a variety of studies have provided evidence of cardiac toxicity. In contrast to the popular view that ethanol has beneficial effects on the heart acutely, doses that are mildly intoxicating have been shown to adversely affect left ventricular function in some circumstances. This effect is in part dependent on prior experience with alcohol; that is, larger doses are required to demonstrate impaired pumping action of the heart in the chronic alcoholic subject without clinical evidence of heart disease (8–13). For instance, 6 oz of scotch fed to normal individuals over a 2-hr period has been found to diminish the force of heart muscle contraction at a mildly intoxicating blood level of 75 mg/100 ml (11,13) (Fig. 1) without affecting cardiac function in the noncardiac alcoholic. This effect progresses as blood levels rise and usually dissipates within a few hours after drinking ceases. That the rate of administration is of importance is illustrated by the observation that 4 oz of whiskey given over 15 min elicits diminished cardiac performance (14). Supporting the view that ethanol is acutely depressant to myocardium is the fact that ventricular dysfunction is rapidly reversed after 15–30 min of hemodialysis (15). The depressant effects of oral alcohol in humans are even more evident when compared with an isocaloric isovolumic solution of sucrose (Fig. 2). In the latter case the systolic time interval ratio is reduced qualitatively opposite to the ethanol response (13).

Variability in the acute response to ethanol in normal subjects may be related to elicitation of a chronotropic response. Two studies in humans

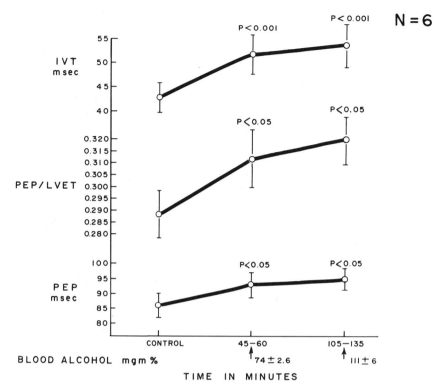

FIG. 1. Response of systolic time intervals to 6 oz of Scotch whiskey in six young normal adults.

showing an enhanced cardiac output were associated with acceleration of heart rate (16,17), which may have been related to the large volume of ethanol and diluent administered orally, as rapidly as 5 min in the latter case. Similarly, when basal sympathetic activity is enhanced, as in the open chest dog (18) or the postexercise state in the human (19), the negative inotropic response may be less evident.

In contrast to findings in alcoholics without clinical evidence of heart disease, the patient who has already had at least one episode of heart failure may exhibit a greater sensitivity to the 6-oz dose of scotch (20) with substantial elevation of left ventricular filling pressure (Fig. 3). The response in cardiac subjects who are not alcoholics may be qualitatively similar (21). An important variation of the acute response to ethanol occurs when combined with other pharmacologic agents. Accidental or suicidal deaths have resulted from the combination with barbiturates. Potentiation of the myocardial depressant effect has been observed experimentally with such a combination (12), which is concurrent with respiratory depression.

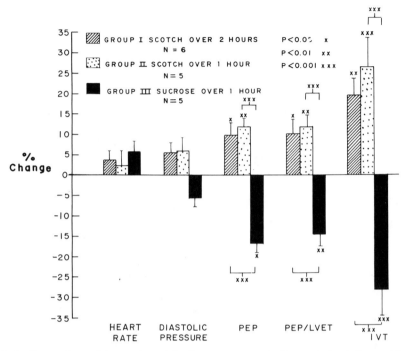

FIG. 2. Comparison of the peak systolic–time responses to the control solution and to alcohol at the two dose rates. Values shown are the mean percent changes from control values at the conclusion of the 1- or 2-hr study. From ref. 13, with permission.

The sympathetic nervous system presumably has an important role in determining the degree of negative inotropic response. Thus blockade of this system has been shown to produce greater depression of left ventricular function during ethanol administration (22) in experimental animals. Similarly in humans, mild abnormality of the left ventricular systolic time intervals was observed at blood levels of 110 mg%, which was substantially intensified by beta-receptor blockade (23). It is noteworthy that the adrenal gland appears to respond with greater secretion of epinephrine, at least after a bolus infusion of ethanol (24) and may participate with cardiac catecholamine stores to modulate the acute depressant effects of ethanol. Intensification of the cardiovascular response to ethanol in animals treated with disulfiram (25), an inhibitor of beta-hydroxylation that lowers levels of endogenous norepinephrine (26), may well be on a similar basis. Since disulfiram is often used therapeutically, it is noteworthy that the interaction with recurrent alcohol use in humans is characterized by hypotension, tachycardia, and hypokalemia. This reaction is quite variable and not solely explicable on the basis of blood acetaldehyde levels or the sympathetic nervous system (27).

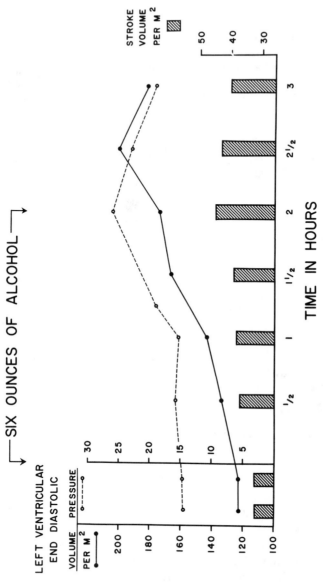

FIG. 3. Effect of ingestion of 6 oz of Scotch on the left ventricular hemodynamics in an alcoholic patient with cardiac decompensation; no such dysfunction is noted with this dose in noncardiac alcoholics. From ref. 20, with permission.

Despite the large number of published observations of the inotropic effects of ethyl alcohol, little has been done to clarify the mechanism by which these effects are produced. In the isolated atrial muscle from guinea pig, concentrations of ethanol at 450 mg/100 ml shortened the action potential due to an increase in the rate of repolarization (8). There was a corresponding fall in isometric force. The authors concluded that part of the fall in isometric force was due to the change in transmembrane action potential, but that the change was too small to entirely account for the magnitude of the inotropic response.

The most consistent results have been obtained in experiments with isolated cardiac tissue. In six different species, developed force declined when ethanol concentration was 100 mg% or above (28). Only the cat showed a decline in developed force at a concentration of 75 mg%.

Concentrations of alcohol that produced a decline in contractile performance shorten the action potential and lower its plateau, which may determine the amount of calcium available for contraction (29–31). It is probable that the decline in contractile force is secondary to the alteration of the action potential by ethanol, since prevention of the latter response also inhibits the effect on contractility (28). The permeability changes that alter the action potential have not been defined.

In considering the direct influence of ethanol on cardiac cells when administered acutely, changes of salts in the muscle are of major importance. The action in reducing force of contraction may well entail altered calcium movement in the cell (32). It is known that potassium and phosphate transiently leak out of the muscle cells after a 12-oz dose (11), an effect that is not attributable to coronary blood flow reduction. The loss of cations may be related to an inhibitory effect of ethanol on active transport of potassium and sodium across cell membranes, which has been suggested as a basic mechanism of action of ethanol upon most cells (33).

Another metabolic change is represented by alteration of lipid transport in the myocardium: the large dose of ethanol reduced the uptake of free fatty acid by the left ventricle, while the increased triglyceride uptake resulted in accumulation of lipid in myocardium (9). This response may contribute to pathologic changes observed in human myocardium at postmortem examination; substantial increases in lipids, presumably triglycerides, have been observed in the alcoholic heart (34).

It is noteworthy that noncardiac striated muscles, including uterine (35) and skeletal muscle (36), are also depressed acutely by ethanol, although in the diaphragm this follows a period of enhanced contractility. With chronic use, the asymptomatic alcoholic may exhibit modest reduction of lactic dehydrogenase, as well as a small reduction in fast-twitch glycolytic fibers and volume of mitochondria (37). The conditions required for acute myopathy and rhabdomyolysis are not well defined, but malnutrition and hypophosphatemia are frequently associated (38).

EFFECTS OF CHRONIC USE

Subclinical Malfunction

With No Hepatic Cirrhosis

Studies of alcoholic subjects with no symptoms or clinical evidence of heart disease or malnutrition suggest that subclinical malfunction may exist (39–43). In one report, 10–15 years of alcoholism and the type of ethanol consumed were documented from the patients' histories or from close relatives. Whiskey was the predominant alcoholic beverage and was consumed several times a week in amounts of 0.5–2.0 pints/day (11). Liver biopsy revealed fatty liver without fibrosis. Left ventricular performance was studied by increasing afterload with infusions of angiotensin. Alcoholic patients without heart failure had abnormally high ventricular filling pressure without a corresponding increase in stroke output, a significantly different response from that of control subjects. This abnormal relationship suggests an adverse effect of chronic ethanolism on the myocardium, confirmed in a subsequent study (11) using an index of contractility at rest (Fig. 4).

Noninvasive studies that measure systolic time intervals confirm that many asymptomatic subjects have modest depression of left ventricular function (42,43) (Fig. 5). Noncardiac alcoholics accumulate alcian-positive material in the myocardial interstitium (44), which may be a basis for the functional abnormality. Some degree of interstitial fibrosis may be present

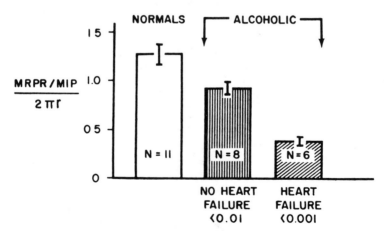

FIG. 4. The left ventricular contractility index at rest in the noncardiac alcoholic was significantly reduced below that of the normal, but is higher in alcoholic subjects who had developed clinical evidence of heart disease. From ref. 11, with permission.

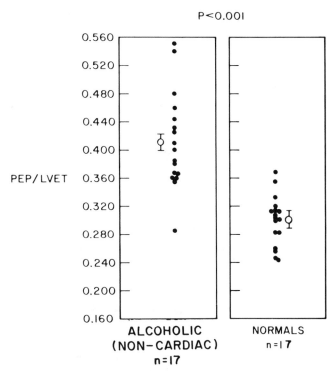

FIG. 5. Systolic time interval ratios (PEP/LVET) in noncardiac alcoholics (**left**) and in normal persons (**right**). *Filled circles* represent individual data points; means are represented by *open circles*. From ref. 122, with permission.

at this state, as suggested by postmortem studies of alcoholics who die without clinical evidence of cardiac disease (45).

In another study, a more advanced form of this subclinical disease was observed: 50% of asymptomatic alcoholic subjects had modest left ventricular hypertrophy, as determined by M-mode echocardiographic criteria, without evidence of decreased myocardial contractility (46). The preclinical state has been subcategorized into an early stage with increased wall thickness without enhanced diastolic internal diameter and a later stage in which internal diameter is increased but wall thickness is not (47).

The high-fidelity electrocardiogram also shows abnormalities not easily seen on the conventional ECG. In one study, the PRc, QRS, and QTc intervals were prolonged in the total alcoholic group (the change in the mean value was significant) and the septal Q wave was frequently absent (43). Enhanced notching and slurs in the QRS are consistent with a primary myocardial disease process. The conduction changes were not likely to be due to increased ventricular mass, as heart size was within normal limits by clincial examination, chest x-ray, and ECG.

With Hepatic Cirrhosis

As the complication of alcoholism with the longest history of recognition, it is noteworthy that alcoholic patients who present with cirrhosis are not usually considered to have significant myocardial pathology or malfunction. However, Lunseth et al. (48) reviewed the cardiovascular status of 108 hospitalized patients dying with fatal cirrhosis and observed associated heart disease in nearly half. Almost one-fourth had arteriosclerotic heart disease, nine were classed as hypertensive and five with valvular disease. Cardiac hypertrophy was present in 30% of the remainder, frequently with pulmonary congestion and edema, which were not definitely defined as cardiac in origin. Pathologic study indicated that hypertrophy was associated with early and moderately advanced cirrhosis, while hearts that were normal or subnormal in weight were associated with advanced cirrhosis, suggesting an effect of malnutrition.

In view of the apparent male predilection for hypertrophy, a recent clinical study is of interest. Patients with biopsy-proven cirrhosis without clinically evident cardiopulmonary abnormalities had a noninvasive study of myocardial performance, using the systolic time interval method of Weissler to determine if in such patients sex is a determinant of cardiac abnormalities. Male cirrhotics, averaging 39 years of age, had significantly abnormal systolic time intervals compared to the age-matched normal controls (43). On the other hand, the female alcoholics with a similar age distribution and an apparent similar intensity of cirrhosis did not exhibit alterations of cardiac function by this test (Table 1). Several studies of cirrhotics have suggested that at least a low-grade cardiac abnormality exists in many such patients, which under appropriate stress may have clinical importance in terms of producing either congestive phenomena or arrhythmias. Interventions with exercise or angiotensin infusion have shown abnormal elevation of left ventricular end-diastolic pressure and subnormal increments of stroke output as well as stroke work (40,41).

One author inferred that the absence of clinical symptoms of heart disease could be attributed to the low systemic vascular resistance characteristic of cirrhosis (40). Data on the responsiveness of the myocardium in terms of the inotropic response to digitalis are in conflict (40).

The variety of cardiac output levels in patients with cirrhosis and portal hypertension have been emphasized by Siegel et al. (49). More recently, Epstein et al. (50) found that half of their subjects were hyperdynamic, apparently unrelated to thiamine deficiency or the withdrawal state. Seven had normal cardiac outputs and three were low; both high and low output patients had similar decrements of renal blood flow. In addition to hypervole-

TABLE 1. Comparison of systolic time intervals in male and female alcoholics

	Normal			All alcoholics			Cirrhosis		
	Male	Female	P	Male	Female	P	Male	Female	P
Number	11	11		22	14		9	10	
Age	34.4 ± 2.6	33.6 ± 3.0	NS	39.4 ± 1.8	35.7 ± 2.1	NS	37.0 ± 3.5	35.0 ± 2.3	NS
Blood pressure									
S	123.5 ± 3.3	111.1 ± 5.1	NS	126.8 ± 3.9	116.9 ± 4.0	NS	123.5 ± 4.6	117.3 ± 5.5	NS
D	79.8 ± 2.0	75.1 ± 3.0	*	81.1 ± 2.2	70.0 ± 2.8	*	81.1 ± 3.7	70.4 ± 3.8	NS
HR/min	64.7 ± 2.4	68.5 ± 2.0	NS	81.6 ± 2.1†	81.2 ± 4.0†	NS	85.3 ± 4.0†	79.5 ± 4.5‡	NS
PEP/LVET	0.316 ± 0.007	0.310 ± 0.01		0.419 ± 0.02†	0.322 ± 0.015	†	0.400 ± 0.023*	0.321 ± 0.017	‡
PEP (msec)	92.4 ± 3.6	92.5 ± 3.1		107.0 ± 4.1‡	90.0 ± 4.4	‡	102.3 ± 6.0	91.4 ± 5.0	NS
PEPI (msec)	118.0 ± 3.1	120.0 ± 3.0		139.6 ± 4.0†	122.4 ± 3.6	*	136.4 ± 6.1‡	123.2 ± 4.4	NS
LVETI (msec)	401.5 ± 5.8	409.1 ± 5.5		397.2 ± 4.8	410.6 ± 4.5	‡	401.3 ± 4.1	413.0 ± 4.6	NS
QS$_2$I (msec)	519.7 ± 8.2	531.1 ± 6.8		536.5 ± 5.5	533.3 ± 5.0	NS	537.8 ± 8.5	536.4 ± 5.4	NS

Superscript symbols indicate statistical significance compared to normals of the corresponding sex; *$p < 0.005$, †$p < 0.001$, ‡$p < 0.05$, unlabelled, not significant.

Column heading P represents a comparison between males and females of the respective groups.

From ref. 43, with permission.

mia, anemia, and hypoxia, a hormonal contribution to the high output state must be considered in patients with high blood glucagon levels related to portal–systemic shunting (51), since this hormone has a positive inotropic action. The hyperdynamic state is associated with a decrease in net vascular tone as well as peripheral oxygen extraction, enhanced pulmonary venous–arterial mixture of oxygen (52), and some degree of myocardial depression.

Patients with this hyperdynamic circulatory state are prone to develop heart failure, which has been correlated with the level of impaired oxygen transport. In addition, in the presence of ascites, venous return and cardiac output are impaired and are normalized with correction of the restriction of venous return to the right heart by removal of ascitic fluid (53).

An important role of albumin has been suggested in view of the twofold increase in plasma clearance observed in patients with cirrhosis (54). Although a considerable amount escapes into the liver, there appears to be leakage in other capillary beds, suggesting a basis for a tendency to pulmonary congestion during acute volume expansion, particularly if renal excretory responses are subnormal (50). In view of the preclinical abnormalities of myocardial function observed particularly in male cirrhotics (43), the heart muscle itself may react subnormally to such circulatory challenges. In addition, the major cardiac neurohormone, norepinephrine, can evoke subnormal responses in the cardiovascular system (55), suggesting another mechanism for impaired cardiac reaction to acute stress in the patient with cirrhosis.

To evaluate cardiac hemodynamics in alcoholic liver disease, left ventricular function in 37 patients with hepatic cirrhosis (group II) was compared with that in 13 normal subjects (group I) matched for age, sex, and cardiac size (56). These groups were contrasted with group III, comprising 32 alcoholics without cirrhosis who had cardiac symptoms but no cardiomegaly or heart failure. Patients with cirrhosis as a group did not differ from normal subjects (group I) in terms of left ventricular filling pressure and cardiac muscle and pump function (cardiac index). However, subgroup IIA ($n = 21$) had a stroke index significantly less than normal, while subgroup IIB had a significantly increased stroke index and myocardial contractility with a diminished systemic arterial resistance (Fig. 6). Similar hepatic abnormalities were present in both subgroups. In group III, left ventricular end-diastolic and aortic mean pressures were significantly elevated compared with values in normal subjects, while cardiac index and indexes of ventricular contraction and relaxation were abnormal (Table 2).

Further examination of patients with cirrhosis indicated that the responses to volume or pressure increments in terms of the level of stroke work for a given filling pressure were most abnormal in group IIA, approximately those of group III. Thus although overt cardiomyopathy is infrequent in patients with cirrhosis, asymptomatic myocardial disease may assume clinical importance during volume or pressure overload (Fig. 7).

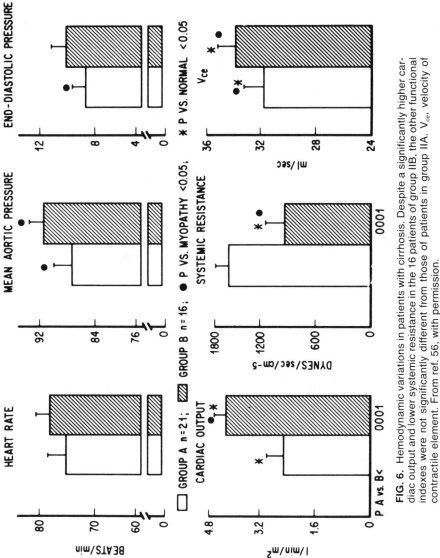

FIG. 6. Hemodynamic variations in patients with cirrhosis. Despite a significantly higher cardiac output and lower systemic resistance in the 16 patients of group IIB, the other functional indexes were not significantly different from those of patients in group IIA. V_{ce}, velocity of contractile element. From ref. 56, with permission.

TABLE 2. *Hemodynamics in normals and alcoholics at rest*

Group	HR	AoM	EDP	SV	CI	SW	S/P	TSR	dP/dt_{max}	V_{ce}	DTES	V_{IR}
Group I: normal subjects (n = 13)	85 ± 5	94 ± 2	9.8 ± 0.5	38.3 ± 2.8	3.17 ± 0.21	51.6 ± 4.9	5.3 ± 0.5	1,403 ± 92	2,000 ± 82	26.4 ± 0.9	20.5 ± 1.1	43.5 ± 4.8
Group II: patients with cirrhosis (n = 37)	77 ± 2	90 ± 2	9.8 ± 0.6	44.4 ± 2.4	3.33 ± 0.17	57.7 ± 3.1	6.6 ± 0.7	1,334 ± 74	2,147 ± 130	30.7 ± 2.2	24.4 ± 1.7	50.9 ± 3.4
p vs. group I	NS	NS	NS	NS	NS	NS	NS	NS	NS	NS	NS	NS
Group III: patients without cirrhosis (n = 32)	76 ± 2	104 ± 3	12.9 ± 1.0	34.9 ± 1.5	2.61 ± 0.10	48.2 ± 2.5	4.4 ± 0.3	1,736 ± 82	1,581 ± 84	18.3 ± 0.9	17.8 ± 0.7	31.7 ± 2.2
p vs. group I	NS	< 0.01	< 0.008	NS	< 0.02	NS	NS	< 0.01	< 0.001	< 0.0001	< 0.05	< 0.04
p vs. group II	NS	< 0.0001	< 0.009	< 0.002	< 0.001	< 0.02	< 0.0001	< 0.001	< 0.001	< 0.0001	< 0.001	< 0.0001

AoM, mean aortic pressure (mm Hg); CI, cardiac output (liters/min/m^2); dP/dt$_{max}$, peak value of first derivative of left ventricular pressure (mm Hg/sec); DTES, ratio of peak negative dP/dt to end-systolic pressure at dicrotic notch (ml/sec); EDP, left ventricular end-diastolic pressure (mm Hg); HR, heart rate (beats/min); S/P, ratio of stroke work to end-diastolic pressure; SV, stroke volume (ml/m^2); SW, stroke work (gm/m^2); TSR, total systemic resistance (dynes·sec/cm^3); V$_{ce}$, velocity of contractile element (ml/sec); V$_{IR}$, rate of relaxation of contractile element (ml/sec).

From ref. 56, with permission.

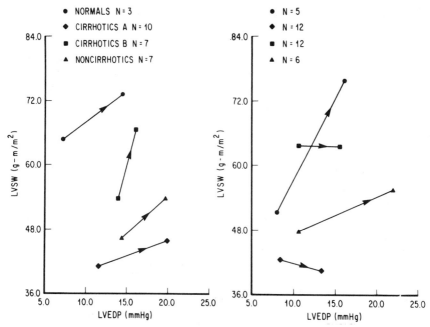

FIG. 7. Effects of increments in volume (**left panel**) and systemic arterial pressure (**right panel**). The latter was increased by an infusion of angiotensin II in the normal subjects (group I) and patients without cirrhosis (group III) and with vasopressin in patients with cirrhosis (group II). In contrast to normal subjects, the two alcoholic groups showed no significant improvement in cardiac work despite a substantial increase in left ventricular filling pressure. LVEDP, left ventricular end-diastolic pressure; LVSW, left ventricular stroke work. From ref. 56, with permission.

Experimental Evidence of Cardiotoxicity of Alcohol

The concept of alcoholic cardiomyopathy has been examined in a variety of animal experiments, with reproduction of myocardial alterations consistent with subclinical heart disease. However, at present, in no animal model has the state of low output heart failure on a chronic ethanol regimen been reproduced successfully. This may be related to greater resistance of the myocardium in subhuman species to the development of heart failure, insufficient duration of alcohol feeding, or the absence of factors present in the human alcoholic, for example, cigarette use, trace metal excess, and other nutritional factors.

While histologic abnormalities have been observed in many alcoholics at postmortem (57), uncertainty as to the quantity of ethanol intake, the nutritional status of the patient (including electrolyte deficits), and the possibility of heart disease from other causes have obscured the relationship of excessive ethanol use and cardiomyopathy. Previous chronic experiments with ethanol have yielded conflicting data in terms of the production of a functional deficit (58). Even in animal models with metabolic or morphologic abnormalities, the fact that heart failure has not been produced has raised a question as to whether the cardiomyopathy observed in human alcoholics is solely attributable to ethanol intake. It should be noted that the long ingestion period of at least 10 years apparently required in humans may be crucial to the development of clinical disease.

The most striking short-term results were reported in the rhesus monkey fed ethanol as 40% of total calories for a period of 4 months (59). Histologically, the heart showed myocytolysis and fibrosis. These changes are somewhat unexpected in view of the relatively brief feeding of ethanol. Quantitation of the changes in terms of fibrous tissue accumulation and loss of myofiber is needed to verify these observations.

To assess longer-term effects, Maines and Aldinger (58) fed alcohol as a 25% solution to rats over a period of 7 months. After 4 months a consistent decrease in ventricular contractile force or isometric systolic tension was observed. Pair-fed controls remained normal and a vitamin supplement did not protect the alcohol-intoxicated animals against myocardial depression. In these open-chest animals aortic pressure was moderately reduced, in contrast to subsequent studies of closed-chest animals. In a subsequent study by Vasdev et al. (59), 40% of total calories were fed as ethanol to a group of rhesus monkeys with a synthetic fluid diet. After a period of 3 months the animals were noted to have marked accumulation of triglyceride and cholesterol ester in the heart. Isotopic studies indicated that the triglyceride increase was at least partially based on enhanced synthesis. Histologically, the heart showed fatty change in the myocardium and evidence of focal myocytolysis, atrophy of muscle fibers, and early fibrosis. These changes are somewhat unexpected in view of the relatively short term of the ethanol feeding. Quantitation of the changes in terms of fibrous tissue and loss of myofiber is needed to verify these observations.

Longer-term studies have been conducted in young adult mongrel dogs (60). These animals were maintained in a relatively normal nutritional state while receiving up to 36% of calories as ethanol, approximating the quantity reported in a population of human alcoholics (61). After an average of 18 months of observation, when evaluation of nutritional status included assay of plasma vitamins, the chronic ethanol and control animals were anesthetized to evaluate left ventricular performance and morphology. Since myocardial lipid alterations have been reported after chronic ethanol intake (34,62), [1-^{14}C]oleic acid metabolism has also been assessed.

While consuming an average of 3.11 ± 0.24 of ethanol/kg daily, the nutritional status of the experimental animals was quite comparable to that of the controls. In addition to a small weight gain that was similar for both groups by the conclusion of the study, the hematocrit, serum protein, and fasting blood glucose in the unanesthetized state remained at control levels. Furthermore, serum albumin determination at the end of the study averaged 3.5 ± 0.2 g/100 ml in five of the controls and 3.4 ± 0.1 g/100 ml in five experimental animals. Plasma vitamins of the B series and other major vitamins were present in similar concentrations at the end of the observation period in the control and alcoholic groups.

To evaluate the degree of intoxication in the chronic state after at least 6 months of alcohol intake, samples for blood ethanol determinations were performed after acute ingestion on at least two occasions in each animal (63) and averaged 213 ± 7 mg/100 ml. Alcohol administration was often associated with some degree of locomotor incoordination and occasional short periods of sleep.

At the onset of the study in the anesthetized state, mean heart rate and aortic pressure were similar in both groups. However, in the chronic ethanol animals there was a significantly higher end-diastolic pressure despite a lower level of end-diastolic volume. Assessment of left ventricular function during afterload increments with angiotensin was undertaken with aortic diastolic pressure evaluations of 16 ± 1.1 mm Hg in the control group and 17 ± 0.9 mm Hg in the ethanol group. Stroke output increased modestly but significantly in the controls, while no such increments occurred in the alcoholic animals. Ejection fraction was similar in both groups before and after angiotensin. Stroke work rose in the normals from 1.39 ± 0.23 to 1.81 ± 0.21 g/kg, but the response was significantly less in the experimental group ($p < 0.01$), 1.03 ± 0.04 to 1.11 ± 0.07 g/kg. The index of contractility revealed no significant difference between normals (1.57 + 0.11) and alcoholics (1.36 + 0.10) before angiotensin; there was a similar decline in both groups during increased afterload.

Normal controls exhibited a moderate rise of end-diastolic pressure and end-diastolic volume during angiotensin infusion. However, a significantly larger rise of end-diastolic pressure occurred in the ethanol group while the end-diastolic volume response was significantly less than in controls. This is presumably the basis for the reduced stroke volume.

To further evaluate the apparent altered stiffness of the ventricle, six of the normal animals and six of the ethanol group were infused at a rate of 50 ml/min for 3–4 min; the normals generally exhibited a proportionate rise of left ventricular end-diastolic pressure and volume. In the ethanol group, there was a significantly higher rise of end-diastolic pressure than in the normals ($p < 0.001$), despite an elevation of end-diastolic volume proportionate to controls.

Heart rate declined and stroke volume rose similarly in both groups without a change in afterload, so that the significantly higher end-diastolic pressure in the experimental group would not appear to be related to these variables.

To examine a potential morphologic basis for the altered diastolic pressure–volume relations attributed to enhanced wall stiffness, apical sections of the left ventricle were examined histochemically. Staining with alcian blue showed distinct accumulation of a glycoprotein-like material in the interstitium of the left ventricular wall in the ethanol group. The degree of staining ranged from 2–3 +, on a scale of 0–4. There was virtually no staining in the normal controls. Periodic acid–Schiff staining was slightly positive in the ethanol group.

Analysis of left ventricular lipids revealed an increment of triglyceride in the ethanol group, which appeared as fine cytoplasmic droplets on oil red O stain. Cholesterol, phospholipid, and free fatty acid levels were not significantly altered in the three layers of myocardium compared with the control group. It is noteworthy that at this stage of chronic alcoholism, the plasma lipid concentrations did not differ from control lipid levels, although transient increases of plasma triglyceride and cholesterol levels were present during the earlier months of the chronic ethanol period.

There was no significant extraction of triglyceride, phospholipid, or cholesterol by the myocardium in the anesthetized state by controls or chronic ethanol animals. In addition to comparable arterial levels of blood glucose, myocardial uptake of glucose did not differ between the groups: 0.44 + 0.04 mM per gram per minute in controls and 0.50 + 0.04 mM/g/min in the ethanol group. Morphologic studies revealed no inflammatory response in heart muscle to complicate the assessment of chemical composition. The changes in lipid metabolism were not accompanied by unequivocal abnormalities of mitochondrial structure on electron micrographs but accumulation of glycogen-type particles was evident. Lysosomal structures were relatively infrequent in both groups. Dilatation of the sarcoplasmic reticulum was a prominent feature in all animals receiving ethanol, and the undifferentiated portion of the intercalated disc was similarly affected. The pathophysiology observed in these chronic alcoholic animals receiving supplementary vitamins is apparently independent of a vitamin deficit, assuming that normal blood levels are indicative of normal tissue concentrations (64). That protein intake was sufficient to meet minimum requirements for adult dog (National Academy of Sciences–National Research Council, 1962) is supported by the fact that the experimental group maintained body weight, serum proteins, and hematocrit. Moreover, the histologic changes of experimental protein deficiency, which may include inflammatory cell infiltrates and hydropic degeneration of myocardial fibers, were not present (65).

The hemodynamic findings in these animals resemble those observed in human alcoholics with preclinical cardiac malfunction (41,42,66). During increased afterload the elevation of filling pressure was significantly higher than in control animals. While stroke volume rose in normals, no increment occurred in the ethanol group presumably related to the lack of end-diastolic volume increase. To evaluate whether the latter was due to diminished myocardial compliance, the filling pressure response to volume expansion during saline infusion was assessed. A significantly greater rise of end-diastolic pressure in the animals receiving ethanol compared with normal controls supports the interpretation of increased diastolic stiffness of left ventricular muscle in the experimental group.

Since left ventricular weights were similar to control hearts, hypertrophy would not seem to contribute to this functional abnormality. Elasticity of muscle has been attributed predominantly to extracellular structures (67), but the relative importance of collagen and glycoprotein in this regard is unknown. Since the former did not appear to be present in increased quantity when tissue was stained with trichrome, histochemical stains were used to assess the potential accumulation of glycoprotein and revealed alcian-blue-positive material. Support for the view that increments of extracellular glycoprotein can diminish diastolic compliance is derived from observations in experimental diabetes where accumulation of periodic acid–Schiff-positive material in the myocardial interstitium was associated with enhanced stiffness (68). In addition, increments of noncollagen material largely limited to the intercellular space may occur in the early stages of amyloid heart disease, a situation that ultimately limits diastolic filling (3,69). While alteration of other myocardial elements such as sarcolemma could contribute to the compliance change in alcoholic animals, the accumulation of glycoprotein in the intercellular space suggests a probable basis for enhanced myocardial stiffness. The glycoprotein composition has not been characterized but presumably has a high content of hyaluronic acid since alcian blue has an affinity for acid mucopolysaccharide (70).

A previous hemodynamic study of chronic ethanol administration in the rat has shown a significant decrease in "potential ventricular force" (58). In contrast, a definite abnormality of ventricular function was not found in the same species fed less ethanol, 15% by volume (71), compared to 25% in the previous series (58). In addition, an important methodologic difference existed, in that ventricular function was tested at the uppermost segment of the ascending portion of the function curve (58), so that the ventricle was not stressed to the same extent as the Lochner study (71). Since caloric equivalents were not provided, it is difficult to compare these data with the present study; moreover, species differences may exist. In a recent study of dogs fed ethanol in a daily quantity similar to that of the present study but for a 14-week period, no hemodynamic abnormality was observed (72). This is consistent with the view that duration of ingestion is an important determinant.

The importance of chronicity is also evident in the reported failure to find morphologic abnormalities of cardiac cell organelles in animals ingesting ethanol for 1–3 months (73,74). Dilatation of the sarcoplasmic reticulum and intercalated disc were the only unequivocal structural abnormalities in the relatively well nourished animals in this current report, findings also observed in two studies of patients with alcoholic cardiomyopathy (75,76). It is problematic whether the extensive abnormalities of myofibrils and mitochondria reported earlier are due solely to toxicity or to coexistent nutritional deficiency, cobalt excess, or other complications (77–79).

The mechanism of altered contractility in the long-term alcoholic groups is not clear; high-energy phosphate levels do not appear to be diminished (80), and total calcium concentrations in the left ventricle were not reduced (81), although intracellular redistribution has been suggested (80). Impaired fluxes of calcium in sarcoplasmic reticulum have been observed in a chronic alcoholic model, and dilatation of this organelle was particularly prominent in the canine model that consumed ethanol for 4 years. Presumably, the significant increase of cardiac cell water and sodium in this group was reflected in the sarcoplasmic reticulum. A resultant distortion of the membranes in this system may be responsible for altered calcium transport and contractility after prolonged feeding of ethanol. An inhibitory effect of long-term ethanol use on myosin adenosine triphosphatase (ATPase) was also demonstrated (82).

Inhibition of sodium/potassium ATPase has been described in several organs as the result of long-term feeding of ethanol (83). However, the steady-state gain by the heart was not associated with potassium loss, in contrast to the situation in which myocardial ATPase is inhibited by digitalis. In addition, accumulation of water contrasts with the typical response to inhibition of this enzyme. Previous observations have indicated an altered fatty acid incorporation (60) as well as composition of phospholipid (84) in animals fed ethanol for a long period. Thus one of the membrane properties limiting permeability of the cell to sodium and water may be affected by the phospholipid alteration without affecting the normal transcellular gradient of potassium.

A potential role of myocardial metabolism of ethanol has been suggested to be a factor in the pathogenesis of cardiomyopathy. In the heart only trace amounts of alcohol dehydrogenase have been found (85), and a microsomal ethanol oxidizing system has not been demonstrated. However, the catalase system has enhanced activity during chronic ethanol administration; this has been interpreted as a protective compensatory mechanism (86). Chronic inhibition of this enzyme in the rat resulted in substantial histologic abnormality, which was largely lacking in animals fed ethanol without the inhibitor.

The question of reversibility of the myocardial abnormality in experimental animals was examined in rats consuming 25% of ethanol daily for up to 8 weeks (87). It was observed that mitochondrial respiration with glutamate or succinate as substrate was depressed, the former more so than the latter. When the animals were returned to a state of abstinence and studied 8 weeks subsequently, respiration with both of these substrates had returned to near control values. In terms of myocardial contractility, the abnormalities of maximum developed time tension to peak tension and the maximum rate of isometric tension development were reversed after 8 weeks of abstinence, although the latter was still reduced to a small extent.

These animal experiments support the view that chronic use of ethanol in substantial quantities can produce myocardial alterations that may be considered an antecedent to heart failure, analogous to the preclinical cardiomyopathy in human alcoholics. Whether development of heart failure in the animal model depends on a longer period of ethanol ingestion or other factors, such as cigarette use common to alcoholism in humans, remains to be elucidated. Intensification of interstitial collagen accumulation and the intracellular cation abnormalities thought to be related to diminished contractility may be critical for progression to cardiac decompensation.

Cardiomyopathy and Heart Failure

Although subclinical cardiomyopathy can be detected in a high proportion of persons who abuse alcohol, symptomatic cardiomyopathy is less common. Factors that determine individual susceptibility to alcohol-related myocardial injury are largely unknown. A relatively high prevalence of alcoholic cardiomyopathy exists in patients attending inner-city and veterans hospitals, and it has been suggested that this could reflect an ethnic or racial predilection to this disorder. No attempts have been made to establish this issue definitively.

No association between alcoholic cardiomyopathy and human leukocyte antigen phenotype has yet been observed (88). Variable organ sensitivity is reflected in clinical reports of cardiac disease unaccompanied by liver disease. This view is supported by the absence of morphologic evidence for alcoholic hepatitis or cirrhosis in patients with heart failure (89). This entity occurs more frequently in men than in women (43). Although this may simply reflect the greater prevalence of alcoholism among the former, a sex difference in susceptibility to the cardiotoxic effects of alcohol may exist. When gender comparisons were restricted to subjects with alcoholic cirrhosis who were under 45 years of age and similar in terms of other relevant parameters, the left ventricular pre-ejection period and ejection time ratio were significantly more prolonged in men than in women. This suggests that the premenopausal woman may be less susceptible to myocardial toxic effects, analogous to the situation in hypertension.

It has been suggested that one or more additional factors, such as systemic hypertension, cigarette smoking, beverage additives, or malnutrition may be needed to ensure clinical expression of alcoholic cardiomyopathy. Even moderate consumption raises arterial pressure to a modest extent, independent of smoking or caffeine use (90).

In an investigation of alcoholics with subclinical heart disease, alcohol abuse was the single most important variable related to cardiac dilatation. The authors concluded that the increases observed in end-diastolic diameter by echocardiography could not be explained on the basis of their potential confounding variables including cigarette smoking (91).

Beverage additives may have a role in some instances in the pathogenesis of alcoholic cardiomyopathy, but the evidence is far from clear. In the mid-1960s, outbreaks of a relatively acute, fulminant cardiomyopathy were described among heavy beer drinkers in a few isolated centers in Belgium and in North America (92,93). It was suggested that the cobalt chloride added to the beer as a foam stabilizer might be the responsible agent, because this disorder had not been described before the use of cobalt salts, and outbreaks stopped when these were withdrawn. Cobalt salts were added to the beer in several other centers, however, where their use was unaccompanied by the development of cardiomyopathy (94). This suggests that other variables, such as nutritional abnormalities, must be present for the toxic effect of cobalt to become manifest. Certain amino acids such as cysteine, for example, decrease the cardiac uptake of cobalt ions so that quantitative or qualitative differences in protein intake might affect the response to the cobalt salts.

Lead has also been implicated in the development of cardiomyopathy, particularly in "moonshine" drinkers (95). More significant changes were observed in myocardial mitochondria in rats during feeding with ethanol and lead than with alcohol alone. The excess myocardial lead can be removed by use of sodium EDTA (96); however, the long-term effects of lead removal on myocardial function have not been assessed.

Severe hypokalemia may affect cardiac function and contribute to cardiac decompensation in some alcoholics (97,98). In dogs, the development of experimental hypophosphatemia is associated with impaired myocardial contractility (99) and in humans profound hypophosphatemia can result in the development of severe congestive cardiomyopathy. It is therefore possible that phosphorus depletion might play a role in the development of cardiomyopathy in some alcoholic individuals. The myocardial abnormalities reverse when the hypophosphatemia is corrected. During the early part of this century, beriberi heart disease was fairly common in the alcoholic population. This phenomenon is rarely seen now, presumably because of the widespread availability of thiamine.

History, Duration, and Quantitation

Clinical experience with congestive cardiomyopathy in alcoholics suggests several factors that need to be considered in making the diagnosis, namely, the quantity, frequency, and duration of alcohol use. These also relate to factors that may be considered as determinants of this disease (Table 3). Clinical reports of cardiomyopathy have emphasized the difficulty in obtaining a history of alcoholism. There is a male predominance, and suggestive diagnostic aspects include social disruption, accident proneness, and a family history of chronic alcohol abuse. The major positive diagnostic feature is the history of ethanol ingestion in intoxicating amounts for many

TABLE 3. *Determinants of cardiomyopathy in alcoholism*

Quantity
Frequency
Duration
Ill-defined variables: nutrition, gender, cigarette use, age of onset

From ref. 213, with permission.

years, frequently marked by periods of spree drinking. Often, the information can be obtained only through persistent questioning over many visits with the patient or by communication with relatives.

Other Variables

In terms of variables that may also affect the development of cardiomyopathy, several factors are considered to be potentially important. In contrast to findings in patients with liver disease, clinically evident malnutrition is usually not present in the cardiac patient. In women the disease is rare prior to the age of menopause. It should also be noted that a genetic predisposition has been evaluated in the terms of the HLA antigens (100). Examination of two loci (A and B) revealed no significant difference from findings in controls. Beverage additives, hypophosphatemia, and cigarette smoking (101) may play a role in the clinical expression of cardiomyopathy.

Major Clinical Manifestations

Congestive cardiomyopathy is typically identified in men between 30 and 50 years of age who have frequently ingested intoxicating amounts of alcohol for a minimum of 10 years (102–104).

The alcoholic individual may first seek medical assistance with varied cardiovascular problems (Table 4). In alcoholics, when cardiac dysfunction progresses to low cardiac output heart failure, pulmonary congestion may lead to exertional or nocturnal dyspnea. With mild degrees of dyspnea, altered pulmonary function must be considered, because impaired alveolar diffusion has been described that is more than can be attributed to cigarette smoking

TABLE 4. *Cardiomyopathy in alcoholic patients: clinical manifestations*

Congestive heart failure
Palpitations, syncopal syndrome
Chest pain (precordial)
Embolism (systemic, pulmonary)
Sudden death

From ref. 213, with permission.

alone (105). Weakness and fatigue presumably resulting from reduced cardiac output are also common.

Physical signs of cardiac decompensation are consistent with other causes of congestive cardiomyopathy (Table 5). Most patients having an element of cardiac decompensation exhibit a diastolic gallop. An atrial gallop is also a frequent finding when there is normal sinus rhythm. In still others, who do not have congestive heart failure, the findings of an atrial gallop in presystole represents an early clue to the presence of myocardial disease (106). When heart failure is long sustained, or after repeated episodes, pulmonary hypertension and right heart failure may become evident. If the patient has not been seen in the earlier stages of the disease, the picture of primary pulmonary hypertension may be mimicked. However, in the patient with left ventricular myocardial disease, pulmonary hypertension commonly develops secondary to long-standing, severe left ventricular failure.

Unless there is complicating papillary muscle insufficiency resulting in mitral regurgitation, cardiomegaly may be moderate in extent; heart rate may revert to near normal after pulmonary congestion is corrected during the initial episode of decompensation. Both pulmonary and peripheral arterial emboli are common features of this disease and sometimes represent the initial manifestation. Systemic emboli may originate from mural thrombi in the left ventricle and left atrium. Factors favoring embolization are cardiac enlargement, congestive failure from any cause, or thrombophlebitis in the venous system. These clinical events frequently seem to be precipitated by intensified drinking, but recurrent illness may occur after a period of abstinence in some individuals.

The thesis that cumulative effects of ethanol over a period of time may result in cardiac abnormalities despite adequate nutrition is illustrated in the following case (Fig. 8). A well-compensated patient was given Scotch whiskey for a period of 5.5 months at a daily dose of 12–16 oz (11). After 6 weeks, the resting heart rate began to increase, circulation time was prolonged, and the venous pressure became elevated without evidence of malnutrition. After 4 months, a ventricular diastolic gallop developed and persisted until the ethanol intake was interrupted. Subsequently, without specific cardiac therapy, there was spontaneous restoration to normal. A major role of ethanol in the production of left-sided heart failure in this person was substantiated

---

TABLE 5. *Physical signs*

Third and fourth heart sounds (gallop rhythm)
Left ventricular hypertrophy
Murmurs (mitral systolic; early, mid, late)
Left ventricular or biventricular failure
Pulmonary hypertension

From ref. 213, with permission.

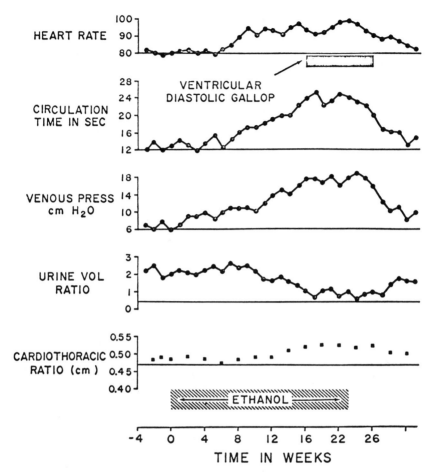

FIG. 8. Observations in a well-nourished patient receiving daily Scotch, which resulted in evidence of heart failure. The failure regressed without medical treatment after interrupting alcohol intake. From ref. 11, with permission.

by gradual reversion of the cardiocirculatory abnormality after alcohol ingestion was interrupted. This observation supports the thesis that the myocardial disease is reversible at certain stages if intake of ethanol is discontinued.

Electrocardiogram

Specific abnormalities of the electrocardiogram have not been found in either preclinical or clinical cardiomyopathy due to alcoholism (Table 6). However, during the former state as well as the latter, a relatively high in-

TABLE 6. *Electrocardiogram*

Tachyarrhythmias—sinus or ectopic
Conduction defects—incomplete bundle branch block (absent Q waves, I, V5, V6), atrioventricular
Left ventricular hypertrophy
Left axis deviation
Infarct pattern
Nonspecific repolarization abnormalities
Normal

From ref. 213, with permission.

cidence of absent septal Q waves has been observed (43). In one reported series with the development of heart failure a variety of nonspecific changes, including ST segment and T wave abnormalities, and evidence of left ventricular and atrial enlargement were frequently observed (107). Twenty-six percent of these patients had left anterior hemiblock, and approximately 10% had left and/or right bundle branch block.

Hemodynamics

Earlier studies of heart disease in patients with alcoholism focused mainly on individuals with cardiomegaly and cardiac decompensation. Hemodynamic assessment indicates that this was a low output form of heart failure distinct from the high output state that may occur in patients with beriberi syndrome (10). In a study of a broader range of addicted patients (108), those whose symptoms included chest pain or palpitations had normal heart size on x-ray examination (groups 1 and 2). In group 3, the symptoms of exertional dyspnea or dyspnea at rest were associated with degrees of cardiomegaly. Despite the substantial difference in physical findings, all three groups exhibited a significant increase in end-diastolic pressure (Fig. 9). However, group 1 was distinguished by the fact that end-diastolic volume was not increased, but actually was somewhat diminished. Groups 2 and 3 were characterized by a significant increase in end-diastolic volume and tension. The latter was enhanced to a significantly greater extent in group 3 and was the most prominent hemodynamic abnormality in this group. A major change in the index of contractility, as well as in the rate of relaxation, occurred in group 1 (Fig. 10). In those with an increased diastolic volume, further moderate depression of these indices was observed. The higher stroke index and lower ejection fraction in group 2, compared to group 1, was presumably due to the higher end-diastolic volume in the former group.

In a separate group with mitral regurgitation, the more severe depression of left ventricular function seen in alcoholics was presumably due to the effect of ethanol on left ventricular performance. Cardiac function in nonalcoholic patients with similar degrees of regurgitant volume was normal (108).

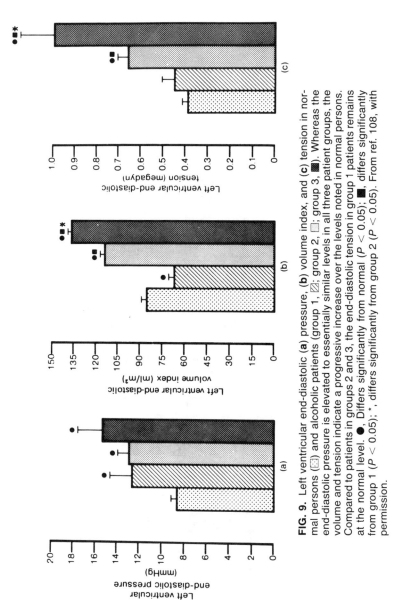

FIG. 9. Left ventricular end-diastolic (**a**) pressure, (**b**) volume index, and (**c**) tension in normal persons (□) and alcoholic patients (group 1, ▨; group 2, ▦; group 3, ■). Whereas the end-diastolic pressure is elevated to essentially similar levels in all three patient groups, the volume and tension indicate a progressive increase over the levels noted in normal persons. Compared to patients in groups 2 and 3, the end-diastolic tension in group 1 patients remains at the normal level. ●, Differs significantly from normal ($P < 0.05$); ■, differs significantly from group 1 ($P < 0.05$); *, differs significantly from group 2 ($P < 0.05$). From ref. 108, with permission.

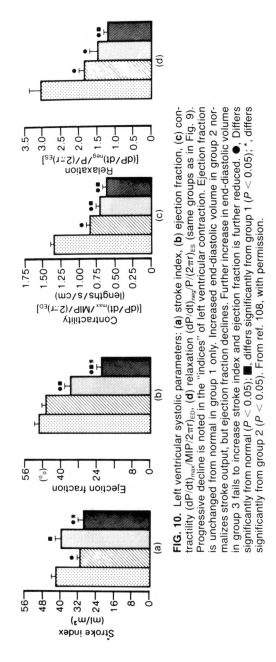

FIG. 10. Left ventricular systolic parameters: **(a)** stroke index, **(b)** ejection fraction, **(c)** contractility $(dP/dt)_{max}/MIP/2\pi r)_{ED}$, **(d)** relaxation $(dP/dt)_{neg}/P/(2\pi r)_{ES}$ (same groups as in Fig. 9). Progressive decline is noted in the "indices" of left ventricular contraction. Ejection fraction is unchanged from normal in group 1 only. Increased end-diastolic volume in group 2 normalizes stroke output, but ejection fraction declines. Further increase in end-diastolic volume in group 3 fails to increase stroke index and ejection fraction is further reduced. ● Differs significantly from normal ($P < 0.05$); ■, differs significantly from group 1 ($P < 0.05$); *, differs significantly from group 2 ($P < 0.05$). From ref. 108, with permission.

It is worth noting that the elevation of end-diastolic pressure without an increase in end-diastolic volume in group 1 is consistent with findings in a prior study of chronic alcoholism in a canine model (60). Increasing the preload enhances this abnormality. However, this model differed, because systolic function was not impaired early. A longer duration of ethanol intake of approximately 4 years was apparently required, as observed in a subsequent study (81). The decrease in systolic function is due presumably to a different process than that leading to the changed compliance in earlier stages of the disease. It is noteworthy that deposition of collagen between cardiac cells in a chronic alcoholic animal, presumed to be a basis for the compliance alteration, did not differ in long- or short-term alcoholic animals. The diminished indices of contractility in long-term alcoholic animals were associated with substantial swelling of the sarcotubular system. This may well be related to changes in the pumping of calcium from the sarcoplasmic reticulum to the contractile protein (80).

Progression to a stage of cardiac decompensation may depend on intensification of processes present in the early stages. At some point, however, there appears to be some degree of impaired synthesis or accelerated degradation of contractile protein, inasmuch as lysis of myofibrils is frequently observed on morphologic study in advanced cardiomyopathy (109). In some patients, the early stage of congestive cardiomyopathy may progress rapidly in terms of serial ultrastructural changes and severe morphologic changes may antecede the appearance of rapid clinical deterioration (109). Clues about the mechanism of this progression are not yet available.

Precipitating Factors

As a rule, there are no clear precipitating events that can readily be identified as inducing heart failure. Outbreaks of cardiomyopathy among heavy beer drinkers were described in the 1960s in a few isolated centers. Cobalt was suggested as a contributory etiologic factor in that heart failure did not appear until some time after cobalt salts were added to the beer and disappeared when the use of cobalt was discontinued (92,93).

Lead has also been implicated, particularly in "moonshine" drinkers, as a factor affecting the development of cardiomyopathy in that particular subgroup of chronic alcoholics (96).

Severe hypokalemia is known to affect cardiac function, and it is likely that there are some patients in whom this may be a contributing element (97,98). Hypophosphatemia is also observed in some alcoholics (110). Its importance is illustrated by the fact that experimentally impaired contractility is reversible with phosphorus repletion (110) and is also corrected in clinical hypophosphatemia (99).

For many years cardiac disease in the alcoholic was recognized principally in those who had associated thiamine deficiency and the syndrome of beriberi. While not readily reproduced in animals, the key features include a high cardiac output associated with arteriolar vasodilatation and peripheral edema (111). This syndrome was described recently in 23 Japanese persons (112). Alcohol was not implicated; rather, the disease resulted from an unorthodox diet of excessive carbonated soft drinks and polished rice. The cardiovascular abnormalities were readily reversed by an adequate diet.

Although it has been the classic view that right ventricular failure is dominant when symptoms develop, several studies have documented a significant elevation of left ventricular end-diastolic and pulmonary capillary wedge pressures (111). Depression of left ventricular function during the acute phase of beriberi heart disease has been described (5). In addition, the persistence of a chronic cardiac abnormality after treatment with thiamine suggests that alcoholism, usually present in persons with beriberi on the North American continent, may be responsible. The reversible nature of the cardiac abnormalities in persons who were apparently not alcoholic was indicated in American prisoners of war in World War II (6). Long-term follow-up failed to reveal a significantly higher incidence of heart disease than in controls.

Differential Diagnosis

Systemic arterial hypertension is perhaps the most common entity in considering differential diagnosis (Table 7). High diastolic arterial blood pressure is found frequently during periods of severe congestive heart failure, which may lead to the false diagnosis of hypertensive heart disease. The blood pressure usually returns to normal after response to therapy. Those patients with minimal clinical disturbance had the greatest elevations of urinary catecholamines, and there was some correlation with the clinical manifestations of sympathetic overstimulation in terms of increased blood pressure and pulse rate as well as urinary catecholamine excretion. The decrease in clinical symptoms was accompanied by a corresponding fall in the level of elevated urinary catecholamines toward normal. Another hormonal factor that may contribute to transient arterial pressure elevation is stimulation of the renin–aldosterone axis, which has been observed to occur some hours after ethanol ingestion (113). Also, the vasoactive hormone vasopressin reached its highest plasma concentrations in the postethanol period (114).

TABLE 7. *What must be excluded*

Sustained systemic arterial hypertension
Mitral valve disease
Coronary artery disease
Pericardial tamponade

From ref. 213, with permission.

A diagnostic entity that often required consideration is mitral valve disease. An apical systolic murmur of mitral insufficiency may more often be observed during a bout of heart failure. However, it is usually not pansystolic and is thought to be related to disease of the posterior papillary muscle and some degree of ventricular dilatation. This is generally not due to rheumatic heart disease when the murmur appears for the first time with onset of heart failure. Also, the murmur has a tendency to disappear as heart failure is corrected. With more advanced disease and right heart failure, tricuspid insufficiency may occur, giving rise to a pansystolic murmur in the third and fourth intercostal spaces that is usually increased by inspiration. When due to cardiomyopathy, this murmur also tends to diminish as cardiac compensation is restored.

Angina pectoris is not an infrequent presentation in male alcoholics without heart failure. This may occur at rest or with exercise and is occasionally associated with a positive exercise stress test despite the absence of significant coronary disease on angiography (115). That this pain is of cardiac, rather than extracardiac, origin is supported by the observation that the left ventricular response to atrial pacing is analogous to that of patients with coronary artery disease during pacing. There is a smaller than normal decline of end-diastolic pressure during pacing and a higher rebound than normal during the postpacing period.

The fourth clinical entity that should be considered in certain patients with advanced cardiomyopathy is pericardial tamponade. There may be considerable cardiac dilatation, the heart sounds may be distant, and a paradoxical arterial pulse may be present. That this is not due to tamponade may be suggested clinically by the presence of a diastolic gallop due to myocardial disease and a palpable apical impulse to the left and below the normal position. The advent of echocardiography for detection and quantification of tamponade is of great aid in differential diagnosis and may preclude the need for invasive tests.

Once the diagnosis of congestive cardiomyopathy is established, some consideration must be given to other potential causes (Table 8), particularly

TABLE 8. *Etiology of congestive cardiomyopathy*

Toxic—ethanol, adriamycin, carbon tetrachloride
Infiltrative—amyloid, collagen diseases, sarcoid, hemochromatosis, neoplastic
Endocrine—diabetes, thyroid disease, acromegaly
Infection—viral (coxsackie, echo), protozoan (Chagas' disease), bacterial (diphtheria), parasitic (trichinosis)
Nutritional—beriberi, obesity (marked), kwashiorkor
Familial
Neuromuscular dystrophies
Postpartum occurrence

From ref. 213, with permission.

in individuals in whom a history of alcohol abuse, at least initially, is difficult to obtain. The prevalence of these entities differs to some extent with age and geographic location. The medical history of the patient is often a major indicator of the correct diagnosis, that is, patients with uremia, those with past evidence of collagen disease, and in individuals with a clear history of marked nutritional abnormalities on physical examination.

Course and Reversibility

In those alcoholic patients who develop cardiac alterations, the earliest abnormality is characterized by diminished left ventricular compliance and a moderate contractility deficit without heart failure. In those who progress, end-diastolic tension is substantially enhanced and further reductions in contractility indices are observed.

Individual case reports have indicated the potential for recovery from mechanical cardiac dysfunction when the patient ceases alcohol consumption. The inherent difficulties of clinical evaluation have precluded a randomized study, but the outlook is generally considered to be poor in those who continue to ingest substantial amounts of ethanol. In a European study of patients with a diagnosis of congestive cardiomyopathy, 50% were considered to be alcoholic and continued to be actively so (115). Two-thirds of these subjects were dead within 3 years, whereas one-third of the nonalcoholics had died.

The effects of abstinence presumably depend on the stage of the cardiac disease at which the patient's behavior is altered. Three studies strongly suggest a beneficial effect of interrupting alcohol intake. In a small series, all 10 patients who stopped drinking survived a decade of follow-up (116). In a study of 31 alcoholics in the United States, follow-up during several years indicated that none of the 12 who stopped alcohol consumption succumbed, whereas there were 19 deaths in those who persisted in their addiction (117). The subjects in both groups had similar degrees of cardiomegaly and congestive heart failure on entrance into the study.

In the only available study of its kind, almost one-third of patients followed on an outpatient basis were found to have apparently maintained abstinence over a 3-year period (118). The majority of these had an improved or unchanged cardiac status, similar to patients with hepatic cirrhosis who become abstinent (119). Deaths occurred preponderantly in those who did not abstain. Some uncertainties exist, since the relative cardiac status on admission to the study was not described. It is noteworthy that more than 20% of those who allegedly were abstinent deteriorated in cardiac status. Presumably at certain stages of the disease, the pathogenetic mechanisms may continue unabated. Whether prolonged bed rest would be advantageous in this subset of patients (104) remains to be demonstrated.

The actual course of congestive cardiomyopathy varies according to the nature of cardiac involvement as well as the severity of left ventricular dysfunction. In general, the outlook is relatively poor in those who continue with substantial amounts of ethanol ingestion. Most striking were results in a series of 108 patients from France hospitalized with a diagnosis of congestive cardiomyopathy. Disease in 42 was attributed to alcohol abuse. Two-thirds of the alcoholic group were dead within 3 years, whereas one-third of the nonalcoholic group had succumbed. In an earlier series of 64 alcoholic patients, a full one-third were apparently persuaded to abstain during a 4-year follow-up period (118). Mortality in this group was 9% after 4 years, in contrast to results in those who remained actively alcoholic; the latter group had a mortality of 57%. Even in the abstinent group, those who improved were a minority. Presumably, at certain stages of the disease, the pathogenetic mechanisms may continue unabated despite traditional pharmacologic management and abstinence from alcohol. Moreover, the encouraging results of abstinence may well have been exaggerated in this investigation by the fact that this group of individuals seemed to have less advanced cardiac disease on entrance into the study.

Management

Recognition of addiction to ethyl alcohol is often difficult and is crucial to effective control of the cardiac problems; the latter involves the same therapeutic modalities as other causes of heart disease. In view of the strong element of denial in such patients, the importance of interview with the next-of-kin is evident. Even the acknowledged alcoholics may subsequently deny recent abuse.

Management of alcoholic cardiomyopathy depends on the state of the disease when the addicted individual is first seen. Even in the absence of cardiac failure or enlargement, patients presenting with unexplained arrhythmias or absent septal Q waves should raise a high index of suspicion requiring verification of a negative history of alcoholism. The key to treatment at all stages involves complete abstinence. The alcoholic with cardiac abnormality may be approached effectively on an individual physician–patient relationship as well as in group therapy.

Pharmacologic management depends on the state of cardiac disease when the patient is first seen. The use of disulfiram for alcoholism and in cardiac patients may be associated with complications in view of the fact that dopamine β-hydroxylase, which is involved in the synthesis of norepinephrine in the heart, is inhibited by this agent (26). During the first episode of heart failure, if the patient has not been symptomatic for a long time and has only modest cardiomegaly without severe pulmonary edema, he/she may be managed initially by diuretics to correct the volume overload; bed rest is also advised. There is presumably a role for preload- and afterload-reducing agents as the disease progresses, but controlled studies on long-term efficacy have not been reported. Digitalis can be most useful in the control of atrial fibrillation or sinus tachycardia and contributes to the management of congestive heart failure in advanced stages of the disease. Although long-term bed rest has been suggested as perhaps aiding in management (104), the most important feature of institutionalization is the enforced abstinence from alcohol.

Vascular Complications

Arrhythmias

An association between alcohol use and cardiac arrhythmias, particularly atrial fibrillation, has long been suspected. However, the role of alcohol is difficult to establish, and the presence of heart disease is doubted if overt cardiomyopathy is not present. Both atrial and ventricular arrhythmias have been observed after the onset of heart failure in the alcoholic (107), but a prevalence different from that for other causes of heart failure is not known to exist. Cardiac arrhythmias have also been shown to occur during ethanol withdrawal (120), and during the preclinical state of alcoholic cardiomyopathy. Among 36 acutely intoxicated chronic alcoholics monitored for arrhythmias over a 12-hr period, only three had no arrhythmia. As expected, sinus tachycardia was common. Ventricular premature depolarizations were the most common significant arrhythmia, occurring in 39% (121).

Thirty-two separate symptomatic dysrhythmic episodes that required hospitalization were seen in 24 patients who drank heavily and habitually with superimposition of especially heavy ingestion before the arrhythmia (122). Overt alcoholic cardiomyopathy was not present and plasma electrolyte levels were usually normal. Because of a rather typical weekend or holiday presentation, this has been termed the "holiday heart" syndrome, defined as an acute cardiac rhythm disturbance with heavy ethanol consumption in a person without other clinical evidence of heart disease, and disappearing without evident residue on abstinence. Ettinger et al. (122) detailed numerous atrial and ventricular arrhythmias. Approximately 1 week after restoration of normal sinus rhythm, patients were assessed by high-speed ECGs. Moderate conduction delays were found and were considered the background for the induction of acute arrhythmias.

The incidence of arrhythmias in the population addicted to alcohol is not known. However, a recent Holter monitor evaluation of patients during intoxication and early withdrawal stages is of interest (123). Subjects were excluded in whom the admission ECG revealed arrhythmias or evidence of cardiac ischemia. Of the 60 patients monitored during the initial 12 or 24 hr,

12 patients were identified who had high composite arrhythmia scores, mainly due to the presence of ventricular premature contractions (Table 9). Biochemical assays of the serum revealed high plasma catecholamine concentrations. Propranolol was effective in controlling arrhythmias, suggesting a role for the sympathetic nervous system.

The mechanism by which these arrhythmias occur is not yet clear. In recent investigations from our laboratory, mild chronic conduction abnormalities, including H-V and QRS prolongation, were induced in otherwise healthy and well-nourished dogs that drank ethyl alcohol in quantity for longer than 1 year (124). In these animals, infiltration of the myocardial interstitium with alcian-blue-positive material and electron microscopic evidence of intercalated disc disruption were observed, either of which alteration could have been responsible for prolonged conduction.

Some cardiac alcoholics in whom magnesium deficiency develops may have serious arrhythmias, apparently related to the use of digitalis, that are responsive to magnesium administration (125,126). Magnesium metabolism in alcoholics is frequently associated with low serum levels or a deficit in total body magnesium, without a high incidence of arrhythmia. Sleep apnea and oxygen desaturation, which have been described in asymptomatic individuals at blood ethanol levels of about 80 mg/dl (127), are also relevant to arrhythmogenesis.

Cardiac conduction delays are believed to play an important role in arrhythmia production by facilitating reentry. Although the PR, QRS, and QT prolongations observed in the above series of patients were of minor degree, it is possible that more severe localized areas of delay are present. Indeed, histologic evaluation of the heart in human cardiomyopathy and after alcoholic ingestion by animals emphasizes a variable patchy distribution of lesions.

Because of the evident ventricular dysfunction in most, we believe this to be an indication of preclinical cardiomyopathy in the majority of these patients. A few had systolic time intervals that were normal. Although we have

TABLE 9. *Alcohol-associated arrhythmias*[a]

Rhythm abnormality	Number
Isolated APCs	4
Atrial fibrillation	12
Atrial flutter	6
Paroxysmal atrial tachycardia[b]	3
Junctional tachycardia	4 (3 in 1 patient)
Isolated PVCs	6
Ventricular tachycardia	1 (after treadmill exercise)

[a]Several patients had more than one arrhythmia. Of atrial arrhythmias, six showed RRBB and three showed LBBB aberration.
[b]One patient with junctional tachycardia showed atrioventricular dissociation.
From ref. 122, with permission.

not yet observed the transition to overt cardiomyopathy in any patient, perhaps because of the limited period of follow-up, this patient group includes at least three patients in whom a diagnosis of possible cardiomyopathy might be entertained because of borderline cardiomegaly.

Experimental Arrhythmogenesis

Using a chronic alcoholic canine mode to test the arrhythmogenic properties of ethanol, an 18-month study was undertaken to test the hypothesis that the electrical properties of myocardium may be altered sufficiently to elicit arrhythmias in response to stimuli that evoke no ectopic beats in normal animals (128). In the fasting state without ethanol in the bloodstream, the alcoholic animal responded during saline infusion as did controls without a change in threshold to electrical stimulation.

The chronic ethanolic animal responded to ethanol (1.5 g/kg), given over 2 hr, with an initial elevation followed by a reduced threshold to electrical stimulation; the threshold diminished progressively as blood ethanol rose to maximal levels. The result is in contrast to findings in a separate group of animals given ethanol for a period of just 1 month. Acute administration of ethanol to these animals was not associated with any change in the electrical threshold; thus recent short-term experience with ethanol is not a necessary condition for electrical instability of myocardium.

Animals having a chronic ethanol intake had normal levels of potassium, sodium, and magnesium in plasma, as well as glucose and free fatty acids. During ethanol infusion, the basal values did not change; thus there was no evident electrolyte or substrate alteration in extracellular fluids that contributed to this phenomenon. The underlying mechanism is not known, but the animals exhibiting a reduced threshold to electrical stimulation had progressive prolongation of QRS and QTc during ethanol, which in certain circumstances could lead to ventricular tachycardia and fibrillation. The suggestion of heterogeneity of conduction delays, as judged from precordial leads, implied that a reentry mechanism may give rise to tachycardia and fibrillation under these circumstances.

Examination of isolated tissue specimens from animals without previous experience with ethanol shows electrophysiologic effects at 200 mg/100 ml. These included reduced resting potential and amplitude of the action potential, as well as allowing of conduction velocity. Muscle cells are more sensitive to ethanol than Purkinje cells (129).

Two previous studies of the myocardial conduction system during acute infusions of ethanol showed conduction delays in nonalcoholic animals (130,131). However, the ethanol infusate was substantially higher in concentration and the blood levels were more rapidly elevated. In one instance, the infusion was into the coronary artery. Studies in animals without prior exposure to ethanol also found elevated thresholds of atrial and ventricular fibrillation during acute administration (132,133) in the presence of acute short-term arrhythmogenic stimuli.

Previous studies of chronic alcoholism in the canine model indicated that, after 8 months of ethanol ingestion, there was dilatation of the specialized portion of the intercalated disc in ventricular muscle (124), as well as changes in the interstitium of the left ventricle marked by accumulation of alcian-blue-positive material (60). These changes may be the basis for conduction abnormalities in the basal state that may be intensified by the myocardial loss of potassium during ethanol infusion (11).

Although not thoroughly authenticated, sudden, unexpected death can occur in alcoholics (134). Kramer et al. (135) indicated that fatty liver was the principal pathologic finding, but there was no detailed histopathologic investigation of the heart. In a series of 100 sudden deaths in which chronic alcoholism was apparently not present, 18 individuals had consumed large amounts of alcohol in the hours preceding death; these amounts were significantly higher than those in persons sustaining nonfatal myocardial infarction (136). More suggestive are results in a series of 50 autopsies, 30 of which involved individuals who died suddenly (137). Historical data indicated that all had been chronic alcoholics for years, and 17 of the 30 had alcoholemia. Compared to results in controls who were considered to have died from lethal alcohol intoxication (138), the sudden death group had greater degrees of myocardial hypertrophy and foci of fibrosis and necrosis, as well mononuclear cell infiltration.

While these clinical reports are in the main circumstantial and other factors require consideration to establish a cause and effect relationship, the multiplicity of reports on arrhythmias in the alcoholic suggest that primary ventricular fibrillation related to chronic alcohol use probably occurs in some individuals.

Hypertension

Although problem drinkers as a group may have higher pressures than controls on random measurement (139), these are usually within the range of normal. Intoxication itself may contribute to blood pressure rise and the withdrawal state is not infrequently associated with transient elevation of arterial pressure. Ethanol administration produces vasoconstriction of skeletal muscle vessels associated with dilatation of vessels to the skin (140). Predominance of the former may account for transient hypertension but there is no clear evidence that chronic hypertension is produced.

A recent report of a large sample of subjects screened in a medical care program indicated that those reporting consumption of three or more drinks per day had a higher prevalence of arterial pressures above 160/95 mm Hg (141). These were based on a single measurement without information on the interval from the last drinking episode. Several reports have noted that after a short period of abstinence in hospital, arterial pressures in noncardiac alcoholics does not appear to differ from a control group (122,142) and usually declines spontaneously in those that had been initially elevated (142). Despite the fact that it appears unlikely that ethyl alcohol is an important factor in chronic hypertension, the role of transient blood pressure elevations needs to be considered in the pathogenesis of the cardiac syndromes associated with alcoholism.

The mechanism of the unstable arterial pressure elevation is of some interest. Noting that certain clinical findings during alcohol withdrawal (i.e., change in blood pressure, pulse, temperature, and pupil diameter) could represent endogenous catecholamine effects, a study was undertaken of the effects of alcohol withdrawal on catecholamine secretion (143). These investigators studied a large group of alcoholics hospitalized after chronic alcohol abuse and suffering from delirium tremens, pure alcoholic hallucinosis, or other withdrawal syndromes.

Those patients with maximal clinical disturbance had the greatest elevations of urinary catecholamines and there was some correlation with the clinical manifestations of sympathetic overstimulation in terms of increase in blood pressure and pulse rate as well as urinary catecholamine excretion. The decrease in clinical symptoms was accompanied by a corresponding fall in the elevated urinary catecholamines toward normal. However, the onset of delirium did not coincide with elevations in catecholamine excretion. During convalescent states, the catecholamine excretion was normal. The authors state that several patients with high excretion values had "low muscular activity and weak tremor." The mechanism of the increase in catecholamine excretion is unknown and may be related more to anxiety (144) and the muscular work (145) associated with tremor and hyperactivity than to a specific alcohol effect. Thyroid hormone levels in blood appear to be normal in alcoholic subjects (146).

Alcohol also may have significant effects on catecholamine metabolism in the central nervous system (147) and these would not necessarily be reflected as changes in the peripheral hormone levels. In addition, alcohol can significantly alter the peripheral metabolism of norepinephrine, decrease in VMA (3-methoxy-4-hydroxymandelic acid) and increase in MHPG (3-methoxy-4-hydrophenylglycol) (148). This change in metabolism presumably reflects an increase in the reductive (MHPG) at the expense of the oxidative pathway (VMA), which could be related to an increased availability of reducing equivalents in the form of NADH, as alcohol is metabolized by alcohol dehydrogenase.

Other hormonal factors that may contribute to transient arterial pressure elevation includes stimulation of the renin–aldosterone axis, which has been reported to occur some hours after ethanol ingestion (113). Another vasoactive hormone, vasopressin, reached its highest plasma concentrations also in the postethanol period (114).

Coronary Blood Flow

Acute response of coronary vasculature to ethyl alcohol apparently varies, at least in part dependent on the rate, route, and dose administered, whether the subject is awake or anesthetized, and the time of flow measurement after ethanol administration. In the conscious dog, 1 g/kg, iv, ethanol resulted in a significant decrease in coronary vascular resistance without heart rate and aortic pressure alterations. This effect was aborted by anesthesia with pentobarbital (149). In humans, 200 mg/kg of ethanol was infused over a 20-min period and measurements were made 10 min later. Blood alcohol levels reached 65 mg% but there was no significant change in coronary blood flow (150). In humans in which ethanol was administered orally over a 2-hr period, sequential measurements of coronary blood flow were found not to change significantly except in proportion to the modest increase in heart rate, at blood levels of approximately 200 mg% (11). Thus the route of administration, as well as the rate, may be critical in determining the response of the coronary vasculature.

Of interest, in view of the tradition that alcohol has a coronary vasodilator effect, are recent observations on the influence of ethanol in nonalcoholic individuals with classical stable angina pectoris and proven coronary artery disease (151). Ten minutes after consuming an alcohol-containing beverage or a noncaloric control, the patients underwent exercise stress testing. Ingestion of either 2 or 5 oz of ethanol was associated with a decreased duration of exercise required to precipitate angina and a significant increase in ischemic ST segment depression.

Coronary Atherosclerosis

It has been a widely held view that chronic alcoholics have less severe atherosclerosis than the rest of the population and more recently it has been claimed that moderate drinking will also reduce the extent and severity of coronary atherosclerosis. An earlier study by Hirst et al. (152) indicated that individuals with cirrhosis and malnutrition had less coronary atherosclerosis than controls but alcoholics without severe liver disease showed no difference from controls. Moreover, a recent postmortem study found that although fatty streaks were less extensive in alcoholics, the extent of atherosclerosis plaques and lesions with coronary stenosis did not differ from that of controls (153).

A recent survey has concluded that moderate alcohol use is associated with a reduced risk of myocardial infarction (154). This conclusion gains support from an angiographic study in subjects presenting with chest pain or prior infarction (155). Significantly less atherosclerotic occlusive disease was found in subjects consuming larger amounts of ethanol, most evident in those over 60 years of age but there was no effect in those under 40. These findings fit with the hypothesis that ethanol enhances the levels of high density lipoproteins, which can facilitate the removal of cholesterol from the arterial wall (156). That ethanol affects the particular subspecies of high density lipoprotein having such action remains to be demonstrated. In addition, the angiographic study of Barboriak et al. (155) revealed no effect of alcohol on the incidence of myocardial infarction. Other prospective studies of cardiovascular disease among problem drinkers have found an apparent increased cardiovascular mortality in individuals consuming substantial amounts of alcohol (139,157,158).

In a preliminary examination by Leathers et al. (159) on the influence of ethyl alcohol in the macaque nemestrina, the nonhuman primates were fed a high cholesterol, high lipid diet for 18 months. In those fed 36% of calories as ethanol, the high density lipoprotein concentrations increased and low density lipoprotein diminished, associated with reduced coronary artery narrowing. In contrast, a report on the spontaneous atherosclerosis of the white carneau pigeon fed 8% ethanol found that cholesterol ester concentrations in the aorta were significantly higher in the ethanol-fed pigeons after 6 months. These results suggested that chronic ethanol feeding in low doses contributed to one of the key events in atherogenesis (160).

Atypical Myocardial Infarction

The occurrence of myocardial infarction traditionally has been attributed to occlusive disease of the coronary arteries and, in patients who succumb, the arterial pathology usually is represented as diffuse atherosclerosis of extramural vessels. However, variations from this general observation have recently been reported during coronary angiography after infarction. Individual cases or reports of small groups have been presented showing little evidence of luminal narrowing of the coronary arteries, usually in subjects without known risk factors. Precordial pain is often observed in myopathies of varied etiology; however, the association of alcoholism with the clinical syndrome of acute myocardial infarction has not previously been observed. Transmural myocardial scar has been found at postmortem examination in subjects with alcoholism and without significant coronary atherosclerosis. To elucidate this relationship, alcoholic subjects admitted to a coronary care unit (CCU) with unequivocal evidence of acute transmural myocardial infarction were investigated (44). Ten of 12 were without traditional coronary risk factors. Those with prior electrocardiograms frequently exhibited absent Q waves in leads 1, V_5, and V_6, which, however, became manifest as the infarction evolved. Examination of the coronary arteries at postmortem or by angiography showed no significant occlusive lesions.

Morphologic examination of the myocardium revealed concentric periarterial fibrosis, which was postulated to restrict coronary flow increments during periods of high blood flow requirements. This phenomenon is considered analogous to cardiac muscle necrosis associated with the periarterial lesions of constrictive pericarditis (161), perhaps conditioned by the abnormal metabolism of cardiac cells in chronic alcoholism.

Demonstration of the factors that precipitate regional necrosis, that is, greater pericoronary fibrosis or myocardial demand, is required to establish this hypothesis. Since extravascular coronary resistance may be acutely enhanced by elevated filling pressure, the increased ventricular end-diastolic pressure that may be present in the chronic alcoholic at rest, or after acute ethanol ingestion, which was the case in most of these patients, may represent a precipitating factor. In this background, enhanced diastolic tension and myocardial oxygen requirements may be associated with inadequate coronary flow increments.

A thromboembolic process was deemed unlikely in this study on the basis of several observations. The patients without previous infarction did not have prior heart failure, cardiomegaly, evidence of arrhythmias, or valvular disease, which appear to be prerequisites for embolization from the left heart chambers (162). Thrombocytosis and drugs affecting platelets were also not present. These patients were considered to have a preclinical form of toxic heart muscle disease prior to infarction, and mural thrombi have not been described at this state.

Crucial to the thromboembolic postulate is the demonstration in such patients that emboli emanating from the left side of the heart are distributed to the systemic circulation in an incidence approximating that of proven mural thrombi. As a clinical model for the distribution of emboli in the arterial circulation, patients with prosthetic valves and a relatively high incidence of embolization show a striking noncoronary preponderance (163). None of the total of 12 patients in this series, representing 20% of CCU admission for the given period, had evidence of embolization to any organ. Since angiography was not feasible during acute infarction, the presence of thromboembolism was assessed indirectly by serial determinations of circulating platelet levels, which are known to be altered during systemic thromboembolic phenomena. The absence of a change in platelet turnover as a reflection of arterial thromboembolism was unlikely in these patients.

Although the pathogenesis of this entity is not known with certainty, an interaction with other consumable substances must be considered. Most ethanol users smoke cigarettes, which have been associated with infarction without significant coronary artery disease. Since alteration of sex hormones may occur in alcoholics (164), it is pertinent to indicate that myocardial infarction has been described in relatively young men with a high estrone to testosterone ratio (165), a situation that may be obtained in these patients with atypical myocardial infarction.

Of interest here is the finding in a prospective epidemiologic study that intemperance might be a risk factor; heavy alcohol consumption appeared to enhance the risk of developing coronary heart disease, but the pathologic nature of the "coronary disease" was not described (158).

Sudden Death

It is important to be aware that a relatively high incidence of sudden unexpected death has been observed in a group of young adult alcoholics (135). These patients had fatty liver as the principal pathologic finding. In this respect, they were similar to alcoholics previously found to have physiologic evidence of cardiac malfunction (11). Additional information in this regard comes from a study of outpatient alcoholics in Oslo, in whom an increased incidence of sudden cardiac death was observed (134). Ventricular fibrillation may have occurred in these patients.

The association of arrhythmias with ethanol use usually has been accompanied by other variables that make the etiologic relationship uncertain. To determine the influence of uncomplicated, habitual use, male mongrel dogs consuming 36% of daily calories as ethanol for 3 years and a nonalcoholic control group were compared before and during a 2-hr intravenous infusion of 15% ethyl alcohol (128). Both were nutritionally normal. After anesthetic induction, a bipolar pacing catheter was positioned in the right ventricular apex via a jugular vein with chest intact. A single 2-msec constant-current pulse with intensity up to 50 mA was synchronized on T to test for repetitive ventricular responses at 15-min intervals during infusion and 1 hr thereafter. In the nonalcoholic group ($n = 7$) the basal heart rate of 128 ± 12 was unaltered. The threshold was reduced from 50 to 40 mA with blood ethanol levels of 110–160 mg/100 ml, but no tachycardia was observed. QRS by high-speed ECG remained the same and the basal heart rate of 115 ± 8 was unchanged. At 60 min, the repetitive ventricular response threshold was reduced to 22 ± 2.1 mA at blood ethanol levels of 110 ± 8 mg/100 ml. By 90 min, all animals responded to 15 ± 1.3 mA, with the ventricular response of 89 ± 3.5 msec further prolonged to 103 ± 7 msec ($p < 0.01$). Blood pH, Po_2, serum glucose, potassium, and magnesium remained unchanged. Isovolumic saline infusion for 2 hr produced no change of threshold or conduction. Thus acute ethanol use in chronic alcoholic animals further delays conduction and may be a basis for electrical instability when there is an underlying conduction aberration. These data support the view expressed in the clinical studies that, in circumstances not yet well defined, the alcoholic individual runs a risk of sudden death due to ventricular fibrillation.

PATHOGENESIS AND CHANGES IN ULTRASTRUCTURE

Metabolic Response

Ethanol is metabolized predominantly in the liver, first as acetaldehyde catalyzed by alcohol dehydrogenase and then followed by a second oxida-

tive step from acetaldehyde to acetate, catalyzed by aldehyde dehydrogenase (166). Since the activation of acetate to acetyl coenzyme A (CoA) is at
least partially inhibited during ethanol oxidation, much of the acetate formed
is released into the circulation (167), reaching levels between 1 and 2 mmol.
The heart can oxidize acetate rapidly (168), approximately 30% on first pass,
and appears to participate in the reduction of the oxidation of fatty acids in
humans (169). In studies of humans, administration of ethanol was associated with increased plasma concentrations of acetate and lactate. The arteriovenous difference of free fatty acid across the myocardium diminished
while the myocardial utilization of acetate and lactate increased nearly proportionate to their arterial concentrations. These two substrates accounted
for an average of two-thirds of the myocardial oxygen extraction. Acetate
itself when present in blood in high concentrations on the order of 12 mmol/
liter can depress myocardial function (170). The mechanism is not clear because similar cardiovascular responses were obtained employing calcium
acetate as compared to sodium acetate.

The mechanism for triglyceride accumulation in heart muscle during acute
exposure to ethanol is not clear since enzymatic activities in the myocardium
have not been shown to be altered (169). Very large doses of ethanol (171)
can increase plasma free fatty acid concentrations. However, the usual situation is for plasma free fatty acids to be reduced, presumably because of
enhanced reesterification in adipose tissue attendant to the increased plasma
concentrations of acetate and lactate. Increased extraction of triglyceride
has been proposed as one mechanism for cardiac lipid accumulation (9). In
the presence of inhibition or diminished fatty acid oxidation, the greater
availability of this substrate may be the major mechanism for the enhanced
triglyceride levels in myocardium. Enhanced lipoprotein lipase activity may
promote this alteration of lipid transport (172).

Fatty acid composition of heart triglyceride is substantially changed (171)
and shows a close resemblance to that of plasma free fatty acid, suggesting
that the source of increased fatty acid in the myocardium is plasma lipid. An
unexpected finding was the observation that the altered composition persisted over a 2-week period after the acute challenge with ethanol. A potential role for the carnitine system in triglyceride accumulation was also suggested by the observation that addition of carnitine to homogenates of rabbit
heart exposed to ethanol substantially restored fatty acid oxidation and esterification rates toward control levels.

The metabolic response to the first metabolite of ethanol, acetaldehyde,
appears to represent an important response. Schreiber et al. (173) had originally shown that the intact heart exhibited no change in cardiac protein
synthesis with ethanol levels at 200–300 mg/100 ml. However, acetaldehyde,
0.8 mM, markedly inhibited cardiac protein synthesis. To further localize
the action of acetaldehyde and to separate this response from that of contractile function, these authors subsequently studied cell-free systems using
isolated cardiac muscle microsomes. At an acetaldehyde concentration of
0.12 mmol, protein synthesis was reduced approximately 50%. Significant

inhibition of synthesis was still observed at acetaldehyde levels of 0.06 mmol. How this response related to the effects of ethanol on calcium transport in the cardiac sarcoplasmic reticulum remains to be delineated.

It has been shown that transport of calcium by the sarcoplasmic reticulum is stimulated by phosphorylation of the membrane protein by cAMP-dependent protein kinase (174). The inhibition of calcium transport in this system by ethanol is significantly potentiated in the presence of phosphorylation. Also, lower concentrations of ethanol, which are consistent with those present *in vivo,* have a demonstrable effect. It is uncertain that interference with calcium transport at this level plays a role in the negative inotropic effect of ethanol since one study has shown no interference by ethanol with the relaxation phase of contraction (175). Additional acute effects of ethanol of isolated components of the cardiac cell include inhibition of Na/K–ATPase activity in plasma membrane in a dose-dependent manner, an effect also produced by acetaldehyde (169). Such an action in itself would not appear to be involved in the negative inotropic action of acute ethanol administration since digitalis, which also inhibits the potassium-dependent portion of ATPase, enhances contractility. Finally, it has been reported by Puskin and Rubin (176) that both ethanol and acetaldehyde can directly influence the activity of the contractile proteins of muscle. An inhibitory effect was achieved by blocking stimulation of contractile activity of ADP rather than an action on myosin ATPase. It was not clear whether this toxic effect was related to a direct action on actomyosin or on the regulatory proteins, troponin and tropomyosin.

The role of acetaldehyde as the first metabolite of ethyl alcohol has been of some interest. Using relatively large concentrations, Walsh et al. (177) observed sympathomimetic response in the isolated left atrium of guinea pigs. The positive inotropic responses were inhibited by propranolol. Release of catecholamines is assumed to be predominantly from the adrenal medulla in a dose-dependent fashion (178). Acute hemodynamic studies of the myocardial effects of acetaldehyde in the experimental animal have indicated that at blood levels of acetaldehyde expected after a moderate dose of ethyl alcohol, acetaldehyde elicits only mild responses in comparison to an infusion of ethanol. This minimal depressant effect can be substantially masked by larger doses of acetaldehyde, which can induce tachycardia and arterial pressure elevations (179,180). Exaggerated production of acetaldehyde can be seen in some Orientals, associated with tachycardia without blood pressure elevation (181). The importance of the observation that chronic alcoholics have higher blood levels of acetaldehyde in response to a given dose of ethanol needs elaboration in terms of its possible importance in the production of chronic disease (182).

Finally, studies of intact animals have observed that acute doses of alcohol can produce hypocalcemia (183). This effect persists for 5 hr after administration of alcohol and is not associated with altered blood levels of phosphate. The moderate hypocalcemia could contribute to the negative inotropic action of ethyl alcohol. In both conscious and anesthetized dogs, doses of 2–4 g/kg induced hypocalcemia. In another study, Peng and Gittleman (184) noted that alcohol administration decreased the ionized fraction of blood calcium. The minimal effective dose of ethanol for this action may not be as low as that for induction of negative inotropic response directly attributable to alcohol.

Myocardial Abnormalities

Myocardial metabolism of alcohol may be important in the pathogenesis of alcoholic cardiomyopathy; however, no appreciable metabolism of alcohol occurs in the myocardium, which has little alcohol dehydrogenase activity (85) and does not appear to contain a microsomal ethanol oxidizing system. Instead, myocardial catalase activity is enhanced in rats fed ethanol chronically; inhibition of this enzyme results in the development of significant histologic abnormalities in the myocardium (86,185).

The long-term effects on the heart have been investigated by several researchers. Vasdev and co-workers (59) daily fed ethanol to rhesus monkeys as 40% of total calories and after 4 months observed myocytolysis and fibrosis in the myocardium. The loss of myofibers and degree of accumulation of fibrous tissue were not quantified, however, and there has not been an attempt to reproduce these findings.

Mongrel dogs (60,81) were fed 36% of their daily calories as ethanol for periods of up to 4 years. Collagen was deposited between the myofibers in perivascular areas of the myocardium at a relatively early stage. Left ventricular compliance showed an early decrease without a change of heart weight, but did not then progress despite continued alcohol intake. Thus the decrease in compliance was attributed to the deposition of collagen in the myocardium, analogous to observations in asymptomatic humans (45,57). Ultimately, left ventricular contractility *in vivo* was reduced only after 5 years of ethanol feeding (81). Cell accumulation of water and sodium was observed only in the long-term alcoholic group, without a reduction of cell potassium (81). In view of the dilatation of sarcoplasmic reticulum and subsarcolemmal regions observed by electron microscopy, it was postulated that edema of cardiac cells may limit the rate of calcium availability to contractile protein and thus affect contractile function in long-term alcoholism.

Sarma et al. (186) studied glycerinated heart muscle preparations from dogs fed ethanol for 2 years and noted that the force–velocity relation (V_{max}) was significantly reduced, although the maximal developed tension, maximal rates of tension rise, and times to peak tension were unchanged. More recently, the coupling of excitation–contraction in the rat fed 40% of calories as ethanol has been analyzed after a 30-week experimental period (187). Using the isolated papillary muscle, these animals demonstrated an inability to develop normal levels of force and a reduced force–velocity relation. A concomitant shortening of action potential duration led the authors to postulate that this electrophysiologic alteration may be the basis for the depressed contractile force.

Alterations of myocardial high-energy phosphate after chronic alcohol consumption have also been examined. The hamster model (188) was fed ethanol at a concentration of 50% for 6 months. The hamsters had a significantly higher inorganic phosphate and lower ATP levels while maintaining normal intracellular pH and phosphocreatine levels. Coronary blood flow and oxygen consumption were maintained at normal levels despite a significant reduction of developed pressure in the ventricle.

The maintained creatine–PO_4 levels contrast with the cardiomyopathy of the Syrian hamster and myocardial ischemia, in which a significant decline of phosphocreatine occurs before the decrease of ATP. Reduction of developed pressure with exposure to alcohol may have helped to preserve the phosphocreatine pool. The normal levels of intracellular pH, coronary blood flow, and oxygen consumption suggested that substrate and oxygen uptake were adequate and that metabolites were removed effectively.

Uncoupling of the phosphorylation potential may have been mediated by a fatty acid metabolite of ethanol. Ethyl oleate has been shown to bind to mitochondria and when hydrolyzed releases free fatty acids that cause uncoupling of oxidative phosphorylation (189). It is noteworthy that the alterations of energy phosphate parallel those that follow acute exposure in hamsters naive to alcohol (190). The significance, therefore, of these changes to the reduction of myocardial performance in the chronic model remains to be demonstrated.

In vitro experiments suggest important acute effects that may ultimately mediate pathophysiology. Thus ethanol initially interacts primarily with the aqueous regions of the membrane surface rather than the bilayer. Each mole of ethanol is bound tightly to each mole of protein comprising the Ca–ATPase pump (191), but the additional interactions with protein are not known. In the sarcoplasmic reticulum, impaired uptake and binding of calcium have been observed in chronic alcohol models at 1 day following the last exposure to ethanol (192). When assayed 2 days after ethanol withdrawal, however, the velocity of calcium uptake by the isolated sarcoplasmic reticulum and whole-heart homogenates did not differ from control in a rat model fed 23% ethanol for 17 weeks (186). These data suggest a time dependency related to the terminal period of ethanol ingestion.

An inhibitory effect of long-term ethanol use of myosin ATPase has also been observed. The relationship of myofibrillar Ca^{2+} ATPase activity to impaired contractility has been ambiguous, however. In a study of rats fed ethanol for 17 weeks, activity of this enzyme was significantly inhibited by 11 weeks, and this effect persisted until termination (193). Unexpectedly, myocardial contractility was not affected at any interval.

Accumulation of water and Na^+ in cardiac cells without a reduction in K^+ has been described in the rat (194) and a long-term canine model (186).

In view of the swollen sarcoplasmic reticulum observed by electron micros-copy, it was postulated that distortion of the tubular membranes may limit the rate of calcium availability to contractile protein and thus diminish con-tractile performance.

Inhibition of Na^+/K^+–ATPase has been observed in the myocardium as a result of the long-term feeding of ethanol; however, the observed gain of sodium and accumulation of water contrasts with the typical response to inhibition of this enzyme (81,195). Previous observations have indicated an altered fatty acid incorporation (81) as well as composition of phospholipid in animals fed ethanol for a long period. One of the membrane properties limiting permeability of the cell to sodium and water may thus be affected by the phospholipid (84) alteration without affecting the normal transcellular gradient of potassium.

Interaction of Cigarette and Alcohol Use on Myocardium

Since most human alcoholics indulge in cigarette smoking as well, nicotine and/or other components of cigarettes may play a role. In previous studies of an animal model exposed to chronic cigarette smoking, left ventricular performance was observed to decline, associated with morphologic evi-dence of collagen accumulation (101,196).

To assess the role of cigarette smoking in the development of heart muscle disease from chronic alcoholism (197), 18-month-old litter male beagles were prepared with a permanent tracheostomy. These were alternately placed into four groups: group 1, a control of 10 animals; group 2, nine animals smoking seven cigarettes per day, 5 days per week as reported earlier (101); group 3, seven animals fed ethanol as 20% of calories; and group 4, six animals re-ceiving ethanol and also smoking cigarettes as the animals in group 2.

Smoking in groups 3 and 4 was performed by the method of Cahan and Kirman (1968). The cigarettes were a standard brand manufactured by the University of Kentucky, Tobacco and Health Research Institute, were unfil-tered, and contained 1.35 mg nicotine per cigarette, excluding the nicotine in the 23-mm butt remaining from the 85-mm cigarette. The smoking was done in two sessions each day and preceded the introduction to ethanol by 1 week.

Both the control and experimental animals were fed approximately 28 cal/lb. The controls and the smokers received a diet sufficient to maintain body weight in the adult animal (National Research Council 989, No. 8, 1962) consisting of 26% of calories as protein, 12% fat, and 62% carbohydrate. The corresponding values in the alcoholic groups were 16.6% of calories as protein, 7.7% lipid, and 39.7% carbohydrate, which met the minimum stan-dard for maintaining a normal nutritional state. All animals received a vita-min supplement twice weekly.

Due to the difficulties of feeding by gastric tube for a prolonged period, the ethanol was administered in drinking water up to a final concentration of 25%. The actual intake per animal was estimated by measuring the residual ethanol solution of the previous day, correcting for evaporation from a separate container. After 4 weeks of progressively increasing doses, animals consuming 20% of calories as ethanol were admitted to the experimental group. The chronic ethanol animals were provided 20% of calories as ethyl alcohol 5 days per week.

The resting hemodynamic values in the anesthetized state at the onset of the study in the four groups are shown in Table 10. Compared with group 1, both the smokers and the animals receiving alcohol alone or in combination with cigarette smoking became hypertensive and had significantly higher systolic and diastolic pressures. The systolic pressure in group 3 animals consuming alcohol only was, however, not significantly different from the control animals of group 1. There were no significant differences in pressures between the three experimental groups. Heart rate, stroke volume, and left ventricular end-diastolic and pulmonary artery pressures did not differ significantly among the four groups. The left ventricular end-diastolic volume was increased in alcoholic smokers of group 4 only. The other three groups had similar end-diastolic volume values.

Left ventricular ejection fraction in the dogs receiving alcohol only (group 3) or in conjunction with cigarette smoking (group 4) was reduced to 27 and 23%, respectively, compared with 44 and 35%, respectively, in groups 1 and 2 (each $p < 0.03$). Both the smoking and the alcohol groups exhibited significant deficit in the contractile function of the left ventricular muscle. This index was 1.41, 1.19, and 1.28 muscle lengths/sec/cm, respectively, versus 2.41 in the normal dogs (each $p < 0.007$). The more readily measured index of contractility, the velocity of contractile element at peak isometric stress (VCE), which is not corrected for end-diastolic fiber length, also showed a similar reduction: 18.8, 17.5, and 19.9 muscle lengths/sec, respectively, versus 30.6 in the normal dogs (each $p < 0.003$). The contractile deficit in the alcoholics did not appear to be exacerbated by the addition of cigarette smoking. The indices of contractility did not significantly correlate with the enhanced arterial pressure in the smoking and the alcoholic groups.

Assessment of left ventricular function during afterload increments with angiotensin were undertaken with aortic diastolic pressure elevation of 16 ± 7 mm Hg in four groups (Fig. 11). Stroke work increased modestly but significantly in the controls at approximately the same filling pressure. No such increment occurred in either experimental group, despite a substantial increase of the end-diastolic pressure in the alcoholics and the smokers. To assess relative myocardial stiffness, saline was infused into the left ventricular chamber. The normal controls exhibited a modest rise of stroke work without increasing the filling pressure. Those dogs receiving alcohol with or without concomitant cigarette smoking showed a significant rise in filling pressure with minimal increase of stroke work (Fig. 10). Significantly, higher

TABLE 10. Left ventricular function in four groups of dogs at rest (mean ± standard deviation

	HR	AoS	AoD	EDP	EDV	SV	EF	dP/dt	V_{CE}	Cy Ix	TSR	SW
Group 1 (controls)	143±20	123±18	76±10	8.4±3.3	2.77±0.41	1.42±0.65	43.9±6.9	2341±815	30.6±9.6	2.41±0.72	3819±1413	2.26±1.24
Group 2 (smokers)	153±15	153±20	109±13	8.4±2.8	3.60±1.1	1.21±0.50	34.8±9.1	2035±417	18.8±4.0	1.41±0.35	4969±1519	2.42±1.12
P vs 1	NS	0.003	0.004	NS	NS	NS	NS	NS	0.002	0.003	NS	NS
Group 3 (alcoholics)	142±23	143±35	109±27	7.0±2.8	4.7±2.40	1.23±0.62	27.2±4.0	1951±862	17.5±4.5	1.19±0.38	4868±1665	2.40±1.47
P vs 1	NS	NS	0.006	NS	NS	NS	0.003	NS	0.003	0.002	NS	NS
P vs 2	NS	NS	NS	NS	NS	NS	0.03	NS	NS	NS	NS	NS
Group 4 (alcoholic smokers)	139±49	160±26	120±13	7.0±2.1	5.17±1.40	1.22±0.55	23.2±6.7	2370±162	19.9±2.8	1.28±0.17	6130±1861	2.58±1.32
P vs 1	NS	0.008	0.0001	NS	0.03	NS	0.0006	NS	0.004	0.001	0.05	NS
P vs 2	NS	NS	NS	NS	0.02	NS	0.006	NS	NS	NS	NS	NS
P vs 3	NS	NS	NS	NS	NS	NS	NS	NS	NS	NS	NS	NS

AoD, AoS = aortic diastolic and systolic pressures, respectively (mmHg); Cy Ix = Frank-Levinson index of contractility (muscle lengths/s per cm); dP/dt = first derivative of left ventricular pressure (mmHg/s); EDP = left ventricular end-diastolic pressure (mmHg); EDV = left ventricular end-diastolic volume (ml/kg); EF = ejection fraction (percent); HR = heart rate (beats/min); NS = not significant; p = probability; SV = left ventricular stroke volume (ml/kg); SW = left ventricular stroke work (g/kg); TSR = total systemic resistance (dynes × s cm^{-5}); V_{CE} = velocity of contractile element at peak dP/dt (muscle lengths/s); wt = body weight (kg).
From ref. 197, with permission.

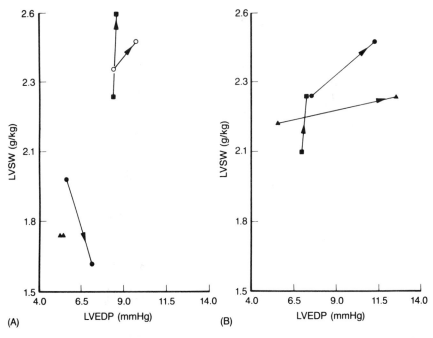

FIG. 11. The response of the left ventricle to pressure and volume increments with (**A**) angiotensin and (**B**) saline infusions. Stroke work increased modestly but significantly in normals at about the same filling pressure. No such increments occurred in either experimental group despite a substantial increase of end-diastolic pressure. *Closed squares* represent normals, *open circles* indicate smokers, *closed circles* indicate animals receiving alcohol alone, and *triangles* represent animals receiving both alcohol and cigarettes. From ref. 197, with permission.

end-diastolic pressure and tension were elicited after saline in the dogs receiving alcohol with or without concomitant cigarette smoking than in controls (Fig. 12). With the large variance, the differences in the two alcohol groups were not significant.

Although this study has revealed no intensification of the effects of chronic ethanol ingestion by simultaneous cigarette use over the 18-month experimental period, the development of cardiomyopathy generally requires a prolonged period of exposure, usually a minimum of 10 years in humans (11). In addition, the daily dose of ethanol as 20% of calories, which was the maximum the beagle consumed spontaneously, may have been an insufficient dose to elicit a toxic interaction with cigarette use. Thus we cannot exclude the potential for longer exposure periods or higher dosages to reveal interactions of these agents that were not observed in this experimental protocol.

While plasma lipids were not altered by any of the chronic interventions, myocardial triglyceride in the chronic ethanol groups was increased signifi-

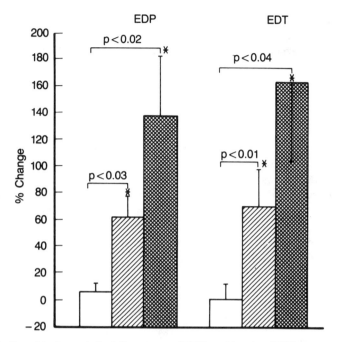

FIG. 12. Left ventricular end-diastolic pressure (EDP) and tension (EDT) response to saline infusion. No change occurred in these two parameters in the normal groups (□). Expressed as percent change from preinfusion values, a significant decrease in left ventricular compliance occurred in alcoholics (▨) and the alcoholic smokers (▓). From ref. 197, with permission.

cantly above that of smokers, but not significantly versus group 1. Presumably, the large variance in the latter is responsible since this lipid class has regularly been found to be increased in prior chronic studies (60,84). This lipid increment was apparently inhibited by simultaneous cigarette use.

It has been postulated from epidemiologic studies that the cardiac risks of long-term smoking are only evidenced when associated with other risk factors (198). Under the conditions of this study, the cardiomyopathic effects of ethanol were not intensified by the use of cigarettes, and, conversely, the effects of smoking were not significantly affected by chronic ethyl alcohol consumption.

Changes in Ultrastructure

The gross anatomic features of the adult in human alcoholic cardiomyopathy include an increase in cardiac weight, cardiac dilatation including all chambers but particularly the ventricles, a high incidence of mural thrombi, and patent coronary arteries (<50% obstruction) (199). Histologically, these hearts are characterized by hypertrophy with increased diameters of the muscle cells, variable degrees of interstitial fibrosis, and small foci of myocytolysis. An increase in lipid droplets and a decrease in the activity of a number of enzymes of oxidative metabolism have been detected by histochemical assay.

Ultrastructural studies have shown evidence of myofibrillar damage and lysis, dilatation of sarcoplasmic reticulum and T tubules, enlargement of nuclei, increased numbers of lipofuscin particles, and areas of partial separation of intercalated discs as well as focal edema of capillary endothelial cells. Although intramyocardial coronary arteries have been reported to exhibit edema, fibrosis, and subendothelial humps (200), significant occlusive disease does not appear to contribute to the myocardial pathology. None of the gross, histologic, histochemical, or electron microscopic changes are sufficiently specific to allow for a morphologic distinction to be made between alcoholic and nonalcoholic patients with congestive cardiomyopathy.

CONCLUSION

The widespread use of ethyl alcohol suggests its potential importance in clinical medicine. There is no proven therapeutic effect in cardiac patients, and its role as an etiologic factor in heart disease has been disputed over the years and attributed to coexistent malnutrition. The latter factor, however, has been disassociated from ethanol use in many patients with cardiomyopathic forms of heart failure.

Major support for the role of ethanol as a toxic agent when used in large amounts for a prolonged period has been obtained in various species of animals, including the subhuman primate.

Abnormalities include depression of ventricular function and metabolic and morphologic changes that parallel the changes in human with preclinical malfunction of the heart. Although the mechanism of progression to heart failure or arrhythmias is not known, several factors may be associated. These include, particularly in males, the cumulative effects of ethanol alone or after intensified drinking episodes, simultaneous exposure to trace metals in excess, and occasional specific nutritional deficiency or superimposed infection. The low prevalence of clinical nutritional deficiency in patients with alcoholic cardiomyopathy and the infrequency of heart disease in patients with cirrhosis or neuropathy support the view that the cardiac abnormality is not commonly dependent on malnutrition. Clinical data indicate that the cessation of alcohol intake may reverse the disease or interrupt its progression in many patients. However, the pathogenetic process may continue unabated in some patients who become abstinent.

TOXIC EFFECTS OF OTHER ALCOHOLS AND RELATED AGENTS

Methanol

Methanol (methyl alcohol or wood alcohol) is a common industrial solvent. It is also used as an antifreeze fluid, a solvent for shellac and some paints and varnishes, and a component of paint removers. Solid, canned fuels contain methanol. As an adulterant, it renders unpotable and tax-free the ethanol that is used for cleaning, paint removal, and other purposes.

The absorption and distribution of methanol and ethanol are similar. In addition, methanol is metabolized in humans by the same enzymes that metabolize ethanol–alcohol dehydrogenase and aldehyde dehydrogenase to formaldehyde and formic acid (201). Oxidation of methanol, like that of ethanol, proceeds at a rate that is independent of its concentration in the blood. However, this rate is only one-seventh that of ethanol and complete oxidation and excretion thus usually require several days.

Methanol has long been recognized as a human intoxicant due to its abuse as a substitute for ethyl alcohol in alcoholic beverages. Although humans are susceptible to methanol poisoning, lower species, such as rats or mice, are not. An asymptomatic latent period of 8–36 hr may precede the onset of symptoms of intoxication. If ethanol is imbibed simultaneously in sufficient amounts, signs and symptoms of methanol poisoning may be considerably delayed or on occasion even averted. In such cases ethanol intoxication is prominent, and ingestion of methanol may not be suspected.

Signs and symptoms of methanol poisoning include headache, vertigo, vomiting, severe upper abdominal pain, back pain, dyspnea, motor restlessness, cold clammy extremities, blurring of vision, and hyperemia of the optic disc. Blood pressure is usually unaffected. The pulse is slow in severely ill patients. No other cardiac effects have been described.

The most pronounced laboratory finding is severe metabolic acidosis—the result of oxidation of methanol to formic acid, which accumulates (202,203). Moderate ketonemia and acetonuria are also evident. Despite the severe acidosis, Kussmaul respiration is not common because of respiratory depression caused by the intoxication. Coma can develop with amazing rapidity in relatively asymptomatic subjects. In moribund patients the respiration is slow, shallow, gasping, and "fish-mouth."

Death, which usually is due to respiratory failure, may occur suddenly, if patients are not treated for metabolic acidosis, and blindness may result even if treatment for metabolic acidosis is performed. Thus a patient may be left partially or totally blind even though he/she may recover from the metabolic acidosis.

Isopropyl Alcohol

Isopropanol is widely used in industry as a solvent and disinfectant and in the home as a constituent of rubbing alcohol, skin and hair products, and antifreeze. For industrial or home applicants, isopropanol may be combined with or used as a substitute for ethanol, methanol, or ethylene glycol. Isopropanol is second to ethanol as the most commonly ingested alcohol (204) and, in one poison control center study, was the fifth most common cause of drug overdose (205). Toxicity results both from ingestion and from inhalation in poorly ventilated spaces, such as that which occurs in young children given isopropanol sponge baths.

Isopropanol is a potent CNS depressant and causes cardiovascular depression in large doses. The metabolite, acetone, may potentiate and lengthen the duration of CNS symptoms. Mild acidosis may develop by conversion of acetone to acetic acid and formic acid. The shift in the NAD/NADH ratio brought about by the action of alcohol dehydrogenase may cause decreased gluconeogenesis and hypoglycemia similar to ethanol.

Isopropanol intoxication has a rapid onset of action (30–60 min), with peak effects within several hours. The clinical picture is similar to that of ethanol intoxication, except that the early elation phase is usually absent, the duration of action is longer because of acetone formation, and the odor of acetone is more prominent.

Severe poisoning presents early with deep coma, respiratory depression, and hypotension. The hypotension results from peripheral vasodilatation. Serious arrhythmias have not been reported. Tachycardia has been the most common finding in a recent series (206).

Cases of acute tubular necrosis, hepatic dysfunction, hemolytic anemia, and myoglobinuria have been reported, but the direct role of acetone is unclear since hypotension and prolonged coma also occurred in each case and could have accounted for the findings (207). Mild hypothermia may occur as a result of CNS depression and peripheral vasodilation.

Ethylene Glycol

Ethylene glycol is a colorless, odorless, sweet-tasting compound that has wide commercial use as an antifreeze, coolant, preservative, and glycerine substitute. As recently as 1960, 40–60 deaths resulting from its use in suicide and as a poor man's alcohol substitute were reported. Ethylene glycol has intoxicating properties similar to those of ethanol, but its metabolites are responsible for CNS, cardiopulmonary, and renal dysfunction together with severe metabolic acidosis.

These central nervous system manifestations are related to the aldehyde metabolites of ethylene glycol, which reach their maximum concentrations

6–12 hr after ingestion (208). The amount of protein and number of leukocytes in the cerebrospinal fluid are frequently increased.

In the second stage, cardiopulmonary symptoms become prominent. These consist of mild hypertension, tachypnea, and tachycardia. Congestive heart failure, pulmonary edema, and bronchopneumonia may occur. The pathophysiology of the cardiopulmonary symptoms is not well known, but widespread capillary damage is assumed to be the primary lesion (209). The pleura, pericardium, and myocardium show petechial hemorrhages upon section. The cardiac histology also includes degenerative myocardial changes.

Effective treatment of ethylene glycol toxicity was first reported in 1959, when Schreiner et al. (210) documented the beneficial effects of early hemodialysis. In 1965, an important treatment compound was added when Wacker et al. (211) introduced the infusion of ethanol that served as a high-affinity competitive substrate for the alcohol dehydrogenase. In 1973, Underwood and Bennett (212) described an aggressive therapeutic approach to ethylene glycol poisoning that combined the use of ethanol with early hemodialysis, followed by vigorous diuretic therapy and urinary alkalinization.

ACKNOWLEDGMENTS

We extend our deep gratitude and sincere appreciation to Ms. Gale Dwyer and Ms. Glenda L. Byrd for typing the manuscript.

REFERENCES

1. Bruun X. Surveys of drinking and abstaining, urban, suburban and national studies. *Q J Studies Alcohol* 1972; suppl 6.
2. Eliaser M, Giansiracus F. Heart and alcohol. *Calif Med* 1964;84:234.
3. Brigden W, Robinson J. Alcoholic heart disease. *Br Med J* 1964;2:1283.
4. Evans W. The electrocardiogram of alcoholic cardiomyopathy. *Br Heart J* 1959;21:445.
5. Attas M, Hanley HG, Stultz D, Jones MR, McAllister RG. Fulminant beriberi heart disease with lactic acidosis: presentation of a case with evaluation of left ventricular functions and review of pathophysiologic mechanisms. *Circulation* 1978;58:566.
6. Alleman RJ, Stollerman GH. The course of beriberi heart disease in American prisoners-of-war in Japan. *Ann Intern Med* 1948;28:949.
7. Brink AJ, Lochner A, Lewis CM. Thiamine deficiency and beriberi heart disease. *S Afr Med J* 1966;40:581.
8. Gimeno AL, Gimeno MF, Webb JL. Effects of ethanol on cellular membrane potentials and contractility of isolated rat atrium. *Am J Physiol* 1962;203:194.
9. Regan TJ, Koroxenidis GT, Moschos CB, Oldewurtel HA, Lehan PH, Hellems HK. The acute metabolic and hemodynamic responses of the left ventricle to ethanol. *J Clin Invest* 1966;45:270.
10. Wendt VE, Ajluni R, Bruce TA, Prasad AS, Bing RJ. Acute effects of alcohol on the human myocardium. *Am J Cardiol* 1966;17:804.
11. Regan TJ, Levinson GE, Oldewurtel HA, Frank MJ, Weiss AB, Moschos CB. Ventricular function in noncardiacs with alcoholic fatty liver. The role of ethanol in the production of cardiomyopathy. *J Clin Invest* 1969;48:397.
12. Newman WH, Valicenti JE Jr. Ventricular function following acute alcohol administra-

tion: a strain-gauge analysis of depressed ventricular dynamics. *Am Heart J* 1971; 81:61.

13. Ahmed SS, Levinson GE, Regan TJ. Depression of myocardial contractility with low doses of ethanol in normal man. *Circulation* 1973;48:378.

14. Gould L, Reddy R, Goswami K, Venkataraman K, Gomprecht RF. Cardiac effect of two cocktails in normal man. *Chest* 1973;63:943.

15. Symbas PN, Tyras DH, Ware RF, Baldwin BJ. Alteration of cardiac function by hemodialysis during experimental alcohol intoxication. *Circulation [Suppl]* 1972;46 (2):227.

16. Riff DP, Jain AC, Doyle JT. Acute hemodynamic effects of ethanol on normal volunteers. *Am Heart J* 1969;78:592.

17. Juchems R, Kobe R. Hemodynamic effects of ethyl alcohol in man. *Am Heart J* 1969;78:133.

18. Mierzwiak DS, Wildenthal K, Mitchell JH. Aute effects of ethanol on the left ventricle in dogs. *Arch Int Pharmacodyn* 1972;199:43.

19. Blomquist G, Saltin B, Mitchell JH. Acute effects of ethanol ingestion on the response to submaximal and maximal exercise in man. *Circulation* 1970;42:463.

20. Regan TJ. Ethyl alcohol and the heart. *Circulation* 1971;44:957.

21. Conway N. Hemodynamic effects of ethyl alcohol in coronary heart disease. *Am Heart J* 1968;76:581.

22. Wong M. Depression of cardiac performance by ethanol unmasked during autonomic blockade. *Am Heart J* 1973;86:508.

23. Child JS, Kovick RB, Levisman JA, Pearce ML. Cardiac effects of acute ethanol ingestion unmasked by autonomic blockade. *Circulation* 1979;59:120.

24. Hirose T, Higashi R, Ikeda H, Tamura K, Suzuki T. Effect of ethanol on adrenaline and noradrenaline secretion of the adrenal gland in the dog. *Tohoku J Exp Med* 1973;109:85.

25. Nakano J, Holloway JE, Schackford JS. Effects of disulfiram on the cardiovascular responses to ethanol in dogs and guinea pigs. *Toxicol Appl Pharmacol* 1969;14:439.

26. Musacchio J, Kopin IJ, Snuder S. Effects of disulfiram on tissue norepinephrine content and subcellular distribution of dopamine, tyramine and their β-hydroxylated metabolites. *Life Sci* 1964;3:769.

27. Sauter AM, Boss D, von Wartburg JP. Reevaluation of the disulfiram–alcohol reaction in man. *J Stud Alcohol* 1977;38:1680.

28. Fisher VJ, Kavaler F. The action of ethanol upon the contractility of normal ventricular myocardium. In: Rothschild MA, Oratz M, Schreiber SS, eds. *Alcohol and abnormal protein biosynthesis: biochemical and chemical.* New York: Pergamon Press; 1975: 187–202.

29. Kavaler F, Hymans PS, Lefkowitz RB. Positive and negative inotropic effects of elevated extracellular potassium level on mammalian ventricular muscle. *J Gen Physiol* 1972;60:351.

30. Reeves JG, Newman WH. Cardiovascular responses to hemorrhage after alcohol in dogs. *Q J Stud Alcohol* 1972;33:464.

31. Beeler GW Jr, Reuter H. The relation between membrane potential, membrane currents and activation of contraction in ventricular myocardial fibers. *J Physiol* 1970; 207:211.

32. Seeman P, Chau M, Goldberg M, Sauks T, Sax L. The binding of Ca^{2+} to cell membrane increased by volatile anesthetics (alcohols, acetone, ether) which induce sensitization of nerve or muscle. *Biochim Biophys Acta* 1971;225:185–93.

33. Kalant H, Israel Y. Effects of ethanol on active transport of cations in biochemical factors in alcohol. In: Maickel RP, ed. *Biochemical factors in alcoholism.* Oxford: Pergamon Press; 1967:25–37.

34. Ferrans VJ, Hibbs RG, Weilbaecher DG, Black WC, Walsh JJ, Burch GE. Alcoholic cardiomyopathy: a histochemical study. *Am Heart J* 1965;69:748–765.

35. Gimeno MAF, Bedners AS, de Vastik FJ, Gimeno AL. Effect of ethanol on the mortality of isolated rat myometrium. *Arch Int Pharmacodyn Ther* 1971;191:213–19.

36. Cooper SA, Dretchen KL. Biphasic action of ethanol on contraction of skeletal muscle. *Eur J Pharmacol* 1975;31:232–236.

37. Kiessling HH, Pilstrom L, Bylund AC, Piehl K, Saltin B. Effects of chronic ethanol

abuse on structure and enzyme activities of skeletal muscle in man. *Scand J Clin Lab Invest* 1975;35:601–607.

38. Knochel JP, Bilbrey GL, Fuller TJ, Carter NW. The muscle cell in chronic alcoholism: the possible role of phosphate depletion in alcoholic myopathy. *Ann NY Acad Sci* 1975;252:274–286.

39. Asokan SK, Frank MJ, Witham AC. Cardiomyopathy without cardiomegaly in alcoholics. *Am Heart J* 1972;84:13.

40. Limas CJ, Guiha NH, Lekagul O, et al. Impaired left ventricular function in alcoholic cirrhosis with ascites. Ineffectiveness of ouabian. *Circulation* 1974;49:755.

41. Gould L, Shariff M, Lilieto M. Cardiac hemodynamics in alcoholic patients with chronic liver disease and presystolic gallop. *J Clin Invest* 1969;48:860.

42. Spodick DH, Pigott VM, Chirife R. Preclinical cardiac malfunction in chronic alcoholism. Comparison with matched normal controls and with alcoholic cardiomyopathy. *N Engl J Med* 1972;287:677.

43. Wu CF, Sudhakar M, Jaferi G, Ahmed SS, Regan TJ. Preclinical cardiomyopathy in chronic alcoholics: a sex difference. *Am Heart J* 1976;91:281–285.

44. Regan TJ, Wu CF, Weisse AB, Moschos CB, Ahmed SS, Lyons NM, Haider B. Acute myocardial infarction in toxic cardiomyopathy without coronary obstruction. *Circulation* 1975;51:453.

45. Hognestad J, Teisberg P. Heart pathology in chronic alcoholism. *Acta Pathol Microbiol Scand* 1973;81:315.

46. Askanas A, Udoshi M, Sadjadi SA. The heart in chronic alcoholism: a noninvasive study. *Am Heart J* 1980;99:9.

47. Matthews EC Jr, Gardin JM, Henry WL, et al. Echocardiographic abnormalities in chronic alcoholics with and without overt congestive heart failure. *Am J Cardiol* 1981;47:570.

48. Lunseth JH, Olmstead EG, Abboud F. A study of heart disease in one hundred eight hospitalized patients dying with portal cirrhosis. *AMA Arch Intern Med* 1958;102:405.

49. Siegel JH, Greenspan M, Cohn JD, Del Guercio LRM. The prognostic implications of altered physiology in operation for portal hypertension. *Surg Gynecol Obstet* 1968;126:249.

50. Epstein M, Schneider N, Befeler B. Relationship of systemic and intrarenal hemodynamics in cirrhosis. *J Lab Clin Med* 1977;89:1175.

51. Sherwin R, Joshi P, Hendler R, Felig P, Conn HO. Hyperglucagonemia in Laennec's cirrhosis. The role of portal–systemic shunting. *N Engl J Med* 1974;290:239.

52. Schomerus H, Buchta I, Arndt H. Pulmonary function studies and oxygen transfer in patients with liver cirrhosis and different degree of portal–systemic encephalopathy. *Respiration* 1975;32:1.

53. Guazzi M, Polese A, Magrini F, Fiorentini C, Oliva MT. Negative influence of ascites on the cardiac function of cirrhotic patients. *Am J Med* 1975;9:165.

54. Parving HH, Ranek L, Lessen NA. Increased transcapillary escape rate of albumin in patients with cirrhosis of the liver. *Scand J Clin Lab Invest* 1977;37:643.

55. Manghani KK, Ginsburgh J, Newman SP, Bernard AG, Lunzer MR, Sherlock S. Proceedings: interference with sympathetic function and catecholamine responsiveness in liver disease. *Gut* 1975;16:399.

56. Ahmed SS, Howard M, ten Hove W, Leevy CM, Regan TJ. Cardiac function in alcoholics with cirrhosis: absence of overt cardiomyopathy—myth or fact? *J Am Coll Cardiol* 1984;3:697–702.

57. Schneider FH. Effects of length of exposure to a concentration of acetaldehyde on the release of catecholamines. *Biochem Pharmacol* 1974;23:223.

58. Maines JE III, Aldinger EE. Myocardial depression accompanying chronic consumption of alcohol. *Am Heart J* 1967;73:55.

59. Vasdev SC, Chakravarti RN, Subramanyam D, Jain AC, Wahi PL. Myocardial lesions induced by prolonged alcohol feeding in rhesus monkeys. *Cardiovasc Res* 1975;8:134.

60. Regan TJ, Khan MI, Ettinger PO, Haider B, Lyons MM, Oldewurtel HA. Myocardial function and lipid metabolism in the chronic alcoholic animal. *J Clin Invest* 1974; 54:740.

61. Neville JN, Eagles JA, Sampson G, Olson RE. The nutritional status of alcoholics. *Am J Clin Nutr* 1968;21:1329.

62. Marciniak M, Gudbjarnason S, Bruce TA. The effect of chronic alcohol administration on enzyme profile and glyceride content of heart muscle, brain and liver. *Proc Soc Exp Biol Med* 1968;128:1021.
63. Roach MK, Greaven PJ. A micro-method for the determination of acetaldehyde and ethanol in blood. *Clin Chim Acta* 1968;21:275.
64. Leevy CM, Baker H, Ten-Hove O, Frank O, Cherrick GR. B-complex vitamins in liver disease of the alcoholic. *Am J Clin Nutr* 1965;16:339.
65. Chaunhan S, Nayak NC, Ramalingaswami X. The heart and skeletal muscle in experimental protein malnutrition in rhesus monkeys. *J Pathol Bacteriol* 1965;90:301.
66. Asokan SK, Frank MJ, Witham AC. Cardiomyopathy without cardiomegaly in alcoholics. *Am Heart J* 1972;84:13.
67. Brady AJ. Active state in cardiac muscle. *Physiol Rev* 1968;48:570.
68. Regan TJ, Khan MI, Jesrani MU, Oldewurtel HA, Ettinger PO. Alterations of myocardial function and metabolism in chronic diabetes mellitus. In: Dhalla NS, ed. *Myocardial metabolism*. Baltimore: University Park Press; 1973:169–178.
69. Buja LM, Khoi NB, Roberts WC. Clinically significant cardiac amyloidosis. *Am J Cardiol* 1970;26:394.
70. Zuguibe FT. The carbohydrates. In: Zugibe FT, ed. *Diagnostic histochemistry*. St Louis MO: Mosby Press; 1970.
71. Lochner A, Cowley R, Brink AJ. Effect of ethanol on metabolism and function of perfused rat heart. *Am Heart J* 1969;78:770.
72. Pachinger OM, Tillmanns H, Mao JC, Fauvel JM, Bing RJ. The effect of prolonged administration of ethanol on cardiac metabolism and performance in the dog. *J Clin Invest* 1973;52:2690.
73. Hall JL, Rolands DJ Jr. Cardiotoxicity of alcohol. An electron microscopic study in the rat. *Am J Pathol* 1970;60:153.
74. Gvozkjak A, Bada V, Kruty F, Niederland TR, Gvozkajak J. Chronic effect of ethanol on the metabolism of myocardium. *Biochem Pharmacol* 1973;22:1807.
75. Bulloch RT, Pearce MB, Murphy ML, Jenkins BJ, Davis JL. Myocardial lesions in idiopathic and alcoholic cardiomyopathy. Study by ventricular septal biopsy. *Am J Cardiol* 1972;29:15.
76. Ferrans VJ, Roberts WC, Shugoll GI, Massumi Ra, Ali N. Plasma membrane extensions in intercalated discs of human myocardium and their relationship to partial dissociations of the discs. *J Mol Cell Cardiol* 1973;5:161.
77. Hibbs Rg, Ferrans VJ, Black WC, Weilbaecher DG, Walsh JJ, Burch GE. Alcoholic cardiomyopathy: an electron microscopic study. *Am Heart J* 1965;69:766.
78. Alexander CS. Idiopathic heart disease. II. Electron microscopic examination of myocardial biopsy specimens in alcoholic heart disease. *Am J Med* 1966;41:229.
79. Auger C, Chenard J. Quebec beer-drinkers' cardiomyopathy: ultrastructural changes in one case. *Can Med Assoc J* 1967;97:916.
80. Sarma JSM, Shigeaki I, Fischer R, et al. Biochemical and contractile properties of heart muscle after prolonged alcohol administration. *J Mol Cell Cardiol* 1967;8:951.
81. Thomas G, Haider B, Oldewurtel HA, et al. Progression of myocardial abnormalities in chronic alcoholism. *Am J Cardiol* 1980;3:335.
82. Segel LD, Rendig SV, Choquet Y, et al. Effects of chronic graded ethanol consumption on the metabolism, ultrastructure, and mechanical function of the rat heart. *Cardiovasc Res* 1975;9:649.
83. Israel Y, Rosenmann E, Hein S, et al. Effects of alcohol on the nerve cells. In: Israel Y, Mardones J, eds. *Biological basis of alcoholism*. New York: Wiley; 1971:53.
84. Reitz RC, Helsabeck W, Mason DP. Effects on chronic alcohol ingestion in the fatty acid composition of the heart. *Lipids* 1973;8:80.
85. Alexander CB, Forsyth GW, Nagasawa HT, et al. Alcoholic cardiomyopathy in mice. Myocardial glycogen, lipids and certain enzymes. *J Mol Cell Cardiol* 1977;9:235.
86. Kino M. Chronic effects of ethanol under partial inhibition of catalase activity in the rat heart: light and electron microscopic observations. *J Mol Cell Cardiol* 1981;13:5.
87. Weishaar R, Sarm JSM, Maruyama Y, et al. Reversibility of mitochondrial and contractile changes in the myocardium after cessation of prolonged ethanol intake. *Am J Cardiol* 1977;40:556.

88. Kachru RB, Proskey AJ, Telischi M. Histocompatibility antigens and alcoholic cardiomyopathy. *Tissue Antigens* 1980;15:398.

89. Lefkowitch JH, Fenoglio JJ Jr. Liver disease in alcoholic cardiomyopathy: evidence against cirrhosis. *Hum Pathol* 1983;14:457.

90. Klatsky AL, Friedman GD, Armstrong MA. The relationships between alcoholic beverage use and other traits to blood pressure: a new Kaiser permanente study. *Circulation* 1986;73:628.

91. Dancy M, et al. Preclinical left ventricular abnormalities in alcoholics are independent of nutritional status, cirrhosis, and cigarette smoking. *Lancet* 1985;1:1122.

92. Morin Y, Daniel P. Quebec beer-drinkers' cardiomyopathy: etiological considerations. *Can Med Assoc J* 1967;97:926.

93. Sullivan J, Parker M, Carson SB. Tissue cobalt content in "beer drinkers" myocardiopathy. *J Lab Clin Med* 1968;71:893.

94. Wilberg GS, et al. Factors affecting the cardiotoxic potential of cobalt. *Clin Toxicol* 1969;2:257.

95. Asokan SK. Experimental lead cardiomyopathy: myocardial structural changes in rats given small amounts of lead. *J Lab Clin Med* 1974;84:20.

96. Asokan SK, Witham AC. Myocardial malfunction of unknown cause. *Cardiovasc Clin* 1972;4:113.

97. Harrison CE Jr, Cooper G, Zujko KJ, Coleman HN. Myocardial and mitochondrial function in potassium depletion cardiomyopathy. *J Mol Cell Cardiol* 1972;4:633.

98. Ledwoch W, et al. The influence of chronic potassium deficiency on energy product, calcium metabolism and phospholipid composition of isolated heart mitochondria. *J Mol Cell Cardiol* 1979;11:77.

99. Fuller TJ, et al. Reversible depression in myocardial performance in dogs with experimental phosphorus deficiency. *J Clin Invest* 1978;62:1194.

100. Kachru RB, Proskey AJ, Telischi M. Histocompatibility antigens and alcoholic cardiomyopathy. *Tissue Antigens* 1980;15:398.

101. Ahmed SS, Moschos CB, Lyons MM, et al. Cardiovascular effects of long-term cigarette smoking and nicotine administration. *Am J Cardiol* 1976;37:33.

102. Burch GE, Giles TD. Alcoholic cardiomyopathy: concept of the disease and its treatment. *Am J Med* 1971;50:131.

103. Koide T, et al. Cardiac abnormalities in chronic alcoholism. An evidence suggesting association of myocardial abnormality with chronic alcoholism in 107 Japanese patients admitted to a psychiatric ward. *Jpn Heart J* 1972;13:418.

104. McDonald CD, Burch GE, Walsh JJ. Alcoholic cardiomyopathy managed with prolonged bed rest. *Ann Intern Med* 1971;74:681.

105. Banner AS. Pulmonary function in chronic alcoholism. *Am Rev Respir Dis* 1973; 108:851.

106. Segal JP, Harvey WP, Stapleton JF. Clinical features and natural history of cardiomyopathy. In: Fowler NO, ed. *Myocardial disease*. New York: Grune & Stratton; 1973:37–57.

107. Bashour TT, Fahdul H, Cheng T. Electrocardiographic abnormalities in alcoholic cardiomyopathy. A study of 65 patients. *Chest* 1975;68:24.

108. Ahmed SS, Levinson GE, Fiore JJ, Regan TJ. Spectrum of heart muscle abnormalities related to alcoholism. *Clin Cardiol* 1980;3:335–341.

109. Kunkel B, Lappy H, Kober G, et al. Correlations between clinical and morphologic findings and natural history in congestive cardiomyopathy. In: Kaltenback M, Logen F, Oldsen EFJ, eds. *Cardiomyopathy and myocardial biopsy*. Berlin: Springer-Verlag; 1978:271.

110. Darsee JR, Nutter DO. Reversible severe congestive cardiomyopathy in three cases of hypophosphatemia. *Ann Intern Med* 1978;89:867.

111. Wagner PI. Beriberi heart disease. Physiologic data and difficulties in diagnosis. *Am Heart J* 1965;69:200.

112. Kawai C, Wakabayashi A, Matsumura T, et al. Reappearance of beriberi heart disease in Japan, a study of 23 cases. *Am J Med* 1980;69:383.

113. Linkola J, Fyhrquist F, Nieminen MM, et al. Renin–aldosterone axis in ethanol intoxication and hangover. *Eur J Clin Invest* 1976;6:191.

114. Linkola J, Yikahri R, Fyhrquist F, et al. Plasma vasopressin in ethanol intoxication and hangover. *Acta Physiol Scand* 1978;104:180.
115. Bory M, et al. *Les myocardiomyopathies ethyliques,* vol 6. Novelle: Presse Medicale; 1977:3295.
116. Koide T, et al. Variable prognosis in congestive cardiomyopathy: role of left ventricular function, alcoholism, and pulmonary thrombosis. *Jpn Heart J* 1980;21:451.
117. Shugoll GI, et al. Follow-up observations and prognosis in primary myocardial disease. *Arch Intern Med* 1972;129:67.
118. Demakis JG, et al. The natural course of cardiomyopathy. *Ann Intern Med* 1974;80:293.
119. Powell WJ Jr, Klatskin G. Duration of survival in patients with Laennec's cirrhosis. *Am J Med* 1968;44:406.
120. Talbott GD. Primary alcoholic heart disease. *Ann NY Med Sci* 1975;252:237.
121. Abbasakoor A, Beanlands DC. Electrocardiographic changes during ethanol withdrawal. *Ann NY Acad Sci* 1976;273:364.
122. Ettinger PO, Wu CF, de La Cruz C Jr, Ahmed SS, Regan TJ. Arrhythmias and the "holiday heart:" alcohol-associated cardiac rhythm disorders. *Am Heart J* 1978; 95:555.
123. Zilm DH, Jacob MS, McCleod SM, et al. Propranolol and chlordiazepoxide effects of cardiac arrhythmias during alcohol withdrawal. *Alcoholism Clin Exp Res* 1980;4: 400.
124. Ettinger PO, Lyons MM, Oldewurtel HA, Regan TJ. Cardiac conduction abnormalities produced by chronic alcoholism. *Am Heart J* 1976;91:66.
125. Iseri LT, Freed J, Bures AR. Magnesium deficiency and cardiac disorders. *Am J Med* 1975;58:837.
126. Jones JE, Shane SR, Jacobs WH, et al. Magnesium balance in chronic alcoholism. *Ann NY Acad Sci* 1969;162(suppl 2):934.
127. Taasan VC, Block AJ, Boysen PG, et al. Alcohol increases sleep apnea and oxygen desaturation in asymptomatic men. *Am J Med* 1981;71:240.
128. de la Cruz CL Jr, Haider B, Ettinger PO, et al. Effects of ethanol on ventricular electrical stability in the chronic alcoholic animal. *Alcoholism* 1977;1:158.
129. Hope RR, Vallone T, Scherlag BJ, et al. Effect of alcohol on cardiac electrophysiology. *Clin Res* 1978;26:5A.
130. Kostis JB, Horstmann E, Mavrogeorgis E, et al. Effect of alcohol on the ventricular fibrillation threshold in dogs. *Q J Stud Alcohol* 1973;34:1315.
131. Goodkind JM, Gerber N Jr, Mellen Jr, et al. Altered intracardiac conduction after acute administration of ethanol in the dog. *J Pharmacol Exp Ther* 1975;194:633.
132. Paradise RR, Stoelting V. Conversion of acetyl strophanthidin-induced ventricular tachycardia to sinus rhythm by ethyl alcohol. *Arch Int Pharmacodyn Ther* 1965; 157:321.
133. Madan BR, Gupta RS. Effect of ethanol in experimental auricular and ventricular arrhythmias. *Jpn J Pharmacol* 1967;117:683.
134. Sundby P. Alcoholism and mortality, in Universitiestforlaget. *Alcohol research in the northern countries,* publication 6. New Brunswick, NJ: National Institute for Alcohol, Stockholm University Center for Alcohol Study; 1967.
135. Kramer K, Kuller L, Fisher R. The increasing mortality attributed to cirrhosis and fatty liver in Baltimore (1957–1966). *Ann Intern Med* 1968;69:273.
136. Myers A, Dewar HA. Circumstances attending 100 sudden deaths from coronary artery disease with coroner's necropsies. *Br Heart J* 1975;37:1133.
137. Velisheva LS, Goldina BG, Boguslavsky VI. *Proceedings: USA–USSR first joint symposium on sudden death.* Washington, DC: DHEW; 1978: Publ No (NIH)78-1470.
138. Mendelson JH, Ogata M, Mello NK. Effects of alcohol ingestion and withdrawal on magnesium states of alcoholics: clinical and experimental findings. *Ann NY Acad Sci* 1969;162:918.
139. Dyer AR, Stamler J, Paul O, et al. Alcohol consumption, cardiovascular risk factors, and mortality in two Chicago epidemiologic studies. *Circulation* 1977;56:1067.
140. Fewings JD, Hanna MJD, Walsh JA, Whelan RH. The effects of ethyl alcohol on the blood vessels of the hand and forearm in man. *Br J Pharmacol* 1966;27:93.
141. Klatsky AL, Friedman GD, Siegelaub AB, Gerad MJ. Alcohol consumption and blood pressure. *N Engl J Med* 1977;296:1194.

142. Koide T, Ozeki K. The incidence of myocardial abnormalities in man related to the level of ethanol consumption. *Jpn Heart J* 1974;15:337.
143. Giacobini E, Izekowitz S, Wagmann A. Urinary norepinephrine and epinephrine excretion in delirium tremens. *Arch Gen Psychol* 1960;3:289.
144. Elmadjian F, Hope JM, Lamson ET. Excretion of epinephrine and norepinephrine in various emotional states. *J Clin Endocrinol Metab* 1957;17:608.
145. Garlind T, Goldbert L, Graf K, Perman ES, Strandell T, Storm G. Effect of ethanol on circulatory, metabolic and neurohormonal function during muscular work in man. *Acta Pharmacol Toxicol* 1960;17:106.
146. Wright J, Merry J, Fry D, Mark V. Pituitary function in chronic alcoholism. *Adv Exp Med Biol* 1976;59:253.
147. Majchrowicz E. Alcohol aldehydes and biogenic animes. *Ann NY Acad Sci* 1973;215:84.
148. Davis VE, Cashaw JL, Huff JA, Brown H, Nicholas L. Alteration of endogenous catecholamine metabolism by ethanol ingestion. *Proc Soc Exp Biol Med* 1967;125:1140.
149. Pitt B, Sugishita Y, Green HL, Friesinger GC. Coronary hemodynamic effects of ethyl alcohol in the conscious dog. *Am J Physiol* 1970;219:175.
150. Mendoza LC, Hellberg K, Rickart A, Tillich G, Bing RJ. The effect of intravenous ethyl alcohol on the coronary circulation and myocardial contractility of the human and canine heart. *J Clin Pharmacol* 1971;11:165.
151. Orlando J, Aronow WS, Cassidy J, Prakash R. Effect of ethanol on angina pectoris. *Ann Intern Med* 1976;84:652.
152. Hirst AE, Hadley GG, Gore I. The effect of chronic alcoholism and cirrhosis of the liver on atherosclerosis. *Am J Med Sci* 1965;249:143.
153. Rissanen V. Coronary and aortic atherosclerosis in chronic alcoholics. *Z Rechtsmed* 1974;75:183.
154. Klatsky AL, Friedman GD, Siegelaub AB. Alcohol consumption before myocardial infarction. *Ann Intern Med* 1974;81:294.
155. Barboriak JJ, Rimm AA, Anderson AJ, Schmidhowser M, Tristani FE. Coronary artery occlusion and alcohol intake. *Br Heart J* 1977;39:289.
156. Castelli WP, Gordon T, Hjortland MC, et al. Alcohol and blood lipids. *Lancet* 1977;2:153.
157. Pell S, D'Alonzo CA. A five year mortality study of alcoholics. *J Occup Med* 1973;15:120.
158. Wilhelmsen L, Wedel H, Tibblin G. Multivariate analysis of risk factors for coronary heart disease. *Circulation* 1973;43:950.
159. Leathers CW, Bond MG, Rudell LL. Effects of ethanol on dislipoproteinemia and coronary artery atherosclerosis in non-human primates. *Circulation* 1978;57,58(II):77.
160. Subbiah MTR. Ethanol and atherosclerosis: effect of chronic ethanol ingestion on plasma cholesterol, cholesterol excretion, and aortic cholesterol accumulation in spontaneously atherosclerosis-susceptible pigeons. *Artery* 1977;3:495.
161. Levine HD. Myocardial fibrosis in constructive pericarditis: electrocardiographic and pathologic observations. *Circulation* 1973;48:1268.
162. Wenger NJ, Bauer S. Coronary embolism. *Am J Med* 1958;25:549.
163. Cleland J, Molloy PJ. Thromboembolic complications of the cloth-covered Starr–Edwards prosthesis No. 2300 aortic and No. 6300 mitral. *Thorax* 1973;28:41.
164. Mendelson JH, Mello NK, Ellengboe J. Effects of acute alcohol intake on pituitary–gonadal hormones in normal human males. *J Pharmacol Exp Ther* 1977;202:676.
165. Phillips GB. Relationship between serum sex hormones and glucose, insulin, and lipid abnormalities in men with myocardial infarction. *Proc Natl Acad Sci USA* 1977;74:1729.
166. Majchrowicz E. Metabolic correlates of ethanol, acetaldehyde, acetate and methanol in humans and animals. *Adv Exp Med Biol* 1975;56:111.
167. Lindeneg O, Mellemgaard K, Fabricius J, Lundquist F. Myocardial utilization of acetate, lactate and free fatty acids after ingestion of ethanol. *Clin Sci* 1964;27:427.
168. Williamson JR. Effects of insulin and starvation on the metabolism of acetate and pyruvate by the perfused rat heart. *Biochem J* 1964;93:97.
169. Williams ES, Li TK. The effect of chronic alcohol administration of fatty acid metabolism and pyruvate of heart mitochondria. *J Mol Cell Cardiol* 1977;9:1003.

170. Kirkendol PL, Pearson JE, Bower JD, Holbert RD. Myocardial depressant effects on sodium acetate. *Cardiovasc Res* 1978;12:127.
171. Kikuchi T, Kako KJ. Metabolic effects of ethanol on the rabbit heart. *Circ Res* 1970;26:625.
172. Mallov S, Cerra F. Effect of ethanol intoxication and catecholamine on cardiac lipoprotein lipase activity in rats. *J Pharmacol Exp Ther* 1967;156:426.
173. Schreiber SS, Briden K, Oratz M, Rothschild MA. Ethanol, acetaldehyde and myocardial protein synthesis. *J Clin Invest* 1973;51:2820.
174. Retig JN, Kirchberger MA, Rubin E, Katz AM. Effects of ethanol on calcium transport by microsomes phosphorylate by cyclic AMP-dependent protein kinase. *Biochem Pharmacol* 1977;26:393.
175. Hirota Y, Bing OHL, Abelmann WH. Effects of ethanol on contraction and relaxation of isolated rat ventricular muscle. *J Mol Cell Cardiol* 1976;8:727.
176. Puskin S, Rubin E. Adenosine diphosphate effect on contractility of human muscle actomyosin: inhibition by ethanol and acetaldehyde. *Science* 1975;188:1319.
177. Walsh MJ, Hollander PB, Truitt EB Jr. Sympathomimetic effects of acetaldehyde on the electrical and contractile characteristics of isolated left atria of guinea pigs. *Pharmacol Exp Ther* 1969;167:173.
178. Schneider FH. Effects of length of exposure to and concentration of acetaldehyde on the release of catecholamines. *Biochem Pharmacol* 1974;23:223.
179. Jesrani MU, Gopinathan K, Khan MI, Oldewurtel HA, Regan TJ. Acetaldehyde and the myocardial depressant effects of ethanol. *Circulation* 1971;44(II):127.
180. Friedman HS, Matsuzaki S, Choe S, Fernando H, Celis A, Zaman Q, Lieber CS. Demonstration of dissimilar acute hemodynamic effects of ethanol and acetaldehyde. *Clin Res* 1976;24:623A.
181. Zeiner AR, Paredes A, Christensen HD. The role of acetaldehyde in mediating reactivity to an acute dose of ethanol among different racial groups. *Alcoholism Clin Exp Res* 1979;3:11.
182. Korstein MA, Matsuzaki S, Feinman L, Lieber CS. High blood acetaldehyde levels after ethanol administration: difference between alcoholic and nonalcoholic subjects. *N Engl J Med* 1975;292:386.
183. Peng T, Cooper CW, Munson PL. The hypocalcemic effect of ethyl alcohol in rats and dogs. *Endocrinology* 1972;91:586.
184. Peng T, Gittleman HJ. Ethanol-induced hypocalcemia, hypermagnesemia and inhibition of the serum calcium raising effects of parathyroid hormone in rats. *Endocrinology* 1974;94:608.
185. Fehimi HD, et al. Increased myocardial catalase in rats fed ethanol. *Am J Pathol* 1980;96:373.
186. Sarma JSM, et al. Biochemical and contractile properties of heart muscle after prolonged alcohol administration. *J Mol Cell Cardiol* 1976;8:951.
187. Tepper D, Capassa JM, Sonnenblick EH. Excitation–contraction coupling in rat myocardium alterations with long term ethanol consumption. *Cardiovasc Res* 1986;20:369.
188. Wu S, et al. The preventive effect of verapamil on ethanol-induced cardiac depression: phosphorus-31 nuclear magnetic resonance and high-pressure liquid chromatographic studies of hamsters. *Circulation* 1987;75:1058.
189. Lange LG, Sobel BE. Mitochondrial dysfunction induced by fatty acid ethyl ester, myocardial metabolites of ethanol. *Clin Invest* 1983;72:724.
190. Auggermann W, et al. Reversibility of acute alcohol cardiac depression: ^{31}P NMR in hamsters. *FASEB J* 1988;2:256.
191. Napolitano CA, Herbette LG. An attempt to correlate the membrane localization of ethanol with functional perturbations in the calcium-pump ATPase of sarcoplasmic reticulum. *Biophys J* 1988;2:256.
192. Segal LD, Rendig SV, Mason DT. Alcohol-induced cardiac hemodynamic and Ca^{2+} flux and dysfunctions are reversible. *J Mol Cell Cardiol* 1981;13:443.
193. Hastillo AH, Poland J, Hell ML. Mechanical and subcellular function of rat myocardium during chronic ethanol consumption. *Proc Soc Exp Biol Med* 1980;164:415.
194. Polimeni PI, Otten MD, Hoeschen LE. In vivo effects of ethanol on the rat myocardium: evidence for a reversible, nonspecific increase of sarcolemmel permeability. *J Mol Cell Cardiol* 1983;15:113.

195. Noren GR, et al. Alcohol-induced congestive cardiomyopathy: an animal model. *Cardiovasc Res* 1983;17:81.
196. Ahmed SS, Moschos CB, Oldewurtel HA, Regan TJ. Myocardial effects of long-term smoking. Relative roles of carbon monoxide and nicotine. *Am J Cardiol* 1980;46:593.
197. Ahmed SS, Torres R, Regan TJ. Interaction of chronic cigarette and ethanol use on myocardium. *Clin Cardiol* 1958;8:129–136.
198. Dick TSB, Stone MC. Prevalence of three cardinal risk factors in a random sample of men and in patients with ischemic heart disease. *Br Heart J* 1973;35:381.
199. Ferrans VJ, Buja LM, Roberts WC. Cardiac morphologic changes produced by ethanol. In: Rothschild MA, Oratz M, Schreiber SS, eds. *Alcohol and abnormal protein biosynthesis, biochemical and clinical*. New York: Pergamon Press; 1975:139.
200. Factor SM. Intramyocardial small vessel disease in chronic alcoholism. *Am Heart J* 1976;92:561.
201. Tephly TR, Makar AB, McMartin KE, Hayreh SS, Martin-Amat G. In: Majchrowicz E, Noble EP, eds. *Methanol: its metabolism and toxicity. Biochemistry and pharmacology of ethanol*, vol 1. New York: Plenum Press; 1979:145–164.
202. McMartin KE, Martin-Amat G, Makar AB, Tephly TR. Methanol poisoning. V. Role of formate metabolism in the monkey. *J Pharmacol Exp Ther* 1977;201:564–572.
203. Jacobson D, McMartin KE. Methanol and ethylene glycol poisonings: mechanism of toxicity, clinical course, diagnosis and treatment. *Med Toxicol* 1986;1:309–334.
204. Litovitz TL, Normann SA, Veltri JC. 1985 annual report of the American Association of Poison Control Centers National Data Collection System. *Am J Emerg Med* 1986;4:427–458.
205. Saracino M, Flower J, Lovejoy FH. The epidemiology of poisoning from drug products. *Am J Dis Child* 1980;134:763–765.
206. Kelner M, Bailey DN. Isopropanol ingestion: interpretation of blood concentrations and clinical findings. *J Toxicol Clin Toxicol* 1983;20:497–507.
207. Kulig K, Duffy JP, Linden CH, et al. Toxic effects of methanol, ethylene glycol and isopropyl alcohol. *Top Emerg Med* 1984;6(2):14–29.
208. Frommer JP, Ayus JC. Acute ethylene glycol intoxication. *Am J Nephrol* 1982;2:1–5.
209. Hagemann PO, Chiffelle TR. Ethylene glycol poisoning. A clinical and pathological study of three cases. *J Lab Clin Med* 1948;33:573–584.
210. Schreiner GE, Maher JF, Marc-Aurele J, Knowlan D, Alvo M. Ethylene glycol: two indications for hemodialysis. *Trans Am Soc Artif Intern Organs* 1959;5:81–89.
211. Wacker WE, Haynes H, Druyan R, Fisher W, Coleman J. Treatment of ethylene glycol poisoning with ethyl alcohol. *JAMA* 1965;194:1231–1233.
212. Underwood F, Bennett WM. Ethylene glycol intoxication: prevention of renal failure by aggressive management. *JAMA* 1973;226:1453–1454.
213. Regan TJ. Alcohol: it is a risk for cardiovascular disease. *Baylor Cardiology Series* 1982;5(4):7–11.

Cardiovascular Toxicology, Second Edition,
edited by Daniel Acosta, Jr.
Published by Raven Press, Ltd., New York, 1992.

14

Cardiovascular Toxicology of Halogenated Hydrocarbons and Other Solvents

Samir Zakhari

Division of Basic Research, National Institute on Alcohol Abuse and Alcoholism, Rockville, Maryland 20857

The use of chemicals has undoubtedly improved the quality of life in the 20th century. For example, the use of fertilizers, pesticides, and herbicides has increased the production of crops up to 80-fold, thereby alleviating the problem of hunger in many parts of the world. Chemicals have been used successfully to combat human diseases and epidemics and to produce new fibers for textiles. Even chemicals that simply add color or flavor to our environment have contributed to our appreciation of life.

Notwithstanding these contributions, exposure to sufficient concentrations of chemicals, voluntarily or involuntarily, on an acute or a chronic basis, can be toxic to various organs. Thus many workers have fallen ill due to occupational exposure—especially at the beginning of the industrial revolution—to chemicals, and several carcinogens have inadvertently been injected into our environment.

Solvents are an integral part of our daily lives. Their use ranges from making ballpoint pen ink to removing paint. They are found in products such as nail polishes, varnishes, adhesives, air fresheners, fire extinguishers, typewriter correction fluids, and plastic coating and are extensively used in industry. Exposure to solvents may occur in conjunction with housekeeping, home maintenance, hobbies, or on the job.

Another kind of exposure to solvents and propellants occurs during the intentional inhalation of the vapors in order to get "high" (1). The practice of inhaling solvents, commonly and erroneously called "sniffing," reached an epidemic proportion in the 1970s in teenagers. It has been reported that about 13% of teenagers (2) and 3–10% of school children (3) are volatile substance abusers; a proportion of these become chronic abusers (4–6). Chronic abusers are just as likely to be female as they are to be male (7).

The content of this chapter does not necessarily reflect the views of the National Institute on Alcohol Abuse and Alcoholism, nor does mention of trade names or commercial products imply endorsement by the Institute.

Chronic abuse of solvents also has been reported in industrial workers (8–10). The most commonly abused solvents are toluene, acetone, typewriter correction fluid (11–15), and alkyl nitrites (16,17). Table 1 lists the composition of abused solvents. Some solvents, halogenated hydrocarbons in particular, have proved to be fatal, when absorbed in sufficient concentration, by inducing myocardial arrhythmia. The failure of autopsy to demonstrate the cause of death suggested that fatality was due to ventricular fibrillation and cardiac arrest (18–20). Thirty-four cases of death related to the deliberate inhalation of various solvents were reported by Garriott and Petty (23). Similarly, cases of sudden death in adolescents who had "sniffed" a typewriter correction fluid were reported (24).

Because of their lipophilicity, organic solvents affect the central nervous system and can cause dermatitis by removing skin lipids or by sensitization. Through inhalation or absorption via the skin, solvents, in high concentrations, are capable of producing acute toxic encephalopathy characterized by headache, irritability, lightheadedness, incoordination, and coma (25).

Chronic exposure to solvents in sublethal doses may result in subtle toxicity that would be manifested only after a prolonged period of exposure. Workers who manufacture or otherwise handle such chemicals often are exposed to low concentrations of these solvents. Armeli and co-workers (26) reported a study in a Milanese factory in which workers were exposed to the solvent methyl isobutyl ketone for over 5 years. The most common symptoms in these workers included asthma, insomnia, headache, diarrhea, and vomiting. In the same year, Tiller and colleagues (27) reported on the association between occupational exposure to carbon disulfide and heart disease mortality. More recently, Wilcosky and Tyroler (28) reported on the prevalence of ischemic heart disease among workers in the rubber industry exposed to carbon disulfide, ethanol, and phenol. Increased awareness of safety precautions in industry, however, has led to the use of protective clothing and suitable ventilation, with a consequent decrease in the number of occupational toxicity cases. Cardiomyopathy due to the chronic ingestion of excessive amounts of ethanol is beyond the scope of this chapter and is discussed elsewhere (see chapter by Ahmed and Regan; 29).

For a comprehensive discussion on the toxicity of solvents in general, the reader is referred to reviews by Andrews and Snyder (30) and by Ayres and Taylor (31). Clinical toxicology of volatile substances of abuse is discussed by Flanagan and colleagues (22) and others (32–36). This chapter is concerned primarily with the cardiotoxic effects of commonly used solvents. Pertinent solvents and the principal target organ(s) for their effects are enumerated in Appendix 1. Toxic effects in humans (including epidemiologic studies, fatalities, and experimental inhalation), arrhythmogenic effects, effects on myocardial contractility, heart rate, cardiac output, blood pressure, and coronary arteries, as well as structural changes and teratogenic effects in the myocardium due to the exposure to solvents are addressed in this chapter.

TABLE 1. *Composition of abused products*

Product	Solvent/constituents
Acrylic paint	Toluene
Aerosols	Fluorocarbons, trichloroethane
Anesthetic	Diethyl ether, halothane
Antifreeze	Ethylene glycol
Cleaning fluid	Naphtha, trichloroethylene, trichloroethane, carbon tetrachloride, ethanol
Deodorants	Fluorocarbons
Dry cleaning agents	Methylene chloride, tetrachloroethylene, methyl chloroform, trichloroethylene
Dyes	Acetone, methylene chloride
Fire extinguishers	Bromochlorodifluoromethane
Gasoline	Hydrocarbons, alkyl lead, benzene
Glues/adhesives	Benzene, xylene, toluene, acetone, carbon tetrachloride, naphtha, *n*-hexane, trichloroethylene, trichloroethane
Lighter fluid	Naphtha, benzene
Local anesthetics	Ethyl chloride, fluorocarbon 11
Nail polish remover	Acetone, amyl acetate
Paint remover	Naphtha, benzene, methylene chloride, acetone, methanol
Paints/varnishes	Toluene, trichloroethylene, methylene chloride
Plastic cement	Methyl ethyl ketone, methyl isobutyl ketone, methyl cellosolve acetate, ethyl acetate
Polystyrene cements	Trichloroethylene, acetone, toluene, hexane
Rubber cement	Benzene, hexane, trichloroethylene
Rubbing fluid	Isopropanol
Room deodorizer	Isobutyl nitrite
Shoe polish	Toluene, chlorinated hydrocarbons
Spot remover	Trichloroethane, trichloroethylene, carbon tetrachloride
Surgical plaster remover	Trichloroethylene
Thinner	Xylene, toluene, ethanol
Tile cement solvent	Trichloroethylene
Typewriter correction fluid	Trichloroethane, trichloroethylene, perchloroethylene

Adapted from ref. 21 and ref. 22.

STUDIES IN HUMANS

The current information on the cardiovascular toxicity of solvents has partly been derived from observations of human subjects who have been exposed occupationally, accidentally, or intentionally in connection with "sniffing." The following section addresses epidemiologic studies, reported fatalities, and experimental studies in humans.

Epidemiologic Studies

Comprehensive critical reviews of the epidemiologic literature on cardiovascular diseases and chemical agents, including solvents (37), and solvents in particular (38) in the work environment, have recently been published. In addition, occupational health hazards due to exposure to solvents have been reviewed by others (39–48).

The first epidemiologic study that called attention to the association between the occupational exposure to a solvent and heart disease mortality was published in 1968. In that study, Tiller and colleagues (27) reported on mortality among Finnish viscose rayon workers exposed to carbon disulfide. The finding of an association between exposure to carbon disulfide and mortality from cardiac disease prompted the adoption of various measures to reduce the levels of carbon disulfide to which workers were exposed. Eight years after the intervention, the relative risk of coronary death was reduced from 5.6 to approximately 1 (49). The association between occupational exposure to carbon disulfide and ischemic heart disease was further confirmed in a very large study in the United States (50).

Methyl chloroform, also known as 1,1,1-trichloroethane, is widely used in the textile industry as a cleaning solvent. An epidemiologic study reported by Kramer and colleagues (51) showed that exposure to 100–350 ppm of methyl chloroform for a period ranging from 1 to 6 years did not cause statistically significant electrocardiographic changes, although the data suggest possible sinus rhythm abnormalities (short-duration arrhythmias and ST segment changes were observed). Of 151 workers in that study, over two-thirds were female and 90% were under 45 years of age.

Another halogenated solvent, methylene chloride, is widely used in manufacturing photographic films and in degreasing and paint stripping. Male workers at Eastman Kodak exposed to 30–125 ppm of methylene chloride for up to 17 years showed no greater incidence of cardiovascular disease than controls (52). However, the same article reported on a retrospective cohort study in the same factory that showed mortality increase in the exposed workers. The Standardized Mortality Ratio (SMR) was 391 for hypertension, a statistically significant number (with 4 deaths) and 115 for ischemic heart disease (IHD) (with 33 deaths). A follow-up study in the same factory (53) reported the results of an epidemiologic study in which 1013 workers were exposed to an average concentration of 26 ppm for 22 years. There were no statistically significant differences between the incidence of ischemic heart disease in these workers and the expected ratio in the general population. Using a different cohort definition, Hearne and colleagues (54) more recently showed that SMRs for cardiovascular disease were below 100.

Two epidemiologic studies in which workers were exposed to a mixture of solvents including methylene chloride were reported. In one study (42), workers in a fiber production plant were exposed to 140–475 ppm of methylene chloride in addition to methanol and acetone. The SMRs for cardiovascular diseases and IHD were 90 and 106, respectively. However, using stratified analysis, the authors suggested a statistically significant twofold increase in cardiovascular disease and a threefold elevation in IHD in exposed workers. In the other study, Wilcosky and Tyroler (28) reported no overall increase in IHD in workers exposed to methylene chloride, although

10 exposed workers in the age group of 40–49 years demonstrated a significant increase in IHD.

An epidemiologic study of 6929 workers occupationally exposed to trichloroethylene (TCE), a solvent extensively used at an aircraft maintenance facility during the 1950s and 1960s, failed to show any significant association between exposure to TCE and cardiovascular disease (55). Although the study focused on lymphoreticular neoplasms as the cause of death, the reported SMRs for IHD were 98 and 90 in exposed men and women, respectively. Although the main health problem associated with chronic exposure to carbon tetrachloride is known to be liver cirrhosis, Teta and Ott (56) reported that the SMR for arteriosclerotic heart disease in workers exposed to carbon tetrachloride for more than 10 years is 136. Except for carbon tetrachloride, epidemiologic studies on chlorinated hydrocarbons demonstrate that acute exposure to high concentrations of these solvents may be more detrimental to the cardiovascular system than chronic exposure to low concentrations (see subsequent section of this chapter on arrhythmogenic effects).

A group of chemicals known as fluorocarbons include fluorine-containing derivatives of methane, ethane, ethylene, and propane that are primarily used as propellants, refrigerants, solvents, and in fire extinguishers. Two major problems are posed by the extensive use of fluorocarbons. The first is their depleting effect on the ozone layer of the stratosphere (57), with a consequent increase in the incidence of skin cancer. The second is the growing number of reported fatalities associated with the use or abuse of such products. Although the use of fluorocarbons has been reduced significantly due to efforts to protect the ozone layer, epidemiologic studies demonstrating the arrhythmogenic properties of these compounds will briefly be discussed. In the same year when the report on the damaging effect of fluorocarbons on the ozone layer was published, Speizer and colleagues (58) reported a significant increase in palpitations in pathology residents (who extensively used fluorocarbons 12 and 22) as compared to unexposed individuals from the radiology department. Furthermore, the pathologists showed a 28% increase in new palpitations acquired after employment versus 14% in radiologists. Electrocardiographic changes induced by fluorocarbons included atrial premature beats, paroxysmal atrial fibrillation, and premature ventricular contractions. Similar findings were reported by Edling and colleagues (59), who studied electrocardiograms in 89 refrigeration repair workers who were exposed to fluorocarbon 22 and fluorocarbon 12. Arrhythmia and sudden bradycardia were reported. A strong association between heart disease mortality and exposure to phenol has been reported (28).

Reported Cases/Fatalities

Cases reported in the literature involve hospitalization or fatalities due to chronic abuse of, or acute accidental exposure to, solvents. A 15-year-old boy who sniffed glue (the principal solvent was toluene) intermittently for 2 years developed dilated cardiomyopathy and pansystolic murmur. Within 10 days he underwent cardiac transplantation. Histological examination of the excised heart showed myocarditis and eosinophilic infiltration (60). Similarly, Cunningham and colleagues (61) reported on a 16-year-old boy who developed anterior infarction and ventricular fibrillation following chronic abuse of toluene. Acute myocarditis that resulted in death from cardiac failure was attributed to chronic solvent abuse (62). Evidence of cardiac toxicity was observed in two patients after chronic exposure to methyl chloroform: a 14-year-old male developed ventricular extrasystole and left ventricular dilatation, and a 54-year-old man who had repeated industrial exposure to the solvent developed atrial fibrillation and congestive cardiomyopathy (63,64). Two fatal cases of workers exposed to the same solvent were described by Jones and Winter (65). An industrial accidental exposure to fluorocarbon 113 resulted in death (66). Five workers in a coal-hydrogenation plant died after chronic exposure to coal-liquid. Their deaths were attributed to cardiovascular disease (67). The pulse rate of a man who was exposed to 200 ppm of toluene for 3 hr was significantly decreased and his diastolic pressure was increased (68). Hantson and colleagues (69) reported on two cases of trichloroethylene toxicity.

Experimental Inhalation in Humans

Experiments performed by Stewart et al. (70) on human volunteers exposed to 0.1%, 0.5%, and 0.025% of trichlorofluoromethane (FC 11) or dichlorodifluoromethane (FC 12) demonstrated no arrhythmogenic effects of these compounds at the concentrations tested. Furthermore, at a concentration of 0.1%, FC 12 did not aggravate the premature ventricular contractions experienced by one subject prior to a 1-hr exposure period. Earlier, Azar (71) also failed to demonstrate electrocardiographic changes in subjects exposed to 0.1% and 1.0% of FC 12 for 2.5 hr.

In other studies, human volunteers exposed to 15% bromofluoromethane (halon 1301) showed electrocardiographic irregularities and revealed sensation of impending unconsciousness (72).

ARRHYTHMOGENIC EFFECTS

Solvents' effects on the cardiovascular system (CVS) are complex. On one hand, they affect various physiological functions of cardiomyocytes such as contractility and energy production, but on the other hand, because of their affinity to lipids, they also act on the central nervous system (CNS). Thus the sympathetic and parasympathetic control of the heart, the sympathoadrenal medullary system, and circulating hormones (e.g., catecholamines, vasopressin, serotonin) that are involved in the central and peripheral control of the heart and blood vessels could contribute to the overall cardiovascular effects of solvents.

Central Neural Mechanisms in the Cardiovascular Effects of Solvents

Chronic occupational exposure to methyl butyl ketone and *n*-hexane are known to cause peripheral neuropathy (73). Furthermore, patients intoxicated by solvents frequently report symptoms of palpitations and vascular instability, which suggest autonomic disturbance. Indeed, Matikainen and Juntunen (74) reported a significant decrease in the function of the parasympathetic division of the autonomic nervous system in workers exposed to carbon disulfide, toluene, or to a mixture of solvents (alipathic and aromatic hydrocarbons, alcohols, ketones, esters, and ethers) for several years.

In order to illustrate the complexity of the cardiovascular responses to solvents, a brief discussion of the central neural and autonomic nervous system mechanisms that contribute to the modulation of the overall cardiovascular response is warranted.

Sensory Receptors and Afferent Fibers Involved in Cardiovascular Reflexes. Three different types of receptors are involved in the control of the cardiovascular function. These receptors, illustrated in Fig. 1, are (a) baroreceptors, located mainly in the carotid sinus and aortic arch; (b) chemoreceptors, located in the carotid and arterial bodies, which are sensitive to changes in blood gases and pH, and in the heart and lungs, which are affected by bradykinin, prostaglandins, and metabolites associated with myocardial ischemia; and (c) mechanoreceptors, located in the myocardial chambers and the coronary vasculature. The afferent impulses from these mechanoreceptors are carried by both myelinated and unmyelinated sympathetic and parasympathetic fibers. The sympathetic afferent fibers have their cell bodies in the dorsal root ganglia and synapse in the dorsal horn of the spinal cord. Activation of receptors subserved by these fibers produces excitation of the efferent sympathetic outflow (75–77) and inhibition of efferent parasympathetic (vagal) activity (78). The sympathosympathetic excitatory reflex mediates cardiac pain due to myocardial ischemia (79–81). Ventricular receptors that discharge during systole and coronary artery receptors are subserved by myelinated parasympathetic fibers (X cranial nerve), which are projected in the nucleus tractus solitarius (NTS) in the medulla oblongata (82).

Central Pathways Contributing to Efferent Activation. The NTS is the first synapse in the supraspinal arc in the cardiovascular reflex pathways (83). Afferents to the CNS synapse to the NTS, which then connects to the nucleus ambiguus, either directly or via the dorsal motor nucleus of the vagus (84,85) and possibly through the raphe nuclei (86). The vasomotor center, located in the ventrolateral medulla, is important in the regulation of

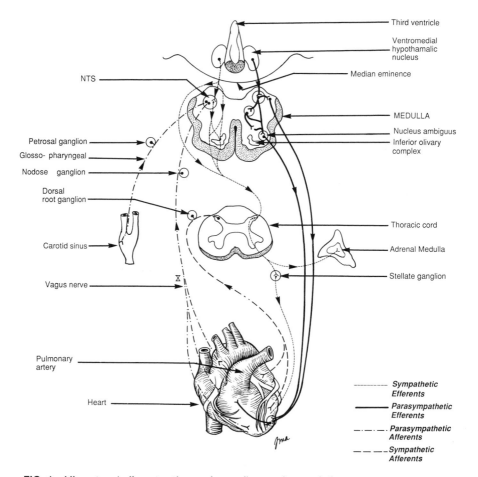

FIG. 1. Afferent and efferent pathways for cardiovascular regulations.

autonomic efferent signals. Input from the hypothalamus (paraventricular nucleus and dorsal, medial, lateral anterior, and posterior regions) and the forebrain are also important for the control of the cardiovascular responses (87–90).

The result of a solvent's actions on the CVS is therefore the algebraic sum of direct effects on the heart and the interference with central mechanisms that control cardiovascular responses.

Animal Studies

In 1911, Levy and Lewis (91) discovered that the sudden death of cats under chloroform anesthesia was due to the sensitization of the myocardium to epinephrine-induced arrhythmia. This discovery was followed by the observation that numerous halogenated solvents possess the same property. Table 2 summarizes the arrhythmogenic properties of various solvents in different species.

Arrhythmogenic effects of halogenated solvents were observed in anesthetized (92–96) and unanesthetized animals (19,71,97): healthy normal dogs (98,99) and those with experimentally induced myocardial infarction (97,100). In addition, sensitization of the myocardium to the arrhythmogenic effect of epinephrine was demonstrated by injecting exogenous epinephrine (19,101,102) or by increasing the levels of endogenous epinephrine by treadmill exercise (71) during exposure to halogenated solvents. Changes in the electrocardiogram included depression of the ST segment and disturbances in atrioventricular and intraventricular conduction (103), changes in repolarizability (104), bradycardia (105,106), ventricular fibrillation (124), and cardiac arrest (105,125).

In the 1970s, the arrhythmogenic properties of fluorinated compounds were studied extensively. Most of those studies were conducted to determine the potential of these compounds for inducing cardiac arrhythmias, in the presence or absence of elevated levels of epinephrine, rather than to investigate the mechanism of the arrhythmogenic effect. Taylor and Harris (116) observed the arrhythmogenic properties of aerosols containing trichlorofluoromethane (FC 11), dichlorodifluoromethane (FC 12), or dichlorotetrafluoroethane (FC 114). Several halogenated compounds were studied for their induction of myocardial arrhythmias or forsensitizing the heart to epinephrine. Spontaneous and epinephrine-induced arrhythmias have been demonstrated by Van Stee and Back (126) in dogs and monkeys exposed to bromotrifluoromethane. Wills (96) reported that spontaneous arrhythmias appeared in cats exposed to 1.7% of FC 11 and 8.8% FC 12, without epinephrine infusion.

The sensitization of the myocardium to the arrhythmogenic effect of epinephrine was demonstrated by injecting exogenous epinephrine (127) during the exposure to the halogenated hydrocarbon, or by factors such as noise or treadmill exercise that increase the levels of endogenous epinephrine in animals (71). Dogs exposed to 80% v/v of monochlorodifluoroethane (FC 142b) in oxygen showed an 8.3% incidence of marked arrhythmias. Simultaneous exposure to loud noise resulted in a 41.7% response (71).

Exposure of the myocardium to a halogenated hydrocarbon does not produce permanent sensitization to the arrhythmogenic effect of epinephrine. Clark and Tinston (98) found that injection of a challenging dose of epinephrine 10 min after the cessation of exposure to a known sensitizing concentration of fluorocarbon did not result in arrhythmias. The lack of permanent sensitizing effect of halogenated compounds was ascribed to their rapid elimination from the bloodstream on cessation of exposure (128). Indeed, Mullin and colleagues (129) found that 5 min after cessation of exposure of dogs to bromotrifluoromethane, the arterial blood level dropped from 32.4

TABLE 2. *Halogenated hydrocarbons studied for their arrhythmogenic properties*

Compound	Species	Concentration (%)	Reference
Carbon tetrachloride	Dog	Unknown	107
Chloroform	Cat	Anesthesia	108
Chloropentafluoroethane	Mouse[a]	20	109
(FC 115)	Dog	15.0–25.0	19, 71
1,2-Dibromotetrafluoroethane	Dog	1.8	96
(halon 2402)	Guinea pig	1.8	96
Dichlorodifluoromethane	Dog	5	19, 71
(FC 12)	Dog	10	99
	Dog	10	110
	Rabbit	10	111
	Monkey	5.0–10.0	112
	Rat	60	113
cis-Dichloroethylene	Dog	25.0–50.0	114
trans-Dichlorethylene	Dog	25.0–50.0	114
Dichlorofluoromethane	Mouse[a]	10.0–20.0	109
(FC 21)	Monkey	2.5–5.0	112
1,2-Dichloropropane	Dog	0.25	115
Dichlorotetrafluoroethane	Mouse[a]	20	109
(FC 114)	Dog	2.5	110
	Dog	2.5–5.0	19, 71
	Dog	5.0–10.0	99
	Monkey	9	116
	Monkey	5.0–10.0	112
Difluoroethane (FC 152a)	Dog	15	19, 71
	Dog	20	110
Ethyl bromide	Dog	Unknown	107
Ethyl chloride	Dog	Anesthesia	107
Fluorocarbon 502	Dog	10.0–20.0	19
Halothane	Dog	0.5–1.53	117
	Dog	2.0–4.0	118
	Cat	2.0–4.0	118
1,2-Hexafluoroethane	Dog	2.2	96
(FC 1166)	Guinea pig	8.7, 33.8	96
	Cat	44	96
Isopropyl chloride	Dog	Unknown	107
Methyl bromide	Dog	Unknown	107
Methyl chloride	Dog	Unknown	107
Methylene chloride	Dog	Unknown	107
	Dog	2.5	119
	Monkey	2.5–5.0	112
	Mouse[a]	40	109
Monochlorodifluoroethane	Dog	5.0–10.0	19, 71
(FC 142b)			
Monochlorodifluoromethane	Mouse[a]	40	109
(FC 22)	Dog	5	19, 71
	Dog	25.0–70.0	120
Octafluorocyclobutane	Mouse[a]	20	109
(FC C-318)	Dog	2.2	96
	Dog	10.0–50.0	19,71
	Dog	20	110
	Guinea pig	2.2	96
Propyl chloride	Dog	Unknown	107
1,1,1-Trichloroethane	Dog	0.5	19
	Monkey	2.5–5.0	112
Trichloroethane	Mouse[a]	40	109

TABLE 2. *Continued*

Compound	Species	Concentration (%)	Reference
Trichlorethylene	Dog	Anesthesia	121
Trichlorofluoromethane	Mouse[a]	10	109
(FC 11)	Dog	0.35–1.21	19
	Dog	1.25	98
	Dog	80	99
	Dog	1.0	110
	Dog	0.87	96
	Dog	0.5–1.0	71
	Guinea pig	0.87	96
	Monkey	2.5–5.0	112
	Rat	2.5–5.0	92
Trichloromonofluoroethylene	Dog	25.0–50.0	114
Trichlorotrifluoroethane (FC	Dog	0.5–1.0	19
113)	Mouse[a]	10	109
	Monkey	2.5–5.0	112
Trifluorobromomethane	Dog	2.2	96
(halon 1301)	Guinea pig	2.2–8.7	96
Trifluorochlorethylene	Dog	25.0–50.0	114
Vinyl chloride	Dog	15.0–90.0	122
	Mouse	20	109
	Dog	5.0	123
	Dog	5.0–10.0	19, 71

[a]Anesthetized.

to 3.0 µg/ml. In addition, it has been suggested that, because of their lipophilic properties, halogenated hydrocarbons are concentrated primarily in fatty tissues and adrenals (130).

Although it is generally agreed that a threshold concentration of halogenated hydrocarbons is necessary to provoke myocardial sensitization to epinephrine, the concentration–response relationship varies significantly. Thus while Wills (96) found that quadrupling the concentration of trifluorobromomethane and hexafluoroethane resulted in an increase of approximately 11% in the number of guinea pigs showing sensitization to the infusion of epinephrine, Azar (71) reported an increase from 8 to 41% in the cardiac sensitization to epinephrine as a result of doubling the concentration of FC 11 from 0.5 to 1.0%. In addition, increasing the concentration of cyclooctafluorobutane (FC C-318) from 25 to 50% resulted in a more than fivefold increase in the incidence of arrhythmias (71). This discrepancy is probably due to differences in species and in the levels of anesthesia.

The threshold concentration is independent of the duration of exposure. This phenomenon was clearly demonstrated by Azar (71), who found that the threshold concentration of FC 12 necessary to produce cardiac arrhythmias in unanesthetized dogs is 5.0% (v/v). Exposure to concentrations of 1.0 and 2.5% of FC 12 for 6 hr/day for 5 days failed to induce arrhythmias in 6 dogs. A concentration of 5.0% on the other hand, produced arrhythmias in 5 of 12 dogs exposed to FC 12 for 5 min. Increasing the concentration to

13.5% produced arrhythmias in 2 of 7 dogs during the 30-sec exposure period.

The arrhythmogenic effect of halogenated hydrocarbons varied from one species to another. For example, difluoroethane, which did not induce arrhythmias in mice and monkeys, produced changes in rat electrocardiograms (100). Furthermore, FC 12 induced arrhythmias in monkeys and rats but not in mice (100). Even when all species developed myocardial arrhythmias, the concentration of halogenated hydrocarbon required to trigger that response varied from one species to another. Aviado (92) reported that dogs and monkeys exhibited arrhythmias upon exposure to FC 11 at a lower concentration than that needed to induce the same response in rats and mice.

To test the effect of solvents on the severity of arrhythmia after coronary insufficiency, a situation that could be experienced by humans with heart problems, Hoffmann (131) occluded the left coronary ascending artery in closed-chest urethane-anesthetized rats. The following solvents were administered by gavage 1 hr before coronary ligation: carbon bisulfide (8.3 mmol/kg), chloroform (5.7 mmol/kg), trichloroethylene (16.7 mmol/kg), and ethanol (174 mmol/kg). Single oral administration of the above solvents reduced the survival rates of the animals to 29, 27, 36, and 24%, respectively. The survival rate in the control group was 59%.

The arrhythmogenic potential is not limited to halogenated hydrocarbons. The aromatic hydrocarbons benzene and toluene were tested in chloralose-anesthetized rats (132). When inhaled, both solvents brought about electrocardiographic changes: benzene decreased the duration of the P wave, whereas toluene increased the duration of the QRS complex and especially the PR interval, indicating a decrease in intraventricular and atrioventricular conduction. While benzene sensitized the heart to the arrhythmogenic effects of epinephrine, toluene did not. Furthermore, toluene reduced ventricular ectopic activity caused by coronary ligation or the administration of aconitine, whereas benzene exacerbated arrhythmia (133).

It should be noted that not all organic solvents induce myocardial arrhythmias. In fact, propylene glycol, a constituent of most pharmaceutical solvent vehicles, displayed pronounced antiarrhythmic properties when injected intravenously (0.2–0.3 ml/kg) into dogs and rats with spontaneous or drug-induced arrhythmias (134). This antiarrhythmic effect, which was attributed to an increase in the refractory period of the heart (135), represents only one facet of the effects of propylene glycol on the myocardium. Intravenous injection of 160–800 mg/kg of propylene glycol into anesthetized dogs caused a powerful reflex stimulation of the cardiomotor vagus and transient inhibition of efferent sympathetic outflow (136).

Arrhythmias Reported in Humans

Electrocardiographic changes have been reported in humans accidentally or voluntarily exposed to solvents. More than 40 years ago, Walter and

Weiss (137) reported that the electrocardiographic changes observed after acute intoxication with methyl chloride persisted for about 800 days. Ten years later, Gummert (138) described Wilson-block-type electrocardiographic changes, characterized by tall, slender R waves followed by a wider S wave, after methyl chloride poisoning. Ventricular arrhythmias were reported in humans who were chronically exposed to methyl chloroform (63,64). Cardiac arrhythmias have also been reported in humans after exposure to 1,2-dichloroethane (139), 1,1,1-trichloroethane (140), trichloroethylene (141), and FC 12 (142).

Mechanisms of the Arrhythmogenic Effects

Generally, rhythm changes in the heart are brought about by disturbances in the automaticity of the impulse-producing cells in the SA node, by disturbances in impulse conduction, or by abnormal mechanisms or factors replacing normal rhythm. These mechanisms, graphically depicted in Fig. 2, are identified as follows:

1. *Disturbances in impulse generation.* Changes in the generation of impulses in the pacemaker cells that are controlled by the autonomic nervous system could result from the following: (a) Interference with the spontaneous changes in the membrane potential of the SA node cells. Increased sympathetic activity results in the acceleration of the rate of sinus discharge, whereas vagal stimulation leads to reduction of impulse generation resulting in bradycardia or cardiac standstill. (b) Variations in the myocardial environmental conditions, such as pH (metabolic acidosis or alkalosis), pCO_2, and ionic gradients and fluxes (K^+, Na^+, Ca^{2+}). (c) Reflexes from upper and lower respiratory tract. Pulmonary stretch receptors mediate Hering–Breuer respiratory reflex, and pulmonary J receptors are subserved by unmyelinated vagal fibers, which cause hypotension and bradycardia. Also, Kratschmer reflex, induced by irritation of the nasal mucosa produce apnea, hypotension, and bradycardia. (d) Local hypoxia, ischemia, or hyperkalemia affect the firing of ectopic pacemaker cells.

2. *Disturbances in impulse conduction.* This effect is due to (a) augmented automaticity in Purkinje fibers; (b) delayed propagation of impulses in Purkinje fibers that results in a gradual decrease in conduction, ultimately leading to heart block and tachyarrhythmia by impulse reentry; and (c) increase in the refractory period of AV node

3. *Mechanisms replacing normal rhythm.* These are (a) impairment of K^+ efflux from cardiomyocytes, or delayed afterdepolarization of cardiac cells; (b) sensitization of the heart to epinephrine; (c) changes in the inotropy of the heart (a decrease in myocardial contractility sufficient to decrease cardiac output and blood pressure will trigger a sympathoadrenal discharge that affects cardiac rhythm); and (d) decrease in the coronary blood flow with concomitant myocardial ischemia that encourages the formation of ectopic foci.

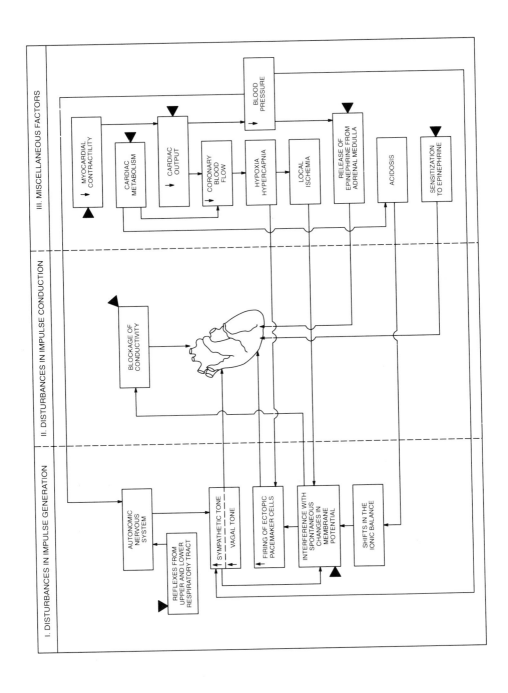

I. DISTURBANCES IN IMPULSE GENERATION | II. DISTURBANCES IN IMPULSE CONDUCTION | III. MISCELLANEOUS FACTORS

REFLEXES FROM UPPER AND LOWER RESPIRATORY TRACT

AUTONOMIC NERVOUS SYSTEM

SYMPATHETIC TONE

VAGAL TONE

FIRING OF ECTOPIC PACEMAKER CELLS

INTERFERENCE WITH SPONTANEOUS CHANGES IN MEMBRANE POTENTIAL

SHIFTS IN THE IONIC BALANCE

BLOCKAGE OF CONDUCTIVITY

MYOCARDIAL CONTRACTILITY

CARDIAC METABOLISM

CARDIAC OUTPUT

CORONARY BLOOD FLOW

HYPOXIA HYPERCAPNIA

LOCAL ISCHEMIA

BLOOD PRESSURE

RELEASE OF EPINEPHRINE FROM ADRENAL MEDULLA

ACIDOSIS

SENSITIZATION TO EPINEPHRINE

Known and hypothesized mechanisms by which solvents may precipitate cardiac arrhythmias are the following:

1. *Reflexes from upper and lower respiratory tract.* Exposure of the upper respiratory tract to different halogenated hydrocarbons produced apnea, bradycardia, and hypotension in the anesthetized dog (143). This phenomenon, also known as the Kratschmer reflex, is due to an increase in the vagal tone, which also triggers myocardial arrhythmias. Blaha and co-workers (144) and Kaufman and colleagues (145) successfully prevented bronchoconstriction due to exposure of the nasopharynx to irritant aerosols by sectioning the trigeminal nerve. The same response was demonstrated in the mouse (146) and in the dog (147). Some halogenated hydrocarbons also stimulate the pulmonary receptors of the lower respiratory tract. Dogs exposed to halogenated solvents exhibited tachycardia that was mediated by the sympathetic nerve (143). Previous work by Lamb and colleagues (148) and Sellick and Widdicombe (149) demonstrated that sensory vagal nerves can be stimulated by chemical irritation.

2. *Interference with spontaneous changes in membrane potential.* It is not clear whether solvents alter the permeability of cardiac membranes to ions with the consequent change in membrane potential that may result in myocardial arrhythmias. Wills (96) showed that halogenated solvents do not facilitate the arrhythmogenic activity of epinephrine by facilitating the efflux of intracellular potassium.

3. *Blockage of conductivity.* The ability of chlorinated compounds to interfere with conductivity has been demonstrated in anesthetized (109) and unanesthetized mice (94). Atrioventricular block and ventricular ectopic beats were observed in animals exposed to methylene chloride and trichloroethane (109). Reinhardt and co-workers (19) suggested that the mechanism of the arrhythmogenic effect resides in the ability of these halogenated solvents to interfere with the conductivity in the myocardium, perhaps through local disturbances in the electrical potential across cell membranes. Second and third degree heart blocks were identified in mice exposed to methyl chloroform (150).

4. *Decrease in myocardial contractility.* A decrease in the inotropy of the heart could result in a decrease in the cardiac output and systemic blood pressure. This, in turn, will trigger a sympathoadrenal discharge that releases epinephrine from the adrenal medulla. In addition, several solvents have been found to sensitize the heart to the arrhythmogenic effect of epinephrine. The extent of the decrease in blood pressure is affected by the tone in various vascular beds. Van Stee and colleagues (151) found that the blood level of halogenated hydrocarbons and the myocardial afterload are detrimental to the arrhythmogenic threshold.

FIG. 2. Schematic representation of mechanisms by which solvents may precipitate cardiac arrhythmias. *Solid triangles* denote possible sites of action.

5. *Hypoxia and myocardial ischemia.* Oxygen deprivation and myocardial ischemia secondary to a decrease in coronary blood flow may play a role in the precipitation of myocardial arrhythmias. Experiments conducted by Kawakami and colleagues (152) showed that hypoxia induced significantly higher atrioventricular conduction disturbances than did fluorocarbon 113 alone. Hypoxia also enhanced the arrhythmogenic properties of trichloroethylene and tetrachloroethylene (153). Since hypoxia or myocardial ischemia may increase the sensitivity of Purkinje fibers to epinephrine, Wills (96) tested the interaction between oxygen and epinephrine. Animals were exposed to 0.87% of trichlorofluoromethane in air enriched by either oxygen or nitrogen. Sensitization to injected epinephrine was found to be enhanced by inhalation of low oxygen and decreased, though not abolished, by high oxygen concentrations. Contrary to expectation, experiments performed on dogs (97) and rats (100) with experimentally induced myocardial infarction showed that there is no difference between these experimental animals and controls in the threshold-inspired levels of halogenated hydrocarbons needed to sensitize the heart to epinephrine. On the other hand, cardiomyopathic hamsters used by Drew and Taylor (154) showed both qualitative and quantitative differences from controls in arrhythmogenic patterns. Myopathic hamsters were more sensitive, that is, developed arrhythmias at lower concentrations than controls; in addition, whereas the myopathic hamsters developed atrial arrhythmias and bradycardia, the controls exhibited ventricular tachycaria.

6. *Metabolic acidosis.* Ingestion of toxic doses of methyl alcohol or ethylene glycol leads to severe metabolic acidosis (30,155). The increase in hydrogen ions in the extracellular fluid results in the movement of hydrogen ions into cells in exchange for K^+, thus leading to hyperpotassemia. Increase in the extracellular K^+ results in idioventricular rhythm and atrial standstill especially in the anoxic heart.

7. *Interference with autonomic control of pacemaker.* Catecholamines are released from the adrenal medulla due to exposure to halogenated solvents (100). These investigators found that adrenalectomy, or prior injection of beta-adrenergic blocking drugs, decreased the incidence of cardiac arrhythmias in rats. Wills (96) examined the role of alpha- and beta-receptors in the precipitation of arrhythmias by halogenated compounds and, after treating animals with a compound that possesses both alpha- and beta-blocking properties, showed that epinephrine failed to induce arrhythmias. On the other hand, prior blockage of cholinergic receptors with atropine did not prevent the arrhythmias (109).

EFFECT ON MYOCARDIAL CONTRACTILITY

In addition to their depressant effects on the central nervous system, a prominent feature of a great number of organic solvents is their ability to attenuate myocardial contractility. This negative inotropic effect has been documented in different species, both *in vivo* and *in vitro*, for the following halogenated hydrocarbons: 1,1,1-trichloroethane (156), methylene chloride (157,158), trichloroethylene (110), tetrachloroethylene (159), dichlorodifluoromethane (160,161), bromochlorodifluoromethane (162), ethylene chloride (163), propylene dichloride (115), acetylene dichloride (164), and bromotrifluoromethane (165); as well as for ethanol (166–170), methanol (171), pentanol (172), isopropanol (173), ethyl acetate (174), methyl ethyl ketone (175), methyl isobutyl ketone (176), and *n*-hexane and 2,5-hexanedione (177). Chronic exposure to trichloroethylene was reported to cause congestive cardiomyopathy in humans (178).

Methylene chloride, an extensively used solvent, has a unique toxicologic feature; it is metabolized to carbon monoxide (179–182). Although methylene chloride is moderately toxic to the heart, patients with myocardial impairment may be especially at risk (183,184). However, *in vitro* experiments conducted by Juhasz-Nagy and Aviado (185) showed no evidence that the formation of carboxyhemoglobin increases the cardiotoxicity of methylene chloride, either in normal or ischemic hearts.

Propylene glycol, a commonly used solvent for pharmaceutical preparations, was tested in conscious calves (186). Intravenous injection of propylene glycol resulted in a transient period (1–4 min) of myocardial depression characterized by asystole, systemic hypotension, and decreased pulmonary arterial blood flow.

Mechanism of Myocardial Depression

The myocardium is influenced not only by its own intrinsic multiple control mechanisms, such as changes in muscle length, but also by autonomic nervous system innervation coupled with various reflexes originating from lungs, adrenals, and various vascular beds. Solvents could affect the force of myocardial contractility by exerting a direct negative inotropic effect on the heart, or by acting on the central nervous system. Effects on the myocardium would depend on the relative contribution of forces that differ in magnitude and direction. To appreciate fully the myocardial depressant effects of solvents, it is essential to understand the metabolic processes that provide the heart with energy. For that purpose, a short review of myocardial metabolism follows.

Olsen (187) divided the processes of energy production and utilization in the myocardium into three phases: (a) energy liberation, (b) conservation of produced energy in the form of the energy-rich compound adenosine triphosphate (ATP), and (c) utilization of energy for mechanical work. These phases are graphically depicted in Fig. 3.

The main substrates for energy production in the heart are glucose and lactate. Esterified and free fatty acids, pyruvate, and lactate, when present

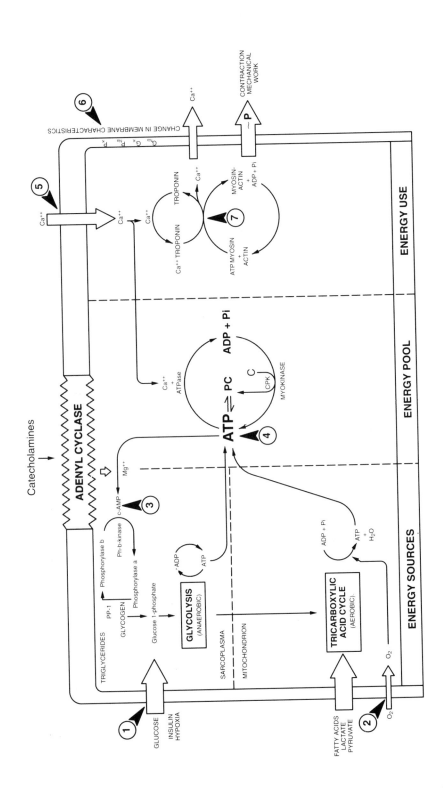

in the arterial blood in sufficiently high concentrations, can be extracted by cardiomyocytes and used as energy sources. Furthermore, the presence of lipase in the myocardium suggests that triglycerides may also be used as a fuel for myocardial metabolism.

1. *Energy liberation.* The myocardium produces energy by (a) glycolysis and (b) the Krebs tricarboxylic acid cycle. Under normal conditions, aerobic metabolism in the Krebs cycle is the main source of energy. However, under stress conditions, the metabolism in the subendocardium may be partly anaerobic. These metabolic pathways are illustrated in Fig. 4. For further details of these processes, the reader is referred to the comprehensive review by Merin (188). The Krebs cycle takes place within the mitochondria and therefore in close proximity of the components of the electron transfer system.

2. *Energy conservation.* This phase involves energy storage in the heart in the form of the energy-rich compounds ATP and phosphocreatine (PC). The rate of aerobic and anaerobic glycolysis is controlled by ATP levels. The rate-limiting step in glycolysis is the conversion of fructose-6-phosphate to fructose 1,6-diphosphate. Another factor that affects energy formation is myocardial hypoxia, which enhances glucose uptake, glycogen breakdown, and glycolysis. The accumulation of adenosine monophosphate and inorganic phosphate in the hypoxic myocardium leads to the activation of phosphorylase and phosphofructokinase enzymes.

3. *Energy utilization.* Cardiac contraction is initiated by the depolarization of the sarcolemma; the generated electrical impulses are responsible for the propagation of the self-perpetuating action potential. This electrical impulse allows calcium ions, sequestered in the cisternae of the longitudinal system, to move out into the myofibrils. The released calcium then activates the myofilaments by binding ATP into reactive sites between the myosin and the actin filaments.

During the action potential in the myocardial cell, three different currents have been identified: (a) a fast inward current of primarily sodium ions, resulting in the upstroke of the action potential; (b) a slow inward current, primarily of calcium ions, during the plateau of the action potential; and (c) a delayed outward current, primarily of potassium ions, which is responsible for repolarization (189). Details of the role of calcium in myocardial contractility are discussed elsewhere (190,191). The molecular events leading to excitation–contraction coupling are depicted in Fig. 5.

FIG. 3. Processes involving energy production and utilization in the myocardium. Possible sites of solvents' actions are: glucose or oxygen extraction, permeability of membrane to calcium or other ions with the consequent interference in the action potential, enzymatic activity, excitation–contraction coupling, or the availability of ATP itself. c-AMP, cyclic adenosine monophosphate; ADP, adenosine diphosphate; ATP, adenosine triphosphate; Pi, inorganic phosphate; C, creatine; PC, phosphocreatine; CPK, creatine phosphokinase.

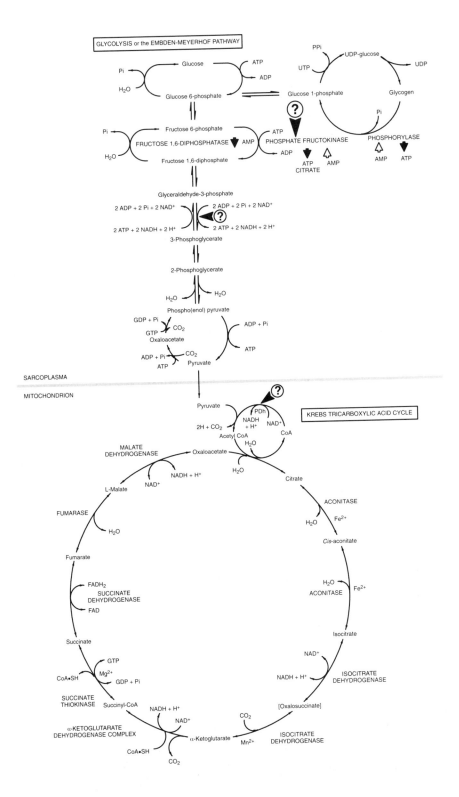

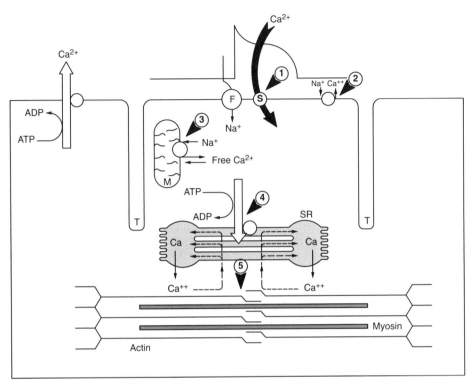

FIG. 5. Potential mechanisms of attenuation of myocardial contractility by solvents (numbers one to five). ATP, adenosine triphosphate; ADP, adenosine diphosphate; M, mitochondria; F, fast channels; S, slow channels; SR, sarcoplasmic reticulum; T, T tubules.

By interfering with the process of energy delivery, liberation, storage, or use, organic solvents could depress myocardial contractility. Several mechanisms have been postulated to explain the negative inotropic effect observed with solvents in general and halogenated hydrocarbons in particular; these mechanisms could involve interference with the autonomic nervous control of the heart, the availability of fuel substrate, oxygen extraction, and metabolic processes for energy production and/or utilization, namely, excitation–contraction coupling.

FIG. 4. Metabolic pathways of the energy liberation in the myocardium. AMP, adenosine monophosphate; ADP, adenosine diphosphate; ATP, adenosine triphosphate; Pi, inorganic phosphate; PPi, Pyrophosphate; UTP, uridine triphosphate; UDP, uridine diphosphate; NAD, nicotine adenine dinucleotide; NADH, reduced NAD, GDP, guanosine-5'-diphosphate; GTP, guanosine-5'-triphosphate; PDh, pyruvate dehydrogenase; CoA, coenzyme A; iCDh, isocitrate dehydrogenase; FMN, flavine mononucleotide; FAD, flavine adenine dinucleotide; FADH, reduced FAD. Possible sites of actions are marked with *solid arrows*. *Solid arrows* pointed downward denote inhibition; *open arrows* pointed upward denote stimulation.

The fact that solvents are lipophilic led Van Stee and co-workers (192) to suggest that the presence of haloalkane molecules in the membrane lipid phase could lead to a disruption of the delicate process of energy production and utilization. This disruption could alter the transmembrane movements of sodium and potassium and the release and reuptake of calcium ions by the sarcoplasmic reticulum.

The availability and uptake by the myocardium of glucose, lactate, pyruvate, and nonesterified fatty acids were not altered when bromotrifluoromethane (27%) was administered by inhalation to anesthetized dogs for 30 min (165). The negative inotropic effect of this compound was ascribed to either a reduction in the rate of oxidative metabolism or to the uncoupling of oxidative phosphorylation. Furthermore, myocardial depression induced by halogenated hydrocarbons was found to be independent of myocardial adrenergic postsynaptic activity, namely, the release of the neurohumoral transmitter epinephrine (151), and was not related to ATP depletion (151,162). Similarly, it was not clear whether halogenated hydrocarbons affect the ability of the myocardium to extract oxygen from the blood, even though Van Stee and colleagues (151) found that hearts from animals exposed to chlorobromomethane and bromochlorodifluoromethane failed to extract a normal amount of oxygen as gauged by the oxygen content of the coronary sinus blood. The determinants of myocardial oxygen consumption are heart rate, blood pressure, ventricular pressure, and the rate of rise of the left ventricular pressure $(dp/dt)_{max}$ (193). Since halogenated solvents cause a decrease in systemic arterial pressure, left ventricular pressure, and left ventricular dp/dt, it would be expected that these compounds decrease the oxygen demand by the myocardium.

Depression of the CNS may contribute to the attenuation of myocardial contractility observed with some solvents. However, this relationship is not clear.

EFFECT ON HEART RATE

Halogenated solvents induced a biphasic response in the heart rate of experimental animals. Thus at low concentrations, a slight increase or no change in the heart rate was observed, whereas higher concentrations resulted in a decrease in the heart rate (92,112). This concentration-dependent response could be explained on the basis of the relative contribution of the direct effect of these solvents on the SA node and the activation of the carotid–aortic reflex mechanisms due to their hypotensive effects. Adrenalectomy or injection of beta-adrenergic blocking agents has prevented cardioacceleration in response to halogenated solvents (194,195).

Experiments performed on F344 rats exposed to solvent refined coal heavy distillate (HD), a mixture of aliphatic and polycyclic aromatic compounds), showed that inhalation of 0.7 or 0.24 mg/L of HD for 6 hr/day for 6 weeks resulted in a concentration-dependent increase in heart rate and mean aortic blood pressure. In addition, angiotensin concentrations were decreased in a dose-dependent manner. The changes in blood pressure and heart rate returned to the control levels 6 weeks after cessation of exposure (196).

Among the ketones studied for their effect on the myocardium, acetone increased the contraction rate of the spontaneously beating rat's atrium at concentrations of 10–210 mM. This was partially ascribed to the release of norepinephrine from sympathetic nerve endings from the atria (197). The positive chronotropic effect was abolished by propranolol (a beta-adrenergic receptor blocker) or by pretreating with reserpine (a norepinephrine depleter). Acetone concentrations above 210 mM caused a gradual decrease in the curve of the atrial contraction rate while still enhancing norepinephrine release. In the anesthetized dog, both methyl ethyl ketone and methyl isobutyl ketone also induced an increase in the heart rate (175,176).

Propylene glycol, a widely used drug solvent, caused a precipitous drop in the heart rate and blood pressure of anesthetized dogs when injected intravenously in doses of 160–800 mg/kg (136). In the same study, atropine prevented these changes whereas sympathetic blocking by bretylium tosylate had little effect. It was concluded that propylene glycol induces a powerful reflex stimulation of the cardiomotor vagus and transient inhibition of efferent sympathetic activity.

EFFECT ON CARDIAC OUTPUT AND BLOOD PRESSURE

The decrease in cardiac output and blood pressure observed after the administration of commonly used solvents could be secondary to the decrease in myocardial force of contraction, a direct relaxant effect on the smooth muscles of various vascular beds leading to a decrease in vascular resistance and pooling of blood in the capacitance vessels, or due to an indirect effect on the central nervous system. To appreciate the complexity of blood pressure control, factors that affect blood pressure are graphically depicted in Fig. 6.

When injected intravenously in anesthetized dogs, methanol caused a progressive decrease in stroke volume, cardiac output, and systemic blood pressure at concentrations of 130 mg/100 ml and higher; cardiac standstill occurred at blood concentrations exceeding 400 mg/100 ml (171). Conversely, chronic ethanol consumption is associated with hypertension (198).

Unlike alcohols, propylene glycol (propane-1,2-diol) produced no effect on dogs' or cats' blood pressure when given intraperitoneally or orally at a dose level of 0.5 ml/kg (199).

Halogenated hydrocarbons produced a decrease in cardiac output and blood pressure secondary to the attenuation of myocardial contractility, with a consequent shift in myocardial performance upward on the Starling ventricular function curve (1).

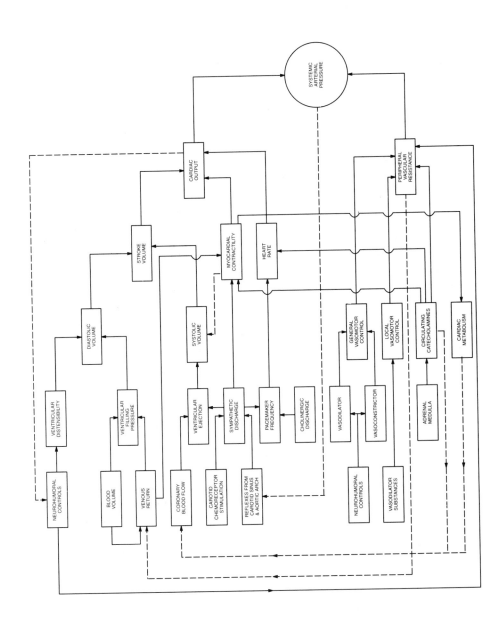

EFFECT ON CORONARY ARTERIES

A decrease in myocardial contractility and cardiac output induced by organic solvents is expected to result in a decrease in coronary blood flow. Indeed, a decrease in blood flow in the left anterior descending coronary artery was demonstrated in dogs exposed to methylene chloride, 1,2-dichloro-2,2-difluoroethane and 1,1,2-trichloro-1,2,2-trifluoroethane (1). Whether this decrease in coronary blood flow is secondary to a decrease in cardiac output or in the myocardial oxygen demand is not clear. The effects of two solvents, namely, carbon disulfide and toluene, on the coronary arteries deserve a special discussion.

Carbon disulfide, an extensively used solvent in the production of rayon, increased the incidence of coronary heart disease and worsened its prognosis (200) and induced vascular changes in the retina and the brain (201). Studies performed in England, Japan, Finland, and the United States documented the association between exposure to carbon disulfide and the occurrence of atherosclerosis in the coronary arteries (41,202). Nurminen and Hernberg (49) conducted a follow-up study on workers exposed to carbon disulfide over a 15-year period (1967–1982). During the first 5 years where workers were exposed to an average concentration of 22 ppm, a four- to sevenfold excess mortality occurred among workers due to ischemic and other heart diseases. In the last 5 years when the level of exposure was reduced to 10 ppm, the relative risk ratio dropped from 3.2 to 1.0. This association was attributed to the effect of carbon disulfide on lipid metabolism (203–205). The low density lipoprotein cholesterol was significantly increased in young men (aged 21–35 years) exposed to 40–116 mg/m^3 carbon disulfide for 8 years; total cholesterol and high density lipoprotein cholesterol levels did not differ significantly from the control group (206). Thus the increase in vascular disease induced by carbon disulfide may be related to the increase in atheroma formation (201).

Although the adverse effects of toluene are manifested mainly as CNS depression, a recent finding by Takahashi and colleagues (207) deserves comment. Takahashi and co-workers administered toluene orally to male New Zealand rabbits at a dose of 0.5 g/kg; the blood toluene levels averaged 12.7 μg/g after 15 min and 13.8 μg/g after 1 hr. This single dose of toluene resulted in a significant increase in plasma triglyceride and free fatty acids concentrations and a temporary elevation of blood glucose levels. Because triglycerides were associated with myocardial infarction (208), it remains to be seen whether chronic exposure to toluene leads to coronary heart disease. Furthermore, alcohol was reported to delay the metabolism and elimination of toluene (31). Because moderate alcohol consumption reportedly

---

FIG. 6. Factors that contribute to the overall control of systemic blood pressure.

protects against coronary heart disease (209,210), and because alcohol increases triglyceride levels, the interaction between concurrent alcohol use and toluene exposure is intriguing.

PATHOLOGICAL CHANGES

Structural effects induced by organic solvents vary with different conditions. Based on the duration and extent of exposure to organic solvents, manifestation of cardiac toxicity could range from subtle functional or biochemical changes to severe structural damage to the myocardium. Because organic solvents are lipid soluble, they dissolve in cell membranes, thereby disrupting processes such as oxidative phosphorylation by the inner mitochondrial membrane with subsequent effects on cytochromes and ATPase.

Two types of cardiomyopathies can be induced by toxic agents: (a) cardiomyopathy secondary to cardiac metabolic imbalance and (b) cardiomyopathy induced by direct cardiotoxic mechanisms (211). Gross and microscopic pathological changes induced in the myocardium by organic solvents are discussed next.

Animals exposed to 1,2-dichloropropane exhibited fatty degeneration of the heart (212,213). Fibrous swelling of the cardiac muscle also was observed in rats exposed to 3000 ppm of trans-1,2-dichloroethylene for 8 hr (214). Myocardial pathological changes due to chronic alcohol consumption, which have been documented in both animals (215,216) and humans, are discussed elsewhere (see chapter by Ahmed and Regan; 29).

Polyethylene glycols of different molecular weights are usually used as vehicles in pharmaceutical preparations. Klugmann and co-workers (217) reported that polyethylene glycol 400 protected the hearts of mice against adriamycin-induced cardiac microscopic alterations.

Cardiomyopathy and degeneration of heart muscles after abuse of toluene were reported (218–220).

TERATOGENIC EFFECTS

Glycol ethers possess special feature for solvent toxicity, namely, their teratogenic effects on the myocardium. When diethylene glycol monomethyl ether was tested in CD-1 mice in doses of 720 or 2165 mg/kg/day, cardiovascular malformations occurred in 4.8 and 71.4% of litters, compared to none in the control group (221). Ethylene glycol monomethyl ether (EGME) also was found to be teratogenic in Sprague–Dawley rats (222,223). In these studies, 25 or 50 mg/kg EGME was administered by gavage to pregnant rats on gestation days 7–13. Results showed a dose-dependent increase in the incidence of fetuses with cardiovascular malformation, primarily right ductus arteriosus and ventricular septal defect, and a prolonged QRS wave in the

ECG. Changes in the QRS waves suggest the presence of an intraventricular conduction delay in the fetuses. Furthermore, the activity of ornithine decarboxylase in the heart was disrupted by EGME (224). In 1984, Nelson and colleagues (225) studied the teratogenic effects of five structurally related glycol ethers or esters in rats. Results indicated that 2-methoxyethanol induced cardiovascular defects in the fetuses when the dams were exposed to 50 or 100 ppm, 7 hr/day on gestation days 7 through 15 (226). Also, 2-ethoxyethyl acetate produced similar results at 390 ppm. However, exposure to 2-butoxyethanol (200 ppm), 2-(2-ethoxyethoxy) ethanol (100 ppm), or 2-methylamino ethanol (150 ppm) resulted in no embryotoxicity. In fact, 2-butoxyethanol produced maternal toxicity at levels below those that produced embryotoxicity. It was concluded that shorter alkyl chain glycol ethers are more embryotoxic than those with longer chains. In addition, effects produced by esters were similar to those induced by ethers.

Alcohols also have been found to be teratogenic. When methanol was administered by inhalation (20,000 ppm, 7 hr/day on days 1–19 of gestation) to Sprague–Dawley rats, it induced a statistically significant number of cardiovascular defects (227,228). Two alcohols, *n*-propanol and isopropanol, showed no teratogenic effect at 3500 ppm (229). Similarly, no teratogenic effect was observed in rats when 1,1,1-trichloroethane was administered at concentrations of 3, 10, or 30 ppm in drinking water (230).

Ethanol also was found to be teratogenic in chick embryos (231) and in mice (232,233) and is known to induce fetal alcohol syndrome (FAS) in humans. FAS, which refers to a pattern of defects in children born to alcoholic mothers, often includes cardiac anomalies and may be due to anoxia, alcohol itself, or its metabolite acetaldehyde (234). Zierler (235) suggested that exposure of embryos to ethanol during cardiogenesis increases the risk of congenital heart disease. A study in Finland of the teratogenic effects of solvents in humans found an association between maternal exposure to solvents during pregnancy and ventricular septal defects in the newborn (236,237). Further epidemiologic study by the same group (238) showed that exposure to organic solvents was more prevalent among mothers whose babies showed ventricular septal defect (12.1%) than among the control mothers (7.8%). In addition, mothers exposed to solvents during pregnancy have four- to ninefold increased risk of hypertension and preeclampsia than unexposed women (239). Another epidemiologic study has implicated the exposure to toluene and benzyl alcohol during pregnancy for cardiac teratogenic effects (240). The teratogenic effects of exposure to halogenated solvents also have been reported (241).

Glycerol formal, a solvent that is commonly used in pharmaceutical and pesticide formulations, also was found to be teratogenic in Sprague–Dawley and Wistar rats when administered orally, subcutaneously, or intramuscularly on days 6 through 15 of gestation (242). Doses of 0.5 or 1 ml/kg induced cardiovascular malformations, particularly ventricular septal defects.

COMBINED EFFECTS OF ALCOHOL/SOLVENTS ABUSE

In a review on volatile substances of abuse (VSA), Linden (17) stated that "concurrent ethanol abuse is extremely common in chronic VSA users." Furthermore, Dinwiddie et al. (243) found that intravenous drug abusers (IVDA) with a history of solvent use were more likely to abuse alcohol and exhibit antisocial personality disorder than IVDAs without history of solvent use. Because alcohol abuse induces cardiomyopathy and arrhythmias (see chapter by Ahmed and Regan; 29), attention should be focused on the combined effects of ethanol and solvents on the cardiovascular system.

In addition, ethanol readily induces the metabolizing enzyme cytochrome *P450 IIE1* (244), which has been shown to metabolize a large number of solvents (see Table 3) (245). Consequently, there is a higher risk associated with exposure to such VSA when alcohol is consumed. By inducing the enzyme *P450 IIE1*, chronic alcohol consumption may increase the rate of sol-

TABLE 3. *Solvents metabolized by cytochrome* P450 IIE1

Solvent	Metabolite measured	Reference
Aromatic compounds		
Pyridine	Pyridine *N*-oxide	253
Benzene	Phenol	254
Phenol	Hydroquinone; catechol	255
Styrene	Glutathione conjugate	256
Halogenated alkanes and alkenes		
Carbon tetrachloride	Lipid peroxidation/chloroform	256, 257
Chloroform	Glutathione conjugate	256, 258
Chloromethane	Formaldehyde	256
Dibromoethane	Glutathione conjugate	256
Dichloropropane	Glutathione conjugate	256
1,2-Dichloropropane	Glutathione conjugate	256
1,1,1-Trichloroethane	1,1,1-Trichloro-2-hydroxyethane	256
Trichloroethylene	Chloral	256
Ethylene dibromide	1,*N*⁶-Ethenoadenosine	256
Ethylene dichloride	1,*N*⁶-Ethenoadenosine	256
Vinyl chloride	1,*N*⁶-Ethenoadenosine	256
Vinyl bromide	1,*N*⁶-Ethenoadenosine	256
Halothane	Trifluoroacetic acid	259
1,1,1,2-Tetrafluoroethane	Fluoride	260
Alcohols/ketones/nitriles		
Ethanol	Acetaldehyde	261
Propanol	Propionaldehyde	261
Isopropanol	Acetone	261
Butanol	Butyraldehyde	261
Pentanol	Valeraldehyde	261
Acetol	Methylglyoxal	261
Acetone	Acetol	261
Ethers		
Diethyl ether	Acetaldehyde	262
Methyl *t*-butyl ether	Formaldehyde/*t*-butanol	263

Adapted from ref. 245.

vent metabolism and hence increase the toxicity of solvents that are metabolically activated. For example, one of the best documented cases of potentiation of a solvent's toxicity by alcohol is the induction of liver cirrhosis by carbon tetrachloride (244). This potentiation of CCl_4 hepatotoxicity is due to the induction by ethanol of *P450* and the consequent increased metabolism of CCl_4 to the active radical (246–250). Also, the induction of the cytochrome *P450* system by ethanol explains the exacerbation in alcoholics of hepatotoxicity due to chloroform and other haloalkanes (251). On the other hand, acute alcohol consumption may increase the toxicity of some solvents that do not require metabolic activation by acting as a competitive substrate. For example, Dossing and colleagues (252) found that human volunteers simultaneously exposed to alcohol and toluene have higher toluene concentrations in their alveolar air than those exposed to toluene alone. Furthermore, urinary excretion of hippuric acid, the major metabolite of toluene, in humans exposed to both alcohol and toluene was only 40% of that excreted by individuals exposed to toluene alone.

Excessive alcohol intake results in chronic myocardial toxicity, characterized by pathological changes, arrhythmias, and even sudden death (169,264–284). For further reading on this subject see the chapter by Ahmed and Regan.

STRUCTURE–ACTIVITY RELATIONSHIPS

Halogenated derivatives of aliphatic hydrocarbons in general are more pharmacologically and toxicologically active than the corresponding unsubstituted hydrocarbons. The overall toxicity of halogenated solvents is determined not only by the number of halogen atoms in a molecule but also by molecular configuration (285), the presence of unsaturated bonds (286), and the physicochemical properties of the solvent (287).

Of the chlorinated methanes, carbon tetrachloride is the most cardiotoxic. In the substituted ethane series, chlorine atoms increased the myocardial depressant effect of the molecule. This effect is true for up to four chlorine atoms; the introduction of a fifth atom resulted in a decrease in toxicity (288). The hypotensive effect of unsaturated chlorinated solvents was less pronounced than that for the corresponding saturated compounds (286).

In the alcohol series, cardiac toxicity is proportional to chain length; that is, on a molar basis, longer chain alcohols (up to C_5) are more toxic than those with shorter chains (289).

CONCLUDING REMARKS

Exposure to organic solvents may occur in conjunction with housekeeping, hobbies, or in industry. Intentional inhalation of solvents by teenagers, commonly and erroneously termed "sniffing," is another method of exposure to these agents. Organic solvents can reach the circulatory system through inhalation or absorption through the skin. Apart from a depressant effect on the central nervous system, these chemicals induce liver injury, kidney damage, irritation of the skin and mucous membranes, and myocardial toxicity.

Solvents in general, and halogenated hydrocarbons in particular, have arrhythmogenic and myocardial depressant effects. They depress myocardial contractility, cardiac output, blood pressure, and coronary blood flow. Numerous members of this class can also sensitize the heart to the arrhythmogenic effect of epinephrine. Indeed, this effect has been identified as the mechanism by which abused halogenated solvents and propellants brought about cardiac arrest and sudden death of healthy individuals who engaged in some form of physical exertion after inhaling these compounds. Electrolyte imbalance, hypoxia, acidosis, myocardial infarction, and blockage of conductivity may also be involved in the pathogenesis of solvent-induced arrhythmias. Furthermore, epidemiologic studies have established a firm association between exposure to carbon disulfide and the genesis of coronary atherosclerosis. The myocardial depressant effect of these solvents could be catastrophic in patients with borderline heart failure or those prone to the development of myocardial arrhythmias by other chemicals such as digitalis. In addition, the interaction between these solvents and other medications, such as tranquilizers, antidepressants, barbiturates, and antihypertensives, to name a few, could be disastrous.

Alcohols, including ethanol, also display a negative inotropic effect on the heart, and its toxicity is proportional to the chain length up to five carbons. Myocardial problems associated with ethanol, especially cardiomyopathy, are related to its chronic abuse as a beverage rather than as a solvent. Since solvent abusers may also tend to abuse alcohol, the effect of solvents on the cardiovascular system could be exacerbated by alcohol. This speculation is based on the fact that chronic alcohol consumption can cause cardiomyopathy and arrhythmias, and that alcohol induces cytochrome *P450 IIEI*, an enzyme that also metabolizes numerous organic solvents. It should be noted, as well, that those who inhale "leaded" gasoline not only develop cardiovascular injury but also acquire severe neurotoxicity due to both gasoline and organic lead.

The studies described in this chapter demonstrate a need for further research into the toxicity of solvents on the cardiovascular system. A particular need is to elucidate the mechanisms underlying the arrhythmogenic and myocardial depressant effects of solvents. Because exposure to solvents may be accompanied by alcohol abuse, more research is needed to elucidate the interactions between these two classes of abused substances.

APPENDIX 1. *Commonly used solvents and their principal effects*

Solvent	BP (°C)	Principal effect
1. Aliphatic hydrocarbons		
Cyclohexane	80.7	CNS depression, dermatitis, conjunctivitis
Methylcyclohexane	98–100	CNS depression
Gasoline	60–120	CNS depression, fatty degeneration of liver and kidneys, chemical pneumonitis
n-Heptane	98.5	CNS depression, dermatitis, pulmonary edema, cardiac sensitization
n-Hexane	69	CNS depression, myocardial sensitization, peripheral neuropathy
Kerosene		CNS depression, pulmonary edema, renal failure
Naphtha		CNS depression, skin irritation, peripheral neuropathy
Turpentine	154	CNS depression, nephritis, eczema
Cyclopentadiene	41–42	CNS depression
2. Alcohols		
Amyl alcohol(s)	118	CNS depression, skin and lung irritation, methemoglobinemia
n-Butyl alcohol	115–118	Skin irritation, Meniere's syndrome
iso-Butyl alcohol	108	CNS depression
sec-Butyl alcohol	98–102	CNS depression
tert-Butyl alcohol	82.8	CNS depression
Ethyl alcohol	78.3	CNS depression, cardiomyopathy
Ethylene chlorohydrin	125–132	CNS depression, hypotension, irritation to eyes and skin, pulmonary edema
Methyl alcohol	65	Optic nerve damage, dermatitis, CNS depression
n-Propyl alcohol	97.3	CNS depression, mild skin irritant
iso-Propyl alcohol	82.4	CNS depression, mild skin irritant
Allyl alcohol	96.6	Liver and kidney damage, skin irritation
Cyclohexanol	160	Eye and skin irritation, CNS depression
Benzyl alcohol	204.7	Bactericidal, local anesthetic, hypotensive
Monochlorohydrin	213–228	CNS depression
3. Glycols and derivatives		
Ethylene glycol	197	Nystagmas, lymphocytosis, respiratory and cardiac failure, renal damage
Ethylene glycol monomethyl ether		CNS depression, pulmonary edema, anemia, hemolysis of erythrocytes
Ethylene glycol monoethyl ether		Renal damage
Ethylene glycol diethyl ether		Kidney damage
Ethylene glycol monobutyl ether		Blood dyscrasia

APPENDIX 1. Continued

Solvent	BP (°C)	Principal effect
Diethylene glycol	244.5	CNS depression, kidney damage
Diethylene glycol monomethyl ether		CNS depression, kidney damage, teratogen
Diethylene glycol monobutyl ether		Kidney damage
Dipropylene glycol		CNS depression
4. Ethers and epoxy compounds		
bis-(Chloromethyl) ether		Carcinogen (lung carcinoma), severe irritant to skin and eyes
Chloromethyl ether		Bronchogenic cancer
Dichloroethyl ether	178	CNS depression, pulmonary edema
Dioxane	94–110	CNS depression, liver and kidney damage
Epichlorohydrin	117.9	Chemical pneumonitis, gastrointestinal discomfort, liver damage
Ethyl ether	34.6	CNS depression, albuminuria
Isopropyl ether	68.7	CNS depression
Propylene oxide	35	
Acetal	102	CNS depression
5. Esters		
Methyl formate	31.5	Eye and skin irritation, CNS depression, pulmonary edema
Ethyl formate	53–57	Eye and skin irritation, CNS depression
n-Butyl formate	96–110	CNS depression
Amyl formate	110–130	CNS depression
Benzyl formate	200–202	
Methyl acetate	57	Eye and skin irritation
Ethyl acetate	77.1	Eye and skin irritation
n-Propyl acetate	101.6	CNS depression
iso-Propyl acetate	92	CNS depression
n-Butyl acetate	126	Eye and skin irritation, CNS depression
sec-Butyl acetate	107–114	
iso-Butyl acetate	110–118	Hemolytic
Amyl acetate	120–145	Eye irritation, CNS depression
Benzyl acetate	215	CNS depression
n-Butyl propionate	146	
Amyl propionate	140–170	
n-Butyl butyrate	160–165	

6. Aldehydes and ketones

Furfural	161.8	Skin sensitization, eye and skin irritation, CNS depression
Acetone	56	Dermatitis, CNS depression
Diacetone		Dermatitis, CNS depression
Methyl ethyl ketone	79.6	Dermatitis, CNS depression
Methyl n-propyl ketone	102	Dermatitis, CNS depression
Methyl n-butyl ketone	127	Peripheral neuropathy
Methyl isobutyl ketone	112–118	Dermatitis, CNS depression
Mesityl oxide	129.5	CNS depression
Cyclohexanone	154–156	CNS depression
Methyl cyclohexanone	160–175	Irritant

7. Aliphatic halogenated hydrocarbons

Carbon tetrachloride	75.7	CNS depression, liver and kidney damage
Chloroform	61.2	CNS depression, liver and kidney damage, myocardial sensitization
1,2-Dibromoethane		CNS depression, liver and kidney damage
1,2-Dichloroethane	80–85	CNS depression, pulmonary edema, liver and kidney damage
1,2-Dichloroethylene	48	CNS depression, skin irritant
Methylene chloride	40–42	Cardiac arrhythmias, CNS depression
1,2-Dichloropropane	96	CNS depression, fatty degeneration of liver and kidneys
Tetrachloroethane	140–150	CNS depression, disappearance of ocular and pharyngeal reflexes, peripheral neuritis, thrombocytosis, fatty degeneration of the myocardium
Tetrachloroethylene	119–121	CNS depression, cardiac arrhythmias, liver injury
1,1,1-Trichloroethane	74.1	CNS and myocardial depression
1,1,2-Trichloroethane	113	CNS depression, liver and kidney damage
Trichloroethylene	86.2	CNS and myocardial depression, liver tumors

8. Fluorocarbons

Bromotrifluoromethane		CNS depression, cardiac arrhythmias
Dibromodifluoromethane		Liver and kidney damage (fluoroalkenes)
Dichlorodifluoromethane		
Dichloromonofluoromethane		
Dichlorotetrafluoroethane		
Fluorotrichloromethane		
1,1,1,2-Tetrachloro-2,2-difluoroethane		
1,1,2,2-Tetrachloro-1,2-difluoroethane		

APPENDIX 1. *Continued*

Solvent	BP (°C)	Principal effect
1,1,2-Trichloro- 　1,2,2-trifluoroethane		
Bromochlorotrifluoroethane		
Chlorodifluoromethane		
Chlorotrifluoroethylene		
Difluoroethylene		
Fluoroethylene		
Hexafluoropropylene		
Octafluorocyclobutane		
Tetrafluoroethylene		
9. Aliphatic amines and coal 　**tar bases**		
Ethylenediamine	116	Cutaneous sensitivity, kidney and liver damage
Cyclohexylamine	134.5	Skin irritant
Dicyclohexylamine	255	Skin irritant, CNS depression
Monoethanolamines	171 @ 150 mm Hg	Liver and kidney damage
Diethanolamines	268	Liver and kidney damage
Triethanolamines	277 @ 150 mm Hg	Liver and kidney damage
Pyridine	115	Irritant to eyes and respiratory tree, liver and kidney injury
Picoline	128	Irritant, liver and kidney damage, CNS depression
10. Cyanides and nitriles		
Acetonitrile	81.6	Eye and skin irritation, CNS depression, hematemesis, shock
11. Aromatic hydrocarbons		
Benzene	80	Eye and skin irritation, CNS depression, myocardial sensitization, leukemogenic, aplastic anemia

Compound		
Ethyl benzene (styrene)	136.5	Respiratory depression
Toluene	109–111	CNS depression, eye and skin irritation
Xylene	138–140	CNS depression, liver and kidney damage, pulmonary edema
Cumene	151–156	CNS depression, pulmonary edema
Tetrahydronaphthalene	205–215	CNS depression, dermatitis, anemia
Decahydronaphthalene	183–192	Skin irritation, liver and kidney damage
12. Chlorinated benzenes		
Monochlorobenzene	131.7	CNS depression
O-dichlorobenzene	179.5	Skin and eye irritation, liver, kidney, and lung damage
13. Nitro compounds		
Nitromethane	100	Irritant, CNS depression
1-Nitropropane	132	Irritant, liver damage
2-Nitropropane	120	Irritant, liver damage
1-Nitrobutane	151	Eye irritant, liver and kidney damage
2-Nitrobutane	139	Irritant
Nitrobenzene	211	CNS depression, methemoglobinemia, jaundice
14. Miscellaneous solvents		
N,N-dimethyl formamide	153	Dermatitis, anorexia, hepatomegaly
N-nitrosodimethylamine	151	Skin irritant, jaundice, anorexia, carcinogen
N,N-dimethylacetamide	163	Liver injury, visual and auditory hallucinations
Carbon disulfide	46.5	Atherosclerosis, coronary heart disease, psychosis, renal damage
Benzaldehyde	179	CNS depression
Butyl carbitol	230.4	Kidney damage
Dimethylsulfoxide	189	CNS depression, kidney damage
Mesitylene	164.7	Bone marrow damage, pneumonia
Cresols	195–205	Corrosive, CNS depression

REFERENCES

1. Zakhari S, Aviado DM. Cardiovascular toxicology of aerosol propellants, refrigerants, and related solvents. In: Van Stee EW, ed. *Cardiovascular toxicology.* New York: Raven Press; 1982:281–327.
2. Gay M, Meller R, Stanley S. Drug abuse monitoring: a survey of solvent abuse in the county of Avon. *Hum Toxicol* 1982;1:257–263.
3. Evans AC, Raistrick D. Phenomenology of intoxication with toluene-based adhesives and butane gas. *Br J Psychiatry* 1987;150:769–773.
4. Evans AC, Raistrick D. Patterns of use and related harm with toluene-base adhesives and butane gas. *Br J Psychiatry* 1987;150:773–776.
5. Anderson HR, Macnair RS, Ramsey JD. Deaths from abuse of volatile substances. A national epidemiological study. *Br Med J* 1985;290:304–307.
6. Anderson HR, Bloor K, Macnair RS, Ramsey J. Recent trends in mortality associated with abuse of volatile substances in the UK. *Br Med J* 1986;293:1472–1473.
7. Hershey C, Miller S. Solvent abuse: a shift to adults. *Int J Addict* 1982;17:1085–1089.
8. Cherry N, McArthy T, Waldron H. Solvent sniffing in industry. *Hum Toxicol* 1982;1:289–292.
9. Munjack D. Sex and drugs. *Clin Toxicol* 1979;15:75–89.
10. Parker SE. Use and abuse of volatile substances in industry. *Hum Toxicol* 1989;8:271–275.
11. Pointer J. Typewriter correction fluid inhalation: a new substance of abuse. *Clin Toxicol* 1982;19:493–499.
12. Greer J. Adolescent abuse of typewriter correction fluid. *South Med J* 1984;77:297–298.
13. Greer WER, Giovacchini RP. Sniffing up trouble: inhalation of volatile substances. *JAMA* 1985;254:1721–1722.
14. Zipp TM. Sniffing up trouble: adhesive tape remover pads (letter). *JAMA* 1986;256:39–40.
15. Wodka RM, Jeong EW. Cardiac effects of inhaled typewriter correction fluid. *Ann Intern Med* 1989;110:91–92.
16. Cohen S. The volatile nitrites. *JAMA* 1979;241:2077–2078.
17. Linden CH. Volatile substances of abuse. *Emerg Med Clin North Am* 1990;8:559–578.
18. Bass M. Sudden sniffing death. *JAMA* 1970;212:2075–2079.
19. Reinhardt CF, Azar A, Maxfield ME, Smith PE Jr, Mullin LS. Cardiac arrhythmias and aerosol "sniffing." *Arch Environ Health* 1971;22:265–279.
20. Boon NA. Solvent abuse and the heart. *Br Med J* 1987;294:722.
21. Goldfrank LR, Kulberg AG, Bresnitz EA. Hydrocarbons. In: Goldfrank LR, Flomenbaum NE, Lewin NA, Weisman RS, Howland MA, eds. *Goldfrank's toxicologic emergencies.* Norwalk: Appleton and Lange, 1990;759–768.
22. Flanagan RJ, Ruprah M, Meredith TJ, Ramsey JD. An introduction to the clinical toxicology of volatile substances. *Drug Safety* 1990;5:359–383.
23. Garriott J, Petty CS. Death from inhalant abuse: toxicological and pathological evaluation of 34 cases. *Clin Toxicol* 1980;16:305–315.
24. King GS, Smialek JE, Troutman WG. Sudden death in adolescents resulting from the inhalation of typewriter correction fluid. *JAMA* 1985;253:1604–1606.
25. Rosenstock L, Cullen MR. Organic solvents and related substances. In: *Clinical occupational medicine.* Philadelphia: Saunders; 1986:214–225.
26. Armeli G, Linari F, Montorano G. Rilievi clinici ed ematochimici in operai esposti allazione di un chetone superiore (MIBK) ripetuti a distanza di 5 anni. *Lav Um* 1968;20:418.
27. Tiller JR, Schilling RSF, Morris JN. Occupational toxic factor in mortality from coronary heart disease. *Br Med J* 1968;4:407–411.
28. Wilcosky TC, Tyroler HA. Mortality from heart disease among workers exposed to solvents. *J Occup Med* 1983;25:879–885.
29. Zakhari S. Vulnerability to cardiac disease. In: Galanter M, ed. *Recent developments in alcoholism: children of alcoholics,* vol 9. New York: Plenum Press; 1991:225–260.
30. Andrews LS, Snyder R. Toxic effects of solvents and vapors. In: Klassen CD, Amdur MO, Doull J, eds. *Casarett and Doull's toxicology: the basic science of poisons,* 3rd ed. New York: Macmillan; 1986:636–668.

31. Ayres PH, Taylor DW. Solvents. In: Hayes AW, ed. *Principles and methods of toxicology*, 2nd ed. New York: Raven Press; 1989:111–135.
32. Keaton BF. Chlorinated hydrocarbons. In: Haddad LM, Winchester JF, eds. *Clinical management of poisoning and drug overdose*. Philadelphia: WB Saunders, 1990;1216–1222.
33. Heiselman DE, Cannon LA. Benzene and the aromatic hydrocarbons. In: Haddad LM, Winchester JF, eds. *Clinical management of poisoning and drug overdose*. Philadelphia: WB Saunders, 1990;1222–1232.
34. Graham DR. Solvent abuse. In: Haddad LM, Winchester JF, eds. *Clinical management of poisoning and drug overdose*. Philadelphia: WB Saunders, 1990;1256–1260.
35. Von Berg R. Toxicology updates. Xylene. *J Appl Toxicol* 1982;2:269–271.
36. Waldron HA. Effects of organic solvents. *Br J Hosp Med* 1981;26:645–649.
37. Kristensen TS. Cardiovascular diseases and the work environment. A critical review of the epidemiologic literature on chemical factors. *Scand J Work Environ Health* 1989;15:245–264.
38. Wilcosky TC, Simonsen NR. Solvent exposure and cardiovascular disease. *Am J Ind Med* 1991;19:569–586.
39. Hogstedt C, Axelson O. Long term health effects of industrial solvents—a critical review of the epidemiological research. *Med Lav* 1986;77:11–22.
40. Grossenbacher J, Lob M. Follow-up study of the long-term effects of occupational exposure to benzene. *Schweiz Med Wochenschr* 1982;112:1858–1859.
41. Fine LJ. Occupational heart disease. In: Rom WN, ed. *Environmental and occupational medicine*. Boston: Little, Brown; 1983:359–365.
42. Ott MG, Skory LK, Holder BB, Bronson JM, Williams PR. Health evaluation of employees occupationally exposed to methylene chloride mortality. *Scand J Work Environ Health* 1983;9(suppl 1):8–16.
43. Kurppa K, Hietanen E, Klockars M. Chemical exposures at work and cardiovascular morbidity: atherosclerosis, ischemic heart disease, hypertension, cardiomyopathy and arrhythmias. *Scand J Work Environ Health* 1984;10:381–388.
44. Rosenman KD. Cardiovascular disease and work place exposures. *Arch Environ Health* 1984;39:218–224.
45. James RC. The toxic effects of organic solvents. In: *Industrial toxicology: safety and health applications in the workplace*. New York: Lifetime Learning Publications; 1985:230–259.
46. Cone JE. Health hazards of solvents: state of the art reviews. *Occup Med* 1986;1:69–87.
47. Hogstedt C, Axelson O. Long-term health effects of industrial solvents—a critical review of the epidemiological research. *Med Lav* 1986;77:11–22.
48. Knight AT, Pawsey CGK, Aroney RS, Lawrence JR. Upholsterers' glue associated with myocarditis, hepatitis, acute renal failure and lymphoma. *Med J Aust* 1991;154:360–362.
49. Nurminen M, Hernberg S. Effects of intervention on the cardiovascular mortality of workers exposed to carbon disulphide: a 15 year follow-up. *Br J Ind Med* 1985;42:32–35.
50. MacMahon B, Monson RR. Mortality in the US rayon industry. *J Occup Med* 1988;30:698–705.
51. Kramer CG, Ott MG, Fulkerson JE, Hicks N, Imbu HR. Health of workers exposed to 1,1,1-trichloroethane: a matched-pair study. *Arch Environ Health* 1978;33:331–342.
52. Friedlander BR, Hearne T, Hall S. Epidemiologic investigation of employees chronically exposed to methylene chloride. *J Occup Med* 1978;20:657–666.
53. Hearne FT, Grose F, Pifer JW, Friedlander BR, Raleigh RL. Methylene chloride mortality study: dose–response characterization and animal model comparison. *J Occup Med* 1987;29:217–228.
54. Hearne FT, Pifer JW, Grose F. Absence of adverse mortality effects in workers exposed to methylene chloride: an update. *J Occup Med* 1990;32:234–240.
55. Spirtas R, Stewart PA, Lee JS, Marano DE. Retrospective cohort mortality study of workers at an aircraft maintenance facility: I. Epidemiological results. *Br J Ind Med* 1991;48:515–530.
56. Teta MJ, Ott MG. A mortality study of a research, engineering, and metal fabrication facility in western New York State. *Am J Epidemiol* 1988;127:540–551.

57. Interdepartmental Committee for Atmospheric Sciences. *The possible impact of fluorocarbons and halocarbons on ozone,* Washington, DC: Federal Council for Science and Technology, National Science Foundation, 1975:1–75.
58. Speizer FE, Wegman DH, Ramirez A. Palpitation rates associated with fluorocarbon exposure in a hospital setting. *N Engl J Med* 1975;292:624–626.
59. Edling C, Ohlson C-G, Ljungkvist G, Oliv Å, Söderholm B. Cardiac arrhythmia in refrigerator repairmen exposed to fluorocarbons. *Br J Ind Med* 1990;47:207–212.
60. Wiseman MN, Banim S. Glue sniffer's heart. *Br Med J* 1987;294:739.
61. Cunningham SR, Dalzell GWN, McGirr P, Khan MM. Myocardial infarction and primary ventricular fibrillation after glue sniffing. *Br Med J* 1987;294:739–740.
62. Mee AS, Wright PL. Congestive (dilated) cardiomyopathy in association with solvent abuse. *J R Soc Med* 1980;73:671–672.
63. McLeod AA, Marjot R, Monaghan MJ, Hugh-Jones P, Jackson G. Chronic cardiac toxicity after inhalation of 1,1,1-trichloroethane. *Toxicol Lett* 1987;37:183–193.
64. McLeod A, Marjot R, Monaghan M, et al. Chronic cardiac toxicity after inhalation of 1,1,1-trichloroethane. *Br Med J* 1987;294:727–729.
65. Jones RD, Winter DP. Two case reports of deaths on industrial premises attributed to 1,1,1-trichloroethane. *Arch Environ Health* 1983;38(1):59–61.
66. Yonemitsu K, Tsunenari K, Kanda M. An industrial accidental death due to freon 113 poisoning—toxicological analysis of its cause of death. *Jpn J Legal Med* 1983;37:428–433.
67. Palmer A. Mortality experience of 50 workers with occupational exposure to the products of coal hydrogenation process. In: *Potential health and environmental effects of synthetic fossil fuel technologies,* CONF-780903. Springfield, VA: NTIS, 1979;235–240.
68. Ogata et al., 1970
69. Hantson P, Vandenplas O, Dive A, Mahieu P. Trichloroethylene and cardiac toxicity: report of two consecutive cases. *Acta Clin Belg* 1990;45:34–37.
70. Stewart RD, Newton PE, Baretta ED, Hermann AA, Forster HV, Soto RJ. Physiological responses to aerosol propellants. *Environ Health Perspect* 1978;26:275–285.
71. Azar A. Cardiovascular effects of fluorocarbon exposure. In: *Proceedings of the second annual conference on environmental toxicology.* Wright-Patterson AFB, Oh: Aerospace Medical Research Laboratory; 1971:41–56.
72. Smith DG, Harris DJ. Human exposure to halon 1301 (CBrF$_3$) during simulated aircraft cabin fires. *Aerospace Med* 1973;44:198–201.
73. Allen N. Solvents and other industrial organic compounds. In: Vinken PJ, Bruyn GW, eds. *Intoxications of the nervous system,* part 1. Amsterdam: North-Holland; 1979:361–389.
74. Matikainen E, Juntunen J. Autonomic nervous system dysfunction in workers exposed to organic solvents. *J Neurol Neurosurg Psychiatry* 1985;48:1021–1024.
75. Peterson DF, Brown AM. Pressor reflexes produced by stimulation of afferent fibers in the cardiac sympathetic nerves of the cat. *Circ Res* 1971;28:605–610.
76. Malliani A, Peterson DF, Bishop VS, Brown AM. Spinal sympathetic cardiocardiac reflexes. *Circ Res* 1972;30:158–166.
77. Malliani A, Parks M, Tuckett RP, Brown AM. Reflex increases in heart rate elicited by stimulation of afferent cardiac sympathetic nerve fibers in the cat. *Circ Res* 1973;32:9–14.
78. Schwartz PJ, Pagani M, Lombardi F, Malliani A, Brown AM. A cardiac sympathovagal reflex in the cat. *Circ Res* 1973;32:215–220.
79. Brown AM. Excitation of afferent cardiac sympathetic nerve fibers during myocardial ischaemia. *J Physiol (Lond)* 1968;190:35–53.
80. Brown AM, Malliani A. Spinal sympathetic reflexes initiated by coronary receptors. *J Physiol (Lond)* 1971;212:685–705.
81. Malliani A, Schwartz PUJ, Zanchetti A. A sympathetic reflex elicited by experimental coronary occlusion. *Am J Physiol* 1969;217:703–709.
82. Brown AM. Mechanoreceptors in or near the coronary arteries. *J Physiol (Lond)* 1965;177:203–214.
83. Cottle MK. Degeneration studies of primary afferents of IXth and Xth cranial nerves in the cat. *J Comp Neurol* 1964;122:329–343.
84. Kalia M, Mesulam M-M. Brain stem projections of sensory and motor components of

the vagus complex in the cat: II. Laryngeal, tracheobronchial, pulmonary, cardiac, and gastrointestinal branches. *J Comp Neurol* 1980;193:467–508.

85. Kalia M, Mesulam M-M. Brain stem projections of sensory and motor components of the vagus complex in the cat: I. The cervical vagus and nodose ganglion. *J Comp Neurol* 1980;193:435–465.

86. Lee TM, Kuo JS, Chai CY. Central integrating mechanism of the Bezold–Jarish and baroreceptor reflexes. *Am J Physiol* 1972;222:713–720.

87. Hilton SM, Spyer KM. Participation of the anterior hypothalamus in the baroreceptor reflex. *J Physiol (Lond)* 1971;218:271–293.

88. Thomas MR, Calaresu FR. Responses of single units in the medial hypothalamus to electrical stimulation of the carotid sinus nerve in the cat. *Brain Res* 1972;44:49–62.

89. Grizzle WE, Johnson RN, Schramm LP, Gann DS. Hypothalamic cells in an area mediating ACTH release respond to right atrial stretch. *Am J Physiol* 1975;228:1039–1045.

90. Ciriello J, Calaresu FR. Role of paraventricular and supraoptic nuclei in central cardiovascular regulation in the cat. *Am J Physiol* 1980;239:R137–R142.

91. Levy AG, Lewis T. Heart irregularities, resulting from the inhalation of low percentage of chloroform vapour, and their relationship to ventricular fibrillation. *Heart* 1911/ 12;3:99–111.

92. Aviado DM. Toxicity of aerosol propellants in the respiratory and circulatory systems. IX. Summary of the most toxic: trichlorofluoromethane. *Toxicology* 1975;3:311–319.

93. Aviado DM, Belej MA. Toxicity of aerosol propellants in the respiratory and circulatory systems. V. Ventricular function in the dog. *Toxicology* 1975;3:79–86.

94. Harris WS. Cardiac toxicity of aerosol propellants. In: *Proceedings of the second annual conference on environmental toxicology.* Wright-Patterson AFB, Oh: Aerospace Medical Research Laboratory; 1971:23–28.

95. Hays HW. Etiology of cardiac arrhythmias. In: *Proceedings of the third annual conference on environmental toxicology.* Wright-Patterson AFB, Oh: Aerospace Medical Research Laboratory; 1972:173–184.

96. Wills JH. Sensitization of the heart to catecholamine-induced arrhythmia. In: *Proceedings of the third annual conference on environmental toxicology.* Wright-Patterson AFB, Oh: Aerospace Medical Research Laboratory; 1972:249–258.

97. Trochimowicz HJ, Reinhardt CF, Mullin LS, Azar A, Karrh BW. Cardiac sensitization studies in dogs with myocardial infarctions. In: *Proceedings of the fifth annual conference on environmental toxicology.* Wright-Patterson AFB, OH: Aerospace Medical Research Laboratory; 1974:135–144.

98. Clark DG, Tinston DJ. The influence of fluorocarbon propellants on the arrhythmogenic activities of adrenaline and isoprenaline. In: Proceedings of the European Society's Study on Drug Toxicity XIII Meeting, pp. 212–217, Berlin.

99. Mullin LS, Azar A, Reinhardt CF, Smith PE, Fabryka EF. Halogenated hydrocarbon-induced cardiac arrhythmias associated with release of endogenous epinephrine. *Am Ind Hyg Assoc J* 1972;33:389–396.

100. Doherty RE, Aviado DM. Toxicity of aerosol propellants in the respiratory and circulatory systems. VI. Influence of cardiac and pulmonary vascular lesions in the rat. *Toxicology* 1975;3:213–224.

101. Reinhardt CF, Maxfield ME. Epinephrine-induced cardiac arrhythmia potential of some common industrial solvents. *J Occup Med* 1973;15:953–955.

102. Carlson GP. Epinephrine-induced cardiac arrhythmias in rabbits exposed to tetrachloroethylene. *Toxicol Lett* 1983;19:113–117.

103. Loscalzo B, Bianchi A, Robertaccio A. Intossicazione sperimentale acute con 1-2 dichoroetano: effetti sul cuore, sulla pressione arteriosa, e sulla attività respiratoria. *Lav Um* 1959;11:554–566.

104. Andreuzzi P, Capodeglio E. Comportamento dell'apparato cardiovascular nell' intossictzione sperimentale acuta, sull'animale in toto e sul preparato suorepolmone, da tetracluoruro di carbonjio e dicloroetano. *Folia Med* 1958;41:1007–1018.

105. Johnson HE, Shanor SP. Electrocardiographic findings in dogs inhaling the vapors of diverse chlorinated hydrocarbons. *Toxicol Appl Pharmacol* 1968;12:297 (abst).

106. Saitanov AO, Arsen'eva SS. Electrocardiographic changes in acute dichloroethane poisoning. *Gig Tr Prof Zabol* 1969;13:49–50.

107. Herman H, Vial J. Nouvelles syncopes cardiaques par association toxique de l'adrenaline et des divers produits organiques volatils. *CR Soc Biol* 1935;119:1316–1317.

108. Meek WJ, Hathaway HR, Orth OS. The effects of ether, chloroform, and cyclopropane on cardiac automaticity. *J Pharmacol Exp Ther* 1937;61:240–252.
109. Aviado DM, Belej MA. Toxicity of aerosol propellants on the respiratory and circulatory systems. I. Cardiac arrhythmia in the mouse. *Toxicology* 1974;2:31–42.
110. Simaan JA, Aviado DM. Hemodynamic effects of aerosol propellants. I. Cardiac depression in the dog. *Toxicology* 1975;5:127–138.
111. Cornish HH, Adefuin J. Ethanol potentiation of halogenated aliphatic solvent toxicity. *Am Ind Hyg Assoc J* 1966;27:57–61.
112. Belej MA, Smith DG, Aviado DM. Toxicity of aerosol propellants in the respiratory and circulatory systems. IV. Cardiotoxicity in the monkey. *Toxicology* 1974;2:381–395.
113. Pantaleoni G, Zoccolillo L. Toxicology of the aliphatic halogenated hydrocarbons containing fluorine. *Ann Inst Super Sanit* 1977;13:343–351.
114. Burgison M, O'Malley WE, Heisse CK, Forrest JW, Krantz JC Jr. Anesthesia XLVI. Fluorinated ethylenes and cardiac arrhythmias induced by epinephrine. *J Pharmacol Exp Ther* 1955;114:470–472.
115. Zakhari S. Cardiovascular effects of propylene dichloride on canine heart. Pp. 1–20. *CPSC Prog Rep* 1977;16(CPSC-C-75-078):1–20.
116. Taylor GJ IV, Harris WS. Cardiac toxicity of aerosol propellants. *JAMA* 1970;214:81–85.
117. Hall KD, Norris FH. Fluothane sensitization of dog heart to action of epinephrine. *Anesthesiology* 1958;19:631–641.
118. Raventos J. The action of fluothane: a new volatile anesthetic. *Br J Pharmacol* 1956;11:394–410.
119. Zakhari S, Aviado DM. Hemodynamic effects of methylene chloride in anesthetized dogs. *CPSC Prog Rep* 1977;5(CPSC-C-75-078):1–25.
120. VanPoznak A, Artusio JF. Anesthetic properties of a series of fluorinated compounds. I. Fluorinated hydrocarbons. *Toxicol Appl Pharmacol* 1960;2:363–373.
121. Morris LE, Noltensmeyer MH, White JM Jr. Epinephrine-induced cardiac irregularities in the dog during anesthesia with trichloroethylene, cyclopropane, ethyl chloride, and chloroform. *Anesthesiology* 1953;14:153–158.
122. Carr CJ, Burgison RM, Vitcha JF. Anesthesia. XXXIV. Chemical constitution of hydrocarbons and cardiac automaticity. *J Pharmacol Exp Ther* 1949;97:1–3.
123. Aviado DM. Toxicity of propellants. *Prog Drug Res* 1974;18:365–397.
124. Capodaglio E, Andreuzzi P. Intossicazione sperimentale acute da tetracloruro di carbonio e dichloroetano (granosan). II. Modificazioni emodinamiche ed elettocardiografiche nel preparato "curore-polmone" di coniglio. *Boll Soc Ital Sper* 1958;34:1374–1376.
125. Barzin J. Nouvelle recherches sur la pharmacologie et la toxicologie des solvants organiques employes dans l'industrie. *Arch Int Pharmacodyn* 1940;64:313–353.
126. Van Stee EW, Back KC. Short term inhalation exposure to bromotrifluoromethane. *Toxicol Appl Pharmacol* 1969;15:164–174.
127. Reinhardt CF, Mullin LS, Maxfield ME. Epinephrine-induced cardiac arrhythmia potential of some common industrial solvents. *J Occup Med* 1973;15:953–955.
128. Shargel L, Koss R. Determination of fluorinated hydrocarbon propellants in blood of dogs after aerosol administration. *J Pharm Sci* 1972;61:1445–1449.
129. Mullin LS, Reinhardt CF, Heminsway RE. Cardiac arrhythmias and blood levels associated with inhalation of halon 1301. *Am Ind Hyg Assoc J* 1979;40:653–658.
130. Trochimowicz HJ. Blood levels of fluorocarbon during and after acute inhalation. In: *Proceedings of the Fourth Annual Conference on Environmental Toxicology*. Fairborn, Oh: Aerospace Medical Research Laboratory; 1973:137–148.
131. Hoffmann P. Cardiotoxicity testing of organic solvents by coronary artery ligation in closed-chest rats. *Arch Toxicol* 1987;61:79–82.
132. Vidrio H, Magos GA, Lorenzana-Jimenez M. Electrocardiographic effects of toluene in the anesthetized rat. *Arch Int Pharmacodyn Ther* 1986;279:121–129.
133. Magos GA, Lorenzana-Jimenez M, Vidrio H. Toluene and benzene inhalation influences on ventricular arrhythmias in the rat. *Neurotoxicol Teratol* 1990;12:119–124.
134. Eichbaum FW, Yasaka WJ. Antiarrhythmic effect of solvents: propylene glycol, benzyl alcohol. *Basic Res Cardiol* 1976;71:355–370.
135. Yasaka WJ, Eichbaum FW, Oga S. Antiarrhythmic effects of solvents: II. Effects of propylene glycol and benzyl alcohol on the effective refractory period of isolated rabbit atria. *Cardiovasc Res* 1979;13:717–722.

136. Al-Khudhairi D, Whitwam JG. Autonomic reflexes and the cardiovascular effects of propylene glycol. *Br J Anaesth* 1986;58:897–902.
137. Walter B, Weiss A. Spafolgen akuter Methylchloridvergifung. [Late complications of acute methyl chloride poisoning.] *Med Welt* 1951;20:987–988.
138. Gummert M. The Wilson-block in methyl chloride poisoning. *Z Gesamte Inn Med* 1961;16:677–680.
139. Prezdziak J, Bakula S. Acute poisoning with 1,2-dichloroethane. *Wiad Lek* 1975; 28:983–987.
140. MacDougall IC, Isles C, Oliver JS, Clark JC, Spilg WG. Fatal outcome following inhalation of Tipp-Ex. *Scott Med J* 1987;32:55.
141. Konietzko H, Elster I, Schomann P, Weichardt H. Field studies in the solvent industry. 4. Arrhythmias due to trichloroethylene. *Zentralbl Arbeitsmed* 1975;25:139–141.
142. Astrom T, Jonsson A, Jarvholm B. Exposure to fluorocarbon during the filling and repair of air-conditioning systems in cars—a case report. *Scand J Work Environ Health* 1987;13:527–528.
143. Aviado DM. Cardiopulmonary effects of fluorocarbon compounds. In: *Proceedings of the second annual conference on environmental toxicology.* Wright-Patterson AFB, Oh: Aerospace Medical Research Laboratory; 1971:31–39.
144. Blaha K, Majkus V, Lukes M, Maracek B. Zur Grade der reflecktorischen Verbindungen der oberen und unteren Luftwege. *HNO* 1970;18:73–74.
145. Kaufman J, Chen JC, Wright GW. The effect of trigeminal resection on reflex bronchoconstriction after nasal and nasopharyngeal irritation in man. *Am Rev Respir Dis* 1970;101:768–769.
146. Alarie Y. Irritating properties of airborne materials to the upper respiratory tract. *Arch Environ Health* 1966;13:433–449.
147. Angell James JE, Daly MDeB. Reflex respiratory and cardiovascular effects of stimulation of receptors in the nose of the dog. *J Physiol* 1972;220:673–696.
148. Lamb LE, Dermksian G, Sarnoff CA. Significant cardiac arrhythmias induced by common respiratory maneuvers. *Am J Cardiol* 1958;2:563–571.
149. Sellick H, Widdicombe JG. Vagal deflation and inflation reflexes mediated by lung irritant receptors. *J Exp Physiol* 1970;55:153–163.
150. Zakhari S, Bianchi A. Acute inhalational, oral and intraperitoneal toxicity of methyl chloroform in mice. In: Goldberg E, ed. *Methyl chloroform and trichloroethylene in the environment.* Boca Raton, FL: CRC Press; 1977:17–29.
151. Van Stee EW, Harris AM, Horton ML, Back KC. Toxic hazards evaluation of new Air Force fire extinguishing agents. In: *Proceedings of the fifth annual conference on environmental toxicology.* Wright-Patterson, OH: Aerospace Medical Research Laboratory; 1974:155–167.
152. Kawakami T, Takano T, Araki R. Enhanced arrhythmogenicity of freon 113 by hypoxia in the perfused rat heart. *Toxicol Ind Health* 1990;6:493–498.
153. Kawakami T, Araki R. Synergistic interaction of tri and tetra-chloroethylene, hypoxia, and ethanol on the atrioventricular conduction of the perfused rat heart. *Ind Health* 1988;26:25–33.
154. Drew RT, Taylor GJ. Cardiophysiological studies with stressed animals. In: *Proceedings of the fifth annual conference on environmental toxicology.* Wright-Patterson AFB, OH: Aerospace Medical Research Laboratory; 1974:121–129.
155. Clay KL, Murphy RC. On the metabolic acidosis of ethylene glycol intoxication. *Toxicol Appl Pharmacol* 1977;39:39–49.
156. Herd PA, Lipsky M, Martin HF. Cardiovascular effects of 1,1,1-trichloroethane. *Arch Environ Health* 1974;28:227–233.
157. Zakhari S, Snyder D. Contractile effects of methylene chloride on isolated canine papillary muscle. *CPSC Prog Rep* 1977;14(CPSC-C-75-078):1–13.
158. Zakhari S, Snyder DL, Aviado DM. Cardiopulmonary and carboxyhemoglobin changes following methylene chloride inhalation in dogs. *CPSC Prog Rep* 1977; 10(CPSC-C-75-078):1–33.
159. Kobayashi S, Hutcheon DE, Regan J. Cardiopulmonary toxicity of tetrachloroethylene. *J Toxicol Environ Health* 1982;10:23–30.
160. Kilen SM, Harris WS. Direct depression of myocardial contractility by the aerosol propellant gas, dichlorodifluoromethane. *J Pharmacol Exp Ther* 1972;183:245–255.
161. Taylor GJ, Drew RT. Cardiovascular effects of chronic and acute fluorocarbon 12 ex-

posures on rabbits, AMRL-TR-73-125. In: *Proceedings of the fourth annual conference on environmental toxicology.* Wright-Patterson AFB, Fairborn, OH: Aerospace Medical Research Laboratory; 1973:117–125.

162. Terpolilli RN, Davis RA, Peterson GR, Back K. The effects of bromochlorodifluoromethane on contractility and cardiac tissue levels of high energy metabolites. *Toxicol Appl Pharmacol* 1978;45:336–337.

163. Zakhari S. Cardiovascular effects of ethylene chloride in anesthetized dogs. *CPSC Prog Rep* 1977;15(CPSC-C-75-078):1–19.

164. Zakhari S. Effects of acetylene dichloride (transform) on the canine heart. *CPSC Prog Rep* 1977;17(CPSC-C-75-078):1–31.

165. Van Stee EW, Diamond SS, Harris AM, Horton ML, Back KC. The determination of the negative inotropic effect of exposure of dogs to bromotrifluoromethane. *Toxicol Appl Pharmacol* 1973;26:549–558.

166. Ahmed SS, Levinson GE, Regan TJ. Depression of myocardial contractility with low doses of ethanol in normal man. *Circulation* 1973;48:378–385.

167. Regan TJ, Koroxenidis GJ, Moschos CB, Oldewurtel HA, Lehan PH, Hellems HK. The acute metabolic and hemodynamic responses of the left ventricle to ethanol. *J Clin Invest* 1966;45:270–280.

168. Fisher VJ, Kavaler F. The action of ethanol upon the action potential and contraction of ventricular muscle. *Recent Adv Stud Cardiac Struct Metab* 1975;5:415–422.

169. Regan TJ. Ethyl alcohol and the heart. *Circulation* 1971;44:957–963.

170. Friedman HS. Cardiovascular effects of alcohol with particular reference to the heart. *Alcohol* 1984;1:333–339.

171. DeFelice A, Wilson W, Ambre J. Acute cardiovascular effects of intravenous methanol in the anesthetized dog. *Toxicol Appl Pharmacol* 1976;38:631–638.

172. Nakano J, Moore SE. Effect of different alcohols on the contractile force of the isolated guinea pig myocardium. *Eur J Pharmacol* 1972;20:266–270.

173. Zakhari S. Hemodynamic effects of isoproterenol in the anesthetized dog. In: Goldberg L, ed. *Isopropanol and ketones in the environment.* Boca Raton, FL: CRC Press; 1977:37–45.

174. Nakano J, Moore SE, Kessinger CL. Myocardial depressant action of ethyl acetate. *J Pharm Pharmacol* 1973;25:1018–1020.

175. Zakhari S. Hemodynamic effects of methyl ethyl ketone after inhalation in the dog. In: Goldberg L, ed. *Isopropanol and ketones in the environment.* Boca Raton, FL: CRC Press; 1977:79–86.

176. Zakhari S. Myocardial and hemodynamic effects of methyl isobutyl ketone in the dog. In: Goldberg L, ed. *Isopropanol and ketones in the environment.* Boca Raton, FL: CRC Press; 1977:121–128.

177. Raje RR. In vitro toxicity of *n*-hexane and 2,5-hexanedione using isolated perfused rabbit heart. *J Toxicol Environ Health* 1983;11:879–884.

178. Kirch W, Schwarz W, Von Gizycki C. Congestive cardiomyopathy due to chronic inhalation of trichlorethylene. *Arch Toxicol* 1983;(suppl)5:322–325.

179. Roth RP, Jia-Ruey Lo R, Drew RT. Dichloromethane inhalation and drug metabolizing enzymes: the effect of chemical treatment with mixed function oxidase inducing and inhibiting agents on carboxyhemoglobin formation. In: *Proceedings of the fourth annual conference on environmental toxicology.* Wright-Patterson AFB, Oh: Aerospace Medical Research Laboratory; 1973:279–289.

180. Kubic VL, Anders MW, Engel RR, Barlow CH, Caughey WS. Metabolism of dihalomethanes to carbon monoxide. I. In vivo studies. *Drug Metab Dispos* 1974;2:53–57.

181. Ratney RS, Wegman DH, Elkins HB. In vivo conversion of methylene chloride to carbon monoxide. *Arch Environ Health* 1974;28:223–226.

182. DiVencenzo GD, Hamilton ML. Fate and disposition of methylene chloride in the rat. *Toxicol Appl Pharmacol* 1975;32:385–393.

183. Stewart RD, Hake CL. Paint-remover hazard. *JAMA* 1976;235:398–401.

184. Browning E. Dichloromethane. *Encyclopedia Occup Health Safety* 1983;1:624–626.

185. Juhasz-Nagy A, Aviado DM. Role of carboxyhemoglobin formation in the cardiac effects of methylene chloride. *CPSC Prog Rep* 1977;11(CPSC-C-75-078):1–45.

186. Gross DR, Kitzman JV, Adams HR. Cardiovascular effects of intravenous administration of propylene glycol and of oxytetracycline in propylene glycol in calves. *Am J Vet Res* 1979;40:783–791.

187. Olsen RE. Contractile proteins of heart muscle. *Am J Med* 1961;30:692–707.

188. Merin RG. Myocardial metabolism for the toxicologist. *Environ Health Perspect* 1978;26:169–174.
189. Reuter H. Exchange of calcium ions in the mammalian myocardium. Mechanisms and physiological significance. *Circ Res* 1974;34:599–605.
190. Brady AJ. Electrophysiology of cardiac muscle. In: Langer GA, Brady AJ, eds. *The mammalian myocardium.* New York: Wiley; 1974:135–161.
191. Zakhari S. Mechanism of action of calcium antagonists on myocardial and smooth muscle membranes. *Drugs Exp Clin Res* 1986¹I:817–829.
192. Van Stee EW, Horton ML, Harris AM, Back KC. The effect of 90-minute exposures to bromotrifluoromethane on myocardial metabolism in the dog. In: *Proceedings of the fourth annual conference on environmental toxicology.* Wright-Patterson AFB, Fairborn, OH: Aerospace Medical Research Laboratory; 1973:65–83.
193. Sonnenblick EH, Ross J Jr, Covell JW, Kaiser G, Braunwald E. Velocity of contraction: a major determinant of myocardial oxygen consumption. *J Clin Invest* 1965; 44:1099.
194. Aviado DM, Smith DG. Toxicity of aerosol propellants in the respiratory and circulatory systems. VIII. Respiration and circulation in primates. *Toxicology* 1975;3:241–252.
195. Belej MA, Aviado DM. Cardiopulmonary toxicity of propellants for aerosols. *J Clin Pharmacol* 1975;15:105–115.
196. Zanger RC, Sasser LB, Mahlum DD, Abhold RH, Springer DL. Cardiovascular effects in rats following exposure to a high-boiling coal liquid. *Fundam Appl Toxicol* 1987;9:659–667.
197 Chentanez T, Tantrarungroj K, Sadavongivivad C. Correlation between positive chronotropic effect and norepinephrine release induced by acetone in the rat right atrium. *Toxicol Lett* 1987;37:183–193.
198. Klatsky AL. The cardiovascular effects of alcohol. *Alcohol* 1987;1:117–124.
199. Singh PP, Junnarkar AY, Seshagirirao C, et al. A pharmacological study of propane-1,2-diol. *Arzneimittelforschung* 1982;32:1443–1446.
200. Tolonen M, Hernberg S, Nurminen M, Tiitola K. A follow-up study of coronary heart disease in viscose rayon workers exposed to carbon disulfide. *Br J Ind Med* 1975;32:1–10.
201. Hanig JP, Herman EH. Toxic responses of the heart and vascular systems. In: Amdur MO, Doull J, Klaassen CD, eds. *Casarett and Doull's toxicology: the basic science of poisons, 4 ed.* New York: Pergamon Press, 430–462.
202. Bello S, Halton DM. Occupational chemical exposures and the heart. Canadian Center for Occupational Health and Safety, Report No. P85-5E, 1985, 12 pp.
203. Cunningham VJ. Effects of a single exposure to carbon disulfide on the rate of urea production and on plasma free fatty acid and glucose concentrations in the rat. *Br J Ind Med* 1975;32:140–146.
204. Cunningham VJ, Holt DE. The turnover of blood glucose and plasma free fatty acids in the rat after acute carbon disulfide intoxication. *Biochem Pharmacol* 1977;26:1625–1629.
205. Wronska-Nofer T. Aortic phospholipid synthesis in experimental carbon disulfide intoxication in rats. *Int Arch Occup Environ Health* 1976;36:229–234.
206. Wronska-Nofer T, Laurman W, Rosloneck W. Selected risk factors of ischemic heart disease in workers under conditions of chronic occupational exposure to carbon disulfide. *Med Pr* 1990;41:299–305.
207. Takahashi S, Tanabe K, Maseda C, Shiono H, Fuku Y. Increased plasma free fatty acid and triglyceride levels after single administration of toluene in rabbits. *J Toxicol Environ Health* 1988;25:87–96.
208. Austin MA. Plasma triglyceride and coronary heart disease. *Arteriosclerosis Thromb* 1991;11:2–14.
209. Klatsky AL, Armstrong MA, Friedman GD. Risk of cardiovascular mortality in alcohol drinkers, ex-drinkers, and nondrinkers. *Am J Cardiol* 1990;66:1237–1242.
210. Rimm EB, Giovannucci EL, Willett WC, Colditz GA, Ascherio A, Posner B, Stampfer MJ. Prospective study of alcohol consumption and risk of coronary disease in men. *Lancet* 1991;338:464–468.
211. Balazs T, Ferrans VJ. Cardiac lesions induced by chemicals. *Environ Health Perspect* 1978;26:181–191.
212. Heppel LA, Neal PA, Highman B, Porterfield VT. Toxicology of 1,2-dichloropropane

(propylene dichloride). I. Studies of effect of daily inhalations. *J Ind Hyg Toxicol* 1946;28:1–8.

213. Heppel LA, Highman B, Peake EG. Toxicology of 1,2-dichloropropane. IV. Effect of related exposures to low concentrations of the vapor. *J Hyg Toxicol* 1948;30:189–191.

214. Freundt KJ, Liebaldt GP, Lieberwirth E. Toxicology studies on trans-1,2-dichloroethylene. *Toxicology* 1977;7:141–153.

215. Alexander CS, Sekhri KK, Nagasawa HT. Alcoholic cardiomyopathy in mice: electron microscopic observations. *J Mol Cell Cardiol* 1977;9:247–254.

216. Vasdev SC, Chakravarti RN, Subrahmanyam D, Jain AC, Wahi PL. Myocardial lesions induced by prolonged alcohol feeding in rhesus monkeys. *Cardiovasc Res* 1975;9:134–140.

217. Klugmann FB, Decorti G, Mallardi F, Klugmann S, Baldini L. Effect of polyethylene glycol 400 on adriamycin toxicity in mice. *Eur J Cancer Clin Oncol* 1984;20:405–410.

218. Matoba R, Funahashi M, Fujitani N, Abe T, Nogi H. An autopsy case of sudden death after toluene sniffing. *Nippon Hoigaku Zasshi* 1987;41:438–441.

219. Claydon SM. Myocardial degeneration in chronic solvent abuse. *Med Sci Law* 1988;28:217–218.

220. Cohr K, Stokholm J. Toluene: a toxicologic review. *Scand J Work Environ Health* 1979;5:71–90.

221. Hardin BD, Goad PT, Burg JR. Developmental toxicity of diethylene glycol monomethyl ether (diEGME). *Fundam Appl Toxicol* 1986;6:430–439.

222. Hardin BD, Niemeier RW, Smith RJ, Kuczuk MH. Teratogenicity of 2-ethoxyethanol by dermal application. *Drug Chem Toxicol* 1982;5:277–294.

223. Toraason M, Stringer B, Stober P, Hardin BD. Electrocardiographic study of rat fetuses exposed to ethylene glycol monomethyl ether (EGME). *Teratology* 1985;32:33–39.

224. Toraason M, Stringer B, Smith R. Ornithine decarboxylase activity in the neonatal rat heart following prenatal exposure to ethylene glycol monomethyl ether. *Drug Chem Toxicol* 1986;9:1–14.

225. Nelson BK, Setzer JV, Brightwell WS, Mathinos PR, Kuczuk MH, Weaver TE, Goad PT. Comparative inhalation teratogenicity of four glycol ether solvents and an amino derivative in rats. *Environ Health Perspect* 1984;57:261–271.

226. Nelson BK, Vorhees CV, Scott WJ Jr, Hastings L. Effects of 2-methoxyethanol on fetal development, postnatal behavior, and embryonic intracellular pH of rats. *Neurotoxicol Teratol* 1989;11:273–284.

227. Nelson BK, Brightwell WS, MacKenzie DR, Khan A, Burg JR, Weigel WW, Goad PT. Teratological assessment of methanol and ethanol at high inhalation levels in rats. *Fundam Appl Toxicol* 1985;5:727–736.

228. Webster WS, Germain MA, Lipson A, Walsh D. Alcohol and congenital heart defects: an experimental study in mice. *Cardiovasc Res* 1984;18:335–338.

229. Nelson BK, Brightwell WS, MacKenzie-Taylor DR, Khan A. Teratogenicity of n-propanol and isopropanol administered at high inhalation concentrations to rats. *Food Chem Toxicol* 1988;26:247–254.

230. George JD, Price CJ, Marr MC, Sadler BM. Developmental toxicity of 1,1,1-trichloroethane in CD rats. *Fundam Appl Toxicol* 1989;13:641–651.

231. Fang TT, Bruyere HJ Jr, Kargas SA, Nishikawa T, Takagi Y, Gilbert EF. Ethyl alcohol-induced cardiovascular malformations in the chick embryo. *Teratology* 1987;35:95–104.

232. Uphoff C, Nyquist-Battie C, Toth R. Cardiac muscle development in mice exposed to ethanol in utero. *Teratology* 1984;30:119–129.

233. Daft PA, Johnston MC, Sulik KK. Abnormal heart and great vessel development following acute ethanol exposure in mice. *Teratology* 1986;33:93–104.

234. Abel EL. Prenatal effects of alcohol. *Drug Alcohol Depend* 1984;14:1–10.

235. Zierler S. Maternal drugs and congenital heart disease. *Obstet Gynecol* 1985;65:155–165.

236. Tikkanen J, Heinonen OP. Cardiovascular malformations and organic solvent exposure during pregnancy in Finland. *Am J Ind Med* 1988;14:1–8.

237. Tikkanen J, Kurppa K, Timonen H, Holmberg PC. Cardiovascular malformations, work attendance, and occupational exposures during pregnancy in Finland. *Am J Ind Med* 1988;14:197–204.

238. Tikkanen J, Heinonen OP. Maternal exposure to chemical and physical factors during pregnancy and cardiovascular malformations in the offspring. *Teratology* 1991;43:591–600.
239. Eskenazi B, Bracken MB, Holford TR, Grady J. Exposure to organic solvents and hypertensive disorders of pregnancy. *Am J Ind Med* 1988;14:177–188.
240. McDonald JC, Lavoie J, Cote R, McDonald AD. Chemical exposures at work in early pregnancy and congenital defect: a case-referent study. *Br J Ind Med* 1987;44:527–533.
241. Mercier M, Lans M, De Gerlache J. Mutagenicity, carcinogenicity, and teratogenicity of halogenated hydrocarbon solvents. In: Kirsch-Volders M, ed. *Mutagenicity, carcinogenicity, and teratogenicity of industrial pollutants*. New York, 1984:281–324.
242. Aliverti V, Bonanomi L, Giavini E, Leonee VG, Mariana L. Effects of glycerol formal on embryonic development in the rat. *Toxicol Appl Pharmacol* 1980;56:93–100.
243. Dinwiddie SH, Reich T, Cloninger CR. Solvent use as a precursor to intravenous drug abuse. *Compr Psychiatry* 1991;32:133–140.
244. Lieber CS. Mechanism of ethanol induced hepatic injury. *Pharmacol Ther* 1990;46:1–41.
245. Koop DR. Oxidative and reductive metabolism by cytochrome P450 2E1. *FASEB J* 1992;6:724–730.
246. Zimmerman HJ. Effects of alcohol on other hepatotoxins. *Alcoholism* 1986;10:3–15.
247. Strublet O. Alcohol potentiation of liver injury. *Fundam Appl Toxicol* 1978;4:144–151.
248. Strublet O. Interactions between ethanol and other hepatotoxic agents. *Biochem Pharmacol* 1980;29:1445–1449.
249. Coon MJ, Koop DR, Reeve LE, Crump BL. Alcohol metabolism and toxicity: role of cytochrome P450. *Fundam Appl Toxicol* 1984;4:234–243.
250. Ishak KG, Zimmerman HJ, Ray MB. Alcoholic liver disease: pathologic, pathogenetic and clinical aspects. *Alcoholism Clin Exp Res* 1991;15:45–66.
251. Plaa GL. Toxic responses of the liver. In: Doull J, Klaassen CD, Amdur MO, eds. *Alcoholic liver pathology*. Toronto: Addiction Research Foundation of Ontario; 1975:199–224.
252. Dossing M, Baelum J, Hansen SH, Lundqvist GR. Effect of ethanol, cimetidine, and propranolol on toluene metabolism in man. *Int Arch Occup Environ Health* 1984;54:309–315.
253. Kim SG, Williams DE, Schuetz EG, Guzelian PS, Novak RF. Pyridine induction of cytochrome P-450 in the rat: role of P-450j (alcohol-inducible form) in pyridine *N*-oxidation. *J Pharmacol Exp Ther* 1988;246:1175–1182.
254. Johansson I, Ingelman-Sundberg M. Benzene metabolism by ethanol-, acetone-, and benzene-inducible cytochrome P-450 (IIE1) in rat and rabbit liver microsomes. *Cancer Res* 1988;48:5387–5390.
255. Koop DR, Laethem CL, Schnier GG. Identification of ethanol-inducible P450 isozyme 3a (P450IIE1) as a benzene and phenol hydroxylase. *Toxicol Appl Pharmacol* 1989;98:278–288.
256. Terelius Y, Ingelman-Sundberg M. Metabolism of *n*-pentane by ethanol-inducible cytochrome P-450 in liver microsomes and reconstituted membranes. *Env J Biochem* 1986;161:303–308.
257. Johansson I, Ingelman-Sundberg M. Carbon tetrachloride-induced lipid peroxidation dependent on an ethanol-inducible form of rabbit liver microsomal cytochrome P-450. *FEBS Lett* 1985;183:265–269.
258. Brady JF, Li D, Ishizaki H, Lee M, Ning SM, Xiao F, Yang CS. Induction of cytochromes P450IIE1 and P450IIB1 by secondary ketones and the role of P450IIE1 in chloroform metabolism. *Toxicol Appl Pharmacol* 1989;100:342–349.
259. Gruenke LD, Konopka K, Koop DR, Waskell L. Characterization of halothane oxidation by hepatic microsomes and purified cytochrome P-450 using gas chromatographic mass spectrometric assay. *J Pharmacol Exp Ther* 1988;246:454–459.
260. Olson MJ, Kims SG, Reidy CA, Johnson JT, Novak RF. Oxidation of 1,1,1,2-tetrafluoroethane in rat liver microsomes is catalyzed primarily by cytochrome P-450IIE1. *Drug Metab Dispos* 1990;19:298–303.
261. Koop DR, Coon MJ. Ethanol oxidation and toxicity: role of alcohol P-450 oxygenase. *Alcoholism Clin Exp Res* 1986;10:44s–49s.
262. Brady JF, Lee MJ, Li M, Ishizaki H, Yang CS. Diethyl ether as a substrate for acetone/ethanol-inducible cytochrome P-450 and as an inducer for cytochrome(s)P-450. *Mol Pharmacol* 1987;33:148–154.

263. Brady JF, Xiao F, Ning SM, Yang CS. Metabolism of methyl *tertiary*-butyl ether by rat hepatic microsomes. *Arch Toxicol* 1990;64:157–160.

264. Regan TJ, Ettinger PO, Haider B, Ahmed SS, Oldewurtel HA, Lyons MM. The role of ethanol in cardiac disease. *Annu Rev Med* 1977;28:393–409.

265. Regan TJ, Ettinger PO. Varied cardiac abnormalities in alcoholics. *Alcoholism Clin Exp Res* 1979;3:40–45.

266. Dyer AR, Stamler J, Paul O, et al. Alcohol consumption, cardiovascular risk factors, and mortality in two Chicago epidemiologic studies. *Circulation* 1977;56:1067.

267. Turner TB, Mezey E, Kimball AW. Measurement of alcohol-related effects in man: chronic effects in relation to levels of alcohol consumption. *Johns Hopkins Med J* 1977;141:273.

268. Koskenvuo M, Kaprio J, Kesaniemi A, Poikolainen K. Alcohol-related diseases associated with ischaemic heart disease: a three-year follow-up of middle-aged male hospital patients. *Alcohol Alcoholism* 1986;221:251–256.

269. Gunnar RM, Sutton GC, Pietras RJ, Tobin JR. Alcohol cardiomyopathy. In: Downing HF, ed. *Disease-a-month*. Chicago: Year Book Medical Publishers; 1971:3.

270. Evans W. Alcoholic myocardiopathy. *Prog Cardiovasc Dis* 1964;7:151.

271. McDonald CD, Burch GE, Walsh JJ. Alcoholic cardiomyopathy managed with prolonged bed rest. *Ann Intern Med* 1971;74:681.

272. Alexander CS. Idiopathic heart disease. *Am J Med* 1966;41:213.

273. Demakis JG, Rahimtoola SH, Sutton GC, Gunnar RM. The natural course of alcoholic cardiomyopathy. *Ann Intern Med* 1974;80:293.

274. Ferrans VJ, Hibbs RG, Weilbaecher DG, et al. Alcoholic cardiomyopathy: a histochemical study. *Am Heart J* 1965;69:748–765.

275. Bulloch RT, Pearce MB, Murphy ML, et al. Myocardial lesions in idiopathic and alcoholic cardiomyopathy. *Am J Cardiol* 1972;29:15.

276. Wendt VE, Wu C, Balcon E, Doty G, Bing RJ. Hemodynamic and metabolic effects of chronic alcoholism in man. *Am J Cardiol* 1965;15:175.

277. Wendt VE, Ajluni R, Bruce TA, Prasad AS, Bing RJ. Acute effects of alcohol on the human myocardium. *Am J Cardiol* 1966;17:804–812.

278. Brigden W, Robinson J. Alcoholic heart disease. *Br Med J* 1964;2:1283–1289.

279. Burch GE, DePasquale NP. Alcoholic cardiomyopathy. *Am J Cardiol* 1969;23:723–734.

280. Mason DT, Spann JF Jr, Hughes JL, Zelis R, Amsterdam EA. Alcohol and the heart. *Heart Bull* 1971;20:1–3.

281. Rubin E, Katz AM, Lieber CS, Stein EP, Puszkin S. Muscle damage produced by chronic ethanol consumption. *Am J Pathol* 1976;83:499–515.

282. Buckingham TA, Kennedy HL, Goenjian AK, Vasilomanolakis EC, Shriver KK, Sprague MK, Lyyski D. Cardiac arrhythmias in a population admitted to an acute alcoholic detoxification center. *Am Heart J* 1985;110:961–965.

283. Singer K, Lundberg WB. Ventricular arrhythmias associated with the ingestion of alcohol. *Ann Intern Med* 1972;77:247–248.

284. Ettinger PO, Wu CF, Cruz CD, Weisse AB, Ahmed SS, Regan TJ. Arrhythmias and the "holiday heart": alcohol-associated cardiac rhythm disorders. *Am Heart J* 1978;95:555–562.

285. Cohen JL, Lee W, Lien EJ. Dependence of toxicity on molecular structure: group theory analysis. *J Pharm Sci* 1974;63:1068–1072.

286. Truhaut R, Boudene C, Jouany JM, Bouant A. Application of the physiogram to the investigation of the acute toxicology of chlorinated solvents. *J Eur Toxicol* 1972;5:284–292.

287. Sato A, Nakajima T. A structure–activity relationship of some chlorinated hydro-carbons. *Arch Environ Health* 1979;34:69–75.

288. Von Oettingen WF. The halogenated hydrocarbons: their toxicity and potential dangers. *J Ind Hyg Toxicol* 1937;19:349–448.

289. Rubin J, Rubin E. Myocardial toxicity of alcohols, aldehydes, and glycols, including alcoholic cardiomyopathy. In: Van Stee VW, ed. *Cardiovascular toxicology*. New York: Raven Press; 1982:353–363.

Cardiovascular Toxicology, Second Edition,
edited by Daniel Acosta, Jr.
Raven Press, Ltd., New York © 1992.

15

Environmental Tobacco Smoke Exposure and Occupational Heart Disease

Domingo M. Aviado

Atmospheric Health Sciences, Short Hills, New Jersey 07078

In 1991, the Occupational Safety and Health Administration (1) requested information on exposures and potential adverse health effects that may be associated with poor indoor air quality in the work environment, including information on exposure to environmental tobacco smoke (ETS). One review article, which focused on heart disease and which was published prior to the agency's request, concluded as follows: "the combination of epidemiological studies with demonstration of physiological changes with exposure to ETS, together with biochemical evidence that elements of ETS have significant adverse effects on the cardiovascular system, leads to the conclusion that ETS causes heart disease" (2). Others, however, have expressed conflicting interpretations of human and animal studies on ETS, concluding that it has not been scientifically demonstrated that ETS exposure increases the risk of heart disease in nonsmokers (3,4). The ongoing debate should not only consider the claimed association between ETS work exposure and heart disease in particular, but also occupational heart disease in general. The primary purpose of this chapter is to review the toxicological basis for identifying chemical substances that may be associated with heart disease in the workplace.

At the outset, it should be emphasized that proof of an association between ETS workplace exposure and heart disease is a complex process. Workers, such as garage attendants, may be exposed to one or more substances (such as carbon monoxide) found both in ETS and in other sources, so the total exposure is the sum of two or more sources, for example, vehicular emissions, ambient air pollution, and ETS. The same group of workers may have varied personal habits that have been reported to be associated with heart disease, such as consumption of cholesterol and fats and xanthine beverages at the employee's cafeteria, physical inactivity on the job, and job-related stress. Outside the workplace, there are additional potential risk factors for heart disease, such as lack of leisure time exercise, dietary cooking fat and salt content, household exposure to cooking gas, gas heaters, and household solvents. Other major risk factors reported for heart disease include the worker's familial history of heart disease, diabetes, hypertension, hyperlipidemia, and obesity. Any conclusion on a possible role of ETS in heart disease necessitates controlling for such risk factors.

INVESTIGATIVE METHODS FOR INDUSTRIAL CHEMICALS

Although there are over 300 potentially hazardous chemicals in the workplace, there are less than three scores of industrial chemicals that have been suggested to be associated with heart disease such as ischemic heart disease, coronary atherosclerosis, and cardiac arrhythmia and cardiomyopathy. Although heart disease is the leading cause of death in the United States, occupational exposure to chemicals is considered less prevalent and less important than risk factors in the diet, in the environment, and in familial or inherited susceptibility to cardiovascular diseases.

Although it is relatively simple to establish a strong association between exposure to halogenated solvents and cardiac arrhythmias, it is more complex to obtain supportive evidence as to whether chemicals play a major role in coronary ischemic heart disease and atherosclerosis. Occupational heart diseases can be grouped into three major categories. These can be subgrouped according to the method of investigation, which may involve clinical studies, pathological observations, or experimental animal studies (Table 1): (a) *ischemic heart disease* (Methods A, B, and C), including mortality studies, exercise testing for angina pectoris, and coronary blood flow indicators; (b) *coronary atherosclerosis* (Methods D, E, and F), demonstrable in patients by angiography and histopathology, atherosclerosis in experimental animals, and *in vitro* studies of hematologic factors; and (c) *cardiac arrhythmia and myopathy* (Methods G and H), both clinically and experimentally induced. The three groups of methods and eight subgroupings (A to H) are carried over to consideration of occupational heart disease associated with exposure to chemicals in the course of manufacturing and processing of industrial products. The chemicals supposedly associated with occupational heart diseases are listed in Table 1 under five classes: one inorganic and four organics. Each compound is identified by notations on investigative methods A to H.

Inorganic Oxides and Metals

Carbon monoxide is most widely discussed as a major substance in the etiology of occupational heart disease. Workplace exposure to carbon monoxide is encountered when it is generated in manufacturing an industrial product. In the steel industry, carbon monoxide is produced in blast furnace

TABLE 1. *Industrial chemicals reported to be associated with occupational heart disease*

Industrial chemicals	Ischemic heart disease	Coronary atherosclerosis	Arrythmias and myopathy
Inorganics: oxides and metals			
Carbon monoxide[a]	A B C	D E F	G H
Carbon dioxide[a]			G
Nitrogen oxides[a]			G
Arsenic	A		
Cadmium[a]	A		H
Cobalt	A		
Lead	A	F	H
Nitrogenous compounds			
Nicotine[a]	A		
Aniline[a]		F	
Catechol[a]			G
Dinitrotoluene	A		
Ethylene glycol dinitrate	A C		G
Hydrazine[a]			G
Hydrocyanic acid[a]	C		
Nitroglycerin	A C		H
Pyridine[a]			G
2-Toluidine[a]		F	G
Polynuclear aromatic hydrocarbons	A		
Benzo[a]pyrene[a]		E	
7,12-Dimethyl (*a,h*) anthracene		E	
3-Methylcholanthrene		E	
Nonhalogenated solvents			
Carbon disulfide[a,b]	A B C	D E	H
Acetaldehyde[a]			G
Acetone[a]			G
Benzene[a]			G
Dimethylamine[a]			G
Methylamine[a]			G
Phenol[a]			G H
Toluene[a]			G
Halogenated solvents			
Methyl chloride[a]			G H
Methyl chloroform			G H
Methylene chloride		F	G H
Trichlorofluoromethane			G H

[a]Sidestream smoke (SSS) constituent.
[b]Metabolite carbonyl sulfide is ETS constituent.
Method A, mortality studies; Method B, exercise testing and angina pectoris; Method C, coronary blood flow indicators; Method D, coronary angiography and histopathology; Method E, atherosclerosis in experimental animals; Method F, *in vitro* hematologic factors; Method G, irregular heartbeat; Method H, experimentally induced cardiomyopathy.

smelting of iron ore, cast welding, and vehicular production. Operators of vehicles, parking attendants, tunnel workers, car emission inspectors, tool operators, and traffic police are constantly exposed to exhaust fumes and elevated levels of carboxyhemoglobin in such workers have been reported. All eight subgroups of methods have been applied to arrive at an extensive cardiac toxicologic profile of carbon monoxide (Methods A to H in Table 1). The two other oxides and four heavy metals listed in Table 1 have been less thoroughly investigated.

Among heavy metals reportedly associated with heart disease are arsenic, cadmium, cobalt, and lead. The pathogenesis of heart disease potentially associated with workplace exposure may vary according to volatility of the metallic compound and its exposure level. Cadmium has not been reported to influence the heart directly but may be related to hypertension, which may lead to cardiac complications. Lead may influence the blood and ultimately interfere with cardiac metabolism and function. Arsenic, cobalt, and lead are cellular poisons and there are experimental heart models to support the occurrence of cardiomyopathy from these metals. Only cadmium has been detected in tobacco leaf and tobacco smoke; traces of cadmium are derived from soil.

Nitrogenous Compounds

The ten examples in this group include the following: nicotine (an alkaloid), hydrocyanic acid, and raw products for the manufacture of explosives such as ethylene glycol dinitrate and nitroglycerin. The other six examples (aniline, catechol, dinitrotoluene, hydrazine, pyridine, 2-toluidine) are necessary in the manufacture of pharmaceuticals, pesticides, and dyes. The cardiac toxicologic profiles for each of these compounds are not completely known and have been studied only by one, two, or three methods. The entry on nicotine refers to handling of tobacco leaf, such as cigar manufacturers, kiln dryers, and warehouse operators.

Polynuclear Aromatic Hydrocarbons (PAH)

These are formed as a result of pyrolysis or incomplete combustion of organic materials. There are several hundred PAHs and only a dozen have been reported to be associated with skin tumors via skin painting in mice. Benzo[a]pyrene is the most widely studied compound and only research scientists are occupationally exposed to this single PAH. Workers potentially exposed to PAH mixtures include coke oven operators, creosote wood applicators, asphalt road pavers and roofers, aluminum smelters, and diesel engine operators. Benzo[a]pyrene and two other PAHs listed in Table 1 have been reported to be associated with atherosclerosis in an experimental model. There are no human studies relating to heart disease other than mortality statistics of workers exposed to PAH mixtures.

Nonhalogenated Solvents

Carbon disulfide is a solvent used in the manufacture of viscose rayon, cellophane film, electronic vacuum tubes, sulfur-containing soil disinfectants, and carbon tetrachloride. This is the only solvent for which there are strong data on an association with ischemic heart disease in workers, as well as coronary atherosclerosis in experimental animals. The cardiac toxicologic profile is complete except for the lack of *in vitro* studies on hematologic factors and cardiac susceptibility to arrhythmia. The seven other solvents have not been studied for occurrence of ischemic heart disease and coronary artherosclerosis.

Halogenated Solvents

The author and his colleagues have written monographs on the cardiotoxicity of chlorinated and fluorinated solvents (5–7). Four solvents are identified in Table 1 from the original list of more than 100 solvents that are considered cardiotoxic. The four selected solvents (methyl chloride, methyl chloroform, methylene chloride, and trichlorofluoromethane) are reported to cause fatal cardiac arrhythmia and sudden death in the course of accidental industrial poisonings. Usually it cannot be proved whether cardiac arrest was caused by a direct cardiac effect or the result of respiratory paralysis and coma, since most halogenated solvents are not only cardiotoxic but also central nervous system depressants. Experimental animal studies have supported the potential role of sublethal doses of solvents in cardiac arrhythmias and myopathies, independently of coronary vessels and central nervous system involvement.

Miscellaneous Compounds

Industrial chemicals potentially related to heart disease, but which appear not to directly influence the heart, blood vessels, and circulating blood, are omitted from Table 1. Insecticides, including organophosphates, are reportedly associated with irregular heart rhythms because of their influence on the autonomic nervous system. Chronic obstructive lung disease associated with inorganic dust particles can cause cor pulmonale. Exposure to nephrotoxins, such as mercury and dyes, has been reported to lead to cardiac complications, including congestive heart failure.

CONSTITUENTS OF ENVIRONMENTAL TOBACCO SMOKE

Environmental tobacco smoke is a diluted and aged mixture of constituents derived from either the burning end or cigarette butt: mainstream smoke inhaled from the filtered or unfiltered tip; and sidestream smoke from the lighted end. Nonsmokers sharing a workroom with smoking workers may be exposed to ETS. Sidestream smoke is not inhaled directly by nonsmokers but is diluted immediately by air in the workplace and continuously by air exchanges. The magnitudes of differences between concentrations of substances in mainstream smoke inhaled by the smoker and ETS exposure of nonsmokers have been summarized in a National Research Council monograph (8). The ranges reported in the literature (parts per million or parts per billion) are as follows:

	Mainstream Smoke	ETS
Carbon monoxide	24,900–57,400 ppm	1–18.5 ppm
Nicotine	430,000–1,080,000 ppb	0.5–7.5 ppb
Benzo[a]pyrene	5–11 ppb	0.0001–0.074 ppb

The dilution factors for peak values are as follows: 3100 for carbon monoxide, 144,000 for nicotine, and 148 for benzo[a]pyrene. There is no uniform dilution for all three because of varied levels in mainstream smoke relative to sidestream smoke. The unpredictable fates of vapor components (e.g., carbon monoxide) and particulates (e.g., nicotine and benzo[a]pyrene) are influenced by humidity, temperature, air movement, and adsorption by machinery and furnishings in the workplace.

Work Standards for Industrial Chemicals

The minute levels of carbon monoxide in ETS, up to 3100 times less than the concentration in mainstream smoke, pose a critical challenge to claims that ETS exposure can cause heart disease in nonsmokers. Proponents of the claimed association between ETS exposure and heart disease in general (occupational and nonoccupational) contend that three ETS constituents underlie this relationship: nicotine, carbon monoxide, and polynuclear aromatic hydrocarbons. For completeness, there are 21 reported constituents of sidestream smoke that are also used as industrial chemicals, which are sometimes discussed as potentially associated with heart disease. These are the same 21 industrial chemicals listed in the first column of Table 1 that are manufactured, processed, or emitted in workplaces and are potentially associated with heart disease (marked with superscript a in first column, Table 1). Most halogenated solvents, heavy metals, and polycyclic aromatic hydrocarbons have not been detected in ETS (no superscript in Table 1).

The list of 21 sidestream smoke constituents inputed to ETS in Table 2 is a revision of the author's listing of suspected pulmonary carcinogens in ETS (9,10). Also listed in Table 2 are corresponding threshold limit values (TLVs) for various substances, defined as the recommended standards for 8-hr daily exposure for the prevention of occupational disease (11). Table 2 includes a column of target organs for acute or initial exposure, as well as for chronic or long-term exposure. When TLV levels are exceeded, early and late signs of toxicity appear in skin, mucosa, lungs, liver, kidneys, blood, blood vessels, and nervous system. Manifestations of cardiotoxicity may occur either in acute lethal concentrations (more than 20 times TLV) or repeated exposure to very high, but sublethal, concentrations (more than two to five times TLV, depending on the compound).

TABLE 2. *Sidestream smoke (SSS) constituents with threshold limit values (TLV)*

Chemical name	Acute/ chronic[a]	Max SSS (mg/cig)	TLV (mg/m³)	Cigarette equivalent
Nicotine	M/N	8.2	0.5	6.6
Carbon monoxide	B/N	108	55	50
Methyl chloride	M/N	0.88	10.3	1,170
Cadmium	M/P	0.0007	0.01	1,430
Acetaldehyde	M/P	1.26	180	1,430
Nitrogen oxides	M/N	2.8	50	1,780
Carbon dioxide	N/N	440	9000	2,040
Pyridine	M/H	0.39	16	4,100
Phenol	M/P	0.25	19	7,600
Hydrocyanic acid	B/N	0.11	11	10,000
Methylamine	M/N	0.1	13	13,000
Benzene	N/B	0.24	32	13,300
Catechol	D/K	0.14	23	16,500
Aniline	B/B	0.011	8	44,000
Dimethylamine	M/H	0.036	18	50,000
Carbonyl sulfide	N/V	0.0546	30b	54,945
Hydrazine	M/H	0.00009	0.13	145,000
Acetone	M/N	1	1780	178,000
Benzo[a]pyrene	c	0.00009	0.2	222,000
2-Toluidine	M/B	0.003	9	300,000
Toluene	N/B	0.000035	375	1,000,000

[a]Target organs: B, blood; D, dermal; H, hepatic; K, kidney; M, mucosal; N, nervous; P, pulmonary; V, vascular.

[b]Metabolite of carbon disulfide with corresponding TLV used to calculate cigarette equivalent.

[c]No TLV for benzo[a]pyrene; TLV for coal tar pitch volatiles used to calculate cigarette equivalent.

Cigarette Equivalents to Attain TLV

The 21 sidestream smoke constituents with established workplace standards are listed in the order of increasing number of cigarette equivalents, defined as the number of cigarettes burned in a sealed enclosure of 100 m³ to attain, but not to exceed, the corresponding TLV (last column, Table 2). The list starts with nicotine, which is a reported mucosal irritant (acute exposure) and an autonomic nervous system stimulant (chronic or repeated exposure). The maximum reported sidestream smoke (SSS) collected from one burning cigarette is 8.2 mg. On the basis of TLV (0.5 mg/m³), it would take 6.6 cigarettes to attain TLV for 100 m³ in a sealed, unventilated enclosure (0.5 × 100 ÷ 8.2). It is unlikely for the nicotine concentration in public places to attain the TLV level. If smoking has been at an extremely high level in poorly ventilated rooms, subjective discomforts would be expected to lead to corrective measures before nicotine levels would approach the TLV. The second SSS constituent listed in the order of increasing cigarette equivalents is carbon monoxide: 50 cigarettes burning in a 100 m³ sealed chamber to attain the corresponding TLV (12).

Other than nicotine and carbon monoxide, the remaining 19 SSS constituents would require more than 1000 cigarettes to attain the corresponding TLV. Such excessively high cigarette equivalents suggest that to attain TLV levels, more than 1000 cigarettes need to be ignited simultaneously in an enclosed space of 100 m³. Consideration of cigarette equivalents clearly indicates that exposure to ETS constituents in workplaces rarely approximates TLVs.

Nicotine as ETS Marker

That nicotine and its major metabolite (cotinine) are detected in blood and urine of ETS-exposed nonsmokers has been utilized by proponents of the ETS–heart disease hypothesis. Their reasoning is as follows: since nicotine is the major cause of heart disease seen in cigarette smokers, it follows that any nicotine derived from ETS can cause heart disease in exposed nonsmokers. However, there is disagreement concerning whether any nicotine absorbed by nonsmokers can influence the heart. The estimates of ETS exposure are as follows: a nonsmoker's exposure might be, at most, the nicotine equivalent of $\frac{1}{100}$ to $\frac{1}{1000}$ cigarette in one hr, which has not been reported to have a significant pharmacologic action. In animal experiments, inhalation, ingestion, parenteral injection, and dermal application of nicotine have been reported to influence cardiac function, coronary circulation, and atherogenesis, but these studies used amounts of nicotine that cannot be attained by ETS exposure. Furthermore, coronary atherosclerosis has not been reproduced in experimental animals by injection of nicotine. High nicotine levels of pipe smokers compared to cigarette smokers are not reportedly associated with an increased incidence of ischemic heart disease (13). Workers processing tobacco leaf (cigar making, leaf curing, and warehouse workers) also have not been reported to show a higher incidence of heart disease, compared to nontobacco workers (14).

Cardiac Toxicologic Profile of Industrial Chemicals

The 21 chemicals listed in Table 2, when individually used in factories below the corresponding TLV, have not been associated with heart disease nor any adverse effect on corresponding target organs, that is, mucosal surfaces, skin, blood, nervous system, lungs, kidneys, and liver (see second column of Table 2). The same 21 ETS constituents also appear in Table 1 of industrial chemicals, together with 11 industrial chemicals *not* reported to be present in ETS. As outlined in Table 1, the existing methods for establishing cardiac toxicologic profiles are as follows: Methods A, B, and C for ischemic heart disease; Methods D, E, and F for coronary atherosclerosis; and Methods G and H for cardiac arrhythmia and myopathy. Most industrial chemicals have been studied by one or two methods, thus contributing to an uncertainty of whether these 21 chemicals are related to heart disease. Those that have been studied by three to eight methods have a stronger basis for claims of a relationship with occupational heart disease, namely, carbon monoxide, ethylene glycol dinitrate, nitroglycerin, carbon disulfide, and methylene chloride. There are review articles on industrial chemicals reportedly associated with heart disease (15–17).

A principal objective of this chapter is to evaluate the potential relationships between occupational chemicals and heart disease, in terms of the extent of the available data from human studies and animal experiments. There are reviews on individual industrial chemicals and the occurrence of diseases not limited to the heart (11,18,19). A standard source of reference is the Registry for Toxic Effects of Chemical Substances available in hard copy (20) as well as on-line in the TOXNET database updated by the National Library of Medicine and National Institute of Occupational Safety and Health. Textbooks on internal medicine and cardiology do not have special chapters devoted to occupational heart diseases so that it has been difficult to interest the medical profession. Because industrial chemicals are potentially associated with heart disease by the inhalational route, a World Health Organization monograph entitled *Air Quality Guidelines for Europe* (21) is a helpful reference source. It discusses the following industrial chemicals in a uniform format: inorganic oxides such as carbon monoxide and nitrogen dioxide; heavy metals such as arsenic, cadmium, and lead; polynuclear aromatic hydrocarbons such as benzo[a]pyrene; nonhalogenated solvents such as benzene, carbon disulfide, and toluene; and halogenated solvents such as methyl chloroform and methylene chloride. These 11 industrial chemicals identify those that have been measured indoors (workplace environment) but also emitted outdoors into the environment. Ischemic heart disease is mentioned under carbon monoxide and carbon disulfide.

ISCHEMIC HEART DISEASE

Ischemic heart disease is represented clinically by angina pectoris, myocardial infarction, cardiac arrhythmia, cardiogenic shock, and sudden death. The epidemiologic and clinical literature on work-associated ischemic heart disease consists of the following: Method A, mortality statistics; Method B, exercise testing for anginal pain; and Method C, coronary blood flow indicators. The plan is to state how each method has been applied to the concept that ischemic heart disease is related to exposure to chemical substances in the manufacture of industrial products. Although ETS levels are unlikely to attain their corresponding TLV, it is important to discuss the existing claim that the mere presence of these chemicals is sufficient to suggest an association between ETS and occupational heart disease.

Method A: Mortality Studies

There are scant data on heart disease in workers differentiated by exposure or nonexposure to ETS in the workplace. Most published studies relate to differences in spousal smoking habits, based on the premise that mortality rates of nonsmokers might be influenced by smoking habits of their spouses. In 1984, Schievelbein and Richter (22) reviewed the available literature and concluded that in concentrations of carbon monoxide and nicotine reportedly present in ETS, it is unlikely for ETS exposure to play any role in the development and progression of ischemic heart disease. The 1986 Reports of the Surgeon General and the National Research Council, after examining the available information, concluded that further studies on the potential relationship between ETS exposure and cardiovascular disease are needed in order to determine whether ETS increases the risk of cardiovascular disease in general, and of ischemic heart disease in particular (8,23). Recent epidemiologic studies were reviewed by Wexler (4), who questioned the reported relationship between household exposure to ETS and heart disease.

Prospective (cohort) and retrospective (case control) studies have been conducted on the potential relationship between ETS exposure and IHD incidence. Although some spousal studies (smoker married to nonsmoker) report a statistically significant association, most studies do not. Lee and his collaborators (24) conducted studies in England consisting of administering a questionnaire to 200 hospital patients and 200 controls for each gender and age group. Patients with ischemic heart disease and controls did not show any statistically significant difference in ETS exposure based on smoking habits of spouses. Exposure to ETS was also evaluated by an index of presence in the workplace, during travel, and at leisure. From the standpoint of worker ETS exposure, the negative results of Lee et al. (24) are more relevant than positive results of spousal studies that do not include ETS exposure outside the home environment.

Carbon Monoxide

Heart disease mortality rates have been reported for workers exposed to high levels of carbon monoxide from vehicular emissions (tunnel workers, bus drivers, parking attendants) and industrial furnaces (steel foundry, coke oven, chemical manufacture) (25,26). However, the results of occupational exposure to high levels of carbon monoxide do not support the argument that this substance contributes to heart disease associated with ETS exposure, in which reported levels of the gas are a tiny fraction of the TLV.

Carbon Disulfide/Carbonyl Sulfide

These two compounds are linked by the fact that the former is an industrial chemical reported to be associated with heart disease among workers producing viscose rayon fibers. This compound is metabolized to carbonyl sulfide, which happens to be a reported SSS constituent. The concentration of carbonyl sulfide is so low that it is unlikely to attain the TLV (Table 2: 54,945 cigarettes to attain TLV). However, it is important to discuss mortality studies of rayon viscose workers, because other than carbon monoxide, carbon disulfide is the only industrial chemical for which there are extensive data on an association with ischemic heart disease. In a critical review of the toxicologic literature on carbon disulfide, Beauchamp et al. (27) reviewed data on the mortality rates of viscose rayon workers. In Finland, where there is a high incidence of ischemic heart disease, a significantly higher mortality rate has been reported among exposed workers compared to a control group. However, in Japan where there is a notably lower incidence of ischemic heart disease, no increased mortality rate has been reported among viscose rayon workers. The excess deaths attributed to carbon disulfide became apparent if predisposing risk factors existed, such as hypertension, hyperlipidemia, and excessive intake of cholesterol and saturated fats (27,28).

The above observations are essential to consider in attempts to interpret mortality studies on ETS exposure. Dietary intakes of cholesterol and fatty food were not considered as a confounding factor in mortality studies relating to workers exposed to the industrial chemicals listed in Table 1 (with Method A notation). The reported higher susceptibility of Scandinavians to heart disease is reflected by the lower TLV (15 mg/m³) compared to the TLV in other European countries and the United States (30 mg/m³) (18,19).

Polycyclic Aromatic Hydrocarbons (PAH)

It has been suggested by proponents of the ETS–heart disease hypothesis that Scandinavian roofers show excess mortality for ischemic heart disease (3). They extrapolate from PAH-exposed roofers to ETS-exposed workers without recognizing the difference in composition of PAH. Exposures to PAH among coke oven workers, creosote wood appliers, and asphalt road builders have not been reported to be associated with excess mortality for heart disease but have been reported to be associated with excess mortality for lung cancer. From the standpoint of chemical composition of PAH exposures determined by nature of product, PAH exposures of roofers are irrelevant to ETS exposure (see also Method F).

Heavy Metals

Mortality studies on work-related exposure have been reviewed by Kristensen (16). Lead and cadmium workers have been reported to show a higher mortality rate from heart disease and hypertension. In the absence of experimental animal studies, heart disease is likely to be a complication of hypertension rather than a direct effect of lead or cadmium on the heart and coronary vessels. The suggestion that heart disease may be associated with workplace exposure to arsenic or cobalt can be traced to instances of beer drinking contaminated with either of these metals, and subsequent death from cardiomyopathy.

Method B: Exercise Testing and Angina Pectoris

Exercise testing is essential for the diagnosis of ischemic heart disease (29). A positive diagnosis is based on the appearance of chest pain or classical angina pectoris after completion of standardized exercise on a treadmill or bicycle ergometer. Exercise testing has also been used to evaluate severity of arteriosclerotic heart disease based on time of onset of an ischemic pattern in the electrocardiogram as well as the appearance of cardiac arrhythmias.

ETS Exposure of Anginal Patients

All available reports on exercise testing do not relate to specific occupational groups comparing two subgroups: with ETS exposure and no ETS exposure. There are two studies on anginal patients that suggested to the investigators that ETS exposure during bicycle ergometry may shorten the time period to onset of chest pain. The first study, reported in 1978, consisted of a group of ten American male veterans (30). For various reasons, the 1978 protocol for exercise testing was evaluated by an ad hoc committee of the Environmental Protection Agency. In 1983, the committee concluded that the method used on American male veterans "did not meet a reasonable standard of scientific quality" (31). In 1987, a second study of exercise testing during ETS exposure was reported by Soviet investigators (32). The results were essentially similar to those reported from American veterans. It is this author's opinion that shortening onset of anginal pain during exercise testing as a result of ETS exposure has not been proved pending evaluation of the Soviet protocol. Anti-anginal drugs sold in the United States are supported by results of exercise testing in European laboratories that have been approved by the U.S. Food and Drug Administration and so far, the list does not include any Soviet laboratories.

Influence of Carbon Monoxide on Exercise Testing

Proponents of the theory that ETS exposure aggravates angina pectoris emphasize the presence of carbon monoxide in ETS, in spite of the fact that the concentration inhaled is 3100 times lower than mainstream smoke. Blood carboxyhemoglobin levels of subjects exposed to ETS in public places range from 1 to 3% among nonsmokers. Slight elevations of blood carboxyhemoglobin level (to 2 and 3.9%) have been reported following administration of carbon monoxide in air (100 and 230 mg/m^3) (33). Exercise testing of heart disease patients was reported to result in an ischemic pattern of electrocardiogram at these blood carboxyhemoglobin levels. However, as indicated in Table 2, this would require more than 100 and 200 cigarettes burning in a sealed enclosure of 100 m^3 for carbon monoxide to attain about 2 and 4 times the TLV, respectively.

ETS Exposure as Risk Factor for Angina Pectoris

Proponents of the claim that ETS exposure aggravates angina pectoris have not considered the complexities of the disease separate from other manifestations or complications of ischemic heart disease (i.e., acute myocardial infarction and sudden deaths). Although prospective and retrospective studies report that cigarette smoking is one of many risk factors for acute myocardial infarction and sudden deaths, the data on angina pectoris are even more complex. The 1983 report of the Surgeon General on cardiovascular disease, referring to risk factors, concluded that "variation in the strength of association between smoking and angina pectoris may be influenced by . . . methodological considerations" (ref. 34, p. 70). More recently, it has been argued that the 30-year results of an ongoing prospective study at Framingham, Massachusetts, indicate that cigarette smoking is a negative risk factor in women (i.e., incidence lower in women smokers compared to women nonsmokers) (35). The results in men have indicated either a positive or no significant relationship between cigarette smoking and angina pectoris, depending on methodological variation. Some studies relating to cardiac patients admitted to hospitals report that after an initial cardiac episode, the prognosis is not influenced by smoking (36,37). After the initial infarction, prior smoking was not associated with the severity of subsequent complications. These observations on cigarette smoking in relation to the prognosis of myocardial infarction and the influence of angina pectoris raise additional questions. How can ETS, a dilute mixture of tobacco smoke components in air, aggravate angina pectoris or influence the prognosis of acute myocardial infarction, in light of recent inconsistencies in data derived from smokers?

Method C: Coronary Blood Flow Indicators

Coronary arteries visualized by angiography can show obstruction that is organic (arteriosclerosis and thrombosis) or nonorganic (vasospasm) in nature. Total coronary blood flow is measured by a tracer clearance technique. Patients with ischemic heart disease show a reduction in coronary blood flow that is limited to an infarcted area. When infarction is detected in workers previously exposed to carbon monoxide or carbon disulfide, it is not possible to isolate the potential association with chemical exposure from other potentially confounding risk factors. Carbon monoxide alone, by increasing carboxyhemoglobin, can increase coronary blood flow, but the result would be an oversupply of blood without reduced oxygen utilization because of poisoning oxidative enzymes. Myocardial metabolism requires the sampling of blood from the coronary sinus and a systemic artery to obtain arteriovenous differences of oxygen, carbon dioxide, lipoproteins, and glucose metabolites. There are more direct methods for measuring coronary blood flow in experimental animals (dog, cat, pig, monkey). The relative importance of metabolic and neurohumoral control has been evaluated in experimental animals [see reference cited by Bove (38)]. It has not been possible to reproduce coronary heart disease by exposure to tobacco smoke, which contains nicotine levels higher than ETS, so it is doubtful that existing animal models can give positive results from ETS exposure.

Nitroglycerin and organic nitrates are useful vasodilators for the relief of angina pectoris. The pharmacologic action of nitroglycerin is manifested in workers who are exposed daily to nitroglycerin and ethylene glycol dinitrate, but after a weekend of nonexposure, develop chest pain on Monday morning. Workers suffer from vasospastic angina as a result of nitrate withdrawal during the weekend and are relieved upon resuming nitrate work exposure. Autopsied workers did not show coronary arterial obstruction, confirming the occurrence of vasospastic angina brought about by weekend withdrawal from nitrate. Workers were acclimatized to the nitrate level in work environment (14–16).

CORONARY ATHEROSCLEROSIS

The term coronary *atherosclerosis* used in this chapter refers to histopathologic changes in arteries leading to *ischemic heart disease* (see preceding section). Although both terms are included in *coronary heart disease,* there are differences in methodology. This section is devoted to progressive organic lesions of coronary arteries, the methods for detection, and their evolution, based on human observations and animal experimentation. The focus is on industrial exposure to carbon disulfide and carbon monoxide, because of the relatively greater amounts of data on these substances. The potential relevance of these industrial chemicals to ETS exposure is also discussed.

The demonstration of coronary atherosclerosis ideally should include histopathologic evidence derived from autopsy (Method D). This has been accomplished for worker exposure to carbon disulfide, which has been supported by the occurrence of hyperlipidemia in exposed workers and coronary atherosclerosis in experimental animals (Method E). On the other hand, some industrial chemicals are associated with the development of coronary atherosclerosis based on animal experiments only or on hematologic changes in workers that in animals contribute to aortic atherogenesis (see entries in Table 1). Some of these observations have been used to support the claim that ETS exposure is involved in coronary atherosclerosis. A distinction is made between concepts derived from human studies (Method D), animal experiments (Method E), and *in vitro* techniques (Method F).

Method D: Coronary Angiography and Histopathology

The most direct method for diagnosis of coronary atherosclerosis is by histopathologic examination and coronary angiogram. Although there are isolated reports that workers exposed to carbon monoxide suffer from increased coronary atherosclerosis (antemortem or postmortem), this exposure is confounded by competing risk factors such as personal habits, familial history, and environmental pollution. Among viscose rayon workers, the occurrence of coronary atherosclerosis reported at autopsy of workers dying of heart disease led to mortality studies (Method A). Workers are also reported to suffer from hyperlipidemia, which is not entirely due to carbon disulfide exposure. It is difficult to replicate earlier studies on workers using modern techniques of diagnosing coronary atherosclerosis, because exposure levels have come under strict regulation.

There are no case reports of coronary atherosclerosis in workers exposed to a single polynuclear aromatic amine because workplace exposure is to mixtures that include benzo[a]pyrene. Only research laboratory workers investigating benzo[a]pyrene are candidates for long-term exposure, and so far there has been no report of a higher incidence of heart disease. There are also no case reports of coronary atherosclerosis from prolonged exposure to the heavy metals and nitrogenous compounds listed in Table 1.

Method E: Coronary Atherosclerosis in Experimental Animals

Repeated attempts to induce coronary atherosclerosis in experimental animals by inhalation of cigarette smoke have failed. Additional feeding with a cholesterol-enriched diet has reportedly led to the development of atherosclerosis not involving coronary arteries. In baboons, after 2–3 years of oral feeding of cholesterol and saturated fat, and daily inhalation of cigarette smoke, arterial lesions were compared between smokers and controls. Among male baboons, the extent of carotid atherosclerosis was greater in smokers than in controls, but there were no significant differences in atherosclerosis of the aorta, coronary arteries, iliac-femoral, and bronchial arteries. Among female baboons, there were no significant differences in atherosclerosis between smokers and controls (39).

The same general remarks apply to experimental testing of carbon monoxide in levels far exceeding those reported for ETS exposure. Rabbits, pigeons, and chickens are reported to need supplementary feeding of cholesterol to show carbon monoxide-induced aortic atherosclerosis (40).

Carbon disulfide is the only industrial chemical reported to cause atherosclerosis in animals without supplemental cholesterol feeding. Coronary and aortic atherosclerosis and myocardial lesions were detected in rats after 4 months of inhalation exposure (28). There were elevations of serum cholesterol, phospholipid, and triglycerides, indicating similarity to the human form of atherosclerosis. Other investigators have tested carbon monoxide and benzo[a]pyrene and have not observed hyperlipidemia and atherosclerosis similar to those reported for carbon disulfide. In the past, research on carbon monoxide, benzo[a]pyrene, and other polynuclear aromatic hydrocarbons has not been directed to a comparison with carbon disulfide.

Polynuclear aromatic hydrocarbons have been reported to induce aortic atherosclerosis in pigeons and chickens (41–44). It has been speculated that these studies in birds relate to human subjects exposed to ETS (2). There are several reasons for the inapplicability of results of these bird experiments to coronary atherosclerosis: (a) 7,12-dimethylbenzo(a,h)anthracene and 3-methycholanthrene are not known to be present in ETS; (b) although benzo[a]pyrene is reportedly present in ETS, the dose administered, 50 mg/kg injection, is farfetched compared to concentration levels in SSS, which is 0.00009 mg/cigarette; (c) hepatic metabolism is essential for atherogenesis in one strain, but not in the other strain, a sequence that applies to oral or injected compounds but not to the inhalation route; and (d) the typical result is aortic atherosclerosis and rarely coronary atherosclerosis. Aortic atherosclerosis is different from coronary atherosclerosis because of myocardial extravascular support in the latter. There are intracardiac mechanisms that influence coronary circulation, which are absent in other arterial beds.

There are long-term animal experiments designed to study carcinogenicity or polynuclear aromatic hydrocarbons and, so far, coronary atherosclerosis has not been reported in sacrificed animals.

Method F: *In Vitro* Studies of Hematologic Factors

Hematologic factors include alterations in hemoglobin oxygen transport such as carbon monoxide and methylene chloride increasing carboxyhemoglobin; and aniline and 2-toluidine leading to methemoglobinemia. The ultimate consequence is a reduced supply of oxygen and presumably atherosclerosis resulting from carbon monoxide. However, prolonged testing with methylene chloride or aniline has not been reported to produce experimental atherosclerosis, suggesting that these two industrial chemicals reduce hemoglobin oxygen transport differently from carbon monoxide.

Several techniques have been developed for the specific purpose of discovering therapeutic agents for the prevention, suppression, and reversal of atherosclerosis. Drugs for influencing blood platelets, blood lipoprotein levels, and endothelial vulnerability evolved from application of *in vitro* testing of blood derived from patients with ischemic heart disease, as well as peripheral vascular diseases. The same techniques for identifying therapeutic agents have also been applied to investigating how carbon monoxide and ETS might play a role in atherosclerosis. The interpretation of results derived from one test has been extended to include the entire progression of atherosclerosis even though the test was intended to show a therapeutic, rather than toxic, effect of chemical agents.

In vitro tests have been applied to blood from ETS-exposed subjects, based on the assumption that any reported effect will contribute to coronary atherosclerosis. It should be pointed out that chemically induced platelet aggregation leads to vascular clot formation, which does not necessarily involve interaction with endothelial cells and the formation of atherosclerotic plaque. Also, in the laboratory, it has not been possible to initiate aortic plaque formation by exceeding the normal level of fibrinogen. Any reported increase in fibrinogen level in the blood of ETS-exposed subjects may not be relevant to a potential relationship with coronary atherogenesis. It is conceivable that, for some people, ETS exposure may be perceived as stressful, with release of catecholamines, and that catecholamines are responsible for *in vitro* testing results. It has not been possible to conduct a double-blind testing of ETS exposure since both investigator and subject can detect ETS presence.

Platelet Aggregation

Exposure of healthy nonsmokers to ETS is alleged to alter results of *in vitro* testing of platelets in platelet-rich plasma. Aggregation of platelets is tested by the following agents added *in vitro:* edetic acid and formaldehyde or prostaglandin. The possibility that ETS exposure increases platelet aggregation is alleged to be an important step in the evolution of coronary atherosclerosis in nonsmokers (2).

In vitro studies of platelet aggregation in blood derived from smokers have reported inconsistent results, which question the applicability of this method to ETS exposure in nonsmokers. Platelet aggregation testing using whole blood reported no statistically significant differences between nonsmokers and smokers (45). Cigarette smoking is reportedly associated with alterations in platelet factors involved in thrombus formation, but the change has been attributed to the presence of carbon monoxide levels higher than those reported in subjects exposed to ETS (46). *In vitro* testing does not necessarily reflect events *in vivo*. Although platelets may be activated *in vivo,* they become attached to erythrocytes or form platelet aggregates during the collection and centrifugation needed to make platelet-rich plasma. There is some evidence that activated platelets are lost from supernatant "platelet-rich plasma," which includes older or less active platelets.

Plasma Fibrinogen Levels

Another *in vitro* test for a clotting factor has been added to the list of reports supporting the ETS–heart disease hypothesis. Patients with ischemic heart disease were questioned about their smoking habits, and nonsmokers were queried for ETS exposure in the workplace and household. Control subjects were derived from the same community in Australia (47). It was reported that the collected blood samples showed higher fibrinogen concentrations among current smokers than nonsmokers. Subjects exposed to ETS had higher levels than those not exposed. The differences were not statistically significant because of the high variability of measured fibrinogen levels. According to the questionnaire responses, levels of ETS exposure at work were reported to be higher than at home, but the estimated odds ratio for heart disease was less than one. The investigators interpreted their results to indicate inaccurate reporting of ETS exposure or the possibility that household exposure to ETS is associated more with heart disease than is workplace exposure. The potential relevance of fibrinogen levels in relation to ETS exposure is further questioned by observations that psychosocial factors may influence the plasma fibrinogen concentration in patients with ischemic heart disease (48).

CARDIAC ARRHYTHMIA AND MYOPATHY

The third and last group of methods for establishing cardiac toxicologic profiles for industrial chemicals relates to alterations in cardiac function.

The methods are intended to detect irregularities in heart beat or rhythm, to measure excitability of the intact heart, and to record electrical properties of excised atrium and papillary muscle. Cardiac output is measured by the tracer dilution technique and ventricular imaging in patients; invasive procedures are required for application of the Fick principle in patients and insertion of blood flow recorders in experimental animals. Perfusion of the excised heart offers an opportunity of measuring myocardial contractility and metabolism. Enzymatic studies and electron microscopy complete the techniques for detecting cardiomyopathy. All these procedures have been applied to determine the occurrence and mechanism for two groups of diseases: irregular heart beat or arrhythmia, and cardiomyopathy.

Method G: Irregular Heart Beat

Industrial chemical poisoning can be manifested by irregularities of heart beat or cardiac arrhythmia, in the order of increasing severity: ranging from tachycardia or bradycardia, atrioventricular block, atrial or ventricular extrasystole, atrial fibrillation, to ventricular fibrillation and cardiac arrest. The benign forms (up to atrial fibrillation) are reversible by stopping chemical exposure, but ventricular fibrillation and cardiac arrest require heroic efforts. Poisonings characterized by cardiac arrhythmias have been reported for the following (see Table 1, Method G): most halogenated and nonhalogenated solvents, some nitrogenous compounds, one heavy metal (lead), and one oxide (carbon monoxide). The arrhythmia results from a direct action of the chemical on the heart, specifically by altering excitability, conduction, and refractoriness of one or more of the following: atrial muscle, atrioventricular node, conducting system, and ventricular muscle. The effects have been reported in appropriate human studies and animal experimentation. The occurrence of poisoning by industrial chemicals does not support the proposition that since the same chemicals may be reported at minute levels in ETS, then ETS also may lead to the development of heart disease in workers.

Method H: Experimentally Induced Cardiomyopathy

The most extreme example of unjustified application of results from animal experiments to ETS exposure of nonsmokers is as follows: in the course of attempting to determine whether long-term cigarette smoking leads to cardiomyopathy, rabbits were exposed in an infant incubator (49). It was reported that all the smoke from three burning cigarettes entered the inlet of the incubator through a mechanical device and rabbits were kept for 30 min. This description appears to this author as a sealed chamber with cigarette smoke entering the inlet for 30-min periods. Several groups of rabbits were sacrificed: controls, after one 30-min exposure, twice daily exposure for 2 weeks, and twice daily exposure for 8 weeks. The heart was studied for mitochondrial oxidative processes. There was a decrease in respiration as well as in phosphorylation rate that was interpreted by the investigators as cardiomyopathy. The investigators recognized that carbon monoxide in the incubator was probably responsible for metabolic changes but they did not monitor air or blood levels.

Hugod and collaborators (50–52) exposed rabbits to one of the following mixtures: carbon monoxide 220 mg/m^3 or four times TLV; carbonyl sulfide 130 mg/m^3 or five times TLV; nitric oxide 6 mg/m^3 or one-fifth the TLV. The rabbits were in air-tight exposure chambers containing freely flowing air or predetermined mixtures in air for periods ranging from 1 to 7 weeks. The results of 140 rabbits sacrificed for electron microscopic examination performed blindly showed no morphological signs of myocardial damage. The four vapor constituents, in levels far exceeding ETS levels, were not associated with ultrastructural changes in rabbit heart, signifying the absence of cardiomyopathy.

The rabbit exposure studies described above were extended to include biochemical and histomorphologic investigation of atherosclerosis. Exposure to each of the four gas–air mixtures was not related to intimal damage of the aorta and coronary arteries. The negative results noted for carbonyl sulfide exposed rabbits do not support the claim that this known metabolite for carbon disulfide is responsible for coronary atherosclerosis reported by other investigators.

Cardiomyopathy has been reported following exposure to halogenated solvents, based on case reports of poisoning and experimental studies on intact and perfused heart. Cardiomyopathy from heavy metals is described in case reports of individuals drinking beer from containers that leached arsenic, cadmium, or lead (16). Cardiomyopathy from hydrocyanic acid is also based on case reports of poisoning and is readily supported by biochemical studies of heart muscle. Carbon monoxide is probably the most frequently encountered industrial and household chemical associated with death by cardiomyopathy. History of exposure to vehicular emissions or household natural gas is verifiable by blood analysis for carboxyhemoglobin. Among nonhalogenated solvents, only phenol has been reportedly related to cardiomyopathy (16).

CONCLUDING REMARKS

Among more than 32 industrial chemicals potentially related to heart disease, only four substances or chemical classes have extensive supportive evidence: carbon monoxide, carbon disulfide, ethylene glycol dinitrate and organic nitrates, and methylene chloride and halogenated solvents. The effects of other industrial chemicals (oxides, nonhalogenated solvents, nitrogenous compounds, and heavy metals) have not been adequately supported by human studies and animal experiments.

Methylene chloride is a solvent prototype for industrial chemicals that may be related to cardiac arrhythmia and myopathy in lethal or sublethal levels. Carbon disulfide is a selected prototype for industrial chemicals that may be related to ischemic heart disease or coronary atherosclerosis. There are no data indicating whether prolonged exposure to low levels of methylene chloride is associated with ischemic heart disease or whether high levels of carbon disulfide are associated with cardiac arrhythmia and myopathy. Methods to establish a cardiac toxicologic profile applied to one prototype need to be applied to the other.

The cardiac toxicologic profile for carbon disulfide is as follows: (A) mortality studies of viscose rayon workers report excess ischemic heart disease deaths, provided predisposing or other risk factors are present; (B) there is a high incidence of angina pectoris reported in workers exposed to carbon disulfide; (C) there is a reduction in coronary blood flow reported in workers developing ischemic heart disease, but there are no published results of myocardial tracer clearance studies; (D) coronary angiogram and postmortem histopathologic studies report coronary atherosclerosis associated with carbon disulfide exposure; (E) coronary atherosclerosis developed in experimental animals exposed to carbon disulfide, with or without dietary cholesterol supplement. There is no information for (F) *in vitro* hematologic factors and (G) cardiac arrhythmia; (H) experimental cardiomyopathy was reportedly not detected by electron microscopy in animals exposed to five times TLV for carbon disulfide.

The cardiac toxicologic profiles for carbon disulfide and ETS are compared in Table 3. There are no comparative studies on workers with and without ETS exposures. The theory that ETS causes ischemic heart disease is based on inferences from the following: (A) epidemiologic studies of household exposures reported for nonsmoking spouses of smokers; (B) exercise studies of anginal patients with ETS exposure, but questionable protocol; (C) coronary blood flow assumed to be insufficient because carbon monoxide present in ETS; (D) coronary atherosclerosis assumed to occur because aortic atherosclerosis reported in animals exposed to carbon monoxide at considerably higher levels than ETS; (E) coronary atherosclerosis supposedly occurs because benzo[a]pyrene reportedly associated with atherosclerosis in cholesterol-fed birds; (F) *in vitro* testing for platelet aggregation and reduced fibrinogen level, suggesting atheromatous plaque formation; (G) cardiac arrhythmia postulated based on ventricular excitability studies of animals exposed to carbon monoxide; and (H) cardiomyopathy inferred from rabbit heart mitochondrial studies.

It is the opinion of this author that the available studies do not support a judgment that ETS exposure is associated with any form of occupation-re-

TABLE 3. *Cardiac toxicologic profile for carbon disulfide and environmental tobacco smoke*

Method	Carbon disulfide	Environmental tobacco smoke (ETS)
Ischemic heart disease A. Mortality studies	Excess ischemic heart disease deaths among rayon viscose workers provided predisposing factors present	No information on workers exposed to ETS
B. Exercise testing and angina pectoris	Higher incidence of angina in rayon viscose workers; exercise testing protocol must meet U.S. agency standards	Anginal patients have shorter time to pain onset when exposed to ETS; cigarette smoking questionable risk factor in angina patients
C. Coronary blood flow indicators	Reduced coronary blood flow in patients with ischemic heart disease	
Coronary atherosclerosis D. Coronary angiography and histopathology		
E. Atherosclerosis in experimental animals	Coronary atherosclerosis in rats without cholesterol feeding	Polynuclear aromatic amines causing aortic atherosclerosis in cholesterol-fed birds
F. *In vitro* hematologic factors	No information	Platelet aggregation, endothelial cell damage and reduced fibrinogen level
Cardiac arrythmia and myopathy G. Irregular heart beat	No information	Ventricle excitability studies of animals exposed to carbon monoxide
H. Experimentally induced cardiomyopathy	No ultrastructural changes in rabbit heart	Heart mitochondria studies from rabbits exposed to ETS

lated heart disease. Although ETS reportedly contains constituents that have been associated with occupational heart disease, the concentrations are so low that it is unlikely for any substance to attain the corresponding TLV in a work environment.

Carbon disulfide can be used as a reference model for testing whether an industrial chemical can be considered as an etiologic factor in ischemic heart disease and coronary atherosclerosis. The most comprehensive and critical review of carbon disulfide has been written by members of the Chemical Industry Institute of Toxicology. The theory that ETS exposure causes heart disease was recently summarized by university scientists who have dismissed valid criticisms as industry-supported. All research results, including industry-funded sources, should be used in evaluating the role of ETS in heart disease.

REFERENCES

1. Occupational Safety and Health Administration (OSHA), Department of Labor. Occupational exposure to indoor air pollutants. 56 FR 47892, September 20, 1991.
2. Glantz SA, Parmley WW. Passive smoking and heart disease. Epidemiology, physiology, and biochemistry. *Circulation* 1991;83:1–12.
3. Simmons WS, Decker WJ, Holcomb LC, Huber GL, Brockie RE. Letters to editor and authors' replies. *Circulation* 1991;84:956–959,1878–1879.
4. Wexler LM. Environmental tobacco smoke and cardiovascular disease: a critique of the epidemiological literature and recommendations for future research. In: Ecobichon DJ, WU JM, eds. *Environmental tobacco smoke: Proceedings of the International Symposium at McGill University 1989.* Lexington: Lexington Books; 1990:139–152.
5. Aviado DM, Simaan JA, Zakhari S, Ulsamer AG. *Methyl chloroform and trichlorethylene in the environment.* Cleveland: CRC Press; 1976.
6. Aviado DM, Zakhari S, Watanabe T. *Nonfluorinated propellants and solvents for aerosols.* Cleveland: CRC Press; 1977.
7. Zakhari S, Liebowitz M, Levy P, Aviado DM. *Isopropanol and ketones in the environment.* Cleveland: CRC Press; 1977.
8. National Research Council. Measuring exposures and assessing health effects. In: *Environmental tobacco smoke,* vol 46. Washington, DC: National Academy Press; 1986:266–267.
9. Aviado DM. Suspected pulmonary carcinogens in environmental tobacco smoke. *Environ Tech Lett* 1988;9:539–544.
10. Aviado DM. Health effects of 50 selected constituents of environmental tobacco smoke. In: Kasuga H, ed. *Indoor air quality.* Berlin: Springer-Verlag; 1990:383–389.
11. ACGIH. *Documentation of the threshold limit values and biological exposure indices,* 5th ed. Cincinnati: American Conference of Governmental Industrial Hygienists; 1986.
12. Aviado DM. Carbon monoxide as an index of environmental tobacco smoke exposure. *Eur J Respir Dis* 1984;133:47–60.
13. Wald NJ, Idle M, Boreham J. Serum cotinine levels in pipe smokers: evidence against nicotine as cause of coronary heart disease. *Lancet* 1981;X:775–777.
14. Ghosh SK, Parikh JR, Gokani VN, Rao NM, Doctor PJ. Occupational health problems among tobacco processing workers: a preliminary study. *Arch Environ Health* 1985;40:318–321.
15. Kurppa K, Hietanen E, Klockars M, Partinen M, Rantanen J, Ronnemaa T, Viikari J. Chemical exposures at work and cardiovascular morbidity. Atherosclerosis, ischemic heart disease, hypertension, cardiomyopathy and arrhythmias. *Scand J Work Environ Health* 1984;10:381–388.
16. Kristensen TS. Cardiovascular diseases and the work environment. A critical review of the epidemiologic literature on chemical factors. *Scand J Work Environ Health* 1989;15:245–264.
17. Rosenman KD. Environmentally related disorders of the cardiovascular system. *Med Clin North Am* 1990;74:361–375.
18. Cook, WA. *Occupational exposure limits—worldwide.* Pittsburgh: American Industrial Hygiene Association; 1987.
19. United Nations. *Occupational exposure limits for airborne toxic substances.* Values of selected countries prepared from the ILO-CIS data base of exposure limits, third edition. Geneva: International Labour Office; 1991.
20. USDHHS, Centers for Disease Control, National Institute for Occupational Safety and Health. *Register of toxic effects of chemical substances,* 1985–86 ed., vols 1–6. Washington, DC: US Government Printing Office; 1988.
21. World Health Organization. *Air quality guidelines for Europe.* Copenhagen: WHO regional publications, European Series No. 23; 1987.
22. Schievelbein H, Richter F. The influence of passive smoking on the cardiovascular system. *Prev Med* 1984;13:626–644.
23. USDHHS. *The health consequences of involuntary smoking.* A report of the surgeon general. Washington, DC: US Government Printing Office; 1986.
24. Lee PN, Chamberlain J, Alderson MR. Relationship of passive smoking to risk of lung cancer and other smoking-associated diseases. *Br J Cancer* 1986;54:97–105.

25. Kuller LH, Radford EP. Epidemiological bases for the current ambient carbon monoxide standards. *Environ Health Perspect* 1983;52:131–139.
26. Stern FB, Haperin WE, Hornung RW, Ringenburg VL, McCammon CS. Heart disease mortality among bridge and tunnel officers exposed to carbon monoxide. *Am J Epidemiol* 1988;128:1276–1288.
27. Beauchamp RO Jr, Bus JS, Popp JA, Boreiko CJ, Goldberg L. A critical review of the literature on carbon disulfide toxicity. *Crit Rev Toxicol* 1983;11:169–278.
28. Wronska-Nofer T, Szendzikowski S, Obrebska-Parke M. Influence of chronic carbon disulphide intoxication on the development of experimental atherosclerosis in rats. *Br J Ind Med* 1988;37:387.
29. Sox HC Jr. Exercise testing in suspected coronary artery disease. *DM* 1985;31:1–93.
30. Aronow WS. Effect of passive smoking on angina pectoris. *N Engl J Med* 1978;299:21–24.
31. US Environmental Protection Agency. *Revised evaluation of health effects associated with carbon monoxide exposure: an addendum to the 1979 EPA air quality criteria document for carbon monoxide.* Final report. Springfield: NTIS, US Department of Commerce; 1984.
32. Khalfen E, Klochkov V. Effect of passive smoking on physical tolerance of ischemic heart disease patients (In Russian). *Ter Arkh* 1987;59:112–115.
33. Allred EN, Bleecker ER, Chaitman BR, et al. Effects of carbon monoxide on myocardial ischemia. *Environ Health Perspect* 1991;91:89–132.
34. USDHHS. *The health consequences of smoking. Cardiovascular disease.* A report of the Surgeon General. Washington, DC: US Government Printing Office; 1983:70.
35. Seltzer CC. The negative association in women between cigarette smoking and uncomplicated angina pectoris in the Framingham heart study data. *J Clin Epidemiol* 1991;44:871–876.
36. Kelly TL, Gilpin E, Ahnve S, Henning H, Ross J Jr. Smoking status at the time of acute myocardial infarction and subsequent prognosis. *Am Heart J* 1985;110:535–541.
37. Robinson K, Conroy RM, Mulcahy R. Smoking and acute coronary heart disease: a comparative study. *Br Heart J* 1988;60:465–469.
38. Bove AE. Physiology of the coronary circulation. In: Giuliani ER, Fuster V, Gersh BJ, McGoon MD, McGoon DC, eds. *Cardiology: fundamentals and practice,* 2nd eds. St Louis: Mosby Year Book; 1991:1131–1149.
39. Rogers WR, Carey KD, McMahan CA, Montiel MM, Mott GE, Wigodsky HS, McGill HC Jr. Cigarette smoking, dietary hyperlipidemia, and experimental atherosclerosis in the baboon. *Exp Mol Pathol* 1988;48:135–151.
40. Kjeldsen K. *Smoking and atherosclerosis.* Copenhagen: Tulein & Koch; 1969.
41. Albert R, Vanderlaan F, Nishizumi M. Effect of carcinogens on chicken atherosclerosis. *Cancer Res* 1977;37:2232–2235.
42. Revis NW, Bull R, Laurie D, Schiller CA. The effectiveness of chemical carcinogens to induce atherosclerosis in the white carneau pigeon. *Toxicology* 1984;32:215–227.
43. Penn A, Batastini G, Soloman J, Burns F, Albert R. Dose-dependent size increases of aortic lesions following chronic exposure to 7,12-dimethylbenz(a)anthracene. *Cancer Res* 1981;41:588–592.
44. Majesky M, Yang H, Benditt E. Carcinogenesis and atherogenesis: differences in monoxygenase inducibility and bioactivation of benzo[a]pyrene in aortic and hepatic tissues of atherosclerosis-susceptible versus resistant pigeons. *Carcinogenesis* 1983;4:647–652.
45. Elwood PC, Beswick AD, Sharp DS, Yarnell JWG, Rogers S, Renaud S. Whole blood impedence platelet aggregometry and ischemic heart disease—the Caerphilly collaborative heart disease study. *Atherosclerosis* 1990;10:1032–1036.
46. Mansouri A, Perry CA. Alteration of platelet aggregation by cigarette smoke and carbon monoxide. *Thromb Haemost* 1982;48:286–288.
47. Dobson AJ, Alexander HM, Heller RF, Lloyd DM. Passive smoking and the risk of heart attack or coronary death. *Med J Aust* 1991;154:793–797.
48. Meade TW, Imeson J, Stirling Y. Effects of changes in smoking and other characteristics on clotting factors and the risk of ischaemic heart disease. *Lancet* 1987;X:986–988.
49. Gvozdjakova A, Bada V, Sany L, et al. Some cardiomyopathy: disturbance of oxidative processes in myocardial mitochondria. *Cardiovasc Res* 1984;18:229–232.
50. Hugod C, Astrup P. Exposure of rabbits to carbon monoxide and other gas phase con-

stituents of tobacco smoke. Influence of coronary and aortic intimal morphology. *Munch Med Wochenschr* 1980;122:S18–S24.

51. Hugod C. Myocardial morphology in rabbits exposed to various gas-phase constituents of tobacco smoke. *Atherosclerosis* 1981;40:181–190.

52. Kamstrup O, Hugod C. Exposure of rabbits to 50 ppm carbonyl sulfide—a biochemical and histomorphological study. *Int Arch Occup Environ Health* 1979;44:109–116.

SECTION V

Vascular Toxicology

Cardiovascular Toxicology, Second Edition,
edited by Daniel Acosta, Jr.
Raven Press, Ltd., New York © 1992.

16

Vascular Toxicology

A Cellular and Molecular Perspective

Kenneth S. Ramos

*Department of Physiology and Pharmacology, College of Veterinary Medicine,
Texas A & M University, College Station, Texas 77843-4466*

Epidemiologic and experimental evidence has continued to accumulate over the past 50 years suggesting that a direct correlation exists between occupational and environmental exposure to toxic chemicals and cardiovascular morbidity and mortality. Such a correlation is best exemplified by the recognition that exposure to tobacco smoke constituents is a major contributor to myocardial infarction, sudden cardiac death, arteriosclerotic peripheral vascular disease, and atherosclerotic aneurysm of the aorta. Unfortunately, however, a comparable level of progress has not yet been accomplished in the elucidation of the mechanisms by which toxic chemicals cause vascular injury. This shortcoming is due, at least in part, to the misconception that cardiovascular toxicity is primarily associated with disturbances of myocardial function. This view has been reinforced by the slow onset and long latency periods often associated with vasculotoxic insult.

Progress in the evolution of vascular toxicology as a distinct area of study has been facilitated by recent advances in the fields of pathology and cell biology. Furthermore, evidence implicating free radicals in the regulation of lipoprotein metabolism and toxicant-induced modulation of vascular cell growth have stimulated interest in vascular toxicology by scientists who would have otherwise dismissed such issues. From the outset it must be recognized that vascular toxins can potentially alter multiple blood vessels including arteries, arterioles, capillaries, venules, and veins. These vessels serve as the circuitry for the transport and delivery of oxygen and nutrients to all tissues throughout the body and the removal of waste products of metabolism. In serving these circulatory functions blood vessels can be exposed to blood-borne toxins and their metabolic by-products.

This chapter surveys some of the most prominent vasculotoxic responses to chemicals of natural and/or anthropogenic origin. A detailed discussion of cellular and molecular mechanisms of toxic action for selected chemicals, with emphasis on basic concepts and generalities, has been presented to provide a comprehensive overview of vascular toxicology.

THE BLOOD VESSEL WALL: STRUCTURAL AND FUNCTIONAL CHARACTERISTICS

In view of the heterogeneity characteristic of the vascular tree, knowledge of blood vessel structure and function is essential to the elucidation of chemical toxicity. Blood vessels are often classified as elastic or muscular vessels based on their relative composition and abundance of extracellular matrix proteins. In primates, arteries vary in size from 300 μm internal diameter for large elastic vessels such as the aorta and the carotid to 30 μm for peripheral vessels such as muscular arterioles. Veins are similar to their arterial counterparts but often are thinner and of larger diameter than arteries. Arterioles, capillaries, postcapillary venules, and venules constitute the microcirculation. In contrast to large blood vessels, which are distinct anatomical entities, microvessels are considered a part of the tissue in which they reside.

Mammalian blood vessels of large and medium-size diameter are organized into three morphologically distinct layers (see ref. 1 for a comprehensive review). The innermost layer, referred to as the tunica intima, consists of a single layer of endothelial cells that rests on a loose layer of connective tissue formed by a thin basal lamina and a subendothelial layer. Luminal endothelial cells are flat and elongated with their long axis parallel to the blood flow. These cells act as a semipermeable barrier between the blood and underlying components of the vessel wall. The subendothelial layer is formed by connective tissue bundles and elastic fibrils in which a few cells of smooth muscle origin may occasionally be oriented parallel to the long axis of the vessel. The subendothelial layer is only seen in large elastic arteries such as the human aorta. The medial layer, or tunica media, is composed of elastin and collagen interwoven between multiple layers of smooth muscle cells. The media is separated from the outmost layer, the tunica adventitia, by a poorly defined external lamina. In the majority of vascular beds smooth muscle cells dominate the media but may also be present in the intima of some arteries and veins, as well as the adventitia of veins. The adventitial layer consists of a loose layer of fibroblasts, collagen, elastin, and glycosaminoglycans.

With the exception of capillaries, the walls of smaller vessels also have three distinct layers that share many of the features described for larger vessels. However, in vessels of smaller diameter the media is less elastic and consists of one to three layers of smooth muscle cells. An interesting feature of these vessels is the presence of myoendothelial junctions. Although the exact role of these structures is unknown, they may serve to enhance the stability of the vessel wall and to facilitate molecular transport and intercellular communication. As described for the muscular arteries, venules are structurally similar to their arteriole counterparts. Because muscular venules are larger than arterioles, a large fraction of blood is contained in these capacitance vessels. Capillaries are endothelial tubes, measuring 4–8 μm in diameter, which rest on a thin basal lamina to which pericytes are often attached. When one capillary converges with another, the vessel formed is referred to as a postcapillary venule. The capillary and the pericystic venule are the principal sites of exchange between the blood and tissues.

VASCULAR CELL BIOLOGY

In humans the development of blood circulation (i.e., vasculogenesis) begins at 4 weeks of gestation when simple diffusion of nutrients is no longer sufficient support growth (2). Developing vessels are formed by cells of mesenchymal origin that become angioblasts, which in turn differentiate into blood cells or endothelial cells. Endothelial cells form capillaries that give rise to larger vessels by the apposition of pericytes and/or fibroblasts, which ultimately differentiate into vascular smooth muscle cells. For many years vascular endothelial cells were considered passive participants in the transport of blood. It is now recognized that endothelial cells play an integral role in the regulation of hemostasis, vascular tone, and angiogenesis. Endothelial cells are also involved in the regulation of macromolecular transport across the vessel wall, attachment and recruitment of inflammatory cells, synthesis of connective tissue proteins, and generation of reactive oxygen species (3–5). Under normal conditions, medial smooth muscle cells are found primarily in a quiescent state of growth that is specialized for muscle contraction (6,7). The responses of smooth muscle cells to contractile agonists are mediated by receptors located on the plasma membrane. Activation of these receptors by endogenous transmitters, hormones, or xenobiotics is associated with changes in ionic conductance that ultimately activate the contractile apparatus. Membrane channels, sarcolemmal pumps, energy-dependent sequestration of calcium by intracellular organelles, and a number of calcium binding proteins participate in the maintenance of ionic transport. In addition to their central role in the regulation of vasomotor tone, smooth muscle cells participate in the synthesis of extracellular matrix proteins during arterial repair, the metabolism and/or secretion of bioactive substances, the regulation of monocyte function, and the generation of reactive oxygen species (6,7). Fibroblasts within the adventitial layer secrete some of the collagen and glycosaminoglycans needed to lend structural support to the vessel wall (8).

Under the influence of various stimuli, smooth muscle cells lose the ability to contract and shift toward a phenotypic state characterized by enhanced synthetic and proliferative activity. Cells in the synthetic state are distinguished from their contractile counterparts by their ability to migrate, proliferate, and secrete extracellular matrix components. Phenotypic modulation of smooth muscle cells occurs during various physiologic processes, such as fetal and postnatal development, regeneration and repair of blood vessels, and myometrial development during pregnancy (9). Modulation of smooth muscle cell phenotype from a contractile to a synthetic state is also observed during atherogenesis. In its early stages, atherosclerosis is characterized by focal intimal thickenings of smooth muscle cells that migrate to the intima and proliferate in an uncontrolled fashion (10). Macrophages, extracellular matrix components, and intra- and extracellular lipids accumulate as the lesion advances. The proliferation of smooth muscle cells and accumulation of extracellular matrix components within the lesion contribute to occlusion of the vessel lumen.

The most popular theory of atherosclerosis as proposed originally by Ross and Glomset (11) and recently modified (12) states that atherosclerosis lesions develop as a result of chronic cycles of vascular injury and repair. Consistent with this hypothesis, mechanical or toxic injury to the endothelium has been associated with initiation of the atherogenic response (13–15). As part of the repair process, smooth muscle cell mitogens and chemotatic agents are released from one or more of the cell types involved in the disease process, including endothelial cells, smooth muscle cells, macrophages, and fibroblasts. An alternate hypothesis is the monoclonal theory of atherogenesis as proposed by Benditt (16). Based on the monotypism of glucose-6-phosphate dehydrogenase, these investigators proposed that smooth muscle cells within the atherosclerotic plaque are the progeny of a single smooth muscle cell. As such, the atherosclerotic process would resemble benign neoplastic growth of smooth muscle tumors (leiomyomas). Upon exposure to a toxic or viral agent, smooth muscle cells may exist in a genetically altered state, which gives rise to lesions upon exposure to chemotatic/growth promoting factors. Alternatively, mutations could induce constitutive production of growth factors within smooth muscle cells themselves, resulting in autocrine stimulation of growth. Recent evidence has shown that DNA isolated from human atherosclerotic plaques is capable of transforming NIH3T3 cells and producing tumors in nude mice (17). These observations have stimulated interest in the study of mechanisms of vascular cell growth and differentiation.

Hypertension is typically characterized by a net increase in peripheral vascular resistance. Such increases of vascular resistance may be due to increased concentration of circulating vasoconstrictors, such as angiotensin II or catecholamines. However, local regulation mediated by metabolic, myogenic, or angiogenic mechanisms may also be involved (18). Increased vascular resistance has been associated with an overall increase in wall thickness and smooth muscle mass (19). These changes appear to be due, at least in part, to hypertrophy of smooth muscle cells. A sustained elevation in blood pressure has also been associated with destruction of capillaries at the tissue level. In recent years, the recognition that local degradation of the basement membrane in parent vessels leads to new capillary growth, and that such alterations may be related to toxic insult, has served as a stimulus for intense study in the area of angiogenesis. The angiogenic process involves the formation of blood vessels *in situ* secondary to migration, proliferation, and differentiation of vascular cells. Thus angiogenesis is a critical process in organogenesis and wound repair, as well as during the pathogenesis of cancer and atherosclerosis.

PRINCIPLES OF VASCULOTOXIC SPECIFICITY

A wide spectrum of chemicals including natural products, drugs, and anthropogenic chemicals have been recognized as potential vascular toxins. Angiotoxicity may be expressed at the mechanical, metabolic, or genetic level. As a general rule, vascular toxicity *in vivo* involves the interactions of multiple cellular elements (Table 1). Endothelial cells represent the first cellular barrier to the movement of blood-borne toxins from the lumen of the vessel to deeper regions of the wall. This strategic location makes them particularly susceptible to toxic insult, a feature that may be targeted for selective toxicity in angiogenesis-dependent disorders. Toxic chemicals that reach the subendothelial space may cause injury to medial smooth muscle cells and/or adventitial fibroblasts. Adventitial and medial cells within large

TABLE 1. *Cell types implicated in the vasculotoxic response*

Cell type	Function
Endothelial cells	First barrier to blood-borne toxins; synthesis and release of endothelium-derived relaxing factor; synthesis of pro- and anti-aggregatory factors; attachment and recruitment of inflammatory cells; synthesis of connective tissue proteins; generation of oxygen-derived free radicals and other radical moieties
Smooth muscle cells	Maintenance of vasomotor tone; synthesis of extracellular matrix proteins including collagen and elastin; synthesis of prostaglandins and other biologically active lipids; regulation of monocyte function; formation of free radicals
Fibroblasts	Synthesis of extracellular matrix proteins including collagens; structural support to the vessel wall
Monocytes/ macrophages	Scavenger potential; synthesis of macrophage-derived growth factor; generation of reactive oxygen species; lymphocyte activation, progenitor of foam cells
Platelets	Synthesis of proaggregatory substances and smooth muscle mitogens such as platelet-derived growth factor
Lymphocytes	Release of activated oxygen species; cellular immunity; production of immunoglobulins

elastic arteries, such as the human aorta, may also be reached via the vasa vasorum, the intrinsic blood supply to the vessel wall. In addition, the vasculotoxic response may be dependent on the influence of (a) extracellular matrix proteins that actively interact with vascular cells to modulate biologic behavior, (b) coagulation factors that dictate the extent of hemostatic involvement, (c) hormones and growth factors that regulate proliferative/differentiation programs, and (d) plasma lipoproteins, some of which modulate cellular metabolism. Acute vascular injury may be associated with local inflammatory reactions that sometimes compromise end-organ function. Chronic vasculotoxic insult involves repeated cycles of injury and repair, which may lead to irreversible changes of blood vessel structure and function. Such alterations may promote the pathologic progression of disorders such as atherosclerosis, hypertension, peripheral vascular disease, and vascular aneurysm.

Some of the most prevalent mechanisms that dictate the nature of the vasculotoxic response are listed in Table 2. These mechanisms include (a) selective alterations of vascular reactivity, (b) vessel-specific bioactivation of protoxicants, (c) erratic chemical detoxification, and (d) preferential accumulation of the active toxin within vascular cells. As illustrated in Fig. 1, multiple mechanisms may operate simultaneously for a given toxic agent. Vascular reactivity, as it relates to the intrinsic ability of blood vessels to respond to biologically active substances, can be regulated at multiple levels including changes in signal transduction from the surface to the interior of the cell and/or modulation of contractile protein structure and function. As described for other organ systems, nontoxic chemicals can be converted by vascular enzymes to highly reactive species capable of causing injury to both intra- and extracellular targets. Enzyme systems present in vascular cells, which have been implicated in the bioactivation of vascular toxins, include amine oxidases, cytochrome P-450 monooxygenases, and prostaglandin synthetase. These enzymes play important roles in the regulation of vascular function under physiologic conditions. For instance, copper-containing amine oxidases are widespread enzymes that catalyze the oxidative removal of biogenic amines from blood plasma, the cross-linking of collagen and elas-

TABLE 2. *Putative mechanisms of vasculotoxic insult*

Mechanism	Prototype toxins
Alterations of vascular reactivity	Metals, catecholamines, carbon monoxide, nicotine
Vessel-specific bioactivation	Allylamine, polycyclic aromatic hydrocarbons
Erratic detoxification	Allylamine, dinitrotoluene, hydrazinobenzoic acid, metals
Preferential accumulation	Allylamine, polycyclic aromatic hydrocarbons, TCDD

tin in connective tissue, and the regulation of intracellular spermine and spermidine levels (20). The existence of several cytochrome P-450 metabolites of arachidonic acid involved in the regulation of vascular tone and sodium pump activity has also been recognized (21). A complex of microsomal enzymes, collectively referred to as prostaglandin synthetase, catalyze the formation of biologically active lipids, including prostacyclin and thromboxane A_2. Prostacyclin, the major arachidonic acid metabolite in blood vessels, is a strong vasodilator and endogenous inhibitor of platelet aggregation, while thromboxane A_2, the major arachidonic acid metabolite in platelets, is a potent vasoconstrictor and promoter of platelet aggregation. Evidence continues to accumulate suggesting that vascular-specific activation of protoxins is a significant contributor to vasculotoxic insult. However, the bioactivation of vascular toxins need not be confined to vascular tissue. Angiotoxic chemicals may be bioactivated by other metabolically active organs such as the liver and the lung. In such instances, migration of activated species from the site of activation to the blood vessel is likely involved. Lipophilic metabolites may be transported and delivered to the vessel wall by association with plasma lipoproteins (22). Vascular toxicity may also be due to deficiencies in the capacity of target cells to detoxify the active toxin. Key components of the endogenous antioxidant defense system operative in vascular cells include the glutathione/glutathione reductase/glutathione peroxidase system, superoxide dismutase, and catalase. However, the extent to which these mechanisms contribute to the regulation of vascular function has yet to be defined. Significant differences in the antioxidant capacity of vascular cells relative to other cell types have been documented. For instance, vascular endothelial cells are more sensitive to oxidative stress than fibroblasts (23), while vascular smooth muscle cells appear to be fairly resistant to peroxide-induced injury relative to hepatocytes (24). Limited information is presently available regarding the cellular bases for the differential response of vascular and nonvascular cells. Finally, vascular toxicity may be due to selective accumulation of chemicals within the vascular wall. Although the mechanisms responsible for preferential accumulation of toxins within the vessel wall are not yet known, receptor-mediated internalization of low density lipoproteins may be critical in this process.

The aforementioned mechanisms are intended as a guide for the study of vasculotoxic responses and by no means represent an exhaustive account of all possibilities. As suggested previously, the consequences of vasculotoxic insult are ultimately dictated by the interplay between vascular and nonvascular cells, as well as noncellular factors such as extracellular matrix proteins, coagulation factors, hormones, immune complexes, and plasma lipoproteins. This concept is exemplified by the lymphocytic and platelet involvement in various forms of toxic injury. Furthermore, the toxic response can be modulated by mechanical and hemodynamic factors such as arterial pressure, shear stress, and blood viscosity. An additional consider-

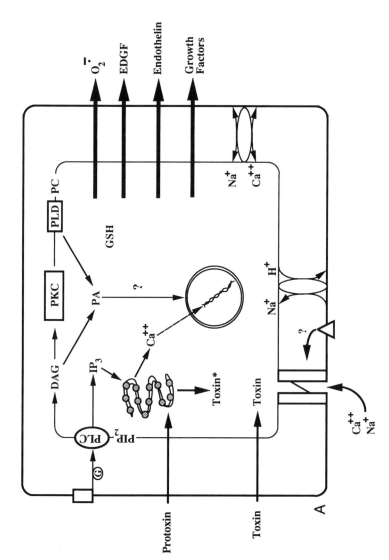

FIG. 1. Selected cellular and molecular targets of vasculotoxic insult in endothelial (**A**) and smooth muscle cells (**B**).

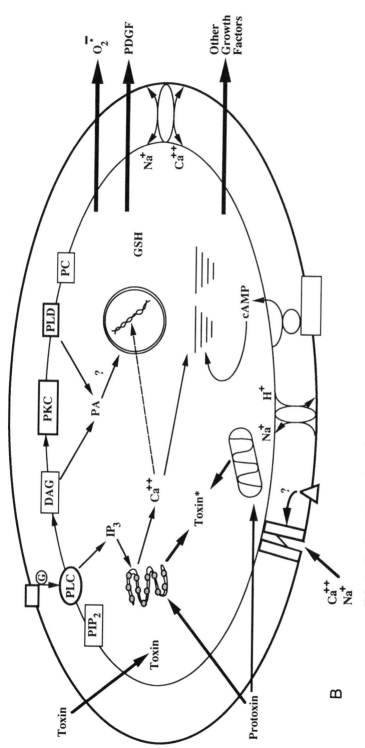

FIG. 1. *Continued.* Alterations of vascular reactivity are often mediated by changes in the distribution of ions across the membrane of vascular endothelial and/or smooth muscle cells. Alternatively, toxicant interference with signal transduction mechanisms at the receptor or second messenger level or structural/functional changes of contractile proteins may also interfere with vascular function. Enzyme systems capable of converting inactive chemicals to reactive forms that cause cell injury have also been identified. Deficient antioxidant capacity in vascular cells has also been suspected as a contributor to enhanced susceptibility to toxic injury. As in other organ systems, accumulation of toxicants within vascular cells has also been implicated in several vascular toxicities.

491

ation is that kinetic and pharmacodynamic differences among different animal species may also alter the toxicologic profile of a given toxicant.

SELECTED VASCULAR TOXINS

Allylamine

Allylamine (3-aminopropene) is an unsaturated aliphatic amine utilized as a precursor in the vulcanization of rubber and the synthesis of pharmaceuticals (25). In addition, several allylamine-type compounds are currently being developed as antifungal agents for human and veterinary use (26). Allylamine is more toxic than other unsaturated primary amines of higher molecular weight (27). Exposure to allylamine by a variety of routes in multiple animal species is associated with selective cardiovascular toxicity (28–31). The specificity of the toxic response may be related to its ability to accumulate in elastic and muscular arteries upon administration *in vivo* (32). Gross lesions are evident in the myocardium, aorta, and coronary arteries of animals exposed to allylamine. Chronic administration is associated with the development of atherosclerotic-like lesions characterized by smooth muscle cell proliferation and fibrosis.

Boor and colleagues first proposed that allylamine toxicity results from bioactivation of the parent compound to a toxic aldehyde (for a review see ref. 33). Although the details of this metabolic conversion have not yet been fully elucidated, vascular-specific bioactivation of allylamine to acrolein and hydrogen peroxide by benzylamine oxidase is considered a prerequisite for the manifestation of toxicity (33,34). Benzylamine oxidase, also known as semicarbazide-sensitive amine oxidase, is a copper-containing amine oxidase found in cardiovascular tissue in higher concentrations than any other tissue (35). Inhibition of this enzyme protects vascular cells from allylamine cytotoxicity. Allylamine preferentially injures smooth muscle cells relative to other cell types within the vascular wall. Although the basis for this selectivity is not yet clear, the localization of benzylamine oxidase within smooth muscle cells appears to be involved (33). However, other mechanisms including deficient detoxification of reactive species, selective accumulation of the parent compound, and/or enhanced susceptibility to toxic metabolic intermediates may also contribute to the specificity of the toxic response. This interpretation is consistent with studies showing that alterations in glutathione levels, a putative target of allylamine toxicity, are not limited to the cardiovascular system (K.S. Ramos and L.R. Cox, *unpublished observations*). The mechanism by which allylamine modulates glutathione levels in multiple organs is not yet clear. Some of our recent work has shown that the enzymatic activity responsible for the metabolic conversion of allylamine to acrolein in aortic tissue is localized in the mitochondrial and microsomal fractions (36). These observations are in agreement with studies by others showing that allylamine, or its metabolites, is sequestered in close proximity to endoplasmic reticulum and mitochondria (37).

Acrolein is an extremely reactive aldehyde that disrupts the thiol balance of vascular cells (38). Although a large number of compounds react with acrolein under physiological conditions, the main reaction products result from nucleophilic addition at the terminal ethylenic carbon. As such, toxicity most likely results from the reaction of acrolein with critical cellular sulfhydryls. Hydrogen peroxide formed during the deamination process may contribute to allylamine-induced vascular injury. However, acute cytotoxicity studies in our laboratory have shown that vascular cells are relatively resistant to hydrogen peroxide, and thus its contribution to the overall cytotoxic injury is likely minimal (34). This interpretation is consistent with the inability of catalase to prevent allylamine-induced cytotoxicity to a significant extent (34). Acrolein can also be converted via NADPH-dependent microsomal enzymes to glycidaldehyde and acrylic acid (39). Although acrolein itself lacks significant transforming potential, glycidaldehyde is cytotoxic and a weak initiator following chemical promotion.

Acrolein itself is a ubiquitous toxic chemical found in engine exhaust and cigarette smoke. Thus a limited number of studies have been conducted to examine the direct vascular toxicity of this aldehyde. Within the context of allylamine-induced cytotoxicity such studies are particularly useful when considering that the toxicologic profile of acrolein need not replicate that of the parent compound. Exogenous acrolein results in extensive injury to the plasmalemma before critical subcellular targets are compromised. In contrast, intracellular formation of acrolein allows simultaneous interaction of the aldehyde with multiple subcellular targets. Using Dahl hypertension-resistant and -sensitive rat strains, Kutzman et al. (40) have demonstrated that exposure to acrolein for 62 days is more toxic to hypertension-sensitive animals than hypertension-resistant counterparts. Since the differences between these strains are not usually manifested in the absence of hypertensive stimuli, the mechanisms responsible for increased susceptibility to acrolein toxicity remain unclear. The indirect sympathomimetic activity of aldehydes including acrolein, acetaldehyde, and formaldehyde may contribute to the enhanced sensitivity of hypertension-prone animals (41).

Because the expression of vasculotoxic insult is often a multifactorial phenomenon characterized by long latency periods, an *in vivo/in vitro* regimen has been used in our laboratory to evaluate the toxicity of allylamine (42,43). Upon completion of defined dosing regimens *in vivo,* aortic smooth muscle cells are isolated and established in primary or secondary culture. This culture system has been used to evaluate the impact of repeated cycles of injury and repair *in vivo* upon smooth muscle cells. Using this approach, we have shown that smooth muscle cells from rats exposed subchronically to allylamine grow more rapidly in primary culture than cells isolated from control animals (42). When seeded on a glass surface, control cells are elongated and spindle shaped, while allylamine cells are more broad and round. In contrast to cells from control animals, smooth muscle cells isolated from allylamine-treated animals do not respond to contractile challenge *in vitro*. Allylamine cells are characterized by numerous ribosomes and rough endoplasmic reticulum. These features are consistent with their enhanced ability to synthesize DNA and collagen relative to cells from control animals. Subsequent studies have shown that allylamine modulates both precursors and products of phosphoinositide metabolism in vascular smooth muscle cells (43). These actions appear to be mediated by enhanced phospholipase-C-mediated turnover of membrane phospholipids. Manipulation of phosphoinositide metabolism upon exposure to dibutyryl cAMP modulates the phenotypic expression of allylamine cells, as judged by changes in morphology, DNA synthesis, and inositol phosphate production (43). Although an intriguing association between cAMP levels and the phenotypic state of vascular smooth muscle cells has been established, the role of cAMP as a regulatory factor in phosphoinositide metabolism and phenotypic modulation is not yet clear.

Carbon Monoxide

Carbon monoxide induces vascular injury in laboratory animals at concentrations to which humans may be exposed from environmental sources such as automobile exhaust, tobacco smoke, and fossil fuels (44). Because most sources of carbon monoxide represent a complex mixture of chemicals, attempts to distinguish the direct effects of carbon monoxide from those of other chemicals such as sulfur oxides, nitrogen oxides, aldehydes, and hydrocarbons have been difficult. Short-term exposure to carbon monoxide has been associated with direct damage to vascular endothelial (45) and smooth muscle cells (46). Injury to endothelial cells increases intimal permeability and allows the interaction of blood constituents with underlying components of the vascular wall. This response may account, at least in part, for the ability of carbon monoxide to induce atherosclerotic lesions in several animal species. Although carbon monoxide enhances total arterial deposition of cholesterol in animals fed a lipid-rich diet (47), its vascular effects appear to be independent of serum cholesterol levels. Carbon monoxide potentiates cellular growth and suppresses collagen synthesis of cultured porcine endothelial cells, but inhibits cellular growth and causes no changes in the collagen synthesis of bovine endothelial cells (45). The mechanisms responsible for such species differences have not yet been defined, but they may serve to explain some of the conflicting reports found in the literature. Smooth muscle cells exposed to carbon monoxide *in vitro* exhibit partial loss of myofilaments and proliferation of intracellular organelles (46). A relative increase in the number of pinocytic vesicles at and below the cell surface and an increase in the number of lysosomes have also been observed. These alterations resemble those observed when smooth muscle cells are grown under hypoxic conditions (46).

The toxic effects of carbon monoxide have been attributed to its reversible interaction with hemoglobin. The formation of carboxyhemoglobin *in vivo* is favored because binding of carbon monoxide to hemoglobin is more cooperative than that of oxygen. As a result of this interaction, carboxyhemoglobin decreases the oxygen carrying capacity of blood and shifts the oxyhemoglobin saturation curve to the left. These actions make it more difficult to unload oxygen and eventually cause functional anemia due to reduced oxygen availability. More recently, evidence has been presented that carbon monoxide exerts toxic effects independent of those associated with carboxyhemoglobin formation. Elevated partial pressures of carbon monoxide in the tissues may lead to the interaction of carbon monoxide with cellular proteins such as myoglobin and cytochrome *c* oxidase (48,49). These metalloproteins contain iron and/or copper centers that form metal–ligand complexes with carbon monoxide in competition with molecular oxygen.

Carbon monoxide elicits a direct vasodilatory response of the coronary circulation (50–52). This response is not mediated by hypoxia, nor by interference with adrenergic, adenosine, or prostaglandin receptors (50). Lin and McGrath (53) have shown that carbon monoxide directly relaxes the rat thoracic aorta. This relaxation is independent of the endothelium and does not appear to be agonist specific. Because norepinephrine-induced contractions are inhibited to a greater extent than those induced by potassium, these investigators have suggested that carbon monoxide preferentially inhibits contractions initiated by calcium release from intracellular stores. More recently, the relaxation of vascular smooth muscle induced by carbon monoxide has been linked to activation of guanylate cyclase in a manner analogous to that of nitric oxide (54). These observations are consistent with studies in this laboratory showing that carbon monoxide increases cGMP levels in cultured aortic smooth muscle cells (55). Because cyanide, a well-known inhibitor of mitochondrial respiration and inducer of cytotoxic hypoxia modulates aortic contractility (56), a role for hypoxia in carbon monoxide-induced alterations of vascular tone should not be dismissed yet.

Catecholamines

Endogenous sympathomimetic amines including epinephrine, norepinephrine, and dopamine exert prominent physiologic effects that are mediated by receptors on the surface of target cells. Acute exposure to toxic concentrations of catecholamines is associated with cardiovascular and hemodynamic changes, some of which are mediated by alterations in peripheral vascular resistance. In addition, repeated exposure to catecholamines induces atherosclerotic lesions in several animal species (57–59). That catecholamines modulate the progression of arterial disease is consistent with the enhanced vascular reactivity to infused norepinephrine observed in essential hypertension (60). The atherosclerotic effect of catecholamines is likely related to their ability to induce endothelial cell injury and/or to modulate the proliferation of vascular cells. Evidence is available suggesting that the proliferative disturbances induced by catecholamines are mediated via α-receptors since prasozin, an α-receptor antagonist, effectively prevents the toxic response (61). However, Pettersson et al. (62) have recently shown that potentiation of the atherosclerotic process by sympathetic activation is inhibited by β-adrenergic receptor blockade. Thus the relative contributions of adrenergic receptors to changes in the proliferation of vascular cells are not yet clear. The observation that both parent compounds and metabolites may be involved in the toxic response further complicates the interpretation of these data (59). Sholley and co-workers (63) have demonstrated that catecholamines inhibit endothelial migration and repopulation of small denuded areas *in vitro*. In this manner, catecholamines may interfere with the repair capacity of blood vessels *in vivo*. Smooth muscle cells exposed to atherosclerotic risk factors, such as diabetes, hypertension, and balloon injury are more susceptible to the effects of catecholamines (64,65). Thus the formation of arteriosclerotic lesions in certain forms of hypertension may be initiated and/or supported by high levels of circulating catecholamines. The atherogenic effect of catecholamines may also be related to their ability to induce contraction of vascular smooth muscle cells. A link may exist between vasoconstrictor and mitogenic mechanisms in vascular smooth muscle cells. This concept is supported by the observation that smooth muscle mitogens are powerful vasoconstrictor agents (66,67). The ability of vasoconstrictor agents to modulate the proliferation of smooth muscle cells may be related to modulation of oncogene expression. Recent studies have shown that angiotensin II, a powerful vasoconstrictor, increases the expression of various oncogenes including c-*fos* and c-*jun* (68).

Oxidative by-products of catecholamines have been implicated in the cardiac toxicity of catecholamines (69,70). The oxidation of catecholamines generates adrenochrome-like products that undergo spontaneous or enzyme-catalyzed oxidation to form oxygen-derived free radicals. Although a similar correlation has not been established for vascular cells, recent studies have demonstrated that 6-hydroxydopa, an oxidative by-product of catecholamines, is present at the active site of serum amine oxidase (20). These observations raise the possibility that oxidative by-products of catecholamines formed under physiologic conditions selectively modulate vascular function. In fact, evidence showing that superoxide anions selectively attenuate the contractile responses to catecholamines has been presented (71). The vascular effects of oxygen-derived radicals have recently been reviewed by Rubanyi (72). Free radicals *in vivo* can be generated secondary to anoxic/reoxygenation injury (73), metabolism of xenobiotics (74), neutrophil-monocyte-mediated inflammation (75), and oxidative modification of low density lipoproteins (76). Superoxide anions inactivate endothelium-derived relaxing factor, while hydrogen peroxide and hydroxyl radicals cause direct vasodilation and stimulate the synthesis and release of relaxation factors. Oxygen radicals are considered important mediators of vascular damage in acute arterial hypertension and experimental brain injury (77–79). Hiebert and Liu (80) have suggested that toxic oxygen metabolites can damage endothelial cells and play an important role in the progression of atherosclerotic lesions. Free radicals generated from the xanthine/xanthine oxidase reaction increase the transfer of albumin across a barrier of endothelial cells *in vitro* (81). Rosenblum and Bryan (82) have presented evidence that hydroxyl radicals mediate the endothelium-dependent relaxation of brain microvessels. It has been suggested that calcium mobilization and activation of protein kinase C play significant roles in the generation and release of superoxide by endothelial cells (83). The release of superoxide from endothelial cells may modulate endothelial functions, as well as that of other constituents of the vascular wall. Within this context, activated endothelial cells have recently been reported to produce and secrete proteases in association with vessel penetration into surrounding connective tissue in response to angiogenic stimuli (84).

Dinitrotoluene

Dinitrotoluene is a nitroaromatic chemical used as a precursor in the synthesis of polyurethane foams, coatings, elastomers, and explosives. The manufacture of dinitrotoluene generates a technical grade mixture, which consists of 75.8% 2,4-dinitrotoluene, 19.5% 2,6-dinitrotoluene, and 4.7% other isomers. Several chronic toxicity studies in laboratory animals have shown that 2,4- and/or 2,6-dinitrotoluene cause cancers of the liver, gallbladder, and kidney, as well as benign tumors of the connective tissues (85–87). In humans, however, retrospective mortality studies in workers exposed daily to dinitrotoluene have shown that dinitrotoluenes cause circulatory disorders of atherosclerotic etiology (88,89). As in other instances of chronic occupational illness, increased mortality from cardiovascular disorders upon exposure to dinitrotoluenes has been related to the duration and intensity of exposure.

Recent studies in this laboratory have shown that repeated *in vivo* exposure of rats to 2,4- or 2,6-dinitrotoluene is associated with dysplasia and rearrangement of aortic smooth muscle cells (90). Marked inhibition of DNA synthesis was observed in medial smooth muscle cells isolated from dinitrotoluene-treated animals. The ability of dinitrotoluenes to modulate DNA synthesis in aortic smooth muscle cells was not due to direct genotoxic or cytotoxic effects (91). Dinitrotoluenes are metabolized in the liver to dinitrobenzylalcohol, which is then conjugated to form a glucoronide excreted in bile or urine. This conjugate is thought to be hydrolyzed by intestinal microflora and subsequently reduced to a toxic metabolite, or the precursor of a toxic metabolite (92,93). Dent et al. (94) have shown that rat cecal microflora convert dinitrotoluene to nitrosonitrotoluenes, aminonitrotoluenes, and diaminotoluenes. *In vitro* exposure of rat aortic smooth muscle cells to 2,4- or 2,6-diaminotoluene modulates' DNA synthesis in a manner that resembles that observed upon dinitrotoluene treatment *in vivo* (90). Interestingly, data have recently been obtained showing that diaminotoluene retards the progression of smooth muscle cells through the G_1 phase of the cell cycle (K.S. Ramos et al., *unpublished observations*). This response resembles that observed upon exposure of smooth muscle cells to other chemical carcinogens (95). However, diaminotoluene has not been detected in metabolism studies upon *in vivo* exposure to dinitrotoluene (93). Because both dinitrotoluene and diaminotoluene must be activated to elicit toxic effects, metabolic intermediates that are common to both of these agents may actually be responsible for the vascular toxicity of dinitrotoluene.

The modulation of DNA synthesis in rat aortic smooth muscle cells by dinitrotoluene may be related to its ability to promote the atherosclerotic process in humans. However, additional studies are required to address this issue since significant species differences in the responses to atherogenic insult have been documented (96). This is particularly important when considering that the rat is relatively resistant to both spontaneous and chemically induced atherogenesis (97).

Hydrazinobenzoic Acid

Hydrazinobenzoic acid is a nitrogen–nitrogen bonded chemical present in the cultivated mushroom *Agaricus bisporus*. McManus et al. (98) have reported that this hydrazine derivative causes smooth muscle cell tumors of the aorta and large arteries of mice when administered over the life span of the animals. These tumors showed the characteristic appearance and immunocytochemical features of vascular leiomyomas and leiomyosarcomas. Smooth muscle cell lysis with vascular perforation apparently precedes malignant smooth muscle cell growth. The ability of hydrazinobenzoic acid to cause vascular smooth muscle cell tumors is shared with other synthetic and naturally occurring hydrazines (99). Although angiomyomas (or vascular leiomyomas) derived histogenetically from the media of blood and lymph vessels occur most commonly in the oral cavity and in the skin (100), evidence that primary leiomyosarcomas occur in the abdominal aorta has been presented (101,102). These observations are particularly significant when considering that transformation of vascular smooth muscle cells is an uncommon event.

We have conducted *in vitro* studies to examine the direct cytotoxic effects of hydrazinobenzoic acid in cultured rat aortic smooth muscle cells. Exposure of smooth muscle cells to hydrazinobenzoic acid (0.1–100 μM) for various times was not lethal to the cells, as reflected by leakage of lactate dehydrogenase (K. Piron and K.S. Ramos, *unpublished observations*). However, significant fluctuations in cellular glutathione content upon exposure to hydrazinobenzoic acid were observed. The impact of such alterations to the *in vivo* toxicity of hydrazinobenzoic acid has yet to be defined. Because free radicals can be generated from hydrazines by oxidizing systems, including metal-catalyzed autooxidation, prostaglandin synthetase, and cytochrome P-450/NADPH (103), the modulation of glutathione by hydrazinobenzoic acid may be mediated by free-radical formation. This suggestion is consistent with previous reports showing that hydrazines bind covalently to macromolecules, promote lipid peroxidation, and induce DNA damage (104,105).

Metals

Although epidemiologic and clinical reports regarding the vascular effects of metals have received some attention in past years (106–108), only a limited number of studies have been conducted to define the cellular and molecular mechanisms of metal-induced angiotoxicity. As in other systems, the vascular toxicity of food- and water-borne elements (selenium, chromium, copper, zinc, cadmium, lead, and mercury), as well as air-borne elements (vanadium and lead), is thought to be due to nonspecific reactions of metals with sulfhydryl, carboxyl, or phosphate groups. In addition, the ability of metals such as cobalt, magnesium, manganese, nickel, cadmium, and lead to interact with and block calcium channels has been recognized for many years (109). More recently, evidence suggesting that intracellular calcium-binding proteins are biologically relevant targets of heavy metal toxicity has been presented. Calmodulin, an ubiquitous calcium-binding protein in eukaryotes, serves as a major intracellular calcium receptor in the regulation of multiple cellular processes. Certain heavy metals, including mercury and lead, effectively substitute for calcium within the calmodulin molecule (110). However, the contribution of this mechanism to the toxic effects of metals has been questioned based on the inability of beryllium, barium, cobalt, zinc, and cadmium to bind readily to calmodulin *in vitro* (111).

To date, most vascular toxicity studies have focused on the effects of cadmium. Cadmium is not preferentially found within blood vessels relative to other tissues. However, when present, cadmium is thought to be localized in the elastic lamina of large arteries, with particularly high concentrations at arterial branching points (112). A large portion of cadmium accumulated in the body is tightly bound to hepatic and renal metallothionein, a mechanism that is considered a means of detoxification (113,114). Thus the low metallothionein levels in vascular tissue may actually predispose to the toxic effects of cadmium (112). Long-term exposure of laboratory animals to low levels of cadmium has been associated with the development of atherosclerosis and hypertension in the absence of other toxic effects (115). Although most experimental studies conducted to date have focused on the putative hypertensive effects of cadmium, some of the critical information required to establish a causal relationship remains elusive.

In 1962, Schroeder and Vinton first reported that exposure of rats to 5 ppm cadmium in the drinking water causes hypertension (116). This observation has been corroborated by several independent laboratories (117,118) and refuted by others (119). To account for such discrepancies, Perry et al. (112) have suggested that cadmium-induced hypertension is only observed in a narrow concentration range of 0.1–5 ppm, above which toxicity without hypertensive effects is only observed. These investigators further proposed that failure to induce hypertension with chronic cadmium may be due to low levels of heavy metal contamination in the water or food supplies used in the course of experiments. This interpretation would be consistent with the observation that selenium and zinc inhibit (120), while lead potentiates, the hypertensive effects of cadmium (121). Concentrations of cadmium that increase blood pressure fail to raise blood pressure in the presence of calcium (115). In contrast, the protective effects of zinc and selenium may be related to their ability to increase the synthesis of cadmium-binding proteins and thus enhance cadmium detoxification.

The mechanism of cadmium-induced vascular toxicity is not yet known. Cadmium has been reported to increase sodium retention (122), induce vasoconstriction (123), increase cardiac output (124), and produce hyperreninemia (125). At the cellular level, cadmium causes vesiculation, vacuolization, widened intercellular junctions, and fragmentation of vascular endothelium (126). *In vitro* exposure to cadmium decreases prostacyclin formation in aortic rings and reduces ADP clearance by arterial tissue (127). The responsiveness of rabbit platelets to nonaggregating concentrations of arachidonic acid or collagen can be potentiated by prior exposure to cadmium chloride (128). In spite of all this evidence, many questions regarding the angiotoxic effects of cadmium remain unanswered. Of particular importance within this context is the study of microvascular responses to cadmium.

Much less work has been conducted to evaluate the vasculotoxic effects of other heavy metals. Because hypertension is not commonly observed during clinical lead intoxication, many investigators consider existing evidence to be conflicting and inconclusive. Epidemiologic studies have shown that a large percentage of patients with essential hypertension have increased body stores of lead (129). Elevated blood pressure has also been observed during childhood lead poisoning (130,131). Although in these children the level of lead burden was not severe, a significant increase in blood pressure was seen on the tenth day of poisoning, which persisted for the remainder of the study. The direct vasoconstrictor effect of lead may be related to the putative hypertensive response (132). This effect can be complemented by lead's ability to activate the renin–angiotensin–aldosterone system (133).

A number of studies have focused on the toxic interactions of metals. For example, lead potentiates the vasopressor response to cadmium (120). In contrast to the protective effects of calcium in cadmium-induced hypertension, calcium is ineffective in reducing the toxic cardiovascular effects of lead (115). However, magnesium promotes the atherosclerotic and hypertensive effects of both lead and cadmium. Mercury and lead cause contraction of aortic smooth muscle *in vitro,* while cadmium is without effect (134). Mercury added to platelet-rich plasma causes a marked increase in platelet thromboxane B_2 production and increased platelet responsiveness to arachidonic acid (135). Although it is unlikely that mercury and lead compete with calcium for intracellular binding sites, their accessibility to the intracellular compartment appears to be calcium dependent (134). Several investigators have proposed that acute lead-induced neuropathy is due to cerebral capillary dysfunction (130,131). This hypothesis is consistent with recent *in vitro* studies showing that lead causes dose- and time-dependent inhibition of cell division and glucose uptake in cerebral microvessel endothelium (136).

Nicotine

Nicotine, an alkaloid found in various plants, mimics the actions of acethylcholine at nicotinic receptors throughout the body. The cardiovascular effects of this potent toxin have been studied within the context of tobacco-associated toxicities, as well as its use as a botanical insecticide. Epidemiologic and experimental studies have suggested that nicotine is a causative or aggravating factor in myocardial and cerebral infarction, gangrene, and aneurysm. Bull et al. (137) have shown that repeated subcutaneous infusion of nicotine for 7 days is associated with reduced prostacyclin production in aortic segments. Reduced prostacyclin production has been observed in isolated rabbit hearts, rabbit aorta, human vein, rat aorta, and umbilical arteries when incubated with nicotine *in vitro* (138–141). It has been suggested that the effects of nicotine are due to competitive inhibition of cyclooxygenase, which precludes the formation of prostaglandin endoperoxides *in vivo.* Alterations in the structural integrity of the aortic endothelium following chronic oral administration of nicotine *in vivo* and upon exposure of cultured aortic endothelial cells *in vitro* have also been noted (142,143). Because nicotine stimulates catecholamine release from sympathetic ganglia and nerve endings, as well as the adrenal medulla, its toxicologic profile may share features in common with those described for catecholamines.

At the cellular level, nicotine modulates the proliferation of vascular endothelial and smooth muscle cells. Nicotine increases the synthesis of DNA in luminal endothelial cells after *in vivo* administration (142). At concentrations lower than those present in blood after smoking, nicotine also increases the rate of DNA synthesis in growth-arrested subcultures of smooth muscle cells (144). This response appears to be independent of those of other mitogens present in the medium and additive to that of serum. Such changes in smooth muscle cell proliferation are consistent with the enhanced rate of phenotypic modulation from a contractile to a synthetic state induced by nicotine. Increased number of lysosomes with incompletely degraded inclusions and/or inhibition of intralysosomal proteolysis in macrophages upon exposure to nicotine have been reported (145). Interestingly, the effect of nicotine on lysosomal structure is shared with other weak bases and amines and may be due to accumulation of the drug within lysosomes. Cytoskeletal changes have also been observed in cultured vascular cells upon exposure to nicotine (146). Although extensive circumstantial evidence is available, the mechanism by which nicotine causes vascular toxicity is not clear.

Polycyclic Aromatic Hydrocarbons

The pioneering work of Benditt and Benditt in the early 1970s paved the way for much of the work focusing on the vascular toxicity of polycyclic aromatic hydrocarbons and their ability to promote the initiation and/or progression of atherosclerosis. These investigators first proposed that atherosclerotic lesions, like benign smooth muscle tumors of the uterus, originate from the mutation of a single smooth muscle cell (147). This proposal was based on the observation that a normal section of the arterial wall contained cells expressing the A and B allele of the glucose-6-phosphate dehydrogenase gene, whereas most plaques were monotypic containing cells expressing only the A or B allele. Although this proposal was received originally with great skepticism, evidence implicating carcinogens (148), radiation (149), and viruses (150) in atherosclerosis has continued to accumulate over the years. Exposure of avian species to benzo[*a*]pyrene and 7,12-dimethylbenz[*a,h*]anthracene causes atherosclerosis without alterations in serum cholesterol levels (148). The ability of these carcinogens to cause atherosclerotic lesions has been associated with cytochrome P-450 mediated conversion of the parent compound to toxic metabolic intermediates. Microsomal monoxygenases, including P-450 forms 2 and 6 and NADPH-cytochrome P-450 reductase, have been identified in rabbit aortic vascular tissue (151). Human fetal aortic smooth muscle cells metabolize benzo[*a*]pyrene and 7,12-dimethylbenz[*a*]anthracene via cytochrome P-450-dependent mechanisms to phenols and 12-hydroxymethyl-7 methylbez[*a*]anthracene, 7-hydroxymethyl-12-methylbenz[*a*]anthracene, 7,12-dihydroxymethyl benz-[*a*]anthracene, and trans-8,9-dihydrodiol-7,12-dimethylbenz[*a*]anthracene, respectively (152). Pretreatment of chickens with Aroclor 1254, 3-methyl-cholantrene and 5,6-benzoflavone, but not phenobarbital or pregnolone 16 α-carbonitrile, results in significant increases in the aortic monoxygenation of polycyclic aromatic hydrocarbons (153). The majority of the activity responsible for the biotransformation of benzo[*a*]pyrene is associated with the smooth muscle layers of the aorta (151). However, cytochrome P-450-dependent monoxygenase activity, which can potentially bioactivate carcinogens, has also been localized in the aortic endothelium (154,155). Interestingly, the activity of aortic aryl hydrocarbon hydroxylase has been correlated with the degree of susceptibility to atherosclerosis in avian species (156).

The generation of phase II metabolites via sulfoconjugation of 3-hydroxybenzo[*a*]pyrene has been demonstrated in aortic tissue (157). This reaction is important in the reduction of toxic phenolics. Sulfation takes place in cultured aortic smooth muscle cells and endothelial cells, in aortic whole organ explants, and in cytosolic fractions of cell-free preparations. The conjugation capacity of avian aortic tissues is 10–20% of the total avian hepatic capacity to sulfoconjugate 3-hydroxybenzo[*a*]pyrene. Avian aortic tissues also contain active UDP-glucuronosyltransferase activity, which catalyzes the glucuronidation of 3-hydroxybenzo[*a*]pyrene (158). In abdominal aortic segments, glucuronosyltransferase activity is eight- to ninefold higher than that of the thoracic aorta. Phenobarbital, but not 3-methylcholanthrene, increases the activity of microsomal fractions in both segments. Although glucuronidation of 3-hydroxybenzo[*a*]pyrene appears to be less active than sulfation in the aortic tissues, the differential distribution of glucuronyltransferase activity may account for differences in the responses of abdominal versus thoracic regions of the aorta to benzo[*a*]pyrene. This concept is supported by studies showing that glucuronidation decreases the mutagenic and carcinogenic effects of polycyclic aromatic hydrocarbons in the Ames test (159) but increases the generation of reactive intermediates in other preparations (160).

Additional studies are required to define the mechanism of vascular toxicity of polycyclic aromatic hydrocarbons. Albert et al. (148) and Penn et al. (161) have reported that treatment with several polycyclic hydrocarbons increases the size, but not the frequency, of atherosclerotic lesions. These observations suggest that polycyclic aromatic hydrocarbons act as promoters of the atherosclerotic process, but argue against their ability to initiate lesion formation. In contrast, Paigen et al. (162) have shown that 3-methylcholanthrene increases both the number and size of lipid-staining lesions in the aorta of animals fed an atherogenic diet for 8 weeks. Furthermore, Majesky et al. (163) have shown that focal proliferation of intimal smooth muscle cells can be produced by an initiation/promotion sequence using 7,12-dimethylbenz[*a*]anthracene and the α-1 selective adrenergic agonist, methoxamine. This discrepancy may be accounted for by regional differences in toxicologic response. Distal segments of aorta have been proposed as preferential sites for promotion, while initiation is thought to be confined to the thoracic region. The final verdict must take into account metabolic, cytotoxic, and genotoxic influences in the expression of toxic insult. Because hydrocarbons associate readily with plasma lipoproteins, Revis et al. (164) have suggested that the atherogenic effect of polycyclic aromatic hydrocarbons is related to the mechanism by which these chemicals are transported in plasma. This proposal was based on the observation that carcinogens that do not associate with lipoproteins, such as 2,4,6-trichlorophenol, are not atherogenic. An interesting area of investigation that has not yet been addressed is whether the vascular toxicity of polycyclic aromatic hydrocarbons is mediated, at least in part, by Ah-receptor mechanisms. In this regard, it is interesting to note that Ah-responsive mice are more susceptible to both 3-methylcholanthrene and atherosclerosis than Ah-resistant mice (165).

Recent studies in this laboratory have shown that *in vivo* exposure of quail to benzo[*a*]pyrene modulates the phosphorylation of medial aortic proteins. Benzo[*a*]pyrene treatment enhances the basal phosphorylation of several medial cytosolic proteins but inhibits C-kinase-mediated phosphorylation of proteins in the particulate fraction of aortic homogenates (166). The inhibitory response appears to be due, at least in part, to loss of protein kinase C activity. The profile of medial protein phosphorylation induced by benzo[*a*]pyrene is altered when *in vitro* phosphorylation measurements are carried out in the presence of endothelial cells. Increased phosphorylation of cytosolic proteins is observed in aortic homogenates containing endothelial and smooth muscle cell proteins (K.S. Ramos and X. Ou, *unpublished observations*). These observations serve to emphasize the concept that multiple cell interactions may be critical to the expression of the toxic response. Because phosphorylation mechanisms are intimately involved with the regulation of vascular smooth muscle cell growth and differentiation, these results suggest that signal transduction pathways involved in the phosphorylation of proteins may be targeted by polycyclic aromatic hydrocarbons. More recently, we have shown that acute benzo[*a*]pyrene exposure causes a modest, but significant, increase in the expression of the *ras* oncogene in naive aortic smooth muscle cells (167). This observation is particularly interesting within the context of carcinogen-induced atherogenesis since expression of the *ras* gene is enhanced during the G_1 phase of the cycle before initiation of DNA synthesis (168).

T-2 Toxin

Trichothece mycotoxins, commonly classified as tetracyclic sesquiterpenes, are naturally occurring cytotoxic metabolites of *Fusarium* species (169). These mycotoxins, including T-2 toxin (4β, 15-diacetoxy-8α-(3-methylbutyryloxy)-3α-hydroxy 12,13-epoxytrichothec-9-ene), are major contaminants of foods and animal feeds and may cause illness in animals and humans. Although the carcinogenic effects of trichothece mycotoxins has been documented for many years, little is known about the vascular toxicity of these agents. Acute parenteral administration of T-2 toxin to laboratory animals induces shock, hypothermia, and death due to cardiovascular and respiratory failure (170). Wilson et al. (171) have reported that intravenous infusion of T-2 toxin in rats causes an initial decrease in heart rate and blood pressure, followed by tachycardia and hypertension, and finally bradycardia and hypotension. These actions may be related to a central effect on blood pressure and catecholamine release (172). Siren and Feuerstein (172) have suggested that while T-2 toxin reduces blood flow and increases vascular resistance in skeletal muscle and mesenteric and renal vascular beds, no changes in mean arterial pressure and heart rate could be detected. Acute T-2 toxin exposure causes extensive destruction of myocardial capillaries, while repeated dosing promotes thickening of large coronary arteries (173). A more generalized atherosclerosis and hypertension are delayed consequences of repeated T-2 toxin exposure (174).

At the cellular level, T-2 toxin is a potent inhibitor of protein synthesis (175). T-2 toxin is thought to bind to the 60S subunit on the ribosome to interfere with peptidyl transferase activity at the transcription site. Inhibition of DNA synthesis is thought to be secondary to the interference with protein synthesis (176). A single large dose of 2 mg/kg or four injections of 0.3 mg/kg T-2 toxin causes necrosis of endothelial cells, accumulation of basement membrane-like material in the intima, and swelling and activation of smooth muscle cells in the media (177). Medial aortic smooth muscle cells decrease in number and increase in size upon exposure to T-2 toxin. Marked inhibition of smooth muscle cell growth is observed in explant cultures of smooth muscle cells. This is followed by stimulation of the proliferative capacity of smooth muscle cells *in vitro*. The fragmentation and increase in basement membrane-like material in these cells suggest that long-term changes occur even after the endothelium has returned to normal.

Miscellaneous Toxins

Exposure of factory workers in rayon plants to carbon disulfide has been associated with a significant increase in mortality from coronary heart disease. Although the mechanism of toxicity is not known, alterations of glucose and/or lipid metabolism and blood coagulation have been suggested (178). Recent studies have shown that 1,3-butadiene, a chemical used in the production of styrene-butadiene, increases the incidence of cardiac hemangiosarcomas, rare tumors of endothelial origin (179,180). Although hemangiosarcomas have also been observed in the liver, lung, and kidney, cardiac tumors are a major cause of death in animals exposed to this chemical.

Tetrachlorodibenzo-*p*-dioxin (TCDD), a widely studied polychlorinated hydrocarbon, induces hyperlipoproteinemia in animals and humans (181,182). In guinea pigs, a single dose of TCDD induces a 19-fold increase in very low density lipoproteins, and a four-fold increase in low density lipoproteins (183). The ability of TCDD to modulate lipid metabolism may be of serious consequences to the preservation of vascular function. Recent studies in our laboratory have shown that TCDD modulates protein phosphorylation in rat aortic smooth muscle cells *in vivo* and *in vitro* (184). Although the significance of these observations is at present unclear, the vascular responses to TCDD resemble some of those described for benzo[*a*]pyrene. This parallelism raises the possibility that the vascular toxicities of these chemicals share common cellular and molecular pathways.

Vitamin D hypervitaminosis causes medial degeneration, calcification of the coronary arteries, and smooth muscle cell proliferation in laboratory animals (185,186). The toxic effects of vitamin D may be related to its structural similarity to 25-hydroxycholesterol, a potent vascular toxin (185). Koh et al. (186) have shown that 1,25-dihydroxyvitamin D binds specifically to surface receptors of rat vascular smooth muscle cells to stimulate proliferation *in vitro*. The toxicity of vitamin D may be related to alterations in cyclic nucleotide metabolism. This suggestion is consistent with studies showing that cyclic nucleotides play a critical role in the regulation of vascular smooth muscle cell function (187). In this regard, recent studies have shown that phosphodiesterase inhibition is associated with toxicity in medium size arteries of the mesentery, testis, and myocardium (188). Other reports showing that theophylline, an inhibitor of phosphodiesterase, causes cardiovascular lesions in mesenteric arterioles (189) and that isomazole and indolidan cause periarteritis of the media and adventitia of small and medium sized arteries have also been presented (190).

From a toxicologic perspective, the recent demonstration that low density lipoproteins are oxidized *in vitro* by oxygen free radicals released by arterial cells is of particular interest. Modified low density lipoproteins attract macrophages and prevent their migration from the tissues (see ref. 84 for a comprehensive review). Oxidation derivatives of cholesterol, such as cholestane-3β, 5α, 6β-triol and 25-hydroxycholesterol are potent inhibitors of 3-hydroxy-3-methylglutaryl coenzyme A (HMG CoA) reductase, the rate limiting enzyme in cholesterol biosynthesis (191). Interestingly, many of the oxidized products of cholesterol that are formed spontaneously are identical to those formed enzymatically by the microsomal and mitochondrial cytochrome P-450 systems (192). However, the significance of these observations *in vivo* remains to be established since serum antioxidants may afford protection against this damage.

CONCLUDING REMARKS

The proposed mechanism of action for the vascular toxins surveyed in this chapter are summarized in Table 3. Although differences in cellular and subcellular targets are noted, many of these toxins share the ability to modulate

TABLE 3. *Selected chemicals with prominent vascular toxicity*

Chemical	Source	Putative mechanism of action
Allylamine	Synthetic precursor/ antifungal analogs	Bioactivation of parent compound by amine oxidase to acrolein and hydrogen peroxide; smooth muscle cell lysis
Butadiene	Synthetic precursor	Endothelial injury
Carbon disulfide	Fumigant, solvent	Metabolic disturbances in glucose/lipid metabolism
Carbon monoxide	Environmental	Carboxyhemoglobin formation with resulting tissue hypoxia; modulation of second messenger systems in vascular smooth muscle cells
Catecholamines	Endogenous amines	Adrenergic receptor-mediated alterations of contractile and proliferative behavior in vascular endothelial and/or smooth muscle cells
Dinitrotoluene	Synthetic precursor	Bioactivation-related changes of DNA synthesis in vascular smooth muscle cells
Hydrazinobenzoic acid	Constituent of *A. bisporus*	Unknown; potential involvement of free-radical-mediated genotoxicity
Metals	Environmental	Interference with cellular sulfhydryl, amino and phosphate residues; interference with calcium-mediated cellular events
Nicotine	Tobacco smoke	Modulation of DNA synthesis in vascular endothelial and/or smooth muscle cells
Polycyclic aromatic hydrocarbons	Tobacco smoke/ environmental	Cytochrome P-450-mediated bioactivation of reactive metabolic intermediates that bind to DNA in vascular smooth muscle cells
T-2 toxin	*Fusarium* mycotoxin	Endothelial and smooth muscle cell injury; modulation of smooth muscle cell proliferation
TCDD	Environmental	Modulation of lipid metabolism and hyperlipoproteinemia, phosphorylation disturbances in vascular smooth muscle cells
Vitamin D	Dietary	Medial toxin, modulation of cyclic nucleotide metabolism

the growth and/or differentiation of vascular cells. Some of these chemicals require metabolic activation for the induction of toxicity, while others cause deleterious effects by virtue of their high chemical reactivity. Not discussed in this chapter were the vascular toxicities mediated by nonspecific alterations of membrane function upon exposure to alcohols and solvents and the hypertensive episodes induced by a variety of autonomic agents. As highlighted throughout the chapter, vasculotoxic insult is potentially associated with injury to one or more of the cell types within the vessel wall. Toxicity often involves the interplay of multiple cellular and noncellular factors. The ultimate consequences of toxic challenge are influenced by the repair capacity of target cells and endocrine/paracrine influences on the tissue.

In recent years, the notion that toxic insult plays a significant role in the pathogenesis of vascular disorders, as well as various target-organ specific toxicities, has fueled interest in vascular toxicology. In attempting to unravel the cellular and molecular mechanisms of vasculotoxic insult, investigators must recognize the large degree of structural and functional heterogeneity characteristic of the vascular system. Such differences add a level of complexity to the study of vascular toxicities that has often been disregarded. A number of exciting new areas in the field of vascular toxicology, such as the study of microvascular toxicities, should be further explored. Future advances will rely on interdisciplinary exchange and cross-fertilization among varied scientific disciplines. Undoubtedly, such efforts must continue to be encouraged.

ACKNOWLEDGMENTS

The research cited in this chapter was supported in part by a grant from the National Institute of Environmental Health Sciences (ES 04849) and from Research Development Funds by the Texas Agricultural Experiment Station. The assistance of Ms. Cindy Hart Thurlow in the preparation of the manuscript is appreciated. I am particularly grateful to Dr. Devaki N. Sadhu and Mr. Russell C. Bowes for their helpful discussions and comments. The contributions of Drs. Lydia R. Cox, Scott L. Grossman, Celestine Alipui, Xiaolan Ou, and Kristien Piron to the unpublished work cited are acknowledged.

REFERENCES

1. Rhodin JAG. Architecture of the vessel wall. In: Bohr DF, Somlyo AP, Sparks HV, Geiger SR, eds. *Handbook of physiology: a critical comprehensive presentation of physiological knowledge and concepts,* vol II. Baltimore: Waverly Press; 1980:1–31.
2. Hudlicka O. Development of microcirculation: capillary growth and adaptation. In: Bohr Dr, Somlyo AP, Sparks HV, Geiger SR, eds. *Handbook of physiology: a critical comprehensive presentation of physiological knowledge and concepts,* vol IV. Baltimore: Waverly Press; 1980:165–216.

3. King GL, Johnson SH. Receptor-mediated transport of insulin across endothelial cells. *Science* 1985;227:1583–1586.
4. Jaffe EA. Physiologic functions of normal endothelial cells. *Ann NY Acad Sci* 1985;454:279–291.
5. Friedl HP, Till GO, Ryan US, Ward PA. Mediator-induced activation of xanthine oxidase in endothelial cells. *FASEB J* 1989;3:2512–2518.
6. Campbell GR, Campbell JH. Smooth muscle phenotypic changes in arterial wall homeostasis: implications for the pathogenesis of atherosclerosis. *Exp Mol Pathol* 1985;42:139–162.
7. Gordon D, Schwartz SM. Arterial smooth muscle differentiation. In: Campbell JH, Campbell GR, eds. *Vascular smooth muscle in culture*, vol I. Boca Raton, FL: CRC Press; 1987:1–14.
8. Sappino AP, Schurch W, Gabbiani G. Differentiation repertoire of fibroblastic cells: expression of cytoskeletal proteins as markers of phenotypic modulations. *Lab Invest* 1990;63:144–161.
9. Campbell GR, Chamley-Campbell JH. The cellular pathobiology of atherosclerosis. *Pathology* 1981;13:423–440.
10. McGill HC. The pathogenesis of atherosclerosis. *Clin Chem* 1988;34:33–39.
11. Ross R, Glomset J. The pathogenesis of atherosclerosis. *N Engl J Med* 1976;295:369–377.
12. Ross R. The pathogenesis of atherosclerosis—an update. *N Engl J Med* 1986;314:488–500.
13. Miano JM, Tota RR, Niksa V, Danishefsky KJ, Stemerman MB. Early proto-oncogene expression in rat aortic smooth muscle cells following endothelial removal. *Am J Pathol* 1990;137:761–765.
14. Nishida K, Abiko T, Ishihara M, Tomikawa M. Arterial injury-induced smooth muscle cell proliferation in rats is accompanied by increase in polyamine synthesis and level. *Atherosclerosis* 1990;83:119–125.
15. Peng S-K, Taylor CB, Hill JC, Morin RJ. Cholesterol oxidation derivatives and arterial endothelial damage. *Atherosclerosis* 1985;54:121–133.
16. Benditt EP. Evidence for a monoclonal origin of human atherosclerotic plaque and some implications. *Circulation* 1974;50:650–652.
17. Penn A, Gargte SJ, Warren L, Nesta D, Mindich B. Transforming genes in human atherosclerotic plaque DNA. *Proc Natl Acad Sci USA* 1986;83:7951–7955.
18. Granger HJ, Schelling ME, Lewis RE, Zawieja DC, Meininger CJ. Physiology and pathobiology of the microcirculation. *Am J Otolaryngol* 1988;9:264–277.
19. Owens GK, Schwartz SM. Alterations in vascular smooth muscle cells in the spontaneously hypertensive rat: role of cellular hypertrophy, hyperploidy, and hyperplasia. *Circ Res* 1982;9:264–277.
20. Janes SM, Mu D, Wemmer D, et al. A new redox cofactor in eukaryotic enzymes: 6-hydroxydopa at the active site of bovine serum amine oxidase. *Science* 1990;248:981–987.
21. Escalante B, Sessa WC, Falck JR, Yadagiri P, Schwartzman ML. Cytochrome P450-dependent arachidonic acid metabolites, 19- and 20-hydroxyeicosatetraenoic acids, enhance sodium–potassium ATPase activity in vascular smooth muscle. *J Cardiovasc Pharmacol* 1990;16:438–443.
22. Ferrario JB, DeLeon IR, Tracy RE. Evidence for toxic anthropogenic chemicals in human thrombogenic coronary plaques. *Arch Environ Contam Toxicol* 1985;14:529–534.
23. Bishop CT, Mirza Z, Crapo JD, Freeman BA. Free radical damage to cultured porcine aortic endothelial cells and lung fibroblasts: modulation by culture conditions. *In Vitro Cell Dev Biol* 1985;21:21–25.
24. Ramos KS, Thurlow CH. Influence of species and growth conditions in vitro upon the toxicologic responsiveness of cultured aortic smooth muscle cells. Submitted for publication, 1992.
25. Sutton WL. Aliphati and alicyclic amines. In: Patty FA, Fassett DW, Irish DO, eds. *Industrial hygiene and toxicology*, vol 2. New York: Interscience; 1963:2038.
26. Ryder NS. Mechanism of action and biochemical selectivity of allylamine antimyotic agents. *Ann NY Acad Sci* 1988;544:208–220.

27. Beard RR, Noe JT. Aliphatic and alicyclic amines. In: Clayton GD, Clayton FE, eds. *Patty's industrial hygiene and toxicology,* vol II. New York: Wiley; 1981:3135–3173.
28. Hine CH, Kodama JK, Guzman RJ, Loquvam GS. The toxicity of allylamines. *Arch Environ Health* 1960;1:343–74/352.
29. Boor PJ, Moslen MJ, Reynolds ES. Allylamine cardiotoxicity: I. Sequence of pathologic events. *Toxicol Appl Pharmacol* 1979;50:581–592.
30. Lalich JJ, Allen JR, Paik WCW. Myocardial fibrosis and smooth muscle cell hyperplasia in coronary arteries of allylamine-fed rats. *Am J Pathol* 1972;66(2):225–233.
31. Guzman RJ, Loquvam GS, Kodama JK, Hine CH. Myocarditis produced by allylamines. *Arch Environ Health* 1961;2:62–73.
32. Boor PJ. Allylamine cardiovascular toxicity: V. Tissue distribution and toxicokinetics after oral administration. *Toxicology* 1985;35:167–177.
33. Boor PJ, Hysmith RM, Sanduja R. A role for a new vascular enzyme in the metabolism of xenobiotic amines. *Circ Res* 1990;66(1):249–252.
34. Ramos K, Grossman SL, Cox LR. Allylamine-induced vascular toxicity *in vitro:* prevention by semicarbizide-sensitive amine oxidase inhibitors. *Toxicol Appl Pharmacol* 1988;96:61–71.
35. Buffoni F. Biochemical pharmacology of amine oxidases. *Trends Pharmacol Sci* 1983;4:313–315.
36. Grossman SL, Alipui C, Ramos K. Further characterization of the metabolic activation of allylamine to acrolein in rat vascular tissue. *In Vitro Toxicol* 1990;3:303–307.
37. Hysmith RM, Boor PJ. Allylamine cardiovascular toxicity: VI. Subcellular distribution in rat aortas. *Toxicology* 1985;35:179–187.
38. Ramos K, Cox LR. Primary cultures of rat aortic endothelial and smooth muscle cells. I. An *in vitro* model to study xenobiotic-induced vascular cytotoxicity. *In Vitro Cell Dev Biol* 1987;21:495–504.
39. Patel JM, Gordon WP, Nelson SD, Leibman KC. Comparison of hepatic biotransformation and toxicity of allyl alcohol and [1,1-2H2]allyl alcohol in rats. *Drug Metab Dispos* 1983;11:164–166.
40. Kutzman RS, Wehner RW, Haber SB. Selected responses of hypertension-sensitive and resistant rats to inhaled acrolein. *Toxicology* 1984;31:53–65.
41. Beckner JS, Hudgins PM, Egle JL. Effects of acetaldehyde, propionaldehyde, formaldehyde and acrolein on contractility, ^{14}C-norepinephrine and [45]calcium binding in isolated smooth muscle. *Res Commun Chem Pathol Pharmacol* 1974;9(3):471–488.
42. Cox LR, Ramos K. Allylamine-induced phenotypic modulation of aortic smooth muscle cells. *J Exp Pathol* 1990;71:11–18.
43. Cox LR, Murphy SK, Ramos K. Modulation of phosphoinositide metabolism in aortic smooth muscle cells by allylamine. *Exp Mol Pathol* 1990;53:52–63.
44. Astrup P, Hellung-Larson P, Kjeldsen K, Mellemgaard K. The effect of tobacco smoking on the dissociation curve of oxyhemoglobin-investigations in patients with occlusive arterial diseases and in normal subjects. *Scand J Clin Lab Invest* 1966;18:450–460.
45. Levene CI, Barlet CP, Fornieri C, Heale G. Effect of hypoxia and carbon monoxide on collagen synthesis in cultured porcine and bovine aortic endothelium. *Br J Exp Pathol* 1985;66:399–408.
46. Paule WJ, Zemplenyl TK, Rounds DE, Blankenhorn DH. Light and electron-microscopic characteristics of arterial smooth muscle cell cultures subjected to hypoxia or carbon monoxide. *Atherosclerosis* 1976;25:111–123.
47. Astrup PK, Kjeldson K, Wanstrup J. Enhancing influence of carbon monoxide on the development of atheromatosis in cholesterol-fed rabbits. *J Atheroscler Res* 1967;7:343–354.
48. Cobarn RF, Mayers LB. Myoglobin oxygen tension determined from measurements of carboxyhemoglobin in skeletal muscle. *Am J Physiol* 1971;220:66–74.
49. Young LJ, Caughey WS. Pathobiochemistry of carbon monoxide poisoning. *FEBS* 1990;272:1–6.
50. McFaul SJ, McGrath JJ. Studies on the mechanism of carbon monoxide-induced vasodilation in the isolated perfused rat heart. *Toxicol Appl Pharmacol* 1987;87:464–473.
51. Graser T, Vedernikov YP, Li DS. Study on the mechanism of carbon monoxide induced endothelium-independent relaxation in porcine coronary artery and vein. *Biomed Biochim Acta* 1990;49(4):293–296.

52. Vedernikov YP, Graser T, Vanin AF. Similar endothelium-independent arterial relaxation by carbon monoxide and nitric oxide. *Biomed Biochim Acta* 1989;48:601–603.

53. Lin H, McGrath JJ. Vasodilating effects of carbon monoxide. *Drug Chem Toxicol* 1988;11(4):371–385.

54. Brune B, Ullrich V. Inhibition of platelet aggregation by carbon monoxide is mediated by activation of guanylate cyclase. *Mol Pharmacol* 1987;32:497–504.

55. Ramos KS, Lin H, McGrath JJ. Modulation of cyclic guanosine monophosphate levels in cultured aortic smooth muscle cells by carbon monoxide. *Biochem Pharmacol* 1989;38:1368–1370.

56. Robinson CP, Baskin SI, Franz DR. The mechanisms of action of cyanide on the rabbit aorta. *J Appl Toxicol* 1985;5:372–377.

57. Helin P, Lorenzen I, Garbarsch C, Matthiessen NE. Arteriosclerosis in rabbit aorta induced by noradrenaline. *Atherosclerosis* 1970;12:125–132.

58. Kukreja RS, Datta BN, Chakravarti RN. Catecholamine-induced aggravation of aortic and coronary atherosclerosis in monkeys. *Atherosclerosis* 1981;40:291–298.

59. Bauch HJ, Grunwald J, Vischer P, Gerlach U, Hauss WH. A possible role of catecholamines in atherogenesis and subsequent complications of atherosclerosis. *Exp Pathol* 1987;31:193–204.

60. Grimm M, Weidmann P, Keusch G, Meier A, Gluck Z. Norepinephrine clearance and pressure effect in normal and hypertensive man. *Klin Worchenschr* 1980;58:1175–1181.

61. Nakaki T, Nakayama M, Yamamoto S, Kato R. α_1-Adrenergic stimulation and β_2-adrenergic inhibition of DNA synthesis in vascular smooth muscle cells. *Mol Pharmacol* 1989;37:30–36.

62. Pettersson K, Bejne B, Bjork H, Strawn WB, Bondjers G. Experimental sympathetic activation causes endothelial injury in the rabbit thoracic aorta via β_1-adrenoceptor activation. *Circ Res* 1990;67(4):1027–1034.

63. Sholley MM, Gimbrone MA, Cotran RS. Cellular migration and replication in endothelial regeneration. *Lab Invest* 1976;36:18–25.

64. Grunwald J, Schaper W, Mey J, Hauss WH. Special characteristics of cultured smooth muscle cell subtypes of hypertensive and diabetic rats. *Artery* 1982;11:1–14.

65. Grunwald J, Haudenschild CC. Intimal injury *in vivo* activates vascular smooth muscle cell migration and explant outgrowth *in vitro*. *Arteriosclerosis* 1984;4:183–188.

66. Berk BC, Alexander RW, Brock TA, Gimbrone MA, Webb RC. Vasoconstriction: a new activity for platelet-derived growth factors. *Science* 1986;232:87–90.

67. Berk BC, Brock TA, Webb RC, Taubman MB, Atkinson WJ, Gimbrone MA. Epidermal growth factor, a vascular smooth muscle mitogen induces rat aortic contraction. *J Clin Invest* 1985;75:1083–1086.

68. Naftilan AJ, Cilliland GK, Eldridge CS, Kraft AS. Induction of the protooncogene c-*jun* by angiotensin II. *Mol Cell Biol* 1990;10:5536–5540.

69. Dhalla NS, Yates JC, Lee SL, Singh A. Functional and subcellular changes in the isolated rat heart perfused with oxidized isoproterenol. *J Mol Cell Cardiol* 1978;10:31–41.

70. Ramos K. Cellular and molecular basis of xenobiotic-induced cardiovascular toxicity: application of cell culture systems. In: Acosta D, ed. *Cellular and molecular toxicology and in vitro toxicology*. Boca Raton, FL: CRC Press; 1990:139–155.

71. Wolin MS, Belloni FL. Superoxide anion selectively attenuates catecholamine-induced contractile tension in isolated rabbit aorta. *Am J Physiol* 1985;249:H1127–H1133.

72. Rubanyi GM. Vascular effects of oxygen-derived free radicals. *Free Radical Biol Med* 1988;4:107–120.

73. McCord JM. Oxygen-derived free radicals in post ischemic tissue injury. *N Engl J Med* 1985;312:159–163.

74. Machlin LJ, Bendich A. Free radical tissue damage: protective role of antioxidant nutrients. *FASEB J* 1987;1:441–445.

75. Babior BM, Curnette JT, McMurick BJ. The particulate superoxide-forming system from human neutrophils: properties of the system and further evidence supporting its participation in the respiratory burst. *J Clin Invest* 1976;58:989–996.

76. Heinecke JW. Free radical modification of low-density lipoprotein: mechanisms and biological consequences. *Free Radical Biol Med* 1987;3:65–73.

77. Kontos HA, Wei EP, Dietrich WD, et al. Mechanism of cerebral arteriolar abnormalities after acute hypertension. *Am J Physiol* 1981;240:H511–H527.
78. Wei EP, Kontos HA, Dietrich WD, Povlishock JT, Ellis EF. Inhibition by free radical scavengers and by cyclooxygenase inhibitors of pial arteriolar abnormalities from concussive brain injury in cats. *Circ Res* 1981;48:95–103.
79. Wei EP, Christman CW, Kontos HA, Povlishock JT. Effects of oxygen radicals on cerebral arterioles. *Am J Physiol* 1985;248(17):H157–H162.
80. Hiebert LM, Liu JM. Heparin protects cultured arterial endothelial cells from damage by toxic oxygen metabolites. *Atherosclerosis* 1990;83(1):47–51.
81. Shasby M, Lind SE, Shasby SS, Goldsmith JC, Hunninghake GW. Reversible oxidant-induced increases in albumin transfer across cultured endothelium: alterations in cell shape and calcium homeostasis. *Blood* 1985;65(3):605–614.
82. Rosenblum WI, Bryan D. Evidence that in vivo constriction of cerebral arterioles by local application of tert-butyl hydroperoxide is mediated by release of endogenous thromboxane. *Stroke* 1987;18:195–199.
83. Matsubara T, Ziff M. Superoxide anion release by human endothelial cells: synergism between a phorbol ester and a calcium ionophore. *J Cell Physiol* 1986;127:207–210.
84. Gross JL, Moscatelli D, Rifkin DB. Increased capillary endothelial cell protease activity in response to angiogenic stimuli *in vitro*. *Proc Natl Acad Sci USA* 1983;80:2623–2627.
85. Chemical Industry Institute of Toxicology. 104 Week chronic toxicity study in rats. Dinitrotoluene. Final Report 1982, Docket # 12362.
86. Ellis HV, Hough CB, Dacre YC, Lee CC. Chronic toxicity of 2,4-dinitrotoluene in the rat. *Toxicol Appl Pharmacol* 1978;45:245.
87. Leonard TB, Graichen ME, Popp JA. Dinitrotoluene isomer-specific hepatocarcinogenesis in F344 rats. *J Natl Cancer Inst* 1987;79:1313–1319.
88. Levine RJ. Dinitrotoluene: human atherogen, carcinogen, neither or both? *CIIT* 1987;7(1):2–5.
89. Levine RJ, Andjelkovich DA, Kersteter SL, et al. Heart disease in workers exposed to dinitrotoluene. *J Occup Med* 1986;28(9):811–816.
90. Ramos KS, McMahon KK, Alipui C, Demick D. Modulation of DNA synthesis in aortic smooth muscle cells by dinitrotoluene. *Cell Biol Toxicol* 1991;7(2):111–128.
91. Ramos K, McMahon KK, Alipui C, Demick D. Modulation of smooth muscle cell proliferation by dinitrotoluene. In: Witmer CM, Snyder RR, Jollow DJ, Kaef GF, Kocsis JJ, Sipes IG, eds. *Biologic reductive intermediates*, vol V. New York: Plenum Press; 1990:805–807.
92. Long RM, Rickert DE. Metabolism and excretion of 2,6-dinitro[¹⁴C]toluene *in vivo* and in isolated perfused rat livers. *Drug Metab Dispos* 1982;10:455–458.
93. Mirsalis JC, Hamm TE, Sherrill JM, Butterworth BE. Role of gut flora in the genotoxicity of dinitrotoluene. *Nature* 1982;295:322–323.
94. Dent JG, Schnell SR, Guest D. Metabolism of 2,4-dinitrotoluene in rat hepatic microsomes and cecal flora. In: *Proceedings of the Second International Symposium on biologically reactive intermediates: chemical mechanisms and biologic effects*. New York: Plenum; 1981:431–436.
95. Sadhu DN, Crum S, Ramos KS. Benzo[*a*]pyrene-induced alterations in [³H]-thymidine incorporation in cultured aortic smooth muscle cells. *Toxicologist* 1991;11:339.
96. Vesselinovitch D. Animal models and the study of atherosclerosis. *Arch Pathol Lab Med* 1980;112:1011–1017.
97. Jokinen MP, Clarkson TB, Prichard RW. Recent advances in molecular pathology. Animal models in atherosclerosis research. *Exp Mol Pathol* 1985;42:1–28.
98. McManus BM, Toth B, Patil KD. Aortic rupture and aortic smooth muscle tumors in mice: induction by *p*-hydrazinobenzoic acid hydrochloride of the cultivated mushroom *Agaricus bisporus*. *Lab Invest* 1987;57(1):78–85.
99. Toth B, Nagel D, Patil K, Erickson J, Antonson K. Tumor induction with N1-acetyl derivative of 4-hydroxy methyl phenyl hydrazine, a metabolite of agaritine of *Agaricus bisporus*. *Cancer Res* 1978;38:177–180.
100. Savage NW, Adkins KF, Young WG, Chapman PJ. Oral vascular leiomyoma: review of the literature and report of 2 cases. *Aust Dent J* 1983;28:346–349.

101. Hernandez FJ, Stanley JM, Ranganath KA, Rubinstein AI. Primary leiomyosarcoma of the aorta. *Am J Surg Pathol* 1979;3:251–254.
102. Milili JJ, LaFlare RG, Nemir P. Leiomyosarcoma of the abdominal aorta: a case report. *Surgery* 1981;89:631–634.
103. Kalyanaraman B, Sinha BK. Free radical-mediated activation of hydrazine derivatives. *Environ Health Perspec* 1985;64:179–184.
104. Noda A, Ishizawa M, Ohino K, Sendo T, Noda H. Relationship between oxidative metabolites of hydrazine and hydrazine-induced mutagenicity. *Toxicol Lett* 1986;31:131–137.
105. Whiting RF, Wei L, Stich HF. Enhancement by transition metals of unscheduled DNA synthesis induced by isoniazid and related hydrazines in cultured normal and xeroderma pigmentosum human cells. *Mutat Res* 1979;62:505–510.
106. Medeiros DM, Pellum LK. Blood pressure and hair cadmium, lead, copper, and zinc concentrations in Mississippi adolescents. *Bull Environ Contam Toxicol* 1985;34:163–169.
107. Voors AW, Johnson WD, Shuman MS. Additive statistical effects of cadmium and lead on heart-related disease in a North Carolina autopsy series. *Arch Environ Health* 1982;37:98–102.
108. Beevers DG, Campbell BC, Goldberts A, Moore MR, Hawthorne VM. Blood cadmium in hypertensives and normotensives. *Lancet* 1976;2:12222–12224.
109. Carafoli E. How calcium crosses plasma membrane including the sarcolemma. In: Opie LH, ed. *Calcium antagonists and cardiovascular disease.* New York: Raven Press; 1984:29–41.
110. Cheung WY. Calmodulin: its potential role in cell proliferation and heavy metal toxicity. *Fed Proc* 1984;43(15):2995–2999.
111. Habermann E, Richardt G. Intracellular calcium binding proteins as targets for heavy metal ions. *Trends Pharmacol Sci* 1986;7:298–300.
112. Perry MH, Erlanger MW, Gustafsson TO, Perry EF. Reversal of cadmium-induced hypertension by D-myo-inositol-1,2,6-triphosphate. *J Toxicol Environ Health* 1989;28:151–159.
113. Georing PL, Klaassen CD. Zinc-induced tolerance to cadmium toxicity. *Toxicol Appl Pharmacol* 1984;74:299–307.
114. Webb M. The metallothioneins. In: Webb M, ed. *The chemistry, biochemistry and biology of cadmium.* Amsterdam: Elseview/North Holland; 1979:195–266.
115. Revis NW, Zinsmeister AR, Bull R. Atherosclerosis and hypertension induction by lead and cadmium ions: an effect prevented by calcium ion. *Proc Natl Acad Sci USA* 1981;78(10):6494–6498.
116. Schroeder HA, Vinton WH Jr. Hypertension in rats induced by small doses of cadmium. *Am J Physiol* 1962;202:515–518.
117. Perry HM Jr, Erlanger MW, Perry EF. Elevated systolic pressure following chronic-level cadmium feeding. *Am J Physiol* 1977;232:H114–H121.
118. Kopp SJ, Glonek T, Perry HM Jr, Erlanger M, Perry EF. Cardiovascular actions of cadmium at environmental exposure levels. *Science* 1982;217:837–839.
119. Shukla GS, Singhal RL. The present status of biological effects of toxic metals in the environment: lead, cadmium, manganese. *Can J Physiol Pharmacol* 1984;62:1015–1031.
120. Perry HM Jr, Perry EF, Erlanger MW. Possible influence of heavy metals in cardiovascular disease: an introduction and overview. *J Environ Pathol Toxicol* 1980;3:195–203.
121. Perry HM Jr, Erlanger MW, Perry EF. Effect of a second metal on cadmium-induced hypertension. *Arch Environ Health* 1983;38:80–85.
122. Doyle JJ, Bernhoft RA, Sandstead HH. The effects of a low level of dietary cadmium on blood pressure, ^{24}Na, ^{42}K and water retention in growing rats. *J Lab Clin Med* 1975;86:57–83.
123. Perry HM Jr, Yunice A. Acute pressor effects of intra-arterial cadmium and mercuric ions in anesthetized rats. *Proc Soc Exp Biol Med* 1965;120:805–808.
124. Perry HM Jr, Erlanger M, Yunice A, Perry EF. Mechanism of the acute hypertensive effect of intra-arterial cadmium and mercury in anesthetized rats. *J Lab Clin Med* 1967;70:963–971.

125. Perry HM, Erlanger MW, Perry EF. Increase in the systolic pressure of rats chronically fed cadmium. *Environ Health Perspect* 1979;28:251–260.
126. Schlaepfer WW. Sequential study of endothelial changes in acute cadmium intoxication. *Lab Invest* 1971;25(6):556–564.
127. Togna G, Togna AR, Caprino L. Vascular endothelium and platelet preparations for the prediction of xenobiotic effects on the vascular system. *Xenobiotica* 1985;15(8,9):661–664.
128. Caprino L, Togna G, Togna AR. Cadmium-induced platelet hypersensitivity to aggregating agents. *Pharmacol Res Commun* 1979;11:731–737.
129. Batuman V, Landy E, Maesaka JK, Wedeen RP. Contribution of lead to hypertension with renal impairment. *N Engl J Med* 1983;309:17–21.
130. Jhaveri R, Lavorgna L, Dube SK, Glass L, Khan F, Evans HE. Relationship of blood pressure to blood lead concentrations in small children. *Pediatrics* 1979;63:674–676.
131. Needleman HL, Schell AS, Bellinger D, Leviton A, Alldred EN. The long-term effects of exposure to low doses of lead in childhood: an 11 year follow-up report. *N Engl J Med* 1990;322:83–88.
132. Chiappino G, Costantini S, Cirla AM. Changes induced by cadmium, zinc, and lead on renal and peripheral vascular resistance in the anesthetized rabbit. *Med Lav* 1968;59:522–533.
133. Fine BP, Vetrano T, Skurnick J, Ty A. Blood pressure elevation in young dogs during low level lead poisoning. *Toxicol Appl Pharmacol* 1988;93:388–393.
134. Tomera JF, Harakal C. Mercury and lead-induced contraction of aortic smooth muscle in vitro. *Arch Int Pharmacodyn Ther* 1986;283:295–302.
135. Caprino L, Togna AR, Cebo B, Dolci N, Togna G. In vitro effects of mercury on platelet aggregation, thromboxane, and vascular prostacyclin production. *Arch Toxicol [Suppl]* 1983;6:48–51.
136. Maxwell K, Vinters HV, Berliner JA, Bready JV, Cancilla PA. Effect of inorganic lead on some functions of the cerebral microvessel endothelium. *Toxicol Appl Pharmacol* 1986;84:389–399.
137. Bull HA, Pittilo RM, Blow DJ, et al. The effects of nicotine on PGI_2 production by rat aortic endothelium. *Thromb Haemostas* 1985;54(2):472–474.
138. Wennmalm A. Nicotine inhibits release of 6-keto prostaglandin F_1 from isolated perfused rabbit heart. *Acta Physiol Scand* 1978;103:107–109.
139. Sonnfield T, Wennmalm A. Inhibition by nicotine of the formation of prostacyclin-like activity in rabbit and human vascular tissue. *Br J Pharmacol* 1980;71:609–613.
140. Stoel I, Biessen WJvd, Zwolsman E, et al. Direct effect of nicotine on prostacyclin in human umbilical arteries. *Acta Therapeutica* 1980;6(4):32–34.
141. Alster P, Wennmalm A. Effect of nicotine on prostacyclin formation in rat aorta. *Eur J Pharmacol* 1983;86:441–446.
142. Zimmerman M, McGeachie J. The effect of nicotine on aortic endothelial cell turnover: an autoradiographic study. *Atherosclerosis* 1985;58:39–47.
143. Tulloss J, Booyse FM. Effect of various agents and physical damage in bovine endothelial cultures. *Microvasc Res* 1978;16:51–58.
144. Thyberg J. Effects of nicotine on phenotypic modulation and initiation of DNA synthesis in cultured arterial smooth muscle cells. *Virchows Arch* 1986;52:25–32.
145. Thyberg J, Nilsson J. Effects of nicotine on endocytosis and intracellular degradation of horseradish peroxidase in cultivated mouse peritoneal macrophages. *Acta Pathol Microb Immunol Scand* 1982;90:305–310.
146. Csonka E, Somogyi A, Augustin J, Haberbosch W, Schettler G, Jellinek H. The effect of nicotine on cultured cells of vascular origin. *Virchows Arch* 1985;407:441–447.
147. Benditt EP, Benditt JM. Evidence for a monoclonal origin of human atherosclerotic plaques. *Proc Natl Acad Sci USA* 1973;70:1753–1756.
148. Albert RE, Vanderlaan M, Burns FJ, Nishizumi M. Effect of carcinogens on chicken atherosclerosis. *Cancer Res* 1977;37:2232–2235.
149. Gold H. Production of arteriosclerosis in the rat: effect of x-ray and high-fat diet. *Arch Pathol* 1961;71:46/268–51/273.
150. Benditt EP, Barrett T, McDougall JK. Viruses in the etiology of atherosclerosis. *Proc Natl Acad Sci USA* 1983;80:6386–6389.
151. Serabjit-Singh CJ, Bend JR, Philpot RM. Cytochrome P-450 monooxygenase system localization in smooth muscle of rabbit aorta. *Mol Pharmacol* 1985;28:72–79.

152. Bond JA, Kocan RM, Benditt EP, Juchau MR. Metabolism of benzo[*a*]pyrene and 7,12-dimethylbenz[*a*]anthracene in cultured human fetal aortic smooth muscle cells. *Life Sci* 1979;25:425–430.
153. Bond JA, Hsueh-Ying LY, Majesky MW, Benditt EP, Juchau MR. Metabolism of benzo[*a*]pyrene and 7,12-dimethylbenz[*a*]anthracene in chicken aortas: monooxygenation, bioactivation to mutagens, and covalent binding to DNA *in vitro*. *Toxicol Appl Pharmacol* 1980;52:323–335.
154. Pinto A, Abraham NG, Mullane KM. Cytochrome P-450-dependent monooxygenase activity and endothelial-dependent relaxations induced by arachidonic acid. *J Pharmacol Exp Ther* 1986;236(2):445–451.
155. Baird WM, Chemerys R, Grinspan JB, Mueller SN, Levine EM. Benzo[*a*]pyrene metabolism in bovine aortic endothelial and bovine lung fibroblast-like cell cultures. *Cancer Res* 1980;40:1781–1786.
156. Majesky M, Yang HY, Benditt E, Juchau M. Carcinogenesis and atherogenesis: differences in mono-oxygenase inducibility and bioactivation of benzo[*a*]pyrene in aortic and hepatic tissue of atherosclerosis-susceptible versus resistant pigeons. *Carcinogenesis* 1983;4:647–652.
157. Yang HYL, Namkung MJ, Nelson WJ, Juchau MR. Phase II biotransformation of carcinogens/atherogens in cultured aortic tissues and cells: I. Sulfation of 3-hydroxy-benzo[*a*]pyrene. *Drug Metab Dispos* 1986;14(3):287–298.
158. Yang HYL, Majesky MW, Namkung MJ, Juchau MR. Phase II biotransformation of carcinogens/atherogens in cultured aortic tissues and cells. II. Glucoronidation of 3-hydroxy-benzo[*a*]pyrene. *Drug Metab Dispos* 1986;14:293–298.
159. Owens IS, Koteen GM, Pelkonen O, Legraverend C. Activation of certain benzo-[*a*]pyrene phenols and the effect of some conjugating enzyme activities. In: Aito A, ed. *Conjugation reactions in biotransformation*. Amsterdam: Elsevier Biomedical; 1978:39.
160. Nemoto N, Kawana M, Tokoyama S. Effects of activation of UDP-glycuronyl transferase on metabolism of benzo[*a*]pyrene with rat liver microsomes. *J Pharmacobiodyn* 1983;6:105–113.
161. Penn A, Snyder C. Arteriosclerotic plaque development is "promoted" by polynuclear aromatic hydrocarbons. *Carcinogenesis* 1988;9(12):2185–2189.
162. Paigen B, Havens MB, Morrow A. Effect of 3-methylcholanthrene on the development of aortic lesions in mice. *Cancer Res* 1985;45:3850–3855.
163. Majesky MW, Reidy MA, Benditt EP, Juchau MR. Focal smooth muscle proliferation in the aortic intima produced by an initiation–promotion sequence. *Proc Natl Acad Sci USA* 1985;82:3450–3454.
164. Revis NW, Bull R, Laurie D, Schiller CA. The effectiveness of chemical carcinogens to induce atherosclerosis in the white carneau pigeon. *Toxicology* 1984;32:215–227.
165. Paigen B, Holmes P, Morrow A, Mitchell D. Effects of 3-methylcholanthrene on atherosclerosis in two congenic strains of mice with different susceptibilities to methylcholanthrene-induced tumors. *Cancer Res* 1986;46:3321–3324.
166. Ou X, Ramos KS. Modulation of aortic protein phosphorylation by benzo[*a*]pyrene: implications in PAH induced atherogenesis. *J Biochem Toxicol* 1992 (in press).
167. Sadhu DN, Ramos KS. Modulation by retinoic acid of spontaneous and benzo-[*a*]pyrene-induced c-Ha-ras expression. In: *Proceedings of the Third International Conference on mechanisms of antimutagenesis and anticarcinogenesis.* 1992 (in press).
168. Sadhu DN, Ramos KS. Steady state mRNA levels of c-Ha-ras protooncogene in rat aortic smooth muscle cells during different phases of the cell cycle. Submitted for publication, 1991.
169. Schiefer HB, Rousseaux CG, Hancock DS, Blakley BR. Effects of low-level long-term oral exposure to T-2 toxin in CD-1 mice. *Food Chem Toxicol* 1987;25(8):593–601.
170. Feuerstein G, Goldstein DS, Ramwell RO, et al. Cardiorespiratory, sympathetic and biochemical responses to T-2 toxin in the guinea pig and rat. *J Pharmacol Exp Ther* 1985;232:786–794.
171. Wilson CA, Everard DM, Schoental R. Blood pressure changes and cardiovascular lesions found in rats given T-2 toxin, a trichothecene secondary metabolite of certain *Fusarium* microfungi. *Toxicol Lett* 1982;10:35–40.

172. Siren AL, Feuerstein G. Effect of T-2 toxin on regional blood flow and vascular resistance in the conscious rat. *Toxicol Appl Pharmacol* 1986;83:438–444.
173. Yarom R, More R, Sherman Y, Yagen B. T-2 toxin-induced pathology in the hearts of rats. *Br J Exp Pathol* 1983;64:570–577.
174. Schoenthal R, Jaffe AZ, Yagen B. Cardiovascular lesions and various tumors found in rats given T-2 toxin, a trichothecene metabolite of *Fusarium*. *Cancer Res* 1979; 39:2179–2189.
175. Ueno Y. Trichothecenes: an overview. In: Rodrickes JV, Hesseltine CW, Mehlmann MA, eds. *Mycotoxins in human and animal health*. Park Forest South, Ill: Pathotox Publications; 1977;189–207.
176. Cannon M, Smith KE, Carter CJ. Prevention, by ribosome-bound nascent polyphenylalanine chains, of the functional interaction of T-2 with its receptor site. *Biochem J* 1976;156:289–294.
177. Yarom R, Sherman Y, Bergmann F, Sintov A, Berman LD. T-2 toxin effect on rat aorta: cellular changes *in vivo* and growth of smooth muscle cells *in vitro*. *Exp Mol Pathol* 1987;47:143–153.
178. Kurppa K, Hietanen E, Klockars M, et al. Chemical exposures at work and cardiovascular morbidity: atherosclerosis, ischemic heart disease, hypertension, cardiomyopathy and arrhythmias. *Scand J Work Environ Health* 1984;10:381–388.
179. Huff JE, Melnick RL, Solleveld HA, Haseman JK, Powers M. Multiple organ carcinogenicity of 1,3-butadiene in B6C3F$_1$ mice after 60 weeks of inhalation exposure. *Science* 1984;227:548–549.
180. Miller RA, Boorman GA. Morphology of neoplastic lesions induced by 1,3-butadiene in B6C3F$_1$ mice. *Environ Health Perspect* 1990;86:37–48.
181. Lovati MR, Galbussera M, Franceschini G, et al. Increased plasma and aortic triglycerides in rabbits after acute administration of 2,3,7,8-tetrachlorodibenzo-*p*-dioxin. *Toxicol Appl Pharmacol* 1984;75:91–97.
182. Walker AE, Martin JV. Lipid profiles in dioxin-exposed workers. *Lancet* 1979;1:446–447.
183. Swift LL, Gasiewicz TA, Dunn GD, Neal RA. Characterization of the hyperlipidemia in guinea pigs induced by 2,3,7,8-tetrachlorodi-benzo-*p*-dioxin. *Toxicol Appl Pharmacol* 1981;59:489–499.
184. Weber TJ, Ou X, Narasimham TR, Safe SH, Ramos KS. Modulation of protein phosphorylation in rat aortic smooth muscle cells by 2,3,7,8 tetrachlorodibenzo-*p*-dioxin (TCDD). *Toxicologist* 1991;11:340.
185. Toda T, Ito M, Toda Y, Smith T, Kummerow F. Angiotoxicity in swine of a moderate excess of dietary vitamin D$_3$. *Food Chem Toxicol* 1985;23(6):585–592.
186. Koh E, Morimoto S, Fukuo K, et al. 1,25-Dihydroxyvitamin D$_3$ binds specifically to rat vascular smooth muscle cells and stimulates their proliferation *in vitro*. *Life Sci* 1988;42:215–223.
187. Murad F. Cyclic guanosine monophosphate as a mediator of vasodilation. *J Clin Invest* 1986;78:1–5.
188. Westwood FR, Iswaran TJ, Greaves P. Pathologic changes in blood vessels following administration of an inotropic vasodilator (ICI 153,110) to the rat. *Fundam Appl Toxicol* 1990;14:797–809.
189. Collins JJ, Elwell MR, Lamb JC, Manus AG, Heath JE, Makovec GT. Subchronic toxicity of orally administered (gavage and dosed-feed) theophylline in Fischer 344 rats and B6C3F$_1$ mice. *Fundam Appl Toxicol* 1988;11:472–484.
190. Sandusky GE, Vodicnik MJ, Tamura RN. Cardiovascular and adrenal proliferative lesions in Fisher 344 rats induced by long-term treatment with type III phosphodiesterase inhibitors (positive inotropic agents), isomazole and indolidan. *Fundam Appl Toxicol* 1991;16:198–209.
191. Naseem SM, Heald FP. Cytotoxicity of cholesterol oxides and their effects on cholesterol metabolism in cultured human aortic smooth muscle cells. *Biochem Int* 1987;14(1):71–84.
192. Hayaishi O. Enzyme hydroxylation. *Annu Rev Biochem* 1969;38:21–44.

Cardiovascular Toxicology, Second Edition,
edited by Daniel Acosta, Jr.
Raven Press, Ltd., New York © 1992.

17

Chemically Induced Injury of Blood Vessels

Pathology Perspectives

*Zadok Ruben, *Reynaldo Arceo, and †Bernard M. Wagner

*Department of Toxicology and Pathology, Hoffmann–La Roche Inc.,
Nutley, New Jersey 07110; †Department of Pathology, New York University School
of Medicine, New York, New York 10016*

Blood vessels are essential for maintaining homeostasis of the tissues and organs they supply and drain. Injury to blood vessels therefore affects not only the vessels but also their associated tissues and organs. Blood vessels are vulnerable to injury by numerous chemicals and drugs. Table 1 lists agents that affect blood vessels (1).

Vascular tissue repair is one of the responses following injury. More importantly, though, is the remarkable structural adaptive response of injured blood vessels for maintaining the required functions of their associated tissues and organs. The structure and function of blood vessels may be altered in disease conditions, and therefore the effect of drugs and chemicals on these blood vessels may be different than in normal physiologic states. It is obvious that correlations between structure and function and elucidating the mechanisms of injury, in addition to determining the nature of the induced changes, are essential for advancing knowledge on the toxic injury of blood vessels. The purpose of this chapter is to highlight some of these aspects of blood vascular injury induced by chemicals and drugs. For more information on toxicologic pathology of blood vessels, the reader may refer to other reviews (2–5).

BLOOD VASCULAR INJURY

The structural responses of the arterial wall to injury depends on the nature of the chemical agent, degree of host exposure, and duration of exposure at the site of injury. Injury may be defined as direct or indirect depend-

TABLE 1. *Agents that affect blood vessels*

Agent	Vascular effect/disease
Heavy metals	
Arsenic	Arteriosclerosis, peripheral vascular disease
Arsine	Pulmonary vascular lesions; pulmonary edema; noncirrhotic portal hypertension
Beryllium	Hemorrhage; decreased hepatic flow; hepatic venous occlusion
Cadmium	Aortic and uterine endothelial damage; renal arteriolar thickening; atherosclerosis; hypertension
Chromium deficiency	Aortic atherosclerosis
Copper toxicity (chronic)	Acceleration of atherosclerosis
Copper toxicity (acute)	Hypotension
Copper deficiency	Aortic aneurysms
Germanium	Hemorrhage; pulmonary and gastrointestinal edema
Indium	Renal and hepatic hemorrhage and thrombosis
Lead	Encephalopathy (damage to endothelial cell with changes in blood–brain barrier permeability; changes in arterial elasticity); effects on vascular ground substance; sclerosis of renal vessels; hypertension
Mercury	Glomerulonephritis (preglomerular vasoconstriction; glomerular immune complex deposits); aortic lesions
Selenium	Atherosclerosis
Thallium	Perivascular cellular infiltration in the brain
Industrial and environmental agents	
Allylamine	Intimal proliferation in renal artery; smooth muscle proliferation in coronary arteries
β-Aminopropionitrile	Aortic atheroma; aneurysm; damage to vascular connective tissue
Boron	Pulmonary edema and hemorrhage
Carbamylhydrazine	Tumors of pulmonary blood vessels
Carbon disulfide	Direct injury to endothelial wall; microvascular effect on ocular fundus and retina; coronary atheroma
Chlorophenoxy herbicides	Hypertension
Dimethyl nitrosamine	Decreased hepatic blood flow; hepatic venous occlusion; hemorrhage and liver necrosis
4-Fluoro-10 methyl 12-benzanthracene	Pulmonary and coronary arterial disease
Glycerol	Renal vasoconstriction, acute renal failure
Hydrochloric acid (aspiration of stomach contents)	Increased microvascular permeability and pulmonary edema
Hydrogen fluoride	Pulmonary edema and hemorrhage
Paraquat	Cerebral and pulmonary edema and hemorrhage
Pyrrolizidine	Pulmonary vasculitis; pulmonary hypertension; hepativ venous occlusion
Organophosphate	Cerebral arteriosclerosis
Vinyl chloride	Portal hypertension; hemangiosarcomas
Gases	
Automobile exhaust	Cerebral hemorrhage and infarct; aortic atheroma
Carbon monoxide	Atherosclerosis
Nitric oxide	Pulmonary edema (vacuolation of arteriolar endothelial cells)

TABLE 1. *Continued*

Agent	Vascular effect/disease
Oxygen	Retinal vasoconstriction and edema; blindness in neonates; decreased visual field in adults; pulmonary edema
Ozone	Pulmonary edema
Drugs and related compounds	
Antibiotic–antimitotics	
Cyclophosphamide	Pulmonary endothelial cell damage
5-Fluorodeoxyuridine	Portal vein thrombosis and gastrointestinal hemorrhage
Gentamicin	Renal vasoconstriction and failure
Vasoactive agents	
Amphetamine	Nonspecific cerebrovascular damage
Dihydroergotamine	Vasoconstriction
Ergonovine	Coronary artery spasm; angina
Ergotamine	Vasospasms; gangrene
Epinephrine	Thrombogenesis
Histamine	Coronary arterial spasm; damage to endothelial hepatic portal vein
Methylsergide	Intimal proliferation; coronary arterial occlusion
Nicotine	Alteration of cytoarchitecture of aortic endothelium and increase in microvilli
Nitrites and nitrates	"Aging" of coronary arteries, recurrent vasodilation
Norepinephrine	Coronary arterial spasms and endothelial damage
Affecters of metabolism	
Alloxan	Microvascular retinopathy, blindness; diabetes
Chloroquine	Retinopathy
Fructose	Microvascular retinopathy; diabetes-like disease
Iodoacetates	Microvascular retinopathy
Anticoagulants	
Sodium warfarin	Hemorrhage, hematomas, and vasculitis
Radiocontrast dyes	
Metrizamide	Thrombosis and necrosis of celiac and renal vessels
Cyanoacrylate adhesives	
2-Cyano-acrylate-*n*-butyl	Arterial granulation tissue formation
Ethyl-2 cyanoacrylate	Thrombosis and degeneration of vascular wall
Methyl-2 cyanoacrylate	Vascular necrosis
Miscellaneous drugs and compounds	
Aminorex fumarate	Pulmonary hypertension; intimal and medial thickening of pulmonary arteries
Aspirin	Damage to endothelial basement membrane; ischemic infarcts; gastric erosions and ulcers
Cholesterol; oxygenated derivatives of cholesterol; noncholesterol steroids	Atherosclerosis
Homocysteine	Atherosclerosis
Oral contraceptives	Thrombosis in cerebral and peripheral vasculature
Penicillamine	Glomerulonephritis; vascular damage in connective tissue
Talc	Pulmonary arteriolar thrombosis; thromboembolism
Tetradecylsulfate Na	Venous sclerosis
Thromboxane A_2	Cerebral vasoconstriction

ing on the access of the agent or its metabolites to the artery. When an injurious chemical enters the arterial wall, regardless of mode of entry, and directly combines with biologically important macromolecules to alter function, direct injury has occurred. If, however, a chemical sets in motion a series of reactions by the cellular components of the arterial wall, which lead to injury through inflammatory cells, immune mediators, or altered homeostasis, then injury may be considered as indirect or secondary. Blood vessels constrict and dilate (Fig. 1). Vasomotion, or the ability of the artery to constrict or dilate, plays a role in determining the nature and severity of chemically induced injury. This critical priority of the artery is under extensive control by the neuroendocrine system and local metabolism affecting the cellular components of the wall (endothelia, connective tissue, and smooth muscle cells), which are integrated functionally by a unique extracellular matrix, elastin, and collagen fibers (6).

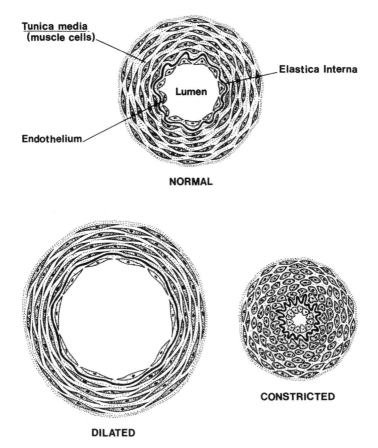

FIG. 1. A schematic diagram illustrating normal, dilated, and constricted blood vessels.

In the mid-19th century, Virchow referred to the vascular endothelium as "a membrane as simple as any that is ever met with in the body." Today, the endothelial cell is regarded as a complex, active regulator of vascular integrity. Endothelium regulates plasma–interstitial fluid exchange and intimal lipids, maintains a nonthrombogenic surface, produces mitogenic factors, and is a crucial element in the inflammatory response. At a physical level, the endothelium is a structural barrier between underlying smooth muscle and substances in the blood. The junctions between endothelial cells are important physical barriers and if the space between endothelial cells widens, fluid and particles may escape from the vascular lumen (Figs. 2 and 3). Toxic compounds are among the circulating substances in the blood, and therefore the endothelium can be viewed as a protectant of the tunica media from injury. The endothelial cell can bind and catabolize certain circulating vasoactive agents (serotonin, norepinephrine, bradykinin), convert inactive precursors into active products (angiotensin I), and directly synthesize a variety of potent autocoids (prostacyclins). To this repertoire, the endothelial cell has now been shown to directly modulate the adjacent smooth muscle cells by secreting second messengers in response to luminal stimuli (7).

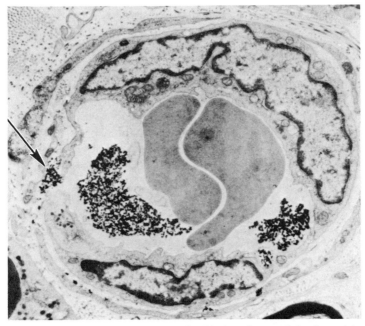

FIG. 2. An electron photomicrograph illustrating black carbon particles (*arrow*) in widened space between two endothelial cells of a mesenteric blood capillary of a dog with constricted mesenteric arterial bed induced by epinephrine.

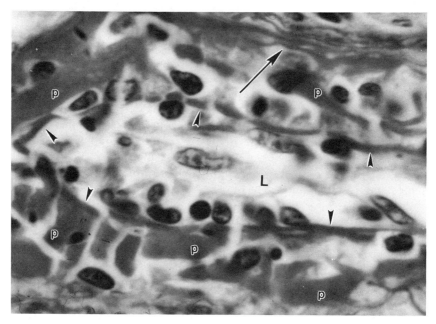

FIG. 3. A histologic photomicrograph at high magnification of a mesenteric arterial wall of a dog with repeated vasoconstriction induced by epinephrine. There is plasma protein (p) leakage into the wall [elastica interna (*arrowheads*) and lumen (L)]. Plasma protein substance is closely associated with extracellular connective tissue fibers (*arrow*); H&E stain.

These messengers, endothelium-derived constricting factor (EDCF) or endothelin and endothelium-derived relaxing factor (EDRF), regulate smooth muscle tone. Vasodilation, however, may not always be dependent on endothelium. In Table 2, examples of agents that cause vasodilation dependent or independent of endothelium are given. The intensive investigation of endothelial cell–smooth muscle cell interactions is yielding new insights into normal and abnormal physiology leading to irreversible injury.

TABLE 2. *Endothelium-dependent and -independent agents that cause vasodilation*

Endothelium-dependent	Endothelium-independent
Acetylcholine	PGI$_2$
Bradykinin	Atrial natriuretic factor
Arachidonic acid	Adenosine
Histamine	Nitroprusside
ADP	Nitrates
ATP	cAMP
Hydralazine	cGMP
Thrombin	

Does cell-to-cell communication exist between the endothelial cell and smooth muscle at a structural level? In 1967, Rhodin (8) was one of the first to investigate this question. It is now well established that in the microvasculature (small artery, arteriole, precapillary sphincter, venule, or small vein), the single layer of endothelial cells is separated from the adjacent smooth muscle layer by an internal elastic membrane. Rhodin showed that extensions of the smooth muscle cell membrane periodically penetrated the basement membrane structure to form an intimate relationship with the abluminal border of the endothelial cell. Termed the myoendothelial junction, it is quite similar to a nexus or gap junction characteristic of junctional complexes that occur between adjacent endothelial cells and adjacent smooth muscle cells. Thus an anatomical basis for chemical intercellular communication between endothelium and smooth muscle does exist. This offers a low-resistance pathway for intercellular signaling via cellular metabolites, ion movement, and voltage-dependent mechanisms.

The transfer of macromolecules across the arterial wall is quite different from the microvasculature. In arteries, the internal elastic lamina acts as a significant barrier to transport of macromolecules across the arterial wall. Studies using horseradish peroxidase or labeled albumin have demonstrated the barrier function of the elastic lamina in normal rat aorta (9). At the microvascular level, macromolecule transport is dependent on the intact endothelial–smooth muscle cell relationship as well as an intact elastic membrane. At a structural level, the microvasculature is capable of extensive vasoactivity. It is now accepted that nitric oxide derived from L-arginine is responsible for the biological activity of EDRF and is a general property of endothelial cell function.

Acetylcholine causes endothelium-dependent dilation of normal arteries in most animals. It is known that coronary angiography can demonstrate focal atherosclerotic lesions. However, histopathology and echocardiography show that atherosclerosis is diffuse. The effect of acetylcholine on "normal" human coronary arteries is controversial. Most studies demonstrate that intracoronary acetylcholine causes vasodilation in keeping with the release of EDRF from normal human coronary endothelium. However, Werns et al. (10) have shown that, in angiographically normal segments of human coronary arteries of patients with discrete coronary artery disease, acetylcholine causes vasoconstriction. The conclusion is that coronary artery disease is associated with a diffuse abnormality of endothelial cell function. Considering mechanisms of drug-induced arterial injury and developing drugs to treat the symptoms of coronary artery disease must take these observations into account.

Pathologists have postulated that recurrent, chronic vasoconstriction plays a role in smooth muscle cell hyperplasia and fibroblast function. It has been shown that endothelin is a very potent stimulus for phosphatidylinositol turnover, diacylglycerol release, and gene transcription in rat fibroblasts and smooth muscle cells. The finding of increased smooth muscle cell replication associated with increased collagen in hypertensive arteries may reflect the effects of endothelin. Endothelin must be considered as a potent and powerful stimulus to the cellular components of the vascular wall.

During vasoconstriction, the circular and longitudinal smooth muscle cells contract, producing a twisting compression of the arterial wall components. The physical characteristics of these components prevent complete obliteration of the lumen. However, the major forces are directed to the luminal surface. This results in a maximum folding and compression of the internal elastic lamina (Fig. 4), forcing endothelial cells to assume an epithelial columnar appearance. Smooth muscle cells immediately adjacent to the internal elastic lamina are squeezed and distorted by the contractile forces and the folds of the lamina. With relaxation, the process reverses and the lamina unfolds with dilation of the lumen.

Thus vasoconstriction, while a normal physiologic process, is associated with structural changes. Failure of these changes to adapt to the contractile forces can result in pathology of the vascular wall (11). This pathology can range from simple loss of endothelial cells to infiltration of plasmatic constituents, smooth muscle cell loss, fragmentation of fibers of the elastica interna (Fig. 5), medial thickening/smooth muscle proliferation (Fig. 6),

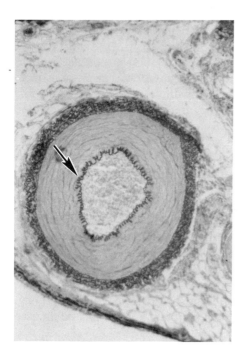

FIG. 4. A histologic photomicrograph at low magnification of a mesenteric artery of a dog with acute constriction induced by epinephrine demonstrating a highly folded elastica interna (*arrow*); elastic Van Gieson's stain.

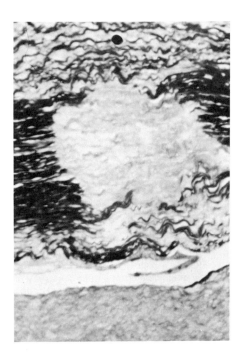

FIG. 5. A histologic photomicrograph at high magnification of elastica interna from a mesenteric artery of a dog demonstrating ruptured elastic fibers following chronic vasoconstriction induced by epinephrine; elastic Van Gieson's stain.

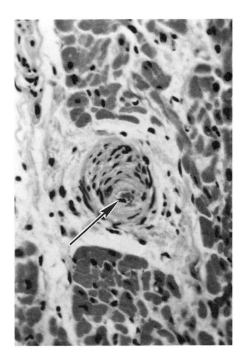

FIG. 6. A histologic photomicrograph at medium magnification of an intramural coronary artery from a human with generalized scleroderma demonstrating a narrow lumen (*arrow*) and proliferative smooth muscle cells following chronic vasoconstriction; H&E stain.

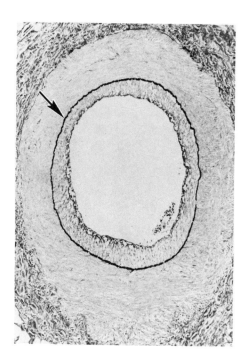

FIG. 7. A histologic photomicrograph at low magnification of a coronary artery of a dog given SK&F 94120 demonstrating intimal proliferation inner to a relatively smooth elastica interna (*arrow*); elastic Van Gieson stain. From ref. 5, with permission.

intimal proliferation (Fig. 7), and inflammatory cell infiltration. With diminished responsiveness to vasoactive agents, the artery increases its vulnerability to further injury.

DRUG-INDUCED VASOCONSTRICTION

Ergot and ergot-derivative drugs are powerful vasoconstriction agents. These drugs have been used in the treatment of migraine, postural hypotension, inadequate venous tone, forms of senile dementia, and, with heparin, as prophylaxis against postoperative thromboembolism. Because of their effect on vascular smooth muscle, these chemicals are prototype vasoconstrictors. There is an extensive clinical literature demonstrating the adverse effects of repeated vascular smooth muscle constriction. While ergot-type agents produce arterial vasoconstriction, they also cause venospasm and can result in venous thrombosis. Of interest is the fact that the vasoconstrictor activity is of long duration and independent of drug plasma levels. There is evidence to suggest that these agents accumulate in smooth muscle and induce constriction through stimulation of 5-HT receptors. However, constriction is maintained by sensitization of the smooth muscle to endogenous vasoconstrictors such as biogenic amines. For dihydroergotamine, the vasoconstriction activity appears to be modulated through a series of active metabolites (12).

Vascular angiography (arteriography and venography) have been helpful in elucidating the pathology (i.e., structural changes) associated with these drugs. A common observation in arteries in patients with vascular complications is segmental stenosis. The vessels are described as having thread-like, thorny, or hour-glass-like narrowing due to spasm. The stenotic arterial segments have smooth margins and no thrombi are present. Thus the toxic effects of ergot drugs on the arterial system may take the form of acute or chronic obstruction. Careful study of serial angiograms and comparison to tissue specimens allow one to postulate a mechanism of drug-induced pathologic changes. With repeated vasoconstriction, there is progressive loss of smooth muscle cells and fragmentation of the internal elastic lamina. The connective tissue stroma condenses and fibroblast activity with increased collagen deposition is induced. At this point, the arterial wall is vulnerable to an arteritis-type response. In the absence of inflammatory cells, smooth muscle cell loss, collagen deposition, and fibroblast hyperplasia continue until a fixed stenosis results.

The segmental pattern of arterial stenosis is in keeping with the anatomy of the wall and the role of the longitudinal smooth muscle cells in constriction. The twisting motion of the longitudinal smooth muscle cells requires segmental anchor points, which are determined physiologically and by receptor density. At the point of maximal vasoconstriction, endothelial cell injury may result in release of other biologically active substances acting on adjacent smooth muscle cells. This serves to accentuate the segmental nature of the stenosis. Vasoconstriction may be a factor in the segmental pathology of panarteritis nodosa and diseases of small, muscular arteries as seen in human generalized scleroderma (Fig. 6) (13).

REGIONAL CONSIDERATIONS IN VASCULAR TOXICITY

Several important organs (e.g., brain, liver, heart, kidney, or lung) have unique vascular beds adapted to the biochemical and physiological requirements of their system. Chemically induced vascular injury can be observed in all organs but its occurrence in the heart, kidney, and lung presents potentially life-threatening situations. The epicardial coronary arteries are capable of significant vasoconstriction resulting in transient reduction of myocardial perfusion. The coronary circulation is divided into three large components based on vascular resistance: there are the large vessels, small resistance vessels, and veins. Under normal conditions, measurements of coronary pressure in different sized arteries and arterioles indicate that 50% of total coronary resistance exists in vessels wider than 100 μm. This distribution of vascular resistance can be changed in a nonuniform manner by a variety of physiological stimuli. Also, many pharmacological stimuli produce similar alterations: norepinephrine, papaverine, dipyridamole, serotonin, vasopressin, nitroglycerin, adenosine, and endothelin. Much more research is needed on the control of the coronary microcirculation regarding vascular resistance. There are extremely complex mechanisms responsible for heterogeneous responses. Coronary arterioles appear to maintain persistent vasomotor tone for longer periods than expected. This may reflect special properties of coronary smooth muscle cells.

RENAL VASCULAR SYSTEM

Understanding the structural and functional complexity of the renal circulation is increasing as new methods of assessment reveal unexpected results (14). In the subcapsular cortical nephron, the efferent arteriole is closely associated with the proximal convoluted tubule of the same glomerulus allowing a large part of the ultrafiltrate to return to the peritubular capillaries coming from the efferent arteriole. The postglomerular efferent arterioles of the mid- and inner-cortical nephrons stand in sharp contrast since they do not necessarily perfuse their own tubules. For juxtamedullary nephrons, the proximal convoluted tubule extends above the glomerulus or origin and is perfused by efferent vessels of glomeruli found in the inner part of the midcortex. There are two distinct groups of glomeruli constituting the juxtamedullary nephrons, each characterized by unique efferent arterioles. For one type, the efferent arterioles are thin walled and divide at once into a capillary network. The other type have straighter and longer efferent arterioles with layers of smooth muscle cells appearing as sphincters.

From detailed studies of the walls of afferent and efferent arterioles, it is clear that the afferent arteriole serves as the major resistance vessel of the renal microcirculation. The efferent arterioles running through the outer medulla branch into dense bundles of vasa recta. Then, at the junction of the outer and inner medulla, the vasa recta form a major capillary network and then join the peritubular plexus. The blood supply of the inner medulla (papilla) comes from the central vessels of the vasa recta bundles. Called the "descending vasa recta," they range in number from 5 to 20 per bundle and course into the papillary tip. At this point, an extensive capillary network surrounds the terminal collecting system and ducts of Bellini. Venous capillaries emerge from the network and become "ascending vasa recta" arranged in countercurrent position to the descending vasa recta.

The urinary concentration process is linked to renal medullary blood flow. While there are minor differences in the microanatomy of the renal circulation between species, the close functional and structural associations are common. Balance of salt and water is crucial to survival, so it is not surprising to note that the regulation of the medullary circulation is under the influence of hormones. Thus the renin–angiotensin and adrenergic nervous systems, prostaglandins, vasopressin, and atrial natriuretic factors play a dynamic role in regulating medullary blood flow. Evidence suggests that the medullary circulation can be regulated separately from overall renal blood flow, an important point in understanding the pathogenesis of papillary necrosis. This means that, for determining the nature and mechanism of chemically induced injury, the pathologist must localize renal vascular injury as precisely as possible. Blood electrolytes and urinary findings can assist in directing attention to the appropriate vascular bed.

THROMBOSIS

The discussion focuses on the three generic categories by which drugs or chemicals increase thrombosis: (a) effects on the blood vessel wall, (b) rheological factors, and (c) blood constituents. The association of blood vascular anatomic sites with factors regulating thrombosis is illustrated in Fig. 8. Table 3 presents examples of agents that increase thrombosis (1,15).

Blood vessel wall. An alteration in the lining endothelium is perhaps one of the most important factors involved in thrombus formation (16). Drugs or

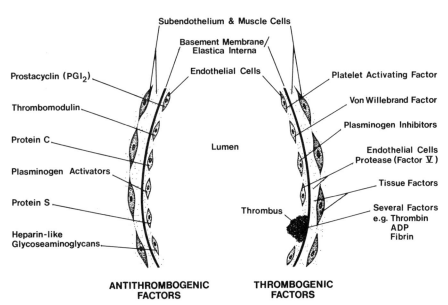

FIG. 8. A schematic diagram illustrating the sites in a blood vessel associated with various factors involved in the control of thrombogenesis.

TABLE 3. *Agents that increase thrombosis*

Agent	Effect
Effect on blood vessel wall	
Homocystine	Deendothelialization
Endotoxin	Deendothelialization
Polyanethol sulfate	Deendothelialization
Rheological factors	
Sodium acetriozate (radiocontrast agent)	Disseminated thrombosis in capillaries and veins; formation of insoluble fibrinogen derivative due to extraction of glycoproteins
Ergotamine	Profound vasoconstriction in peripheral arteries
Pitressin	Profound vasoconstriction in coronary and mesenteric arteries
Oral contraceptives	Venous stasis in lower extremities
Acetylcholine and autonomic blockers	Hypovolemic hypotension and stasis
Sympathomimetic agents	Elevated blood pressure and turbulence at bifurcations; distensions of vessels to produce endothelial damage
Effect on platelets	
Serotonin	Symptomatic thrombocythemia
Progesterone	
Testosterone	
Somatotropic hormone	
Vinblastine	
Vincristine	
Congo red	Increase in platelet aggregation
Ristocetin	
Serotonin	
Thrombin	
Epinephrine	
Adenosine diphosphate	Increase in platelet adhesiveness
Epinephrine	
Thrombin	
Evans blue dye	
Effects on clotting factors	
Epinephrine	Increase in factors VIII and IX
Guanethidine	Secondary effects due to release of epinephrine
Debrisoquin	
Tyramine	
Lactic acid (iv infusion)	Activation of Hageman factor
Long-chain fatty foods (iv infusion)	Activation of contact factors
Catecholamines	Elevation in circulating levels of fatty acids
ACTH	
Thymoleptics	
Nicotine	
Oral contraceptives	Decrease in antithrombin III levels
Mercuric chloride	Inhibition of fibrinolysis
Prednisolone	
ε-Aminocaproic acid	Plasminogen antiactivator
Tranexamic acid	
Aprotinine	Proteinase inhibitors
Iniprol	

chemicals may directly or indirectly damage the vascular endothelium, cause vascular spasms, or produce intimal proliferations; thrombus formation (Fig. 9) may be the result of either case. Once a thrombus is formed, a variety of consequences may occur. Alterations in luminal surface may occur allowing plasma proteins to enter the wall, interfering with the normal response of the wall to endogenous vasoactive substances. The thrombus may become a nidus for infectious contamination, focal calcification or lipid deposition. In time, the thrombus may be organized by fibrosis. A common finding in intravenous toxicity studies is a local venous thrombus formation from damage to the vascular wall at the injection site.

Rheological factors. Stasis of blood, regardless of its cause, may result in thrombus formation. Physical changes such as decreased blood velocity, hypotension, and vasodilation (17) are examples. It should be emphasized that rheological considerations are more applicable to the microcirculation than to the larger vascular beds.

Blood constituents. Blood cells and chemical components of the coagulation cascade are the two major groups of factors involved in thrombus formation. Of blood cells, platelets appear to be the most important. The function and integrity of platelets are under rigid control of vascular factors. The life span of platelets from their generation into the circulation by megakaryocytes to their removal from the circulation by the mononuclear phago-

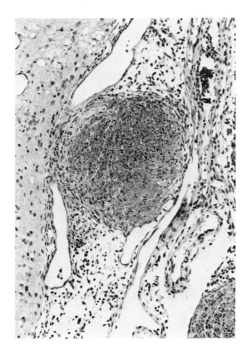

FIG. 9. A histologic photomicrograph at medium magnification of an acute meningeal thrombus of a rabbit with experimental meningitis; H&E stain. Histologic specimen courtesy of Dr. Carol Meschter.

cytic system is different in various species. Endogenous agents such as platelet activating factor and platelet-derived growth factor determine whether a thrombus will occur and to what extent adjacent cells in the vascular wall become activated.

The role of platelet adhesion and aggregation had been a subject of a number of studies, especially its involvement in both the vascular and clotting aspect of hemostasis (18–20). Platelet adhesion is initiated by contact with extravascular components such as collagen. In time, a number of antithrombotic and prothrombotic factors, apparently by the endothelial cells, come into play. The endothelial cells metabolize and release endogenous adenosine diphosphate (ADP), which causes firm platelet aggregation, although its metabolites have antithrombotic properties. PGl_2 (prostacyclin) secreted by the endothelial cells also plays a minor role in thrombogenesis (21,22). Other substances such as serotonin, histamine, and thromboxane A_2 may also regulate platelet aggregation. On the other hand, the endothelial cells may limit coagulation and thrombus formation by synthesis of plasminogen activators, vasoactive amines, and a cofactor on the endothelial cell surface that inactivates thrombin (23–26). Thus injuries to the surface of blood vessels stimulates platelet adhesions to the vessel wall, with spontaneous degranulation and release of their contents, promoting platelet aggregation. This is further enhanced by the release of Von Willebrand factor, ADP, and thromboxane A_2 (27).

A number of drugs/chemicals have the property of inhibiting the release of endogenous ADP and thus preventing platelet aggregation. Aspirin, for example, produces such an affect after oral ingestion for about 4–6 days. While this therapeutic effect is desirable, excess inhibition of endogenous ADP release by aspirin may lead to toxicity characterized by hemorrhages. Salicylates may also have transplacental toxic effect on platelet function in the newborn manifested as neonatal hemorrhages.

Certain changes in blood constituents may enhance thrombogenesis (28,29) by (a) increasing the number and the adhesiveness of platelets (as may occur in postoperative states; (b) increasing blood viscosity (as may occur in polycythemia vera); (c) release of thromboplastin-like substance (as may occur in visceral carcinomas); (d) increasing fibrinogen and other clotting factors in the blood (as may occur in disseminated intravascular coagulopathy); and (e) increasing catecholamine secretion (as may occur in hemorrhagic shock).

Finally, following vascular injury alterations in stasis lead to organization of the thrombus. The organized thrombus may remain as a permanent structure in the blood vessel wall. Depending on the size of the vessel involved, a thrombus may produce partial or complete occlusion and, occasionally, a part of the thrombus may break into the circulation (a complication known as embolism or thromboembolism).

HEMORRHAGE

Chemically induced defects in blood clotting mechanism or a direct action on vascular smooth muscle can produce hemorrhagic tendencies (30). Chemicals can decrease platelet number by direct toxic effect (e.g., anticancer drugs), or indirectly by immune-mediated mechanisms. There are agents that can inhibit synthesis of clotting factors (e.g., coumarin) inhibiting synthesis of prothrombin. Drugs may directly damage vascular smooth muscle, disrupting the vasa vasorum and allowing hemorrhage into the wall to occur. Minoxidil or dopaminergic agents may operate by this mechanism. Dopaminergic receptors on smooth muscle cell membranes appear to be involved in the mechanism. Another mechanism leading to vascular wall hemorrhage is dependent on disruption of the extracellular matrix resulting in reduction of vascular wall tension, thus allowing hemorrhage to take place. Lathyrogenic agents act by this mechanism. Petechial hemorrhage and aneurysm are the main manifestation of toxicity by lathyrogenic agents.

Minoxidil is a potent, long-acting vasodilator primarily used as an antihypertensive agent (31). It lowers blood pressure in experimental animals and humans by a direct action on arteriolar smooth muscle cells (32). In laboratory animals it induces myocardial and arterial lesions, of which the myocardial changes occur at earlier stages. Segmental medial hemorrhage (Fig. 10) and fibrinoid necrosis occur in coronary arteries at the earlier stages of vascular toxicity; this is followed by fibrosis (Fig. 11) and intimal thickening. In addition, there is epicardial and endocardial hemorrhage. The

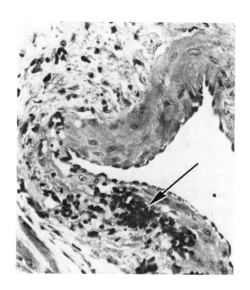

FIG. 10. A histologic photomicrograph at medium magnification of a coronary artery of a dog demonstrating medial hemorrhage (*arrow*) induced by minoxidil; H&E stain. From ref. 32a, with permission.

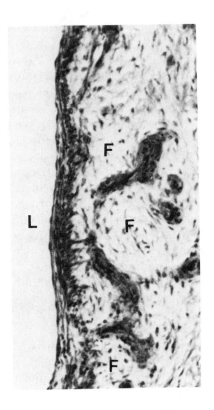

FIG. 11. A histologic photomicrograph at medium magnification of a coronary artery of a dog demonstrating fibrosis (F) in the outer tunica media (a vascular tissue response to injury induced by minoxidil), L, Lumen; Masson's trichrome stain. From ref. 32a, with permission.

above vascular changes accompany the myocardial damage that the drug induces (32–35).

TOXIC VASCULITIS

Chemicals and drugs such as inorganic arsenicals, gold, bismuth, sulfonamides, or methamphetamine are associated with injury known either as toxic vasculitis or toxic necrotizing vasculitis. The main morphologic features, depending on duration of injury, are necrosis, inflammation, and processes of repair particularly fibrosis. The end result may be vessels with narrow lumen and a thickened wall due to endothelial proliferation, fibrosis, and chronic inflammatory cellular infiltrate. Thrombi may occur. Morphologically, toxic vasculitis may not be distinguished from panarteritis nodosa, which is rarely associated with chemicals or drugs. The etiology of panarteritis nodosa is obscure, although multifactorial causes such as heredity, gender, older age, fecundity, hypertension, and nutritional, hormonal, and immune factors have been implicated. The mechanisms of toxicity by chemicals or drugs leading to toxic vasculitis are largely unknown. However, agents that alter endothelial–smooth muscle cell relationships are likely to be associated with toxic vasculitis.

HYPERSENSITIVITY VASCULITIS

Many drugs are associated with hypersensitivity vasculitis. Capillaries, venules, small veins, and arterioles are primarily affected. The response is primarily perivascular and, strictly, it is not a "vasculitis." Thus in the case of venular involvement, for example, perivenulitis (Fig. 12) may be a more adequate descriptive representation of the change than vasculitis. The response in hypersensitivity vasculitis is inflammatory and, compared to toxic vasculitis, there is no necrosis. The predominant inflammatory infiltrate is mononuclear cells. Polymorphonuclear leukocytes, of which eosinophils predominate, may also occur. There is no relationship between the occurrence of hypersensitivity vasculitis and duration of drug exposure nor the length of time following exposure. Hypersensitivity vasculitis in humans is commonly associated with skin rash, which disappears following drug withdrawal. Systemic hypersensitivity vasculitis is extremely difficult to diag-

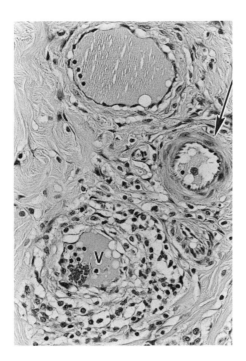

FIG. 12. A histologic photomicrograph at high magnification of perivenulitis (V = venular lumen) in the skin representing drug-induced allergic vasculitis. Muscular artery (*arrow*) is unaffected; H&E stain.

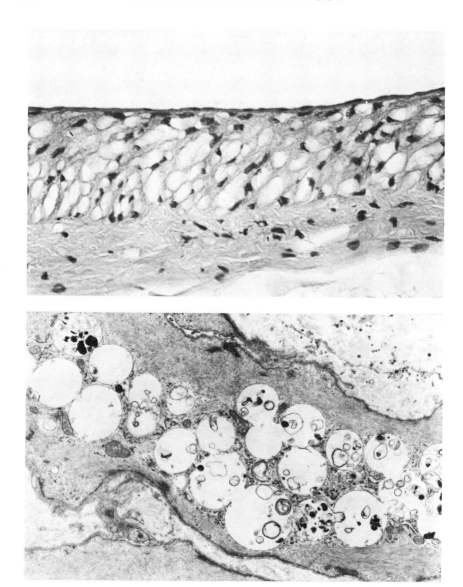

FIG. 13. Clear cytoplasmic vacuoles induced by disobutamide in muscle cells of dog coronary arteries: **above:** a histologic photomicrograph at high magnification (lumen at the top, H&E stain); **below:** an electron photomicrograph of a muscle cell with clear cytoplasmic vacuoles shown in the histologic photomicrograph.

nose clinically. Although the term hypersensitivity vasculitis and the presence of mononuclear inflammatory cells imply an immune mechanism, the evidence to support such an implication remains indefinite.

STRUCTURAL AND FUNCTIONAL CORRELATIONS

Is a morphologic change induced by a drug or a chemical a sign of toxicity (functional impairment)? The answer to this question is essential for determining the biologic and toxicologic significance of structural changes observed in safety assessment studies (36). When the induced morphologic change occurs in blood vessels, the answer to the above question is particularly important: blood vessels maintain the nutritional circulation of the tissues and organs they supply; and blood vessels have a remarkable structural adaptive capacity to preserve their function.

Clear cytoplasmic vacuoles induced in coronary arteries of dogs by disobutamide are a marked morphologic change (Fig. 13), in a highly important blood vessel, which was not accompanied with an overt functional impairment (37). Smooth muscle cells were the main cells whose cytoplasm contained the induced vacuoles. Vacuoles (distended acidic vesicles) occupied almost the entire cytoplasmic area on the microscopic sections examined, yet there was no indication of anticipated functional impairment such as poor myocardial perfusion, ischemia, infarct, or thrombosis. Furthermore, there was no evidence of necrosis, inflammation, atrophy, dysplasia, hyperplasia, or other evidence of vascular damage. Research has shown that vacuoles are a sign of intracellular storage of drug, associated with elevated intracellular phospholipid and monosaccharides, and not a sign of cell degeneration (38,39).

Not all functional impairments of blood vessels are associated with morphologic alterations. The best example is drug-induced acute hypotension. Therefore correlations (and, in some cases, lack of correlations) between structural and functional alterations are important for the integrative approach to toxicology of blood vessels.

SPONTANEOUS PATHOLOGIC CHANGES

There may be morphologic changes not associated with drugs or chemicals in blood vessels of laboratory animals (40–42). These changes may complicate the interpretations of the effects of a drug or a chemical tested. The most common among these pathologic changes are arteritis in beagle dogs and panarteritis nodosa in rats (Fig. 14). Drugs or chemicals may induce arteritis (Fig. 15) in nonsusceptible animals or, more importantly, increase the incidence in susceptible animals. Another point of concern is the possibility of high incidence of such vascular changes in certain colonies. About

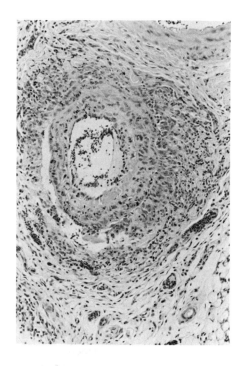

FIG. 14. A histologic photomicrograph at low magnification of a mesenteric artery of a rat with spontaneous panarteritis nodosa; H&E stain.

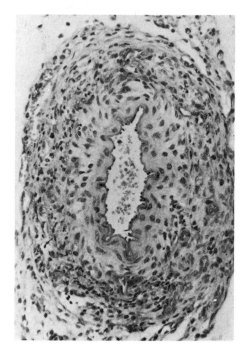

FIG. 15. A histologic photomicrograph at medium magnification of a mesenteric artery of a rat given SK&F 95654 demonstrating drug-induced arteritis. Inflammatory cells are primarily in the tunica adventitia, and hyperplastic muscle cells are in the thickened tunica media; H&E stain. From ref. 4, with permission.

one-third of beagle dogs from a supplier, for example, may have arteritis (43). It is possible therefore that 2–3 dogs of the high-dosage groups in a study in which 8–10 dogs are used may have arteritis. Such results may unnecessarily implicate the drug or chemical tested as the cause of arteritis. Clinical detection and monitoring of arteritis is an enigma, and an implication that a drug may cause arteritis may be detrimental to further development of the investigated drug. For further details, the reader is referred to *Toxicologic Pathology*, Volume 17, Number 1 (Part 2), 1989, for a symposium on arteritis and arterial drug toxicity in the safety assessment of drugs.

CONCLUDING REMARKS

The endothelium and smooth muscle cells are the major structural components of the wall of blood vessels that are affected in the processes of chemically induced injury. Connective tissue cells and components of the extracellular matrix also play a role in the response of blood vessels to injury. Blood constituents, particularly platelets and components of the coagulation cascade, are primary participants in vascular injury.

Structural alterations are limited whereas the mechanisms of injury are numerous, complex, and often poorly understood. Nonetheless, characterization of the morphologic changes often provide important directions for investigating the nature and mechanisms of injury. It is therefore essential that pathologists provide as accurate as possible an anatomic/morphologic description of the changes observed.

Physiologic factors and altered homeostasis in disease conditions should be taken into account when considering the mechanisms of toxic injury to blood vessels. Furthermore, not all structural alterations induced by drugs or chemicals in toxicologic evaluation studies are signs of toxicity. The borderline between physiology (limits of normal functions) and toxicity (functional impairment) is not often clearly defined.

ACKNOWLEDGMENTS

The support of Hoffmann–La Roche, Inc. and the assistance of Mrs. Diane Stolarz in manuscript preparation are greatly appreciated.

REFERENCES

1. Balazs T, Harrig J, Herman E. Toxic responses of the cardiovascular system. In: Klaassen CD, Amdur MD, Doull J, eds. *Toxicology.* New York: Pergamon Press; 1986:387–411.
2. Van Vleet JF, Ferrans VJ, Herman E. Cardiovascular and sketetal muscle systems. In: Haschek WM, Rousseaux CG, eds. *Handbook of toxicologic pathology.* Orlando: Academic Press; 1991:539–624.

3. McAllister HA, Mullick FG. The cardiovascular system. In: Riddell RH, ed. *Pathology of drug induced and toxic diseases.* Naperville: Churchill Livingstone; 1982:201–228.
4. Kerns WD, Joseph EC, Morgan DG. Drug-induced lesions, arteries, rat. In: Jones TC, Mohr U, Hunt RD, eds. *Cardiovascular and musculoskeletal systems* (ILSI Monographs on pathology of laboratory animals). Heidelberg: Springer-Verlag; 1991:76–83.
5. Kerns WD, Joseph EC. Drug-induced lesions of the coronary artery. In: Jones TC, Mohr U, Hunt RD, eds. *Cardiovascular and musculoskeletal systems* (ILSI Monographs on pathology of laboratory animals). Heidelberg: Springer-Verlag; 1991:84–90.
6. Markstein R. Hydergine: interaction with the neurotransmitter systems in the central nervous system. *J Pharmacol* 1985;3:1–17.
7. Highsmith RF, FitzGerald OM. Endothelial cell regulation of vascular smooth muscle. In: Sperelakis N, ed. *Physiology and pathophysiology of the heart,* 2nd ed. Orlando: Academic Press; 1989:755–771.
8. Rhodin JAG. The ultrastructure of mammalian arterioles and precapillary sphincters. *J Ultrastruct Res* 1967;18:191–223.
9. Penn MS, Koelle MR, Schwartz SM, et al. Visualization and quantification of transmural concentration profiles of macromolecules across the arterial wall. *Circ Res* 1990;67:11–22.
10. Werns SW, Walton JA, Hsia HH, et al. Evidence of endothelial dysfunction in angiographically normal coronary arteries of patients with coronary artery disease. *Circulation* 1989;79:287–291.
11. Goldstein RE, Ezra D, Laurindo FRM. Coronary artery spasm: pathophysiology. In: Virmani R, Forman MB, eds. *Nonatherosclerotic ischemic heart disease.* New York: Raven Press; 1989:63–85.
12. Muller-Schweinitzer E. What is known about the action of dihydroergotamine on the vasculature in man? *Int J Clin Pharmacol Ther Toxicol* 1984;22:677–682.
13. Utzmann O, Barret F, Cassan P, et al. Distal mesenteric arteritis: a rare complication of methylsergide treatment. *J Radiol* 1981;62:257–261.
14. Chou S, Porush JG, Faubert PF. Renal medullary circulation: hormonal control. *Kidney Int* 1990;37:1–13.
15. Zbinden G. Evaluation of thrombogenic effects. In: Elliot HW, George R, Okun R, eds. *Annual review of pharmacology and toxicology,* vol 16. Palo Alto, CA: Annual Reviews Inc; 1976:177–188.
16. Furchgott RF. Role of endothelium in response of vascular smooth muscle. *Circ Res* 1983;53:557–573.
17. Mustard JF, Rowsell HC, Murphy EA. Review of thrombosis. *Am J Med Sci* 1964;248:469–496.
18. George JN, Nurden AT, Phillips DR. Molecular defects in interaction of platelets with the vessel wall. *N Engl J Med* 1984;311:1084–1098.
19. Jackson CM, Nemerson Y. Blood coagulation. *Annu Rev Biochem* 1980;49:765–811.
20. Marcus AJ. Platelet function. *N Engl J Med* 1969;280:1213–1220, 1278–1284, 1330–1335.
21. Moncada S. Prostacyclin and arterial wall biology. *Arteriosclerosis* 1982;2:193–207.
22. Moncada S, Vane JR. Pharmacology and endogenous roles of prostaglandin endoperoxidases, thromboxane A_2 and prostacyclin. *Pharmacol Rev* 1979;30:293–331.
23. Esmon CT. The regulation of natural anticoagulant pathways. *Science* 1987;235:1348–1352.
24. Ross R, Glomset J, Kariya B, Hasker L. A platelet-dependent serum factor that stimulates the proliferation of arterial smooth muscle cells in vitro. *Proc Natl Acad Sci USA* 1974;71:1207–1210
25. Schwartz CJ, Sprague EA, Valente AJ, Kelly JL, Edwards EH. Cellular mechanisms in the response of arterial wall to injury and repair. *Toxicol Pathol* 1989;16:66–71.
26. Stern I, Brett J, Harris K, Nawroth P. Participation of endothelial cells in the protein C, protein S anticoagulant pathway: the synthesis and release of protein S. *J Cell Biol* 1986;102:1971–1978.
27. Rogers GM. Hemostatic properties of normal and perturbed vascular cells. *FASEB J* 1988;2:116–123.
28. Rosenberg RD, Rosenberg JS. Natural anticoagulant mechanisms. *J Clin Invest* 1984;74:1–6.

29. Sherry S, Brinkhouse KM, Genton E, Stengle JM, eds. *Thrombosis*. Washington, DC: National Academy of Science; 1969.
30. Davies PF. Current concepts of vascular endothelial and smooth muscle cell communication. *Surg Synth Pathol Res* 1986;4:357–373.
31. Carlson RG, Feenstra ES. Toxicologic studies with the hypotensive agent, Minoxidil. *Toxicol Appl Pharmacol* 1977;39:1–11.
32. Mesfin GM, Piper RC, Carlston RG. The cardiovascular toxicity of minoxidil in experimental animals. In: *Proceedings of the 12th scientific symposium of the BGA, 1984*, Berlin.
32a. Mesfin GM, Piper RC, DuCharme DW, et al. Pathogenesis of cardiovascular alterations in dogs treated with minoxidil. *Toxicol Pathol* 1989;17:164–189.
33. Kerns WD, Arena E, Maeia RA, Bugelski PJ, Mathews WD, Morgan DG. Pathogenesis of arterial lesions induced by dopaminergic compounds in the rat. *Toxicol Pathol* 1989;17(1):203–212.
34. Sobota JT. Review of cardiovascular findings in humans treated with minoxidil. *Toxicol Pathol* 1989;17(1):193–202.
35. Sobota JT, Martin WB, Carlson RG, Feenstra ES. Minoxidil: right atrial cardiac pathology in animals and man. *Circulation* 1980;62:376–387.
36. Ruben Z, Rousseaux CG. The limitations of toxicologic pathology. In: Haschek WM, Rousseaux CG, eds. *Handbook of toxicologic pathology*. Orlando: Academic Press; 1991:131–142.
37. Ruben Z, Dodd DC, Rorig KJ, et al. Disobutamide: a model agent for investigating intracellular drug storage. *Toxicol Appl Pharmacol* 1989;97:57–71.
38. Ruben Z. The pathobiologic significance of intracellular drug storage: clear cytoplasmic vacuoles. *Hum Pathol* 1987;18:1197–1198.
39. Ruben Z. Changes in saccharide and phospholipid content associated with drug storage in cultured rabbit aorta muscle cells. *Lab Invest* 1991;64:574–584.
40. Ayers KM, Jones SR. The cardiovascular system. In: Benirsche K, Garber FM, Jones TC, eds. *Pathology of laboratory animals*. New York: Springer-Verlag; 1978:1–70.
41. Carlton WW, Engelhardt JA. Polyarteritis, rat. In: Jones TC, Mohr U, Hunt RD, eds. *Cardiovascular and musculoskeletal systems* (ILSI Monographs on pathology of laboratory animals). Heidelberg: Springer-Verlag; 1991:71–76.
42. Mitsumori K. Blood and lymphatic vessels. In: Boorman GA, Eustis SL, Elwell MR, Montgomery CA, KacKenzie WF, eds. *Pathology of the Fischer rat*. Orlando: Academic Press; 1990:473–484.
43. Ruben Z, Deslex P, Nash G, et al. Spontaneous disseminated panarteritis in laboratory beagle dogs in a toxicity study: a possible genetic predeliction. *Toxicol Pathol* 1989;17:145–152.

Subject Index

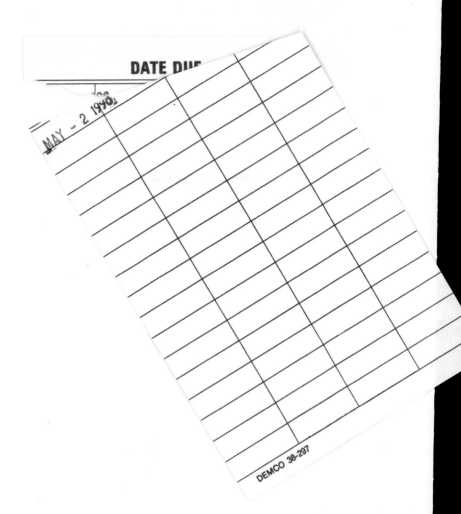

DATE DUE

MAY - 2 1976

DEMCO 38-297